D1271075

Compliments of W.B. Saunders Company

Reproduced from Ars Medica by permission of the Philadelphia Museum of Art

EX LIBRIS

Village Surgeon
A 17th century Dutch etching.

КГМ

BARBARA N.W. WEISSMAN, M.D.

Associate Professor of Radiology,
Harvard Medical School
Chief, Section of Skeletal Radiology,
Brigham and Women's Hospital,
Boston, Massachusetts

CLEMENT B. SLEDGE, M.D.

John B. and Buckminster Brown
  Professor of Orthopedic Surgery,
Harvard Medical School
Orthopedic Surgeon-in-Chief,
Brigham and Women's Hospital,
Boston, Massachusetts

ORTHOPEDIC RADIOLOGY

Drawings by MARCIA L. CHAPIN

1986
W. B. SAUNDERS COMPANY

Philadelphia ○ London ○ Toronto ○
Mexico City ○ Rio de Janeiro ○
Sydney ○ Tokyo ○ Hong Kong

W. B. Saunders Company: West Washington Square
                           Philadelphia, PA   19105

Library of Congress Cataloging in Publication Data

Weissman, Barbara

Orthopedic radiology.

1. Radiography in orthopedia.   I. Sledge, Clement B.,
    1930-   II. Title. [DNLM: 1. Bone and Bones—
    radiography. WE 141 W4330]

RD734.5.R33W45 1986   617′.3   84–13877

ISBN 0–7216–9185–4

Designer: Bill Donnelly
Manuscript Editor: Lorraine Zawodny
Illustration Coordinator: Peg Shaw
Page Layout Artist: Louise Lange

The illustrations in this book, including those used on the cover and chapter openings were done by Marcia L. Chapin.

Orthopedic Radiology   ISBN   0–7216–9185–4

© 1986 by W. B. Saunders Company. Copyright under the Uniform Copyright Convention. Simultaneously published in Canada. All rights reserved. This book is protected by copyright. No part of it may be reproduced, stored in a retrieval system, or transmitted in any form or by any means, electronic, mechanical, photocopying, recording, or otherwise, without written permission from the publisher. Made in the United States of America. Press of W. B. Saunders Company. Library of Congress catalog card number 84-13877.

Last digit is the print number: 9   8   7   6   5   4   3   2   1

PREFACE

As in all areas of successful communication, effective consultation depends on having a common language and a shared body of information. This book is intended to provide these tools to both radiologists and orthopedists. It is hoped that such communication will lead to advances in both fields and to improvement in patient care.

Emphasis has been placed on the implications of radiologic findings with regard to clinical outcomes and treatment decisions. Various treatment methods are mentioned but are not stressed, and the interested reader is referred to additional sources for further detail. The indications and rationale for, and the complications of, many commonly performed orthopedic procedures are reviewed, again with the intention of providing the knowledge necessary to utilize radiographic studies effectively.

This text has been organized to make the information readily accessible so that it can be used at the x-ray viewing area. It is divided by region and subdivided into sections on essential anatomy (including normal radiologic anatomy) and abnormal conditions. All radiographs have been reproduced as though they were of the right side, to facilitate comparison between cases. The graphics in the upper corner of each page are intended to provide quick access to each anatomic section.

The authors sincerely hope that an ancillary benefit of this text will be a harmonious and productive working relationship between radiologists and clinicians involved in treating disorders of the musculoskeletal system.

BARBARA N. WEISSMAN

CLEMENT B. SLEDGE

With eternal love and gratitude
to my family:
Irving, Matthew, and Abigail Weissman
and Lillian and Morris Warren

B. N. W.

ACKNOWLEDGEMENTS

Innumerable individuals have helped to make this textbook possible. We would like to thank our colleagues in Radiology and Orthopedics, especially Doctors J. Leland Sosman, Piran Aliabadi, Ethan Braunstein, Vera Stewart, Harry Z. Mellins, Herbert L. Abrams, and J. Drennan Lowell for their continued encouragement and support. Doctors Douglass Adams, Peter Doubilet, Donald Harrington, B. Leonard Holman, Barbara J. McNeil, Calvin Rumbaugh, Steven Seltzer, Sabah S. Tumeh, Hooshang Poor, Arthur L. Boland, Michael A. Drew, Frederick E. Ewald, Steven J. Lipson, Robert Poss, Donald T. Reilly, Richard D. Scott, Barry Simmons, William H. Thomas, Thomas S. Thornhill, and Joseph Zuckerman provided valuable consultation and reviewed portions of the text. Faith Hulse, Judy Lopez, Linda Evans, Carole Ashe, Phyllis White, Jane Beigley, and Jo-Anne Polack provided invaluable secretarial and research assistance. Donald Sucher and John Buckley reproduced the illustrations. Chris O'Brien, Ken Fallon, David Morse, Gary Lawson, William O'Rourke, Steve Lorenzetti, and Robert Kasparian provided the orthopedic appliances for photography. The support of the W. B. Saunders Company is also greatly appreciated. Particular thanks go to Lisette Bralow and Suzanne Boyd (Editors), Lorraine Zawodny (Copy Editor), and Robert Butler (Production Manager) for their indefatigable efforts.

BARBARA N. WEISSMAN

CLEMENT B. SLEDGE

CONTENTS

Chapter 1

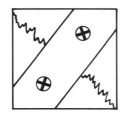

GENERAL PRINCIPLES

RADIOLOGICAL PRINCIPLES AND TECHNIQUES

Since the discovery of x-rays 90 years ago, the use of radiological techniques has soared, leading to the performance of more than 15 million skeletal radiological studies per year in the United States.[10] In addition, the current high tech era of medical imaging offers a wide variety of complex and expensive techniques and makes it essential that the referring physician and the radiologist choose the most appropriate technique in a given clinical situation. Throughout this book there will be references, to the types of radiological studies that *may* be utilized in a given situation. Which of these methods is chosen depends on a wide range of considerations, including medical, socioeconomic, and even medicolegal factors. It is the intent of these introductory pages to provide an overview of some of the currently available techniques so that their applicability to a particular clinical situation can better be evaluated. This discussion presents only the basics. The interested reader will find greater detail in References, noted throughout this section.

X-Rays and Radiation Protection

X-rays are a form of electromagnetic radiation differing from other forms primarily by their shorter wavelengths. Thus the wavelengths of visible light range from 390 to 750 nanometers (nm), and ultraviolet radiation ranges from 2 to 390, but diagnostic x-rays range from 0.01 to 0.1 nm (1 nm = 10^{-9} m).[4] The shorter the wavelength, the higher the energy of the radiation. The relatively high energy of x-rays makes them capable of producing ionization (loss of electrons) of atoms and molecules; therefore, x-rays are a form of ionizing radiation.

Terms frequently used in radiology include the following:[4, 5]

Radiation absorbed dose (rad): a measurement of absorbed energy or absorbed dose; equal to 100 ergs of absorbed energy per gram of tissue (0.01 joule per kilogram).

Roentgen (R): a measure of the amount of radiation exposure (the incident energy per unit area).

Roentgen equivalent man (rem): a unit representing the absorbed dose (in rads) multiplied by a quality factor reflecting the biological effects of that form of radiation in comparison with x-rays. For x-rays this quality factor is one, and 1R of radiation exposure produces about 1 rad of absorbed dose, or 1 rem dose-equivalent.

Gray (Gy): equal to 100 rads, or 1 joule of energy per kilogram.

Sievert (Sv): equal to 100 rems, or 1 joule of energy per kilogram.

Sources of Radiation

The major source of radiation to the general population is from natural sources, including cosmic rays and terrestrial radioactive materials; the dose from these sources averages 0.125 rem per year.[5] Diagnostic radiology is second to natural background radiation as a source of radiation exposure to the population. Doses for selected examinations are shown in Table 1–1. Although the recommended maximum permissible dose for radiation workers has been set at 5 rems per year (dose to whole body or to gonads, bone marrow, or eyes), no limit is set for medical radiation. Thus the value of each examination in which ionizing radiation is used must be weighed against the potential risks of the procedure. On the other hand, the risks of radiation are not so great that diagnostic studies need be forfeited if the examination is necessary. For example, the risk of death from radiation

Table 1–1. Doses of Selected Examinations (Average 1970 Values, in mrads)

Examination		Skin†	Mean BM Dose	Gonad Dose Male	Gonad Dose Female
Skull	PA	666	14	*	*
	LAT	420	17	*	*
	Series	—	78	*	*
Cervical Spine	AP	514	19	*	*
	LAT	288	9	*	*
	Oblique	365	15	*	*
	Series	—	52	*	*
Chest	PA	36	4.6	—	—
	LAT	132	10	—	—
	Overall	—	10	*	1
Thoracic Spine	AP	1050	120		
	LAT	2890	120		
	Series	—	247	3	11
Ribs	Series	—	143	?	?
Upper gastrointestinal series (UGI)	AP	902	79	—	—
	LAT	2420	76	—	—
	AP Spot	902	8.8	—	—
	LAT Spot	2420	13	—	—
	Fluoro	—	167	—	—
	Overall	—	535	1	171
Barium enema (BaE)	AP	1030	109	—	—
	LAT	6220	231	—	—
	AP Spot	1030	14	—	—
	LAT Spot	6220	91	—	—
	Fluoro	—	268	—	—
	Overall	—	875	175	903
Oral cholecystogram (OCG)	—	—	168	*	78
Intravenous pyelogram (IVP)	Overall	—	420	207	588
Abdomen (KUB)	—	951	92	97	221
Lumbosacral (L–S) spine series	—	—	384	218	721
Pelvis	—	—	93	364	210
Hips	—	—	72	600	124

Source: Doubilet PM, Judy PF: Postgrad Radiol 1:309, 1981, with permission.
*< 0.5
†For single views

exposure from a lumbar spine series (0.75 rad) has been equated to the risk of traveling 313 miles by car or smoking 1212 cigarettes.[6]

Effects of Low Levels of Radiation

The effects of low levels of radiation in humans are difficult to quantify. Possible ill effects include the following:

Genetic mutations: Animal studies suggest that doses between 20 and 200 rems to the gonads double the existing mutation rate.[8]

Shortening of life span: Prior to 1955 radiologists had about a 5-year average shorter life span than did other physicians. This is no longer the case, presumably because of decreased radiation exposure. No general aging effect has been shown in Japanese A-bomb survivors.[8]

Carcinogenesis: The dose-response curve for tumor induction with low levels of radiation is still debated. One estimate of risk is 50 to 150 excess cancer deaths per million persons per rem.[5]

Cataracts: The lens of the eye is relatively resistant to x-irradiation–induced cataract formation; several hundred rads are necessary to produce a demonstrable effect.[8]

Embryological effects: Because of possible ill effects, it is recommended that radiological procedures for females of childbearing age be limited to the 10 days following the onset of menstruation in order to avoid the exposure of an embryo to radiation.

Methods of Reducing Radiation Dose

Methods of reducing the radiation dose from diagnostic procedures include changes in radiographic procedures and instrumentation (Table 1–2). An example would be the use of intensifying screens to markedly amplify the film-blackening effect of x-rays, thus reducing patient dose 60 to 80 times. The need for eliminating unnecessary examinations and views is also to be stressed. Since doses are relatively high during fluoroscopy (i.e., 0.4 rads per minute), the feasibility of using video disc recorders should be considered. These recorders can significantly reduce radiation exposure, since the image generated during a short interval of fluoroscopy can be displayed for as long as necessary for viewing without further patient exposure.[2, 4]

Magnification Radiography[15–22]

Two techniques have been used to produce images that are or may be magnified (Fig. 1–1). *Direct* magnification is so named because the final image is enlarged. This enlargement is

Table 1–2. Methods of Dose Reduction in Diagnostic Radiology

Decrease Unnecessary Radiation
Eliminate unnecessary examinations and views
Use shielding
Use collimation
Reduce retake rate
Modify radiology practiced by nonradiologists
Decrease Patient Exposure Required to Produce Image
Decrease exit dosage required to produce image
  Maximize film-screen speed
  Use grids properly
  Use 70- (or 100-) mm spot films in GI studies
  Use x-ray scanning systems
Increase transmission ratio
  Maximize source-to-skin distance
  Optimize mean photon energy
    Maximize tube potential
    Maximize filtration
    Use multiphase generators

Source: Doubilet PM, Judy PF: Postgrad Radiol 1:309, 1981, with permission.

accomplished by increasing the object-to-film distance; it requires the use of both a small focal-spot x-ray tube and a high-resolution recording system. Direct magnification techniques are useful because they theoretically improve resolution, decrease image noise, decrease scattered radiation reaching the recording system, and have an improved visual impact. Thick as well as thin body parts can be examined. According to Genant and colleagues, these advantages lead to the more accurate assessment of small changes in bone structure (Table 1–3). The disadvantages of direct magnification include, first, increased radiation dose to the skin—as much as four times higher than the exposure with conventional film screen radiographs—although the radiation is delivered to a smaller area. A second disadvantage is the relatively circumscribed anatomical region that can be included on the film.

Optical magnification consists of the enlargement by a lens, projector, or microscope of

Table 1–3. Magnification

	Optical	Direct
Disadvantages	High radiation dose	Need for microfocus tube
	Possible motion artifact	
	Manual processing of industrial film	Long exposure
Advantages	Standard x-ray tube	Thick or thin parts may be examined
		Lower exposure than with optical

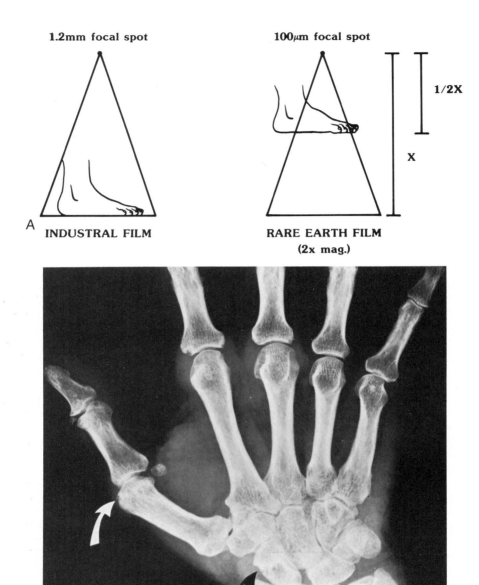

Figure 1–1. Magnification Radiography. *A,* Two methods of producing images that are or may be magnified are shown. On the left is optical magnification, in which the film obtained is magnified by means of a lens or a projector. On the right is direct magnification, in which the object-film distance is increased to achieve the desired magnification, 2 times in this case. *B,* This radiograph of a hand was obtained using direct magnification technique and magnification of about 2.5 times. The erosions due to rheumatoid arthritis are well seen at the wrist (black arrow), the thumb MCP (white arrow), and the index MCP. (*B* is from Seltzer SE, Weissman BN, Finberg HJ, Markisz JA: Semin Arthritis Rheum 11:315, 1982, with permission.)

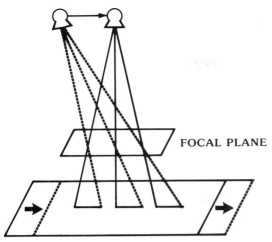

FOCAL PLANE

Figure 1–2. Tomography. The position of each point shown in the focal plane moves the same distance as does the x-ray film (arrow), and therefore the points remain sharply defined. Points above or below this plane will appear blurred. (Redrawn from Curry TG et al: Christensen's Introduction to the Physics of Diagnostic Radiology. Philadelphia, Lea & Febiger, 1984.)

radiographs obtained using fine-grained film. Disadvantages of this technique include the relatively high radiation dose, the need for manual or industrial film processing, and the requirement for special viewing apparatus. Either of these techniques is applicable primarily to the hands and feet for the evaluation of arthritic and metabolic[16, 18, 21] disorders.

Tomography

Standard radiographic techniques superimpose one structure upon another. Tomography was developed to demonstrate structures more clearly at particular levels without this superimposition. The technique involves the synchronous motion of film and x-ray tube in order to produce blurring of all objects except those on the focal plane (Fig. 1–2). Objects farthest from this plane are the most blurred, while objects on the focal plane remain sharply seen, since their images move precisely the same distance as does the film. The tube and film may move linearly (linear tomography) or in a variety of patterns, including circular, hypocycloidal, and trispiral. With linear tomography linear objects parallel to the direction of tube motion will not be adequately blurred. With other tube motions blurring is more uniform (Fig. 1–3). Increasing the distance of tube travel produces thinner sections (thinner focal planes) but also decreases contrast, so that thin-section tomography is applicable only to areas with high contrast, such as the elbow after contrast medium injection.

Patient dose is increased with tomography, but the dose is not prohibitive for occasional examinations if the information that can be obtained is relevant to diagnosis or treatment.

Computed Tomography

Computed tomography (CT) has emerged as an important technique for evaluation of the musculoskeletal system. Advantages of CT scanning over conventional radiography include its much greater ability to discriminate low-contrast objects (i.e., gray and white matter), the cross-sectional display and possible reconstruction of the image in additional planes, and the ability to measure attenuation coefficients. The spatial resolution of CT is less than that of conventional radiography, and the radiation dose is considerably higher (usually 3 to 5 rads to the skin of a tightly collimated area per study) (Table 1–4).

CT scanning is a complex process involving a narrowly collimated x-ray source, detectors, and a data processing system. The x-ray source, the detectors, and the accompanying electronics are mounted on a frame (gantry) that encircles the patient. Early brain scanners (first generation machines) consisted of a pencil beam of x-rays coupled to a single sodium iodide detector (Fig.

Table 1–4. **Radiation Dose from CT Studies**

Site	Area Imaged	Dose (mrads)
Skin	Head or body (multiple scans)	Range: 2000–10,000 + Usual: 3000–5000
Lens	Head (single scan through eyes)	1500
	Head (single scan not through eyes)	40
Ovaries	Head (single scan)	0.1
	Thorax (single scan)	0.4
	Upper abdomen (single scan)	2
	Through ovaries (single scan)	150–450
	Abdomen (multiple scans, including ovaries)	500–1000
Testes	Abdomen (multiple scans)	50–100

Source: Doubilet PM, Judy PF: Postgrad Radiol 1:309, 1981, with permission.

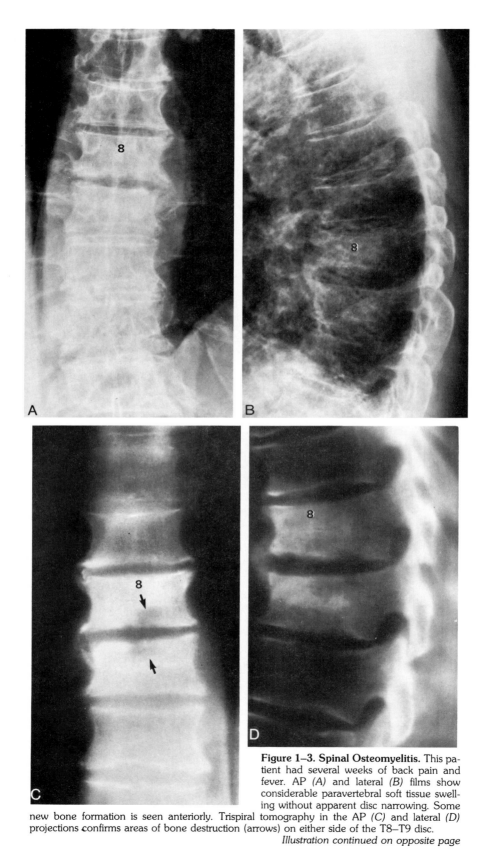

Figure 1–3. Spinal Osteomyelitis. This patient had several weeks of back pain and fever. AP (A) and lateral (B) films show considerable paravertebral soft tissue swelling without apparent disc narrowing. Some new bone formation is seen anteriorly. Trispiral tomography in the AP (C) and lateral (D) projections confirms areas of bone destruction (arrows) on either side of the T8–T9 disc.

Illustration continued on opposite page

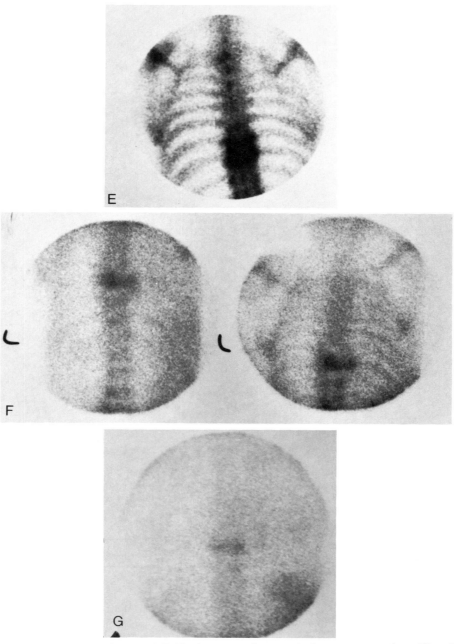

Figure 1–3. Spinal Osteomyelitis *Continued. E,* The bone scan shows marked increase in uptake at T8 and T9. *F,* Two posterior views from the gallium-67 scan obtained 72 hours after isotope injection show uptake in the region of the T8–T9 disc and in the adjacent lateral soft tissues, indicating an inflammatory process. *G,* Follow-up gallium scan 3 weeks later shows less intense uptake and a decrease in lateral extension of the isotope consistent with resolving infection.

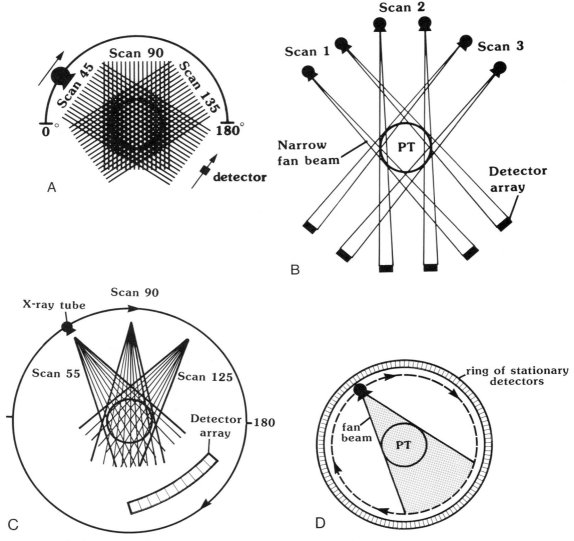

Figure 1–4. CT Scanners. *A,* First generation scanners had a single pencil beam x-ray source and a single detector. Linear motion (translation) of the tube and detector (arrows) was followed by rotation of the unit. *B,* Second generation scanners couple a narrow fan beam of x-rays with multiple detectors so that fewer rotations are necessary. *C,* Third generation (rotate only) scanners have a wide fan beam, and translational motion is therefore unnecessary. *D,* Fourth generation scanners have a rotating fan beam of x-rays and a fixed ring of detectors. (Redrawn from Curry TG et al: Christensen's Introduction to the Physics of Diagnostic Radiology. Philadelphia, Lea & Febiger, 1984.)

1–4).[39] The tube moved in a linear fashion, and multiple readings of x-ray transmission were made at the detector placed opposite. The entire unit (tube and detector) was then rotated, and the linear scan was repeated until 180 degrees of tube motion had been obtained. All the while, measurements of incident and transmitted radiation intensity were recorded and stored in the computer for analysis. The major disadvantage of this system was the long scanning time required (about 5 minutes), which limited use of the technique to immobile areas such as the brain.

Second generation scanners made the examination faster (1 to 3 minutes) by coupling a narrow fan beam of x-rays to multiple detectors.[39, 68] The linear motion (translation) followed by angular motion (rotation) was still used, but the number of rotations could be decreased because of the increased number of detectors, making scanning time faster.

Third generation (rotation only) scanners used a single x-ray source consisting of a wider fan beam that exposed the entire cross-section of the part to be studied at one time, thereby eliminating the need for translational motion.

Scanning occurred as the gantry was rotated over 360 degrees. Scanning time with these units was reduced to 1 to 10 seconds.[39, 68]

Fourth generation scanners use a rotating fan beam and a fixed ring of detectors. Scan time averages 2 seconds.[68]

After the completion of all scans in a particular plane, a computer-generated image based on the x-ray attenuation of each volume of matter within the plane is produced. The attenuation of each volume element (voxel) depends on the atomic number and the density of the tissue.[39, 63] The attenuation coefficients are converted to CT numbers (also called Hounsfield numbers) by comparison with the attenuation of water. The CT number for water is designated 0, that of air −1000, and that of dense bone +1000. The CT values for various tissues are shown in Figure 1–5.

CT images are displayed pictorially in two dimensions (although they were derived from a three-dimensional slice of tissue), and the numerical CT values of each picture element (pixel) are shown as shades of gray. The quantity of CT numbers assigned to each shade of gray can be selected (termed selecting a window). A narrow window-width contains fewer shades of gray and generally produces an image with increased contrast. The window level, the number at which the gray scale is centered, can also be chosen. Typically, for visual evaluation of bone lesions, a wide window-width (approximately 1000 Hounsfield units) and a high window-level (approximately 200 Hounsfield units) are used.

Computed tomography has been used in a wide variety of musculoskeletal disorders, including those related to trauma (spine, acetabulum, and glenoid in particular);[31, 32, 37, 42, 47, 64] back pain (herniated nucleus pulposus and facet joint arthritis);[67] metabolic bone disease (measurement of spinal bone mineral);[30, 40, 70] tumor (soft tissue lesions and soft tissue extension);[27, 33–35, 43, 44, 50, 51, 54, 59, 65, 66] congenital abnormalities (femoral anteversion, talocalcaneal coalition);[55] and the evaluation of multiple surgical procedures, bone grafting among them.[71] Still to be solved is the problem of large metal objects (such as hip prostheses) that produce major artifacts on the CT scan.[52]

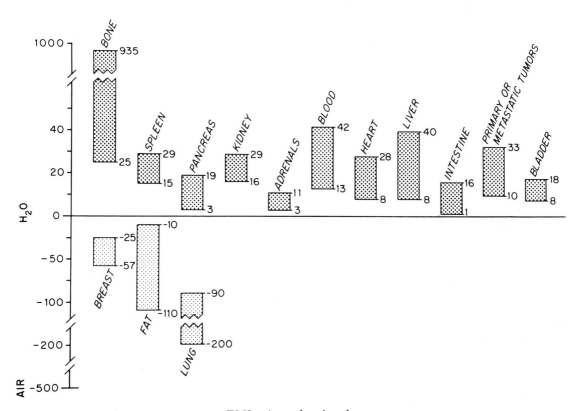

EMI values of various human organs.

Figure 1–5. EMI Numbers. The EMI numbers of various tissues are shown. In general, 1 EMI unit is equal to 2 Hounsfield units. (Reprinted from Alfidi RJ, MacIntyre WJ, Meaney TF, et al.: AJR 124:199, 1975, with permission.)

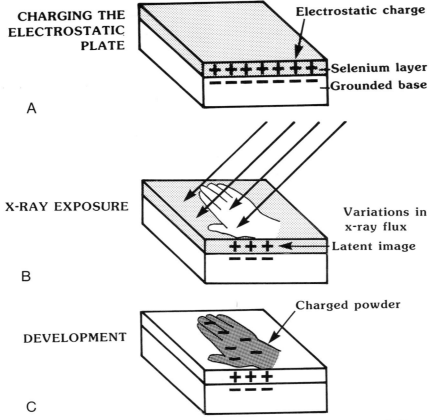

CHARGING THE ELECTROSTATIC PLATE

Electrostatic charge

Selenium layer
Grounded base

A

X-RAY EXPOSURE

Variations in x-ray flux
Latent image

B

DEVELOPMENT

Charged powder

C

Figure 1–6. The Xeroradiographic Process. *A,* The selenium-coated plate is positively charged. *B,* The part to be imaged is placed on the plate and exposed to x-rays. The x-rays discharge the plate in proportion to the amount of radiation reaching its surface, and a latent image is produced. *C,* Negatively charged particles are then sprayed onto the plate and accumulate in proportion to the residual charge. These particles are then fused to paper. (Modified from Wolfe, JN: Xeroradiography of the breast. Springfield, Ill, Charles C Thomas, 1972, by permission.)

Xeroradiography

Xeroradiography is a technique in which the x-ray film utilized in conventional radiography is replaced by a xeroradiographic plate on the surface of which is a thin layer of a photoconductor (selenium).[77] The plate is contained within a cassette and is made ready for radiography by the placing of a positive electrostatic charge on its surface. The part to be radiographed is then placed on the cassette and exposed to x-rays, the x-rays discharging the photoconductor in proportion to the amount of radiation reaching the surface of the plate (Fig. 1–6). Thus, in an area in which dense bone limits the photons reaching the plate, the charge will remain, whereas in areas under soft tissue, a larger portion of x-ray photons will reach the plate and discharge the photoconductor. The resulting pattern of charges is called the electrostatic latent image. To make this latent image

visible, a negatively charged blue plastic powder (toner) is sprayed onto the plate, where it accumulates in proportion to the residual charge. The image depicted in powder is transferred to plastic-coated paper and fixed to it, usually by heating. The xeroradiographic plate can then be reused after heating and cleaning to remove any residuum of the latent image. The final xeroradiograph contains unexposed background areas that are deep blue, exposed background areas that are white, soft tissues that are shades of blue, and calcifications that are deep blue (Fig. 1–7). This coloring can be reversed if desired.

Advantages of Xeroradiography

One advantage of xeroradiography is the *edge effect,* in which the margins between areas of different density are exaggerated. This is caused by the presence of fringe fields, which attract

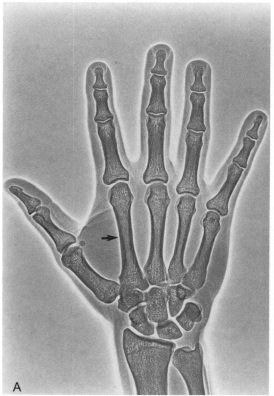
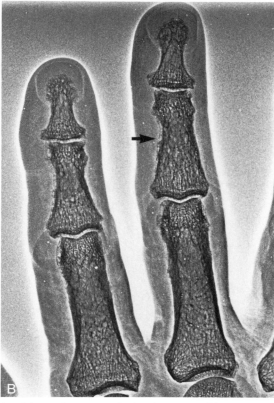

Figure 1–7. Xeroradiography. *A,* Normal examination. Note the ability to demonstrate both soft tissues and bony structures on a single examination. The halo effect (arrow) around the bony corticies is an example of edge enhancement. *B,* Hyperparathyroid bone changes shown on xeroradiography. The subperiosteal bone resorption (arrow) and distal tuft erosion are well seen. (*B* is reprinted from Seltzer SE, Weissman BN, Finberg HJ, Markisz JA: Semin Arthritis Rheum 11:315, 1982, with permission.)

more toner to the side of higher charge and less toner to the side of lower charge. This property facilitates the detection of microcalcification on mammographic studies.

Another advantage of xeroradiography is its *wide latitude,* in which areas of low and high density are well shown on the same view. Thus a lateral view of the neck will show the air-containing trachea, the soft tissue, and bony structures—all with one exposure. The wide latitude also lowers the likelihood of repeated examinations resulting from poor technique.

Disadvantages of Xeroradiography

Large areas of relatively uniform density may be difficult to distinguish from one another. This *broad-area contrast suppression* can be altered by technical manipulations, but large masses (such as a mass in the breast) may be overlooked.

The *radiation exposure* required for xeroradiography is higher than that needed for radiography using film-screen combinations but lower

than that required for nonscreen film radiography (Table 1–5). The high radiation dose needed for xeroradiographic examination of thick parts, such as the hip, sharply limits the use of the examination in these areas. For

Table 1–5. **Doses of Xeroradiography Compared with Screen and Nonscreen Techniques**

	Xero-Radiograph (mrads)	Screen (mrads)	Nonscreen (mrads)
Hand-elbow	76	41	225
Shoulder	464	82	—
Foot	85	18	525
Ankle	192	21	426
Leg (tibia)	208	25	672
Knee	463	68	872
Hip	3370	1770	—

Source: Wolfe JN: Radiology 93:583, 1969, with permission.

Table 1–6. Some Benign Conditions That May Produce Positive Bone Scans

Calcific tendinitis
Surgery
Ectopic bone formation
Osteomyelitis
Fracture
Arthritis
Paget's disease
Renal osteodystrophy
Osteitis pubis
Fibrous dysplasia
Hyperostosis frontalis interna
Aseptic necrosis
Osteoid osteoma

Table 1–8. Radiation Doses from Various Scanning Procedures

	Technetium-99m Bone Scanning Agents	Gallium-67 Citrate
Usual dose	10–20 mCi	3–6 mCi
Radiation dose/ millicurie		
Skeleton	35 mrads/mCi	440–600 mrads/mCi
Bone marrow	15–20	440–600
Kidneys	60–80	
Whole body and gonads	10	260
Bladder	500–1000*	
Colon		900†

Soure: Data from Kirchner PT, Simon MA: J Bone Joint Surg (Am) 63:673, 1981.
*Decreased by frequent voiding and hydration
†Dose can be reduced by using laxatives

thinner parts, such as the hand, doses are relatively comparable to conventional radiographic examinations.

Radionuclide Imaging

Bone Scanning

Currently used technetium-99m labeled phosphorous complexes (polyphosphates, pyrophosphates, and diphosphonates) are excellent agents for bone scanning, combining the superior imaging characteristics of technetium-99m with the affinity for bone of the phosphate compounds. The low radiation dose and sensitivity of the method have led to its use in a wide range of benign as well as malignant disorders (Table 1–6).

Following intravenous injection there is rapid clearance of these isotopes from the blood, with about 50 percent localizing to the skeleton in areas of early osteoid mineralization.[85, 93] Uptake of isotope by bone is dependent on blood flow to the region and on the extraction of isotope, which is related to metabolic activity, capillary permeability, and extracellular fluid volume.[85]

Situations in which a bone scan should be

Table 1–7. Indications for Bone Scanning

Evaluation of bone pain when radiographs are normal or equivocal
Evaluation of patients with known malignancies for staging, selection of biopsy sites, planning radiation treatment, and follow-up after therapy
Evaluation of patients with suspected metastatic disease on radiographs
Evaluation of possible early osteomyelitis
Early diagnosis of stress fracture
Evaluation of joint disease
Evaluation and detection of Paget's disease
Detection of early avascular necrosis
Evaluation of painful total-joint prostheses
Evaluation of bone graft

considered are listed in Table 1–7. Radiation doses accruing from bone and gallium scans are listed in Table 1–8.

The Normal Scan. Images are usually obtained 2 to 3 hours after injection to allow clearance of the isotope from the blood. Images obtained immediately after injection (first transit images) by serial 3-second exposures of the area display regional perfusion. Blood pool images, obtained 60 to 90 seconds after injection, reflect regional blood volume.[85]

Since uptake of the agents by the skeleton depends on the *rate* of mineralization, areas of normally increased bone formation such as the epiphyses, costochondral junctions, sacroiliac (SI) joints, and sternoclavicular joints show increased isotopic uptake. About one third of the injected dose is excreted through the kidneys into the urine,[86] and the kidneys and bladder should therefore be visible. Adequate hydration and frequent voiding in order to lower the radiation dose to the bladder are suggested. In addition, bone scanning agents are taken up in the soft tissues of the pharynx, the glandular tissue of the breast, and the lacrimal system.[85]

Gallium Scanning. Gallium-67 scanning is used in the evaluation of certain tumors and infections. The isotope is administered intravenously as a citrate in doses of 3 to 6 mCi. Almost all the injected dose binds to transferrin and other iron-binding molecules (lactoferrin, ferritin, and siderophores),[131] with 10 to 25 percent of the isotope excreted by the kidneys within the first 24 hours and slower excretion via the bowel. The remaining gallium is distributed largely to the liver (in lysosomes), the bone, and the soft tissues, with skeletal uptake paralleling the uptake of technetium-labeled bone scanning agents. Scanning is delayed at least 24 hours and usually 48 to 72 hours after isotope injection so that blood concentrations are low enough to allow discrimination between areas of uptake and background activity.

The mechanism of localization in tumors is unknown, although transferrin may play a key role.[131] Gallium has been shown to accumulate in various tumors, including Hodgkin's disease, malignant lymphoma, lung cancer, hepatoma, and many soft-tissue and bone sarcomas.[85]

Uptake of gallium into areas of infection has been postulated to result from incorporation of the isotope into leukocytes, binding to the fluid around the leukocytes that have been stimulated to secrete lactoferrin, and direct uptake by bacteria.[131]

Indium Scanning. This technique involves labeling leukocytes that are separated from a specimen of the patient's venous blood with indium-111 (In 111) and then reinjecting the labeled leukocytes intravenously. In normal circumstances 20 percent of the indium-labeled white cells are taken up by the spleen, 20 percent by the liver, and 60 percent by the bone marrow. In 111–labeled white cells will also accumulate in areas of active infection but not in areas of chronic osteomyelitis or in most tumors. The technique has been used for the detection of acute infectious processes,[140, 142] including the evaluation of suspected infection after total joint replacement.[141] Chronic osteomyelitis and tumors do not attract leukocytes, and therefore do not show increased isotope uptake.

Radionuclide Scanning in the Evaluation of Osteomyelitis

Radiographic evidence of acute osteomyelitis is typically delayed. Focal deep soft-tissue swelling, obliteration of deep fat lines, and later subcutaneous swelling, may occur, beginning within 3 days after the onset of symptoms. However, periosteal reaction and bone destruction are not seen for at least 10 days. With use of bone scintigraphy, osteomyelitis may be detected 24 hours after the onset of symptoms, before radiographic changes occur.[129] When it is detected and treated early, radiographic abnormalities may not develop. The area of osteomyelitis is typically seen on bone scan as an area of increased radionuclide uptake with a corresponding area of hyperemia shown on early blood pool scans (see Fig. 1–3). Occasionally, decreased isotopic uptake may be present in acute osteomyelitis because of a decrease in blood flow to the area.[135] In one such instance, increased uptake of gallium was noted, however.[137]

Bone scanning allows the differentiation of acute osteomyelitis from cases of cellulitis or septic arthritis (Table 1–9).[129] It should be emphasized, however, that the diagnosis of septic arthritis should be made by immediate joint aspiration and fluid analysis rather than by imaging methods. A normal bone scan performed more than 24 hours after onset of symptoms essentially excludes the diagnosis of acute pyogenic osteomyelitis.[130, 133]

Despite the importance of the technetium bone scan in the diagnosis of acute osteomyelitis, bone scanning cannot be used to follow the course of osteomyelitis during treatment because increased isotope uptake may persist for many months after appropriate therapy is begun.[125]

Gallium-67 scanning also is useful in acute osteomyelitis and, in addition, is of help in evaluating acute exacerbations of chronic osteomyelitis. Animal experiments have confirmed gallium-67 uptake into areas of infection 24

Table 1–9. Usual Scan Findings in Osteomyelitis, Cellulitis, Septic Arthritis, and Infarction

	Blood Pool Image	Bone Scan	Gallium-67 Scan
Acute osteomyelitis	Focal ↑ bone and ST* ↑	Focal ↑ ± diffuse ↑	↑ Uptake
Cellulitis	Diffuse ↑	Normal or diffuse ↑ bone and ST*	↑ ST uptake*
Septic arthritis	Diffuse ↑ periarticular	Diffuse ↑ periarticular	↑ Uptake in joint
Infarction	No focal ↑	↓ Patchy or ↑ uptake or ↓ activity with rim of ↑ activity	
Chronic osteomyelitis		± ↑ Uptake	Minimal uptake
Acute exacerbation of chronic osteomyelitis		↑ Uptake	↑ Uptake

Sources: Gelfand ML, Silberstein EB: JAMA 237:245, 1977; Gilday DL, Eng B, Paul DJ, et al.: Radiology 117:331, 1975; Lisbona R, Rosenthall L: J Can Assoc Radiol 29:188, 1978; Majd M, Frankel RS: AJR 126:832, 1976.
*ST: Soft tissue

hours old or less. Advantages of gallium scanning over bone scanning in the evaluation of infection include the following: (1) A gallium scan more accurately reflects the area of bone involved with osteomyelitis than does a bone scan because adjacent hyperemia may produce excessively large areas of bone agent uptake. (2) Marked gallium uptake indicates acute infection and can be used to document an acute flare of osteomyelitis superimposed on chronic changes. (3) Gallium scanning may be useful for following response to treatment of osteomyelitis.

Indium-111–labeled leukocytes localize in areas of acute infection and inflammation. In one series of orthopedic conditions studied after injection of indium-111–labeled leukocytes, the sensitivity of the method was 98 percent, the specificity 89 percent, and the overall accuracy 93 percent.[142] Because of technical factors relating to the energy of emitted gamma rays, gallium and indium scans cannot be performed concurrently. It is thought, however, that the indium-labeled white cell scans are more specific for acute infection than are gallium scans.

Ultrasonography

Diagnostic ultrasound has largely been applied to evaluation of the abdomen, but because of its noninvasive nature and the fact that there is no known deleterious effect from medical ultrasound, a number of musculoskeletal applications of this method have developed.

Ultrasound is a form of energy that, by definition, has a frequency greater than 20,000 cycles per second (the maximum frequency of audible sound waves). Frequencies of 1 to 20 million cycles per second (1 to 20 megahertz) are used in diagnostic imaging. In the most basic terms imaging with ultrasound consists of the emission (via a piezoelectric crystal within a transducer) of an ultrasound beam and the subsequent detection (also via the transducer) of the ultrasound beam as it is reflected from internal structures. Unlike x-rays, which travel in a vacuum, ultrasound (and sound waves) require a medium for transmission, and the velocity of transmission varies with the qualities of that medium, primarily with its elasticity and density. Diagnostic ultrasound images result from the reflection of ultrasound waves at tissue interfaces. How much of the beam is reflected at an interface depends on the angle of incidence of the beam and the acoustic impedance of the tissues. At a soft tissue–air interface almost all the ultrasound is reflected; therefore, imaging cannot be performed through the lung, through bowel gas, or through an air gap between the patient and the transducer. Similarly, at bone–soft-tissue interfaces most of the ultrasound beam is reflected, making it necessary to use multiple oblique projections to see beyond bony surfaces. In contrast, at soft tissue–fat

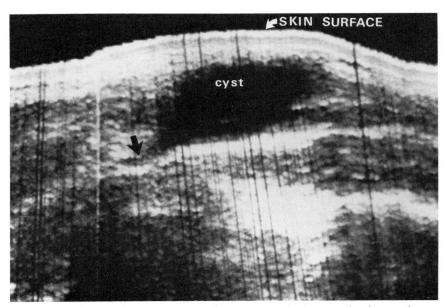

Figure 1–8. Ultrasound Demonstration of a Popliteal Cyst. A longitudinal gray-scale ultrasound examination of the popliteal fossa in the midline shows a 1.8 by 3.2 cm echo-poor region posterior to the knee joint that represents a popliteal cyst. The tubular connection to the joint (black arrow) is shown. (Reprinted from Seltzer SE, Weissman BN, Finberg HJ, Markisz JA: Semin Arthritis Rheum 11:315, 1982, with permission.)

interfaces some of the beam is reflected and some passes through the interface and therefore is available for imaging deeper structures.

Most structures are defined as being cystic, solid, or complex (mixed). Structures are said to be cystic if they are completely echo free. Strong echoes emanate from the interface between the cystic area and the adjacent tissue deep to the cyst. In contrast to cysts solid masses usually reflect echoes within their substance.

The results of ultrasound can be displayed in a number of ways. B-mode scanning is the method most often used for diagnostic imaging. The display represents the echoes from a slice of tissue obtained by moving the transducer along a plane of the body. Early studies were displayed as areas of black or white representing regions of echogenicity. Echoes below a set threshold were not included in the image. With newer gray-scale imaging echoes of various intensities are displayed in proportionate shades of gray. High-speed real-time ultrasonography provides dynamic information (analogous to that provided by radiographic fluoroscopy).

Applications of ultrasonography to the musculoskeletal system include the definition of normal soft tissue anatomy,[162] the detection of intraarticular and periarticular fluid collections (including joint effusion and popliteal cysts), and the evaluation of soft tissue masses (Fig. 1–8).

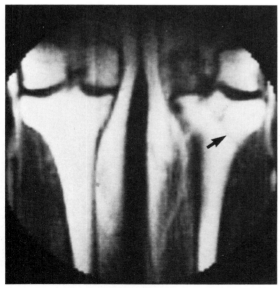

Figure 1–9. Nuclear Magnetic Resonance Image of the Knee. This image of the knees shows a proximal tibial fracture (arrow). Note that the cortex of the bone is of low signal intensity (black), whereas the marrow cavity appears white. (Courtesy of Drs. R. C. Hawkes and D. Kean, QMC, Nottingham University, U.K.)

Nuclear Magnetic Resonance

Nuclear magnetic resonance (NMR; magnetic resonance imaging; MRI) is an imaging technique in which magnetic fields are applied to tissue, and images of the spatial distribution of various nuclei (especially hydrogen) are obtainable. The advantages of NMR include the facts that no ionizing radiation is used, the procedure is not invasive, and the images produced are based on the chemical content and metabolism of a structure as well as on its morphology. Possible skeletal applications of NMR include the evaluation of bone and soft tissue tumors,[167] of avascular necrosis, of herniated nucleus pulposus, and of osteomyelitis (Fig. 1–9).

ORTHOPEDIC PRINCIPLES AND PROCEDURES

Fractures

When to X-Ray

The answer to this question is difficult and is colored by a number of nonmedical issues, including medicolegal ones. Several studies have attempted to develop criteria for high-yield radiography. Of particular note is the study by Brand and associates, in which clinical signs and symptoms of patients entering a busy emergency room after musculoskeletal trauma were reviewed and correlated with the presence of fracture on subsequent radiographs.[170] It was determined that the most accurate predictors for the presence of a fracture was bony deformity, instability, or crepitation (gross signs) at the fracture site. The next most reliable indicator was the presence of point tenderness. Using the presence or absence of these signs and others, patients were assigned to high- or low-risk categories, and it was found that if only the high-risk group had been radiographed (50 percent of the total group), 225 of 235 fractures would have been identified (Table 1–10). In only 2 of the 10 missed fractures (a nondisplaced distal radial and a lateral malleolar fracture) might the treatment have been altered by earlier detection.

In addition to the question of who should have radiographic examinations, the method of tailoring the radiographic examination appropriately is under study. It has been found, for example, that only 2 projections (the AP and the lateral) are necessary for the detection of ankle fractures, although additional oblique views did show some of the fractures to advantage and the mortise view was a useful film in some cases for treatment planning.[171]

Table 1–10. **Distribution of Injuries According to Protocol Classification (High- or Low-Risk) and X-ray Findings (Positive or Negative for a Bone Abnormality)**

Risk Category	X-ray Findings	
	Positive	*Negative*
High*†	225‡	393
Low	10	607

Source: Brand DA, Frazier WH, Kohlhepp WC, et al.: N Engl J Med 306:333, 1982.

*High risk: Gross signs (bone deformity, bone instability, crepitation); point tenderness; ecchymosis or severe swelling in an upper extremity; moderate to severe pain with weight bearing in a hip or thigh; any positive finding in a knee.

$$\dagger\text{Referral fraction} = \frac{225 + 393}{1235} = 50\%$$

$$\ddagger\text{Sensitivity} = \frac{225}{235} = 96\%$$

Where to X-Ray

Patients suffering massive trauma often need chest, cervical spine, and pelvic radiographs in addition to views of obviously injured areas.

Examinations of the most vital areas should be carried out first so that they will be available if the clinical situation deteriorates and additional examinations are necessarily postponed.[173]

Examination of suspected extremity fractures should include at least AP and lateral views. If the shaft of a long bone is the site of possible fracture, the joints on either end of that bone should be included on the radiograph. If the metaphyseal or the epiphyseal area is the site of suspected injury, then only that area and the adjacent joint should be examined so that optimal detail can be provided.

Terminology[183, 197, 198]

A *fracture* is a complete or incomplete break in the continuity of bone or cartilage.[198] Usually, fractures result from a single episode in which excessive stress is applied to normal bone. The stress may be due to the direct application of force or to indirect trauma in which force is applied at a distance from the fracture site. *Open fractures* are associated with a defect in the overlying soft tissues, whereas in *closed fractures* the skin is intact. *Incomplete fractures* are stable injuries in which one side of the bone is broken.

Table 1–11. **Fracture Configurations in Relation to Applied Force**

	Type of Force	Description of Force	X-ray Appearance of Fracture Line	Diagram*
Direct Trauma	Tapping	Small force applied to small area	Transverse fracture line with only one bone fractured, e.g., nightstick fracture	A
	Crushing	Large force on large area	Comminuted or transverse fractures involving both bones if forearm or lower leg involved	B
	Penetrating	Large force applied to small area, e.g., bullet		C
Indirect Trauma	Traction	Avulsion by muscle pull	Transverse fracture	D
	Angulation		Transverse fracture with splintering of cortex on the concave side	E
	Rotation	Rarely occurs alone; usually combined with axial loading	Spiral fracture at 45° to shaft; fracture ends sharp and pointed	F
	Compression	Rare as isolated mechanism	T or Y fracture or longitudinal shaft fracture without displacement	G
	Angulation and axial compression		Curved fracture line with oblique and transverse components and, often, butterfly fragment	H
	Angulation and rotation		Oblique fracture with short blunted ends	I

Adapted from Harkess JW: Principles of fractures and dislocations. *In* Rockwood CA Jr, Green DP, eds. Fractures in Adults, vol. 1. Philadelphia, JB Lippincott, 1984:1–95 by permission.

*See Fig T-1–11, parts A to I.

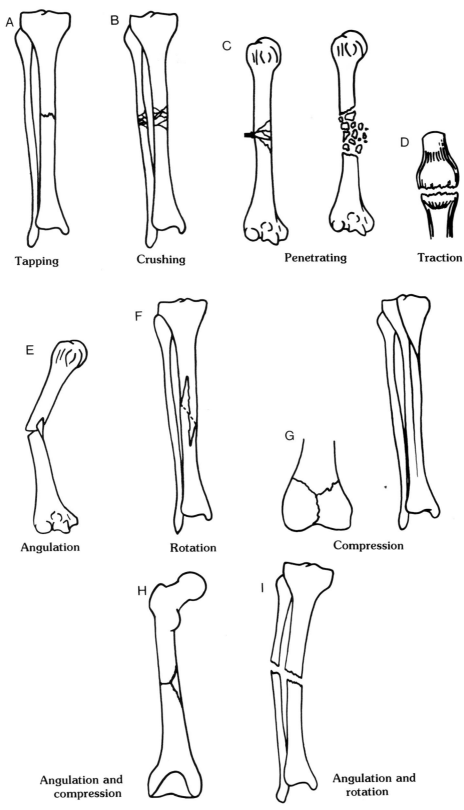

A Tapping

B Crushing

C Penetrating

D Traction

E Angulation

F Rotation

G Compression

H Angulation and compression

I Angulation and rotation

Figure T1–11

These are unusual fractures in adults. *Comminuted* fractures have more than two fracture fragments.

Fracture Configuration.[183] Fracture configuration is largely dependent on the magnitude, type, and site of applied force (Table 1–11).

Fractures Due to Direct Trauma. A *transverse* fracture, especially if it involves only one bone of a forearm or leg, suggests an initiating direct force of small magnitude. With greater force both bones are broken, comminution may be present, and more extensive soft-tissue damage occurs.

Penetrating trauma, usually due to bullets, may be the result of high- or low-velocity missiles. Low-velocity missiles may fracture the bone and become embedded in it but produce relatively little soft-tissue damage in comparison with high-velocity missiles, which cause extensive soft-tissue and bony injury.

Fractures Due to Indirect Trauma. Avulsion fractures are due to the pull of a muscle or tendon and are typically transverse in configuration and near the site of ligamentous insertion. Angular stress may also produce a transverse fracture that is usually angulated or displaced and may have comminution on the side of the bone that has been under compression.

A *spiral* fracture results from rotational stress (torque). The upper and lower ends of the fracture are long and sharp and are connected by a vertical segment. With nondisplaced, true spiral fractures, the fracture line itself is not sharply seen, since it is never completely in profile on any projection.

Pure vertical compression theoretically results in an *oblique* fracture at about 45 degrees to the shaft or in a longitudinal fracture. Since pure compression alone is rare, and since bones are not purely cylindrical in shape, it is more likely that the shaft of a long bone will be driven into the metaphysis, resulting in a T or a Y fracture. Oblique fractures also result from a combination of angulation and rotational stress.

Description of Fracture Deformity

Location. Long-bone fractures are usually described by visualizing the bone as divided into thirds and stating at or between which thirds the fracture has occurred. Joint involvement must be specifically stated.

Type. The fracture is described in terms of its configuration (i.e., spiral, oblique, or transverse). The presence of comminution (more than two fracture fragments) is noted. Two types of comminution include the *butterfly* fragment, in which a triangular bony fragment is present along one side of a long-bone fracture, and the *segmental* fracture, in which two fracture lines isolate a

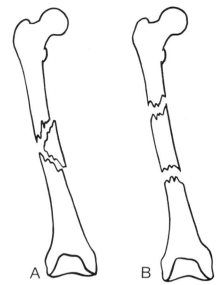

Figure 1–10. Comminution. Two types of comminution are shown. *A,* A triangular "butterfly" fragment is present. *B,* Two fracture lines isolate a segment of the shaft (a segmental fracture).

segment of the shaft of a long bone (Figs. 1–10 and 1–11).[198] Impaction of fracture fragments occurs when one of the fragments is driven into the other. Impaction is suggested on radiographs by increased density along the fracture line. At least two views are needed to make this assessment, since overlap of fragments may produce similar findings.

Position. The position of a fracture is described by relating the position of the distal segment (fragment) to the proximal one. When an extremity fracture is described, the term *distal fragment* includes the entire limb distal to the fracture site.

Alignment. Good alignment refers to the absence of angular or rotational deformity. Angular deformity is generally described (particularly by radiologists) by the direction in which the distal fragment deviates. In the medial-lateral plane, the terms *varus* and *valgus* are often used.*

---

*A short discussion regarding the terms *varus* and *valgus* is in order. Houston and Swischuk note that the current use of these terms is directly opposite to their original meaning and conclude that it would be best to omit these terms altogether. In current practice, however, *varus* refers to a tilt toward the midline of the bone beyond the joint, regardless of whether the prefix is the name of the joint or the bone beyond it.[185] *Valgus* refers to lateral deviation of the distal part. Thus the term *genu valgum* refers to a knock-knee deformity. When fracture deformity is being described, the reference point becomes the fracture site, with the result that, for example, medial angulation of the femur distal to an intracapsular hip fracture is designated *varus deformity.*

fragment is deviated anteriorly. Alternatively (and more often used by orthopedists), angular deformity may be described by the direction of the apex of the angle formed between the fracture fragments (e.g., there is posterior angulation of the fracture apex). Thus the same fracture may be described as having posterior angulation of the fracture apex or anterior angulation of the distal fragment. As long as the description is clear, either terminology is acceptable (Fig. 1–12).

Apposition. *Apposition* refers to the relationship between the fracture ends. If the fracture ends are in contact, complete apposition is present. Partial apposition (displacement) is described by the proportion of the proximal shaft that is no longer in contact with the distal fragment (e.g., there is one half a shafts width lateral displacement of the distal fragment; Fig. 1–13). If the fracture margins are not apposed and one fragment is displaced by more than one shaft-width, shortening (overlapping) may occur. A rough estimate of the number of centimeters of shortening that has occurred should be noted. Bayonet apposition refers to the particular instance in which shortening has occurred without angular deformity. *Distraction* of the fracture describes the pulling apart, or separation, of the fracture fragments.

Rotation. Rotation about the longitudinal axis is difficult to define radiographically. One clue to differences in rotation between proximal and distal fragments is a difference in the width of the bone fragments or the cortices at the fracture site.[194] Evaluation of the joints proximal and distal to the fracture may help in evaluating

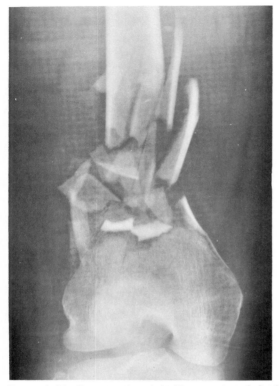

Figure 1–11. Comminution. A highly comminuted distal femoral shaft fracture is present. Several dense cortical fragments are present. An external fixator was used to maintain position during healing.

Varus angulation and medial angulation of the distal fragment are synonymous. Anterior angulation (angular deformity) of the distal fragment refers to malalignment in which the distal

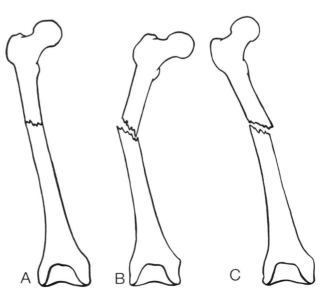

Figure 1–12. Alignment. *A,* There is no angular deformity; hence the alignment is anatomical. *B,* There is medial angulation of the distal fragment (or lateral angulation of the fracture apex). *C,* There is lateral angulation of the distal fragment (or medial angulation of the fracture apex).

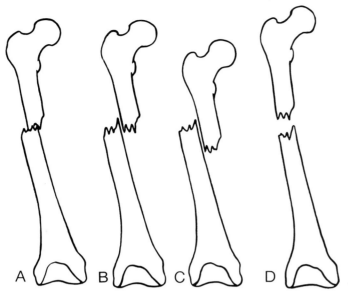

Figure 1–13. Apposition. *A,* The degree of displacement is stated in terms of the proportion of the proximal shaft that is no longer in contact with the distal fragment. Thus in *A* there is half a shaft-widths lateral displacement of the distal fragment. *B,* There is a one shaft-widths lateral displacement of the distal fragment. *C,* Shortening accompanies the full shaft-widths lateral displacement of the distal fragment. This configuration is termed bayonet apposition. *D,* Distraction. The fracture margins are separated.

rotational abnormalities, but clinical evaluation is often most accurate (Fig. 1–14).

Reporting. Thorough description of the location of a fracture, its alignment, its apposition, and any rotational deformity is important (Table 1–12; Figs. 1–15 and 1–16). Value judgments, such as *excellent alignment* or *poor position,* should be omitted. An exception is the use of the term *anatomical position* if the anatomy is essentially restored.

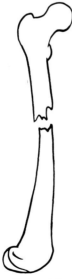

Figure 1–14. Rotation. This rotational abnormality is obvious because of the differences in the rotation of the knee as compared with the hip. Often, rotational abnormalities are difficult to define radiographically.

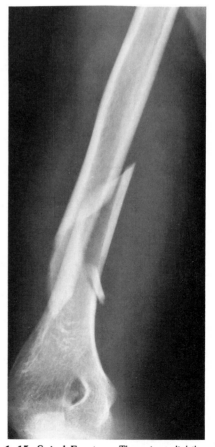

Figure 1–15. Spiral Fracture. There is a slightly comminuted spiral fracture at the junction of the mid- and distal thirds of the humerus with a quarter shaft-widths medial displacement of the distal fragment. No evidence of healing is apparent.

Table 1–12. Essentials of the Radiographic Report in Patients with Skeletal Trauma

Date (plus time if available) of examination
Type of examination (e.g., portable)
Date of report
Projections obtained
Appliances present (e.g., cast)
Description of fracture
  Which bone
  Where in bone
  Type of fracture (e.g., stress fracture, pathological
    fracture)
  Fracture configuration (transverse, oblique, segmental)
  Fracture alignment
  Displacement
  Apposition
  Comparison with previous examination
  State of healing
Final impression

Sources: Kaye JJ: Terminology and reportage of skeletal trauma. *In* American Roentgen Ray Society. Syllabus for the Categorical Course on Musculoskeletal Trauma, Atlanta, 1983; Pitt MJ, Speer DP: Med Radiogr Photogr 58:14–18, 1982.

Fracture Healing

Fracture healing is a complex process in which a number of events take place that result, not in scar, but in the re-formation of bone necessary for structural stability.

Three types of fracture healing have been described: primary union, secondary repair, and healing of membranous bone.

Primary Union. *Primary union* refers to direct bony union across a fracture site (Fig. 1–17). This type of healing is not seen clinically but has been produced experimentally by creating a fracture after a compression plate is in place and then maintaining compression.[198] In these cases healing is said to result from bone resorption, followed by replacement that begins in the cortex of one fragment and continues across the fracture site into the apposing fragment, forming new, continuous haversian systems.[192, 198] No periosteal reaction is visible in this circumstance.

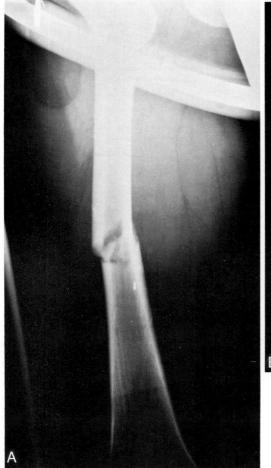
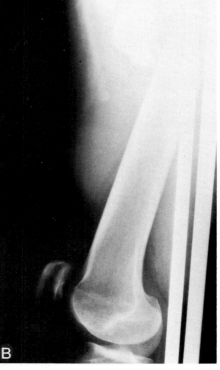

Figure 1–16. Femoral Fracture. AP *(A)* and lateral *(B)* view. There is a midshaft femoral fracture with 5 degrees varus angulation, a shaft-widths posterior displacement of the distal fragment, and 2-cm of shortening.

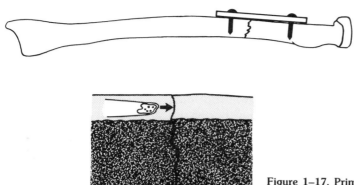

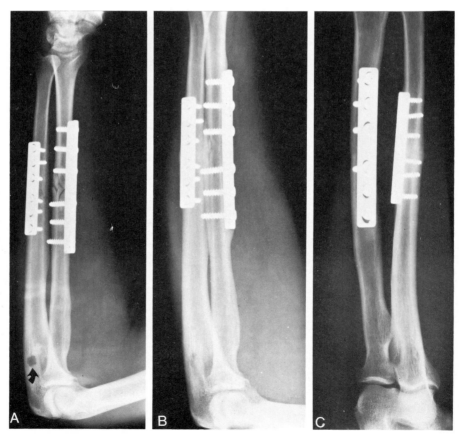

Figure 1–17. Primary Union. This type of union is theoretically possible when fracture fragments are held in apposition by a compression plate. Bone resorption, followed by new bone formation, extends from one fracture fragment to the other (arrows).

In practice, however, compression plating of a fracture does not result in primary union, although the amount of periosteal reaction demonstrable radiographically may be minimal or nonexistent (Fig. 1–18). Thus the absence of visible periosteal reaction after compression plating does not conclusively indicate that primary union has occurred.

Figure 1–18. Fracture Healing after Plating. *A,* A lateral view immediately after plating and bone grafting shows anatomical reduction of the radial and ulnar fracture sites. The radial fracture lines are clearly seen. The proximal ulnar defect (arrow) is the donor graft site. Lateral *(B)* and AP *(C)* views 6 months later show the radial and ulnar fractures to have healed. The minimal callus is typical of fracture healing with compression plating. The graft defect is filling in with bone.

Secondary Repair. Secondary repair is the usual mode of healing of cortical bone and involves the laying down of *callus,* consisting of fibrous tissue, cartilage, and bone. This process is also called endochondral repair, since the changes that occur are similar to, although less organized than, those seen in the epiphyseal plate of growing individuals. This type of healing has been subdivided into stages, depending on the predominant histological picture (Fig. 1–19).

Inflammatory Stage. At the time fracture occurs, there is tearing of the soft tissues around the fracture site. The periosteum opposite the point of impact is torn, but the periosteum on the side of impact may remain intact, creating a soft-tissue hinge. The surrounding muscles are damaged, and blood vessels are torn, with bleeding under the periosteum and between the fracture ends. Lacunar osteocytes die because of interruption of the interosseous channels that supply them with nutrients. Thus the bone at the fracture margins and that extending to the level of the next collateral channel is dead and does not participate in the healing process. The avascular segments may be extensive, with as much as 1 to 5 cm of avascular cortex noted in displaced fractures of the femoral and tibial shafts.[199] The accumulation of necrotic material (marrow, periosteum, and adjacent soft tissue) incites an acute inflammatory response with

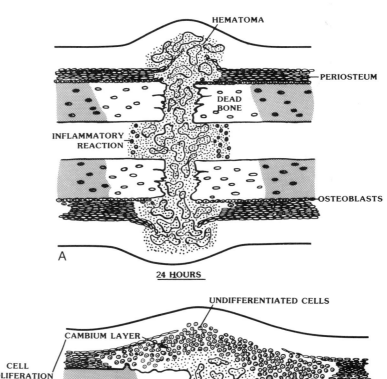

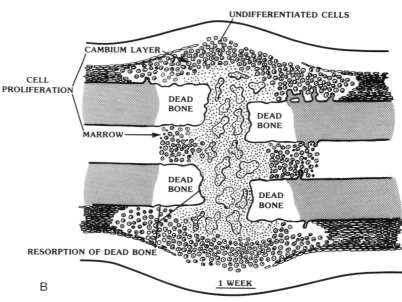

Figure 1–19. Secondary Repair. *A,* Twenty-four hours after fracture. There is hematoma and necrosis of soft tissue elements with an associated inflammatory reaction. The bony margins on each side of the fracture line are dead. *B,* One week after fracture. There is hyperplasia of the combial layer of the periosteum and proliferation of undifferentiated cells in the adjacent connective tissue. New, woven, bone formation has occurred along endosteal and periosteal surfaces. There is some resorption of dead bone.

Illustration continued on following page

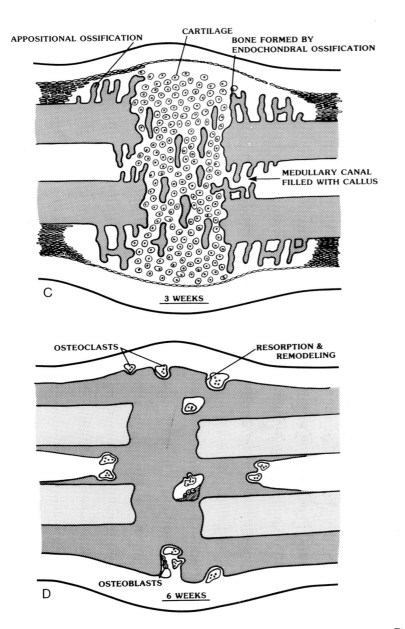

APPOSITIONAL OSSIFICATION
CARTILAGE
BONE FORMED BY
ENDOCHONDRAL OSSIFICATION

MEDULLARY CANAL
FILLED WITH CALLUS

C   3 WEEKS

OSTEOCLASTS

RESORPTION &
REMODELING

OSTEOBLASTS

D   6 WEEKS

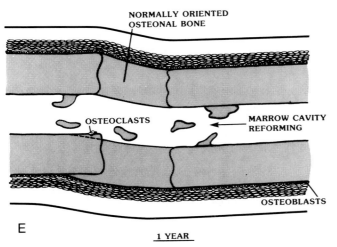

NORMALLY ORIENTED
OSTEONAL BONE

OSTEOCLASTS

MARROW CAVITY
REFORMING

OSTEOBLASTS

E   1 YEAR

Figure 1–19. Secondary Repair *Continued. C,* Three weeks after fracture. Increased amounts of bone have formed under the periosteum. The medullary canal is filled with hyaline cartilage and bone (produced at the edges of the cartilage by endochondral bone formation). This combination of bone and cartilage is early callus. *D,* Six to 12 weeks after fracture. A preponderance of the cartilage has been removed and replaced by bone, which plugs the marrow cavity (darkly stippled). Remodeling has begun. *E,* One year after fracture. Further remodeling has occurred, with reconstitution of the marrow cavity. (Adapted from Kenzora JE: Repair of bone and fracture healing. *In* Cave EF, Burke JF, Boyd RJ, eds. Trauma Management. Copyright © 1974 by Year Book Medical Publishers, Inc., Chicago.

associated vasodilatation; plasma exudation; and infiltration by polymorphonuclear leukocytes, histiocytes, and mast cells.

Reparative Stage. The hematoma that has formed surrounds the fracture site. Within hours fibrin is precipitated within the clot and organization begins, first at the periphery and later centrally. Fibroblasts from the adjacent mesenchyme and blood vessels invade the hematoma, converting it into a mass of granulation tissue. Mesenchymal cells differentiate to form cells capable of producing collagen, cartilage, or bone in amounts that depend on local factors such as the oxygen tension, pH, and stress at the fracture site. Low-oxygen tension is associated with increased cartilage formation, whereas high-oxygen tension in well-vascularized areas favors bone formation. Thus if the callus outgrows its blood supply, cartilage that temporarily bridges the fracture site will be formed.[192] This cartilage will eventually be resorbed and replaced by bone. Bone is also formed from osteoprogenitor

cells derived from the inner (cambium) layer of the periosteum and from the endosteum. These cells have the appearance of normal fibroblasts but have the capacity to divide and give rise to osteoblasts.[192] Thus two sources of bone production are possible: (1) the osteoprogenitor cells of the periosteum or endosteum and (2) fibroblasts in the adjacent soft tissues that, under the influence of certain environmental stimuli, develop the capacity to produce bone—a process termed induction.

From these areas a fusiform mass of fibrous tissue, cartilage, and immature fiber bone, collectively called *primary callus,* develops. The mass of callus immobilizes the fracture fragments sufficiently so that fixation can be discontinued without change in the position of fracture fragments. This corresponds to the stage of *clinical union* (Fig. 1–20).

Remodeling Stage. The bone present in callus is immature (fiber) bone. This type of bone is gradually replaced with adult lamellar bone

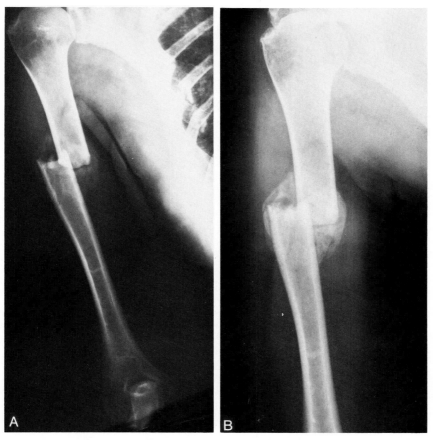

Figure 1–20. Healing Humeral Fracture. *A,* Three weeks after fracture there is early callus formation. *B,* Three weeks later (6 weeks postinjury) there is well developed callus. Minimal tenderness was present at the fracture site, and use of the arm was permitted as tolerated. This corresponds to the stage of clinical union.

25

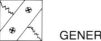

appropriate to withstand normal stress. Radionuclide studies have documented that such bone remodeling may continue for years after a fracture has occurred. It has been suggested that the sites of bone removal and production are determined by an electrical stimulus initiated by stress applied to bone,[179] electropositivity occurring on the convex surface, and electronegativity on the concave aspect of the bone. Electropositive areas are associated with bone resorption and electronegative areas with bone production. Since stress is borne primarily by cortical bone, the medullary callus is gradually resorbed, and the medullary cavities of the major fracture fragments again become continuous.

Healing of Membranous Bone. Where the fracture surfaces are in direct contact, membranous bone unites rapidly via the process of creeping substitution, in which bone apposition or replacement occurs on the surface of trabec-

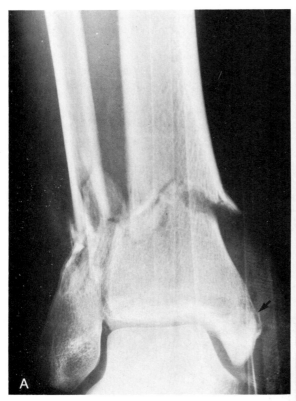

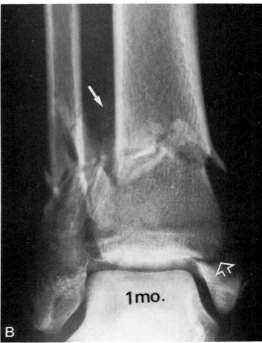

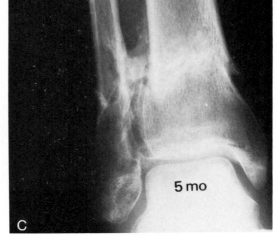

Figure 1–21. Healing Distal Tibial Fractures. *A,* The initial examination shows an almost transverse distal tibial fracture with mild valgus angular deformity. There is a comminuted fibular fracture with angular deformity. The medial malleolar fracture is just visible because of the minor irregularity of the medial cortex (arrow). *B,* At 1 month there is lateral early callus formation (arrow), and some endosteal callus is suggested by the increased density at the fracture line. The medial malleolar fracture line (open arrow) is now more apparent because of bone resorption from the fracture margins. *C,* At 5 months marked healing has occurred, with the distal tibial, the medial malleolar, and the lateral malleolar fracture lines almost obliterated. There is apparent fusion across the tibiofibular syndesmosis.

ulae.[192] Where surfaces are not in contact, there is proliferation of granulation tissue capable of osteogenesis.[199] A minimum of periosteal reaction is noted.

Radiological Correlates (Table 1–13; Figs. 1–20 to 1–22). Initially, the fracture lines are sharp. There is soft-tissue swelling due to hemorrhage and edema. Later, as the hematoma organizes, the soft-tissue swelling decreases. By 10 to 14 days, bone resorption occurs at the fracture margins, and the fracture line, which may have been difficult to see, is now more readily visible.[201] Separated, avascular fracture fragments will become apparent, since their density will remain normal in contrast to the osteo-

penia that develops in vascularized bone with disuse.

Periosteal callus is first identified as an area of faint increase in density in the soft tissues on either side of the fracture line. The rapidity of formation and the amount of periosteal callus formed vary. In young individuals callus may be formed rapidly. In certain areas, such as the patella and the femoral neck, where periosteum is either absent or nonfunctional, periosteal callus does not occur (see Fig. 1–31). In contrast, relatively large amounts of periosteal callus may be seen around fractures that occur in areas covered by muscle, such as the femoral shaft (see Fig. 1–20). Motion at the fracture site

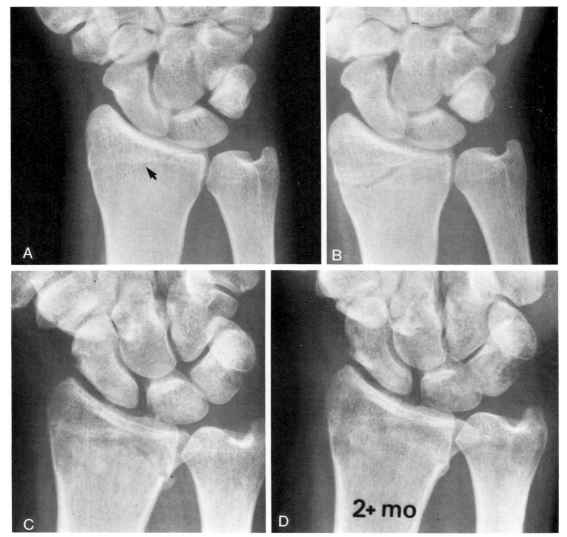

Figure 1–22. Healing of a Colles' Fracture. *A*, The initial PA radiograph shows a faint distal radial fracture line (arrow). *B*, Three weeks later the fracture line is much more apparent because of bone resorption from its margins. *C*, Another patient. At 1 month the fracture line is visible with sclerosis (endosteal callus) on either side. A small amount of periosteal reaction is present. *D*, At about 2½ months the fracture has united.

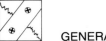

Table 1–13. **Fracture Healing**

Approximate Time	Histological Change	Radiographic Changes
Immediate	Hematoma	Sharp fracture line Soft tissue swelling
+ 6 hours	Fibroblasts penetrate outer margins of hematoma	
+ 2 days	Proliferation of cambium layer of periosteum	
+ 3 days	Capillaries extend into clot; collagen production in clot with organization of hematoma from periphery inward	Soft tissue swelling
+ 6 days	Osteoid produced by cambium layer of periosteum	Subperiosteal bone production
+ 9 days	Metaplasia of fibroblasts in clot to chondroblasts → cartilage across fracture ends that merges with the	Osteopenia
+ 11 days	ring of cartilage that forms around the periphery of the fracture ends (derived from the periosteum)	Bone resorption from fracture margins
+ 16 days	Osteoid produced from endochondral bone formation	Callus visible
+ 30 days	"Good" endosteal osteochondroid callus	
2–3 months	Abundant callus beginning to organize (clinical union)	Callus with sharp margins bridging fracture; fracture line begins to disappear
Months–years	Replacement of fiber bone with lamellar bone (bony union)	Marrow cavity continuous; re-formed cortices

stimulates the formation of periosteal callus, whereas stable fixation considerably limits the amount of callus produced. With time periosteal callus matures, its outer margin becomes more distinct, and eventually the callus merges with the normal cortex.

As healing progresses, *endosteal* as well as periosteal callus is being formed. The endosteal callus, however, may be obscured by the periosteal reaction and by the surrounding cortex. Eventually, however, the fracture line becomes indistinct, disappears, and is replaced by a zone of increased density formed by endosteal callus. During remodeling endosteal callus is removed, and the marrow cavity is re-formed.

When Is the Fracture Healed? The time for healing varies depending on a number of factors, including the age of the patient and the site of fracture (Tables 1–14 and 1–15). A single fracture of a long bone, such as the femur, takes about 4 months to heal, whereas a humeral fracture may take only 2 months. Oblique fractures with greater surface area tend to heal more rapidly.

As summarized by Juhl, the amount and character of periosteal callus may be used as a guide for the removal of traction or a cast, provided that the site and nature of the fracture are taken into account.[187] For example, an upper extremity fracture in which hazy periosteal callus is seen may be stable enough to allow some use. In lower extremity fractures, however, more

Table 1–14. **Factors Influencing the Rate of Fracture Healing**

Faster Healing
  Youth
  Long oblique or spiral fracture configuration
  Impaction

Slower Healing
  Diastasis
  Intraarticular extension
  Limited blood supply

Table 1–15. **Periods of Immobilization of Common Fractures**

Phalanges	A few days to 2 weeks
Metacarpals	2–3 weeks
Carpal bones, other than scaphoid	3–6 weeks
Scaphoid	10–16 weeks
Forearm bones	
Adults	8–14 weeks
Humeral shaft	8–12 weeks
Clavicle	
Adults	4–6 weeks
Metatarsals	3–4 weeks
Tarsals	6–8 weeks
Tibia	
Without fracture of the fibula	
Older children and adults	8–16 weeks
With fracture of the fibula	
Older children and adults	12–20 weeks
Femur	
Older children and adults	12–24 weeks

solid and mature callus, with the outer margins sharp and continuous across the fracture site, is necessary before the extremity can be used. The position of the fracture fragments should have remained constant on serial films before any active use is permitted. The fracture line itself, however, may still be visible.

In cases in which the fracture margins have been apposed and there is little periosteal callus, it is often difficult to know when enough endosteal callus has formed to prevent motion. Sometimes, enough bone resorption will have occurred along the fracture line to make the line more apparent; then gradual fading of this line indicates healing.[187] Finally, the trabecular pattern across the fracture line will become continuous. This, too, may be difficult to assess, since impaction produced at the time of internal fixation may produce apparent trabecular continuity from the outset.

Radionuclide Bone Scanning

Fracture Detection. Studies have shown increased uptake of bone scanning agents at fracture sites as early as 7 hours after injury. Matin noted that within 24 hours of fracture, 80 percent of patients reviewed had abnormal bone scans.[190] Of the 4 patients with false negative scans, 1 examination was technically suboptimal and 3 were in patients older than 65. By 3 days all patients under 65 years and 95 percent of older patients had abnormal scans (Table 1–16). Therefore, in younger patients a negative scan at 24 hours essentially excludes an acute fracture. In older patients a fracture is most unlikely if the bone scan remains negative at 3 days after injury.

Evaluation of Fracture Healing. Uptake patterns on bone scan vary with the age of the fracture. An acute phase of diffuse activity centered at the fracture site persists for 2 to 4 weeks, followed by a subacute phase of well-defined linear uptake lasting 8 to 12 weeks, which is followed by a gradual decrease in isotope uptake.[191] Uptake may remain increased at the fracture site for years, but in general, recent fractures show intense isotopic activity, although older fractures have mildly increased or normal uptake. Matin showed that by 3 years most areas of prior fracture exhibited normal uptake (Table 1–17). The bone scan does not indicate the point at which clinical union is established; it may, however, be helpful in documenting complications such as nonunion.

Abnormalities of Fracture Healing
(Table 1–18)

In the average situation (e.g., fracture of the tibia), union by primary callus is seen in 2 to 3 months and consolidation of callus occurs in 4 to 5 months.[203] Many factors influence the rate of fracture healing, including patient age, fracture configuration, the presence of impaction, diastasis at the fracture site, intraarticular involvement, and the blood supply to the fracture (Table 1–14).

Slow Union. Certain fractures heal slowly even under ideal circumstances.[198] The fracture line remains visible on radiographs, but there is no cavitation of the fracture margins or sclerosis.[203]

Table 1–17. Incidence of Normal Bone Scans at Fracture Site

Fracture Site	% Normal 3 Years After Fracture
Vertebrae	97
Long bones	95
Ribs	100
Miscellaneous	95

Source: Matin P: J Nucl Med 20:127, 1979, with permission.

Table 1–16. Time After Fracture at Which Bone Scan Becomes Abnormal

Time After Fracture	Patients Studied	Number with Abnormal Scans	Percent Abnormal	Percent Abnormal Under Age 65
1 day	20	16	80	95
3 days	39	37	95	100
1 week	60	59	98	100

Source: Matin P: J Nucl Med 20:1227, 1979, with permission.

Table 1–18. Abnormalities of Fracture Healing

	Definition	Radiographic Appearance
Slow Union	Normal slow healing of certain fractures	Fracture line clearly seen No cavitation No sclerosis
Delayed Union	Fragments fail to unite in expected time	Resorption of fracture ends Cavitation along fracture margins No sclerosis
Nonunion	Fragments joined by dense scar or false joint Healing has stopped	Atrophic Fracture line persists No callus No change with long follow-up Hypertrophic Elephant foot Horse foot Oligotrophic Lucency between fracture ends
Malunion	Fracture united in unacceptable position	

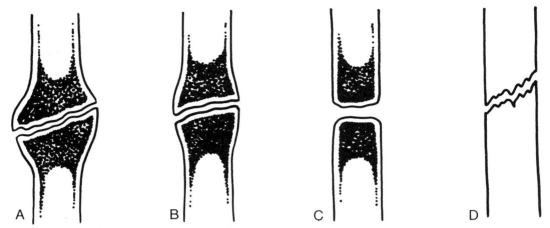

Figure 1–23. Nonunion. The hypertrophic forms—elephant foot *(A)*, horse foot *(B)*, and oligotrophic *(C)*—and the atrophic form *(D)* of nonunion are shown. (Adapted from Naimark A et al: Skeletal Radiol 6:21, 1981, by permission.)

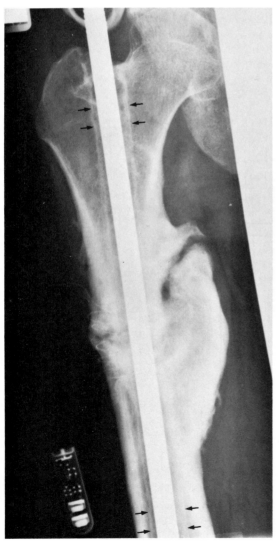

Figure 1–24. Hypertrophic Nonunion with Loosening of the Intramedullary Rod. The coned view of the fracture site shows considerable sclerosis and periosteal reaction. The fracture line remains clearly visible. Proximal and distal bone resorption about the intramedullary rod (arrows) attests to its loosening. A helical cathode device has been inserted for elecrical stimulation.

Delayed Union. This refers to a failure of bony union to occur within the expected time.[198] Fibrous tissue or fibrocartilage remains between the fracture fragments for a protracted period but is eventually replaced by bone.[200] The diagnosis of delayed union is based on clinical assessment.[197] A number of factors predispose to delayed union, and if these factors continue, they also predispose to nonunion. The factors include

1. Fractures in large tubular bones
2. Inadequate immobilization
3. Severe soft tissue damage
4. Extensive necrosis of fracture margins
5. Distraction of fracture edges
6. Comminution
7. Infection
8. Inadequate reduction
9. Surgical intervention, especially with stripping of the periosteum

Radiographic findings include resorption of the fracture margins, with irregular cavities that have been shown on histological examination to be filled with granulation tissue. There is no sclerosis.[203]

Nonunion. The designation of nonunion indicates that healing has stopped before bony continuity has been reestablished. The gap between fracture fragments contains dense fibrous tissue. A variant of nonunion, pseudarthrosis, in which a false joint containing serum forms inside the scar tissue, may occur. This is most often seen in the clavicle, humerus, or tibia.

Radiological Findings of Nonunion. Radiological investigation in patients with suspected nonunion should include multiple views of the fracture site (i.e., anteroposterior, lateral, and both oblique views) so that the diagnosis is not obscured by overlapping bone. Occasionally, fluoroscopy may be helpful (see Fig. 1–26). Findings include smoothing and rounding of the fracture margins and increasing sclerosis of the bone ends in about 25 percent of patients.[184] Motion may be demonstrated on films taken during the careful application of stress. Absence of healing on three successive monthly radiographic examinations is said to indicate nonunion.[182] Progressive bowing deformity at the fracture site and absence of remodeling also suggest the diagnosis.

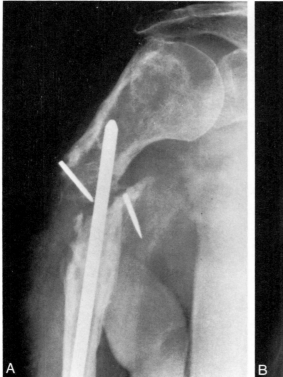
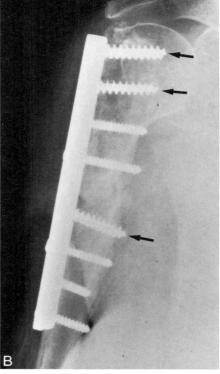

Figure 1–25. Humeral Nonunion Treated wth Bone Grafting and Dynamic Compression (DC) Plate with Cortical and Cancellous Screws. *A,* There had been two surgical attempts to unite this fracture, but union did not occur, and varus deformity developed despite the intramedullary rod. *B,* A third attempt at bone grafting resulted in healing. Both cortical and cancellous (arrows) screws were used.

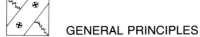
As summarized by Naimark and associates, two radiographically discrete types of nonunion can be distinguished (Fig. 1–23).[194] The first, *hypertrophic nonunion,* is thought to be caused by continued motion at the fracture site (Figs. 1–24 to 1–26). The fracture line persists, and there is buildup of external callus, widening the diameter of the bone ends (the elephant foot or the smaller horse foot appearance). Bone resorption of the fracture margins, termed oligotrophic nonunion, may also occur. Each of these radiographic appearances is said to indicate viability of the bone ends.[194] Hypertrophic nonunion may heal with immobilization alone. The second type of nonunion seen radiographically, *atrophic nonunion,* is thought to result from extensive bone death. The radiographic appearance is that of a persistent fracture line with no demonstrable callus and no change over long periods of time (Fig. 1–27). The fracture ends may be minimally molded. Immobilization alone

is generally ineffective and must be supplemented, in most instances, by bone grafting.

Radionuclide Studies of Nonunion. The diagnosis of nonunion may be suggested by serial quantitative bone scans. Thus Muheim noted an increased ratio of isotopic uptake (fractured leg:nonfractured leg) in comparison with normal healing in a patient with hypertrophic nonunion and a decreased ratio in another patient with atrophic nonunion.[193] Esterhai and co-workers used technetium-99m bone scans to classify patients with nonunion into those with nonunion alone and those with nonunion and false joint formation.[182] This differentiation seems clinically relevant, since nonunions associated with pseudarthrosis usually did not heal after electrical stimulation, whereas those nonunions without pseudarthrosis often healed with this treatment. Nonunions were found to have three patterns of isotopic uptake:

1. Intense focal uptake at the site of non-

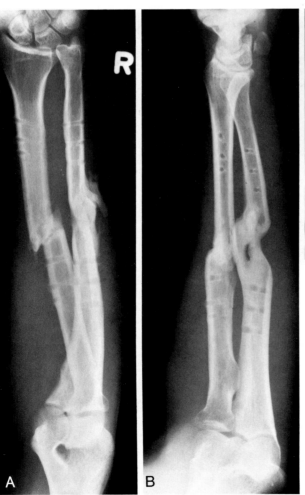

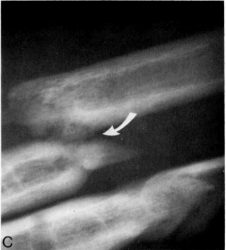

Figure 1–26. Nonunion Demonstrated on Fluoroscopy. Two views *(A and B)* show deformity from prior midshaft radial and ulnar fractures and evidence of prior internal fixation. Little callus is seen about the radial fracture site. Fluoroscopy *(C)* confirms nonunion of the radial fracture (arrow).

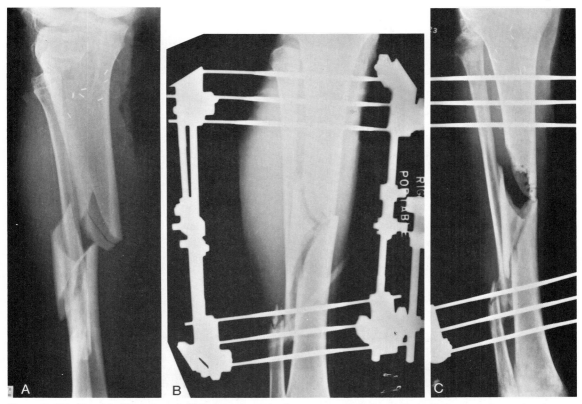

Figure 1–27. Atrophic Nonunion. *A,* This patient sustained comminuted tibial and fibular fractures and vascular damage that was surgically repaired. *B,* The fracture fragments are held in adequate position by a Hoffman apparatus. *C,* Four months later, after debridement and drilling, there is no evidence of healing. The fracture fragments are distracted. Amputation was eventually necessary.

union. These patients usually responded to electrical stimulation. Failures were due to occult infection or inadequate immobilization rather than to pseudarthrosis formation.

2. Two intense areas of isotopic uptake separated by a "cold" zone. This pattern usually indicated the presence of a pseudarthrosis, and most of these fractures did not heal with electrical stimulation.

3. Indeterminate pattern. In this pattern a definite cold zone could not be seen.

It is noteworthy that in this study no patient with a nonunion had a completely cold scan. Matin, however, noted that atrophic nonunion may exhibit a generalized decrease or an absence of radionuclide uptake at the fracture site.[191]

Reduction

The objectives of fracture treatment include allowing the bone to heal in a functional position with return to usual activities in the shortest time, with the least expense, and with minimal cosmetic alteration.[183]

When is reduction adequate? This is a complex question without a single answer. Although healing occurs fastest when the fracture ends are apposed, anatomical reduction is not always possible or necessary in order to achieve a satisfactory clinical result. One important factor in judging the adequacy of reduction is the location of the fracture. Thus, although anatomical reduction is required in treating forearm fractures, considerable deformity may persist in humeral fractures without untoward functional or cosmetic effects. An overlap of 2 cm is tolerable in femoral or tibial fractures and can be compensated by pelvic tilt. Healing of tibial fractures with as much as 5 degrees of varus or valgus angular deformity is acceptable, whereas rotational abnormalities are not acceptable. Anterior or posterior bowing deformities may be compensated by adjacent hinge joints. A final fracture position that is unacceptable functionally or cosmetically is termed malunion (Fig. 1–28; see also Fig. 1–65).

Closed Reduction. Closed reduction is accomplished by traction or manipulation without

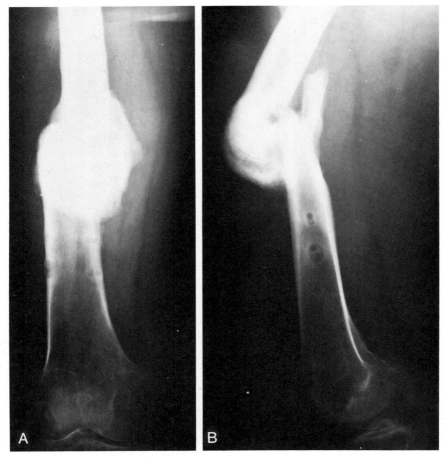

Figure 1–28. Malunion. At the midfemoral fracture site AP *(A)* and lateral *(B)* views show marked angular deformity, for which osteotomy was necessary. Resorption about the distal pin track, indicating prior infection, is present.

surgical intervention. Reduction is usually achieved by applying traction in the long axis of the limb, reversing the mechanism that produced the fracture, and aligning the fragment that can be controlled (the distal fragment) with the one that cannot. The results of closed reduction depend on an intact soft-tissue bond between the fracture fragments. This soft-tissue hinge links the fracture fragments, allows the fracture to be reduced, and, if tension is maintained, stabilizes the fracture after reduction. Once reduction is achieved, it may be maintained by casting, traction, or splinting. Casts may be made of plaster of Paris, in which case the fracture itself may be partially obscured on conventional radiographs—although xerography allows the underlying fracture to be seen to advantage. Fiberglass casts made of light-curing plastics are lightweight, cannot be damaged by water, and are relatively radiolucent.

Traction. Continuous traction may be applied by exerting a pull on the skin or on pins inserted through bone distal to the fracture site. Radiologically demonstrable complications include overdistraction of the fracture site (sometimes leading to delayed union or nonunion) and local complications at the pin sites. Traction may also be produced by means of a plaster cast (e.g., the hanging cast for treating humeral fractures).

Open Reduction. Open reduction refers to the manipulation of fracture fragments after incision of the skin and the soft tissues over the fracture site. Open reduction carries with it the increased hazard of infection and therefore is not undertaken lightly. Standards for open reduction (usually followed by internal fixation) are not universal. The following criteria, however, are suggested by Sisk:[213]

1. Fractures that are not reducible by manipulation or closed methods
2. Displaced intraarticular fractures
3. Certain epiphyseal fractures
4. Major avulsion fractures

5. Nonunions

6. Replantations of extremities

Relative indications include the following:

1. Delayed union

2. Multiple fractures

3. Loss of reduction (a second trial of closed treatment should also be considered)

4. Pathological fracture of a major long bone

5. Facilitation of nursing care

6. Decrease of mortality and morbidity associated with prolonged immobilization

7. Treatment of fractures known to be ineffectively treated by closed means

Contraindications. Open reduction is often contraindicated in the presence of active infection or osteomyelitis, although this is a controversial issue. Severe osteopenia, the presence of fracture fragments of insufficient size to allow solid fixation of the hardware, and the presence of severe soft tissue abnormalities, such as extensive burns, are other contraindications. As in most surgical procedures, general medical contraindications also apply.

Fixation

Fixation refers to the method of holding fracture fragments in position after reduction. *Internal fixation* refers to the placement of hardware across the fracture site. *External fixation* may include the use of casts or specially constructed devices that are affixed to the adjacent bone.

Internal Fixation. Internal fixation of fracture fragments may involve wires, screws and plates, or intramedullary devices. According to the Association for the Study of the Problem of Internal Fixation (AO or ASIF), perfect internal fixation means (1) anatomic reduction, (2) stable internal fixation, (3) preservation of blood supply to the bone fragments and local soft tissues, and (4) early active pain-free motion.[208]

Open reduction is usually followed by internal fixation, although internal fixation may be used even when open reduction is not done. For example, wires may be inserted percutaneously to hold a fracture that has been reduced by closed methods.

Pinning. Smooth or threaded pins or Kirschner wires (K-wires) may be used to hold fracture fragments in position while healing occurs (Fig. 1–29). This method is frequently used to maintain the position of fracture fragments involving the small bones of the hands or feet. The pins are inserted obliquely in relation to the fracture lines. Threaded pins may require general anes-

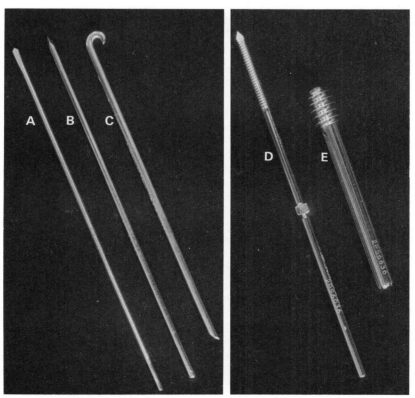

Figure 1–29. Some Pins for Holding Fractures in Position. *A,* Threaded Kirschner wire (K-wire). *B,* Smooth Kirschner wire (K-wire). *C,* Rush pin. *D,* Knowles pin. *E,* Richards compression screw.

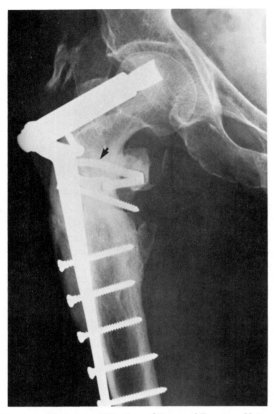

Figure 1–30. Internal Fixation of Femoral Fracture Using a Parham Band. No history is available. A nail and plate have been used, apparently to hold an intertrochanteric-subtrochanteric fracture. A circumferential (Parham) band (arrow) was used; medially, there is considerable bone resorption beneath it.

thesia for their removal, whereas smooth pins may be removed using local anesthesia.[213]

Wires. Circumferential wires may be used as the major mode of fracture treatment or to supplement intramedullary nailing, as in the femur when a butterfly fragment is present. These wires are thin and do not interfere with periosteal blood supply or periosteal callus. The thicker Parham bands, however, may interfere with periosteal circulation (Fig. 1–30).

The concept of *tension-band wiring*, or *plating*, refers to an AO technique based on the principle that an eccentrically loaded bone is subjected to bending stresses, with tension on the convex side and compression on the concave side. A tension band consisting of a wire or a plate absorbs the tensile forces, and the bone is then subjected primarily to axial compression that increases as the part is used. Thus the hardware absorbs the tension, and the bone absorbs the compression (Figs. 1–31 and

1–32).[208] Kirschner wires may be added to increase rotational stability and to help anchor the wires. Since the bone will be subjected to compression stresses, it cannot be grossly deficient or bending will occur that will fracture the wires.

Screws.[183, 213] Two types of screws are used, cortical and cancellous (Fig. 1–33). Cortical screws are threaded throughout their length and have blunt ends. They are usually used to secure bone plates or nail-plate devices. Cortical screws can be used as lag screws (to produce compression) by drilling a hole in the near cortex that is wider than the threads of the screw (overdrilling) so that the threads engage only the far cortex (Fig. 1–34).

Cancellous screws (lag screws) are only threaded distally, and the threads are wider than those in the cortical screw to provide better purchase in cancellous bone. A washer may be placed under the screw head to help prevent its

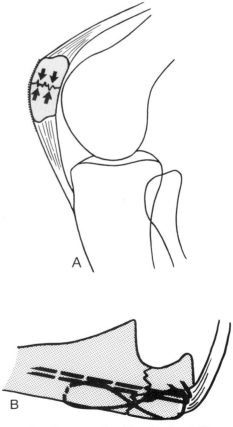

Figure 1–31. The Principle of Tension-Band Wiring. The wire absorbs the tension, and the bone the compression. *A,* The knee. The anteriorly placed tension band (dashed line) and the compression forces on the fracture (arrows) are shown. *B,* The same principle in the elbow produces compression at the fracture site.

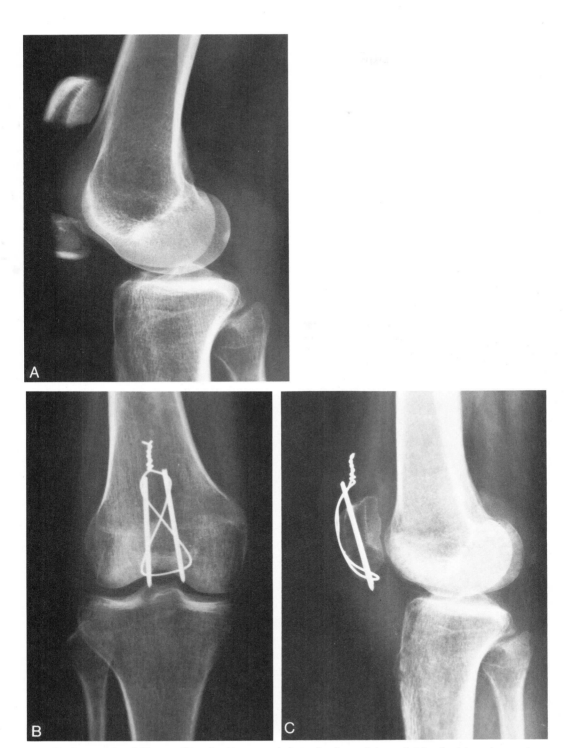

Figure 1–32. Tension-Band Wiring of Patellar Fracture. *A,* Lateral radiograph immediately after injury shows a transverse patellar fracture with wide separation of fracture fragments. AP *(B)* and lateral *(C)* views after tension-band wiring show only minor step-off at the patellar articular surface and 1 mm anterior separation of the fracture fragments. There is moderate osteopenia. Complete healing occurred without complication.

CORTICAL SCREW   CANCELLOUS SCREW

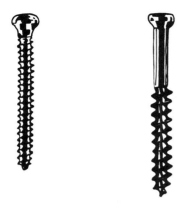

Figure 1–33. Types of Screws.

penetration through the cortex in patients with osteopenia. Malleolar screws are sharply pointed and have distal threads. Because of their sharp points, they can be inserted without predrilling a hole.

Screw fixation alone may be used to treat fractures of the medial malleoli and the medial epicondyle and to treat long oblique or spiral diaphyseal fractures.[185, 213] More often, screws are used in combination with other types of internal fixation. The threaded portion of a cancellous screw should be placed in the distal fragment and should not cross the fracture line lest the threads interfere with compression across the fracture site.

When a cortical screw is used for the fixation of a plate to bone, any screw that crosses a fracture line should be inserted as a lag screw.

Others should engage both the near and far cortices. The presence of a screw or a screw hole makes the bone more liable to fracture (see Fig. 1–37).

Plates. Plates fulfill one or more of the following functions.[208]

Static compression: Appropriate bending of the plate ("tensile prestress") results in axial compression across the fracture.

Dynamic compression: A plate used in this way neutralizes all the tensile stresses so that pure compression stresses are present at the fracture site (Fig. 1–35). According to the ASIF/AO group, this technique may be used in the treatment of pseudarthrosis, after osteotomy, or after attempted fusion. Tension across the device is generated by attaching the plate to one side of the reduced fracture and screwing a tension device into the bone at the other end of the plate, which is then tightened, producing compression across the fracture site.

Another means of providing the dynamic compression is the dynamic compression plate (DCP), which can provide any of the functions of a plate. Rather than round holes, DCP plates have holes with beveled edges (Fig. 1–36). As a screw head is tightened, it slides down the inclined cylinder of the screw hole, producing a horizontal movement of the underlying bone with respect to the plate and compression along the fracture site.

Neutralization: When used in this way, the plate neutralizes most of the torsional, shearing, and bending forces that are present and protects the fixation achieved by lag screws inserted separately or through the plate.

Buttressing: When used for buttressing, the

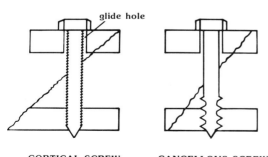

CORTICAL SCREW   CANCELLOUS SCREW
(used as lag screw)

Figure 1–34. Lag Screw and Cortical Screw Used as Lag Screw to Produce Compression Across a Fracture. To use a cortical screw as a lag screw, the hole in the near cortex must be wider than the screw threads so that the threads engage only the far cortex.

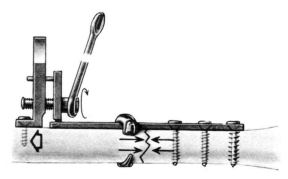

Figure 1–35. Use of the AO Tension Device to Produce Compression at the Fracture Site. As the screw of the tension device is tightened (curved arrow), compression occurs at the fracture site. After the remainder of the screws are inserted into the plate, the tension device is removed, leaving an empty screw hole at the site (open arrow). (Reprinted from Muller ME, et al.: Manual of Internal Fixation: Technique Recommended by the AO Group. Heidelberg, Springer-Verlag, 1979, with permission.)

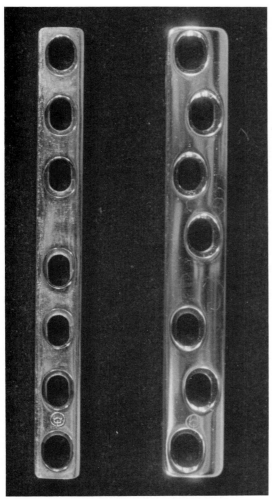

Figure 1–36. Dynamic Compression Plates (DCP). As the screws are tightened in the beveled holes, horizontal movement of the bone with relation to the plate occurs, producing compression at the fracture site.

plate functions to protect a cortical or cancellous bone graft from collapsing or to bridge a long diaphyseal defect while bone graft is being incorporated.

AO plates.[208] Several plates have been developed by the AO group to provide axial compression at the fracture site. After the fracture is reduced, the plate (tension-band) is applied to the side of the bone under tension (the convex side of an angular deformity or the side opposite the soft-tissue hinge). One cortical screw is positioned to hold the plate down. A tension device is then applied to the opposite end of the plate and tightened until the fracture is compressed. The remainder of the screws are inserted into the first fragment, perfectly centered within the holes in the plate. The screw of the tension

device is turned, further increasing the compression across the fracture site. The remaining screws are then inserted, the tension device is removed, and finally, a screw is inserted through the endhole of the plate—usually through only one cortex to provide a more gradual transition of forces between plated and unplated segments.

The dynamic compression plate (DCP) introduced by AO differs from the standard AO plates in that, because of the shapes of the holes and the corresponding screw heads, the fracture fragments are brought together as the screws are tightened. The tension device is not needed to achieve axial compression, and the screws may be angled.

Ideally, fractures treated with compression plating should heal with revascularization and endosteal bone formation and no apparent periosteal callus. The amount of external callus produced reflects the degree of motion at the fracture site.

Other plates. Other plates (Bagby, Hirschhorn, Kondo, and Marumo plates) are in use, and each has advantages.[204]

Complications. With all plates the bone under the plate atrophies, and this predisposes the bone to refracture. The presence of a rigid plate also predisposes the bone to fracture at the lower end of the plate because of differences in the elasticity of the plate and the bone (Fig. 1–37). In order to decrease the propensity to fracture, the end screws may be inserted through only one cortex. After the plates have been removed, fracture may occur through the screw holes. Although these holes fill with woven bone in about 6 weeks,[183] the screw tract remains visible on radiographs considerably longer.

Intramedullary Rods, Nails, and Pins (Figs. 1–38 to 1–43). There are no good definitions that separate the terms *rod, nail,* and *pin,* although rods are generally considered the thickest, whereas nails are thinner, and pins the thinnest. The following remarks apply primarily to rods and to a lesser extent to intramedullary nails and pins.

Intramedullary rods have been used in the treatment of almost all types of diaphyseal fractures, although they are particularly suited for transverse midshaft fractures. Rods are not used for treating open fractures. They generally protect against angular deformity but resist torque poorly. They must be strong enough to maintain alignment and should allow compression to occur at the fracture site.

Since rods interfere with the blood supply to the endosteum and the inner two thirds of the

Text continued on page 44

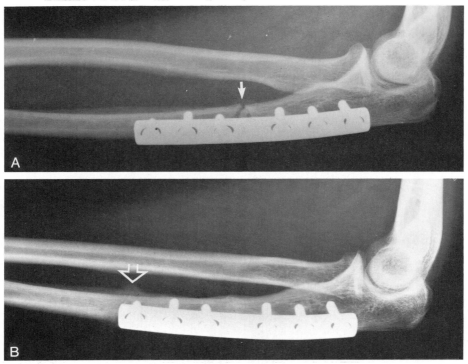

Figure 1–37. Fracture near the End of a Compression Plate. *A*, A compression plate with six screws holds an ulnar fracture in almost anatomical position. Faint periosteal reaction (arrow) is noted. *B*, Ten months later (1 month after another fall and the onset of new pain) the ulnar fracture has healed. Faint periosteal reaction and a faint lucency (open arrow) confirm the presence of a new fracture at the end of the plate.

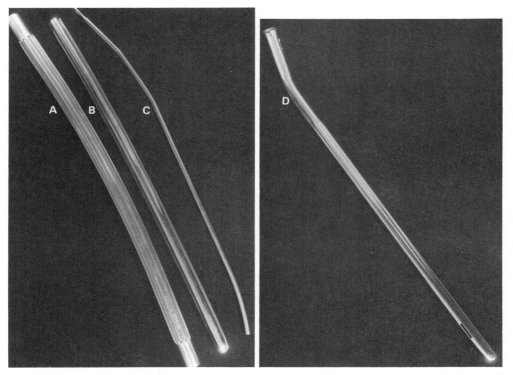

Figure 1–38. Intramedullary Rods. Sampson *(A)*, Küntscher *(B)*, Ender *(C; the distal end is up)*, and AO tibial *(D)* rods.

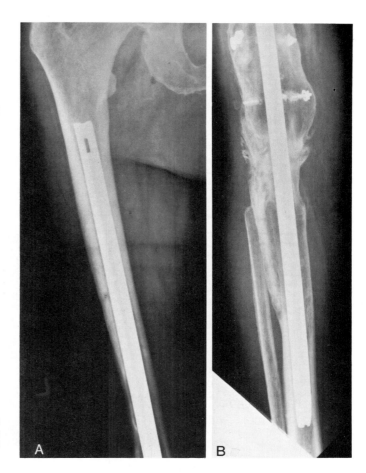

Figure 1–39. Küntscher Nail. AP views of the distal femur *(A)* and the knee *(B)* show the Küntscher nail that was used for immobilization during knee fusion.

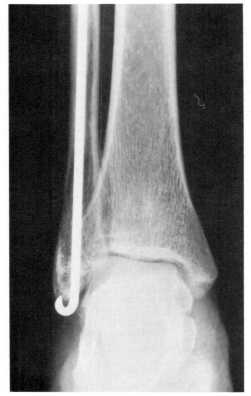

Figure 1–40. Rush Pin. The hooked end facilitates removal and prevents migration.

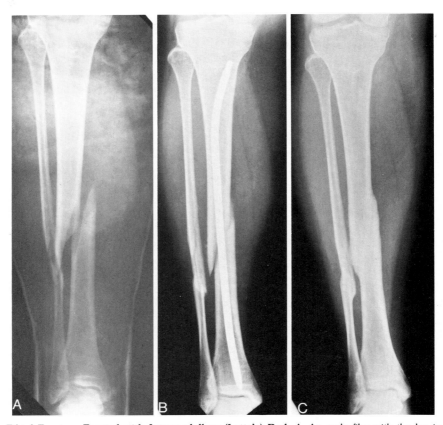

Figure 1–41. Tibial Fracture Treated with Intramedullary (Lotte's) Rod. *A,* An early film with the leg in a plaster cast shows a spiral fracture of the tibia with three quarters of a shaft-widths medial displacement of the distal fragment and about 2 degrees of varus. A fibular fracture is present. *B,* Open reduction and bone grafting were performed, and a rod was advanced across the fracture site. The displacement is markedly reduced. *C,* The intramedullary rod was removed 18 months later, after solid union was established.

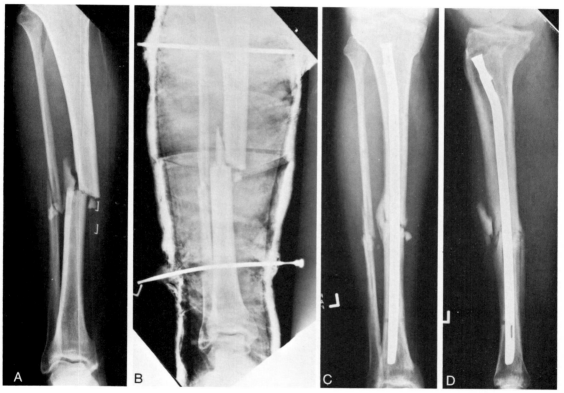

Figure 1–42. Tibial Fracture Treated with Pins in Plaster and Then with Intramedullary Rodding. *A,* There are comminuted fractures of the midtibial and the fibular shafts with 8 degrees of valgus angulation and half a shaft-widths lateral displacement of the distal tibial fragment. *B,* An attempt was made to improve deformity by closed manipulation and by fixation with pins in plaster. Mild varus angular deformity and three-fourths of a shaft-widths lateral displacement of the distal tibial fragment are noted. AP *(C)* and lateral *(D)* views following intramedullary (AO) rod placement. Angular deformity and displacement have been corrected. Moderate callus is noted about both fractures.

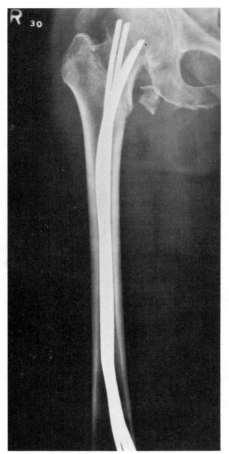

Figure 1–43. Ender Rods. Multiple Ender rods were used for internal fixation after closed reduction of an intertrochanteric fracture.

Table 1–19. **Possible Complications of Intramedullary Rodding**

Poor positioning or incorrect size of rod
Splitting of shaft or separation of fracture fragment
Inadequate fixation, with motion at fracture site
Loosening, bending, or breaking of the rod
Fat embolization
Corrosion of the rod
Spread of infection throughout the shaft

cortex, any healing that occurs is the result of periosteal new bone formation and of the organization of fracture hematoma. When rigid fixation is achieved, periosteal callus is noted to be confined to the fracture site. In contrast, when the rod is loose and motion occurs at the fracture site, periosteal callus is abundant and extends the entire length of the rod (see Fig. 1–24).[213]

After healing has occurred the nail should be removed. Removal is usually done about 18 months after lower extremity fractures.

Possible complications of intramedullary rodding include difficulties in positioning, which may lead to the splitting of the shaft longitudinally, to the inability to advance or withdraw the nail, or to the separation of previously inconspicuous fracture fragments. The nail must be of correct size. If it is too long, it may impinge on an adjacent joint or present a prominent proximal end that may be a source of pain. If the nail is too short, it may not stabilize the fracture sufficiently, or it may become completely embedded in the intramedullary cavity, making it difficult to remove. A too-thin nail may bend or break instead of adequately immobilizing the fracture site.

There may be other complications (Table 1–19): Motion at the fracture site is suggested by bone resorption about the lower end of the rod (the windshield-wiper sign) (see Fig. 1–24). Eventually, the rod may bend or break. The potential for spread of infection throughout the shaft is present.

Types of rods. The *Küntscher nail* has a cloverleaf-shaped cross section; it is hollow and is split longitudinally for part of its length so that it is compressible but can expand when bone resorption occurs (Fig. 1–39).[216] Küntscher emphasized that the entire width and most of the length of the medullary canal should be filled by the rod and that the rod should remain "absolutely immovable" during healing. The *Rush pin* has a sled-runner point that helps guide the pin through the medullary cavity and a hooked proximal end that prevents distal migration of the pin and allows it to be removed after healing has occurred (Fig. 1–40).[214, 215] Although the pin may be inserted after closed reduction of the fracture, exposure of the fracture site has been recommended. The canal is not reamed and is not filled by the pin. For a discussion of *Ender rods*, see the treatment of intertrochanteric fractures in Chapter 8.[43]

External Skeletal Fixation.[217, 218] External skeletal fixation is used principally in the treatment of fractures in which infection or extensive soft-tissue damage is present. The modern era of external skeletal fixation began in the 1930s when workers in the United States and Switzerland developed devices that could provide both immobilization and the possibility of further reduction of fracture deformity after application. Subsequent improvements included increasing the rigidity of fixation by increasing both the strength of the external frame and the number of frames used. Depending on the clinical necessity, unilateral, bilateral, and complex configurations are possible.

Indications. External skeletal fixation has been used for maintenance of compression during attempted fusion, for distraction during limb lengthening, and for immobilization during fracture healing. Indications for use of these devices include the following:

1. Treatment of complex comminuted open fractures, especially if there is segmental bone loss and soft-tissue disruption

2. Fracture stabilization when there is major vascular damage requiring repair

3. Severe osteoporosis when internal fixation may be inadequate

4. Severe epiphyseal and metaphyseal comminution; distraction across the joint may produce realignment of fracture fragments

5. Free vascularized bone graft

6. Infected nonunions, especially if active infection and cellulitis are present.

Relative indications include (1) certain simple fractures, (2) attempted arthrodesis, (3) limb lengthening, (4) certain soft-tissue problems such as extensive burns, and (5) segmental spinal immobilization.

Complications. Pin tract infection: The incidence of pin tract infection has declined with improvements in the materials used. Its incidence increases as the thickness of soft tissue traversed by the pins increases (see Fig. 1–48).

Soft-tissue damage: Damage to adjacent muscles and soft tissues may occur, producing pain or contracture.

Some of the Available Systems. For review of most of the available systems, the reader is referred to the books by Mears and by Seligson and Pope.[217, 218] Some of the more frequently used systems include the following (Figs. 1–44 to 1–48):

The AO (ASIF) system is used primarily in the lower extremities. It may be used as a unilateral device (e.g., for compression of certain stable fractures) or as a bilateral (mediolateral) frame to hold a comminuted fracture—for example, in the tibia—or in a triangular configuration for fractures with segmental bone loss.

The Charnley apparatus may be used for distraction or compression, although it was originally developed for compression following attempted surgical fusion at the knee or ankle (Fig. 1–44). Two smooth or threaded Steinmann pins are inserted in parallel, separated by 2.54 cm, into each of the proximal and distal fragments. These are connected to a bilateral frame

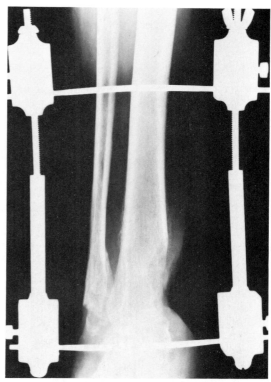

Figure 1–44. Charnley Compression Device. The compression across the site of attempted ankle fusion is shown by the bending of the transfixation pins.

through which compression or distraction is applied.

The Hoffmann device is a versatile system that may be used in both the upper and the lower extremities, in the pelvis, and in the spine, since it can be constructed in a large variety of configurations (Fig. 1–46). Threaded pins are used, and the frame is quadrilateral in configuration.

The Wagner device consists of a strong unilateral frame that is more rigid than the other appliances (Fig. 1–47). It is used particularly for limb lengthening.

Various types of fixation pins are used for the previously discussed devices. Those pins with greatest diameter contribute more to the strength and rigidity of the overall apparatus than do the thinner pins. The former are used particularly in patients with osteopenia. Threaded pins may be used to improve anchorage in bone. Transfixing pins are threaded centrally so that the threads will contact both cortices, the pins being held on each end by the apparatus. Half pins have one end attached to the frame; the other end is threaded. Other pins have two centrally threaded areas and an intervening smooth por-

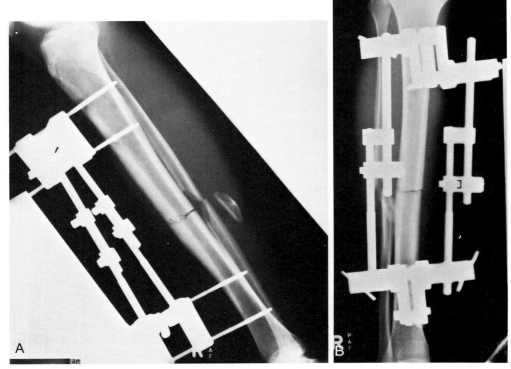

Figure 1–45. External Fixation. This was an open fracture. External fixation was used to hold the tibial fracture fragments in almost anatomical position during fracture healing. A posterior butterfly fragment that originated from the fibula is present.

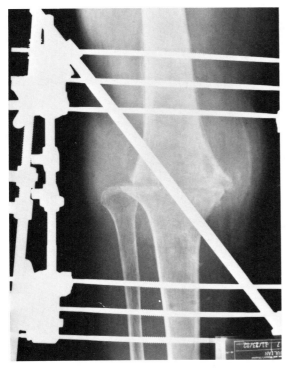

Figure 1–46. Hoffmann Apparatus. Use of a Hoffmann apparatus to achieve fixation during healing of knee fusion was necessitated by the removal of an infected total knee prosthesis. Ideally, the threads of the transfixing pins should engage both cortices. The proximal periosteal reaction was present before this device was inserted.

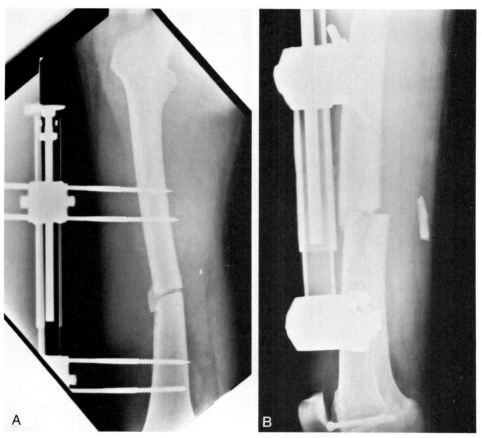

Figure 1–47. Wagner External Fixator. AP *(A)* and lateral *(B)* views show the femoral fracture held in valgus alignment by the fixation apparatus. The threaded portion of the pins should engage both medial and lateral cortices.

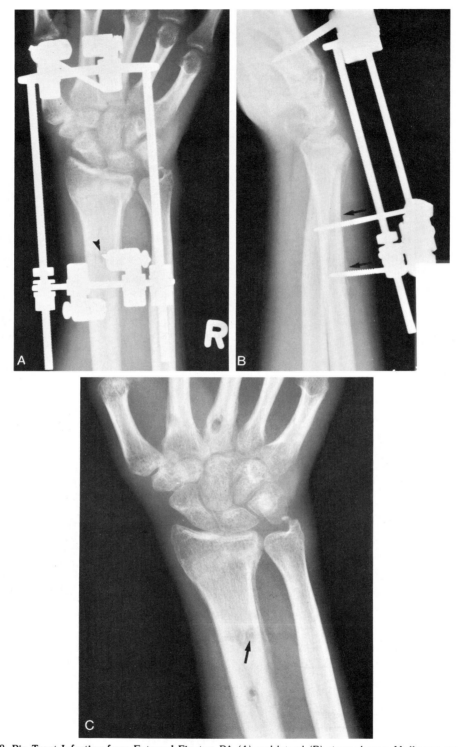

Figure 1–48. Pin Tract Infection from External Fixator. PA *(A)* and lateral *(B)* views show a Hoffmann external fixator maintaining the position of a comminuted Colles' fracture with extension into the joint. There is sclerosis along the fracture, indicating healing. Periosteal reaction (arrows) and bone resorption (arrowhead) indicate pin tract infections. *C,* After hardware removal it is easier to see the ring sequestra (one is indicated by an arrow), adjacent bone resorption, and periosteal reaction involving the index and middle fingers and the radius. Uneventful healing occurred.

tion. Each of the threaded areas should contact a cortex.

Depending on the device, the pins may be placed parallel, transversely, or obliquely and in convergent or divergent paths.

Electrical Stimulation

The application of small electrical currents to bone stimulates osteogenesis at the cathode.[219] Thus currents of 5 to 20 microamperes will result in bone formation, but weaker currents do not have this effect, and stronger currents result in tissue necrosis. These techniques are primarily utilized for the treatment of nonunion.

Two general methods of obtaining electrical stimulation are available: direct current stimulation or pulsing electromagnetic fields.

Direct Current Stimulation. Brighton and a multicenter group use stainless steel Kirschner wires that are insulated except for their tips.[219] The wires are placed percutaneously into the site of nonunion. The anode is placed on the skin, and current is applied for 12 weeks, after which the electrodes are removed, and immo-

bilization is continued for an additional 12 weeks.

Paterson used a surgically implanted apparatus with a helical titanium cathode (Fig. 1–49).[222] The device was left implanted for 6 months, and then the anode and as much of the cathode as possible were removed, leaving the helical portion of the cathode and its adjacent wire within the bone. Overall healing occurred in 86 percent of patients.

Pulsing Electromagnetic Fields. Pulsing electromagnetic fields (PEMF) do not require surgical or percutaneous implantation of cathodes, and the treatment has no known risk. The apparatus is placed externally over the fracture site and is connected to household current for 10 to 12 hours per day. Patient cooperation is therefore necessary. Radiographic examination should confirm that the locator block directly overlies the fracture site (Fig. 1–50).

Contraindications. Contraindications to electrical stimulation include the presence of a true pseudarthrosis with a fluid-filled cavity, active infection (although low-grade infection may be

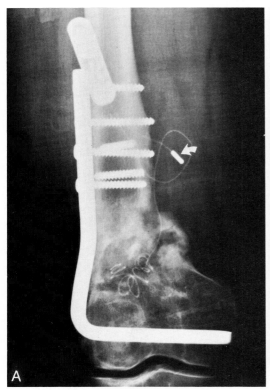
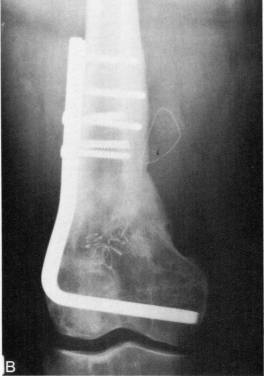

Figure 1–49. Healing after Electrical Stimulation. *A,* A femoral osteotomy had been done but had not healed, even after bone grafting and repeated internal fixation. A surgically implanted helical cathode has been inserted at the osteotomy site. An arrow indicates the anode. *B,* Complete healing has occurred. The anode and a portion of the cathode wire have been removed, but the helical wire remains embedded at the osteotomy site.

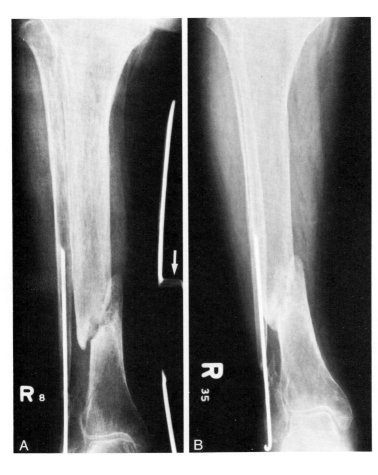

Figure 1–50. Nonunion of Tibial Fracture, Healing with Electrical Stimulation. *A,* Radiograph through a plaster cast shows an unhealed tibial fracture with sclerotic margins, indicative of nonunion. A Rush rod in the fibula maintains the displaced position of the fracture fragments. The locator block (arrow) of the pulsing electromagnetic field stimulator is slightly low in position. *B,* Considerable healing is shown on examination 9 months later.

cured during this treatment), and a large gap at the fracture site.[219]

Results. Healing using electrical stimulation occurs in about 6 months in contrast with bone grafting procedures, which require about 3 months.[219] The overall success rate of about 80 percent is generally comparable to that of bone graft surgery.[219, 220]

Complications. Methods that require surgical or percutaneous insertion of cathode pins may be complicated by infection.

Stress Fractures

Stress fractures, or *fatigue fractures,* result from the repeated application of abnormal stress on normal bone. The activity producing the fracture is often a new and strenuous one. In contrast, the term *insufficiency fracture* is used to describe fractures that occur when normal or physiological stress is applied to abnormally weakened bones.[228] The latter fractures include those occurring in patients with rheumatoid arthritis or with metabolic diseases such as osteoporosis or hyperparathyroidism. Pathological *fracture* spe-

cally refers to fractures in areas of bone replaced by tumor (Fig. 1–51).

Mechanisms of Production. Normally, bone remodeling occurs in response to applied stress and consists of bone resorption followed by new bone formation. Bone resorption is the more rapid process. When the remodeling process is complete, strong osteonal bone will be present along the lines of stress. If the applied stress is increased or is continuous during the period in which bone resorption predominates, a stress fracture may occur.

In describing tibial stress fractures, Sweet and Allman note that the first pathological change consists of cortical bone resorption, which continues for 2 to 3 weeks.[240] Periosteal reaction occurs during the second week and reaches its maximum at about 6 weeks. The cortical areas of resorption begin to fill in at 3 or 4 weeks, but months may be required before the remodeling process is complete.

Radiological Examination. The site of stress fracture reflects the underlying activity and the applied stress (Table 1–20). In the feet the

distinguished. In some cases the fracture line may be demonstrated by CT.

Bone Scanning. Because radiographic diagnosis of stress fractures may be delayed, bone scanning has been suggested as an earlier means of detection. Geslien and associates noted that rapid bone resorption begins 2 or 3 days after the onset of excessive stress and continues for several weeks.[231] Accumulation of technetium-99m–labeled phosphate compounds increases soon after this accelerated remodeling begins, pro-

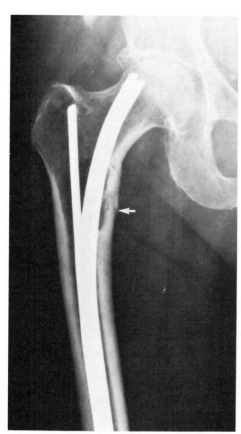

Figure 1–51. Pathologic Fracture with Ender Nails. There has been a fracture (arrow) through a metastatic focus of breast carcinoma. Ender nails were used for fixation.

Table 1–20. **Stress Fractures**

Location	Activity
Sesamoids of metatarsals	Prolonged standing
Metatarsal shaft	Marching, stamping
	Prolonged standing
	Ballet dancing
	Bunionectomy, postoperative
Navicular	Marching, stamping
	Long-distance running
Calcaneus	Jumping, parachuting
	Prolonged standing
	Recurrent immobilization
Tibia: mid- and distal shaft	Ballet dancing
	Long-distance running
Tibia: proximal shaft	Running
Fibula: distal shaft	Long-distance running
Fibula: proximal shaft	Jumping, parachuting
Patella	Hurdling
Femur: shaft	Ballet dancing
	Long-distance running
Femur: neck	Ballet dancing
	Marching
	Long-distance running
	Gymnastics
Pelvis: obturator ring	Stooping
	Bowling
	Gymnastics
	Long-distance running
Lumbar vertebra: pars interarticularis	Ballet dancing
	Heavy lifting
	Scrubbing floors
Lower cervical, upper thoracic spinous process	Shoveling clay
Ribs	Carrying heavy pack
	Golfing
	Coughing
Clavicle	Radical neck surgery
Coracoid of scapula	Trap shooting
Scapula	Assembly work
Humerus: distal shaft	Throwing a ball
Ulna: coronoid	Pitching a ball
Ulna: shaft	Using pitchfork
	Propelling wheelchair
Hook of hamate	Holding golfclub, tennis racquet, baseball bat

Source: Modified from Daffner RH: Skeletal Radiol 2:221, 1978.

calcaneus and the second or third metatarsals are the most frequent sites of involvement.[232, 233]

Radiological findings depend on the site of the fracture and the age of the injury at the time of examination. Fractures that particularly involve cancellous bone, such as those occurring in the metaphyses of long bones, are often first seen as a thin zone of sclerosis (Figs. 1–52 and 1–53). In areas where cortical bone predominates, a thin cortical lucency may be the first sign, followed by localized periosteal reaction (Fig. 1–54).[232, 238]

If the initial films appear negative but clinical suspicion of a stress fracture is high, follow-up radiographs in 1 to 2 weeks may demonstrate either the thin zone of sclerosis or the development of periosteal reaction.

When periosteal reaction predominates, the differential radiographic diagnosis includes osteoid osteoma, chronic osteomyelitis, malignant bone tumors (such as osteogenic sarcoma) and osteomalacia with Looser zones (Fig. 1–55). Tomography will often allow these entities to be

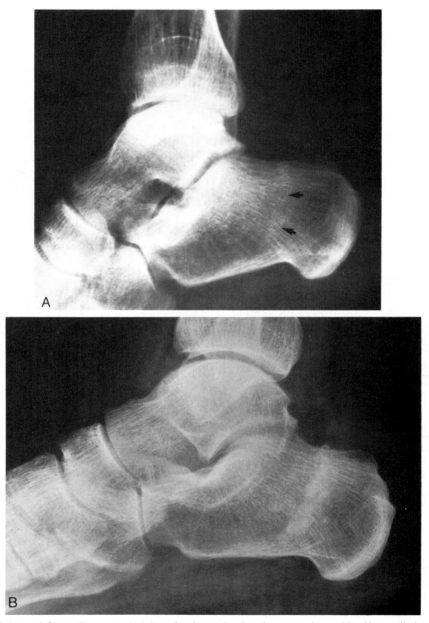

Figure 1–52. Calcaneal Stress Fracture. *A,* A lateral radiograph taken for a complaint of "ankle pain" shows a faint band of increased density in the calcaneus (arrows). This finding was overlooked. *B,* Two weeks later the zone of increased density is more pronounced, and slight periosteal reaction is seen.

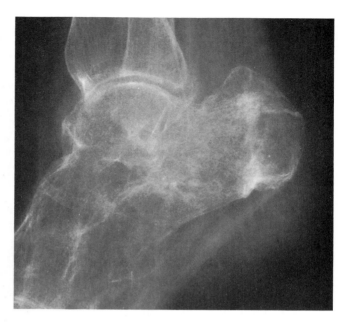

Figure 1–53. Calcaneal Insufficiency Fracture. This patient with severe rheumatoid arthritis and osteopenia complained of heel pain. The calcaneal deformity and the linear sclerosis attest to the presence of a calcaneal insufficiency fracture.

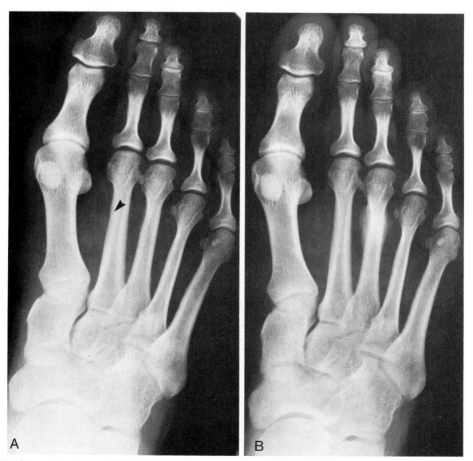

Figure 1–54. Stress Fracture of Third Metatarsal. *A,* Examination about 1 week after symptoms began shows faint periosteal reaction along the third metatarsal shaft. No definite cortical fracture line is seen. The oblique lucency in the second metatarsal (arrowhead) is a vascular canal. *B,* Two weeks later the periosteal reaction has increased.

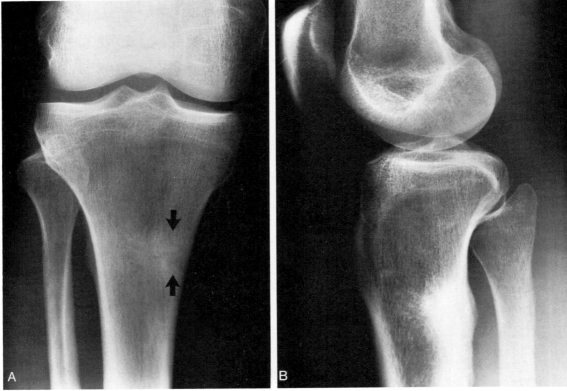

Figure 1–55. Tibial Stress Fracture. *A,* Medially, a thin irregular lucency with surrounding sclerosis (arrows) is present. *B,* The posterior new bone formation is striking, but the fracture line is not seen. The appearance of this view mimics that on an osteoid osteotoma.

ducing a positive bone scan. A normal bone scan in the clinical setting of a suspected stress fracture essentially excludes this entity. The meaning of a positive scan is less clear, since some patients with abnormal scans and clinical suspicion of stress fracture never develop radiological changes. Believers in the method attribute this lack of radiographic change to prompt recognition of the injury and institution of appropriate therapy.[232, 241] In support of this theory, Roub and colleagues noted no increase in isotope uptake on scans of the lower extremities in athletes imaged during the peak of their training.[236] Thus strenuous activity alone does not produce focal increase in isotope uptake.

Bone Grafts

Grafts may be classified according to their origin, their structure, or their function. In general, grafts may be used to fill bony cavities or defects; to bridge areas of pseudarthrosis, delayed union, fresh fracture, or osteotomy; and to replace larger segments of bone removed as a conse-

quence of trauma or surgery. Bone grafting is also used to achieve arthrodesis.

Origin of Bone Grafts

Grafts are categorized according to origin as (1) autografts, in which individuals provide their own grafts; (2) allografts, in which bone is obtained from other persons (Fig. 1–56); and (3) xenografts, in which the graft material is obtained from another species.[247]

Banked Bone. Bone may be obtained under sterile conditions, then preserved and made nonantigenic by freezing, freeze drying, or freeze drying and irradiation sterilization.[247] This bone is stored in bone banks. Although grafts from this bone provide no viable cells, they possess the ability to induce local bone formation.[243]

Types of Bone Grafts According to Function and Structure[247]

Grafts may consist of primarily cancellous bone (e.g., from the ilium), cortical bone (e.g., from the tibia), or combinations of the two. In general, cancellous bone is used when osteogenesis is

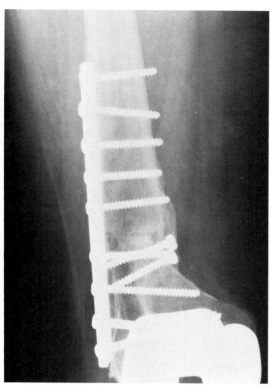

Figure 1–56. Distal Femoral Allograft. Resection of the distal femur was necessary for removal of a bone tumor. The removed segment was replaced by a cadaver allograft, and union between the graft and the proximal host bone is complete.

the primary objective, whereas cortical grafts are primarily used when stability is required.

Onlay Grafts (Fig. 1–57). Onlay grafts are so named because the graft material (primarily cortex) is laid along the existing bone rather than depressed within it. The recipient bone is prepared by removing scar tissue and sclerotic bone that may be present at a pseudarthrosis and by drilling or removing the host cortex at the graft site. The cortical graft is laid across the fracture or nonunion site and held by compression screws. Single onlay grafts were developed prior to current methods of internal fixation and were used for treating nonunion. Dual onlay grafts were developed for treating congenital pseudarthrosis. Both methods have for the most part been eclipsed by the use of compression plates and cancellous bone graft.

Inlay Grafts (Fig. 1–58). Inlay grafts involve the removal of a rectangular piece of cortex, which is then set into a corresponding recess created at the recipient site. In the sliding inlay graft technique, a rectangular piece of cortex is removed and a second, longer rectangular graft is cut and then slid distally to bridge the bony

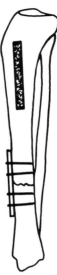

Figure 1–57. Onlay Graft. The bone graft is laid along the existing bone. (Redrawn from Heppenstall RB: Fracture Treatment and Healing. Philadelphia, WB Saunders, 1980:105.)

defect. The piece of cortex that was removed is inserted into the area exposed by the sliding inlay graft (Fig. 1–59). These methods are occasionally used for arthrodesis or for supplementation of internal fixation.[245, 247]

Muscle Pedicle Grafts. This method has been used particularly in the treatment of femoral neck fractures. In that technique bone graft, including the insertion of the quadratus femoris muscle, is removed from the posterolateral as-

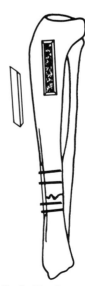

Figure 1–58. Inlay Graft. The bone graft is set into the surgically created recipient site. (Redrawn from Heppenstall RB: Fracture Treatment and Healing. Philadelphia, WB Saunders, 1980:107.)

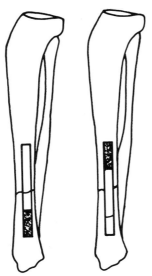

Figure 1–59. Sliding Inlay Graft. The bone graft is slid distally to bridge a bony defect. (Redrawn from Heppenstall RB: Fracture Treatment and Healing. Philadelphia, WB Saunders, 1980:107.)

pect of the intertrochanteric region. The bone, with the muscle insertion, is transplanted to the posterior aspect of the femoral neck, across the fracture site.

Dowel (Peg) Grafts (Fig. 1–60). This graft consists of a long, rounded piece of cancellous bone inserted across the site of a fracture or a nonunion to promote osteogenesis. Since the graft is composed of relatively weak cancellous bone, supplementation by metal internal fixation must also be used in all areas except the medial

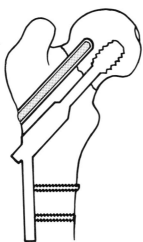

Figure 1–60. Dowel Graft. A core of cancellous bone (stippled area) is inserted to promote osteogenesis. (Redrawn from Heppenstall RB: Fracture Treatment and Healing. Philadelphia, 1980:108.)

malleolus and the small bones of the hands and the feet.

Strut Grafts. These grafts, which most often consist of bone from fibula or rib, provide both stability and potential osteogenesis. They are used in the spine, where immediate stability is essential.

Clothespin (H) Grafts. This technique is also used for spinal grafts. Bone removed from the iliac crest is slotted proximally and distally so that it can be fitted between the processes of the appropriate vertebrae.

Free Vascularized Bone Grafts. These grafts may be used in the reconstruction of large, long bone defects created by excision of aggressive tumors or by traumatic bone loss (see Fig. 1–64).[249] Microvascular techniques are used to anastomose the vascular structures at the graft site to the vascular pedicle of the graft.

Cancellous Bone Grafts. Strips of cancellous bone are often used in conjunction with compression plating for the treatment of nonunion.

Donor Sites

Typical donor sites include the ilium, the tibia, and the fibula.

The Ilium. Iliac graft is generally obtained from the lateral surface of the ilium, below the crest and the anterior superior iliac spine (Fig. 1–61). The lateral cortex and strips of cancellous bone are removed. The medial cortex of the ilium is preserved so that muscular herniation does not occur. If needed, graft may also be removed from the posterior ilium, but the sacroiliac joint should be avoided.

The Fibula. Up to one half of the fibula, in the midsection, may be removed without unfavorable consequences, but the distal fibula and the syndesmosis should not be disturbed.

The Tibia. In cases in which iliac crest graft cannot be used, bone may be taken from the anteromedial tibia, but the tibia is weakened postoperatively, and protected weight-bearing is necessary for several weeks.

Other common donor sites include the greater trochanter, the posterior elements of the spine, and the distal radius when graft is needed for the hand or wrist (see Fig. 1–62).

Healing

As stated by Heppenstall, it is currently believed that although the superficial cells of a bone graft remain viable, most of the graft dies, is resorbed, and is replaced by new bone.[247] This process occurs in three stages, an initial inflammatory stage, a repair stage, and a stage in which active bone marrow is formed within the graft.

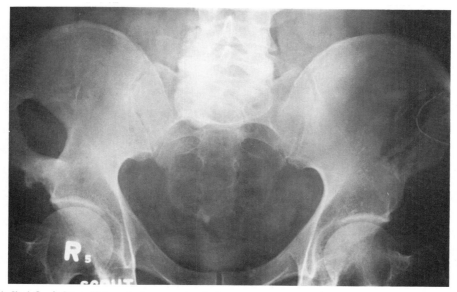

Figure 1–61. Ilial Graft Sites. This patient was supine during two operations to close a sternal wound. The initial defect on the right has sclerotic margins, indicating healing. On the left the irregular margins, bony fragmentation, and surgical drains show the recent postoperative status. Both inner and outer cortices have been removed from each side.

Initially, edema and inflammation occur in response to the necrotic material present within the deep haversian canals and in the marrow. Macrophages remove the necrotic material. The *repair* stage follows, with ingrowth of granulation tissue composed of capillaries and primitive mesenchymal tissue. In *cancellous* grafts new bone derived from the differentiation of host primitive mesenchymal cells is laid down along the necrotic trabeculae. Thus the available bone forms a scaffold for new bone production. With *cortical* grafts the ingrowth of granulation tissue takes longer. Resorption occurs first along the haversian canals and is then followed by repair. This process of bone resorption results in structural weakening of the graft. Thus Enneking and associates noted that at 6 weeks cortical bone graft in an animal model was markedly weakened by bone resorption and remained weak for 6 months, with recovery occurring at about 1 year.[24] At 1 year more than half of the bone graft had been replaced by new bone.

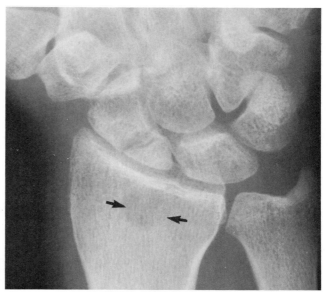

Figure 1–62. Distal Radial Donor Site. Graft bone was removed from the distal radius (arrows) for the grafting of a scaphoid nonunion.

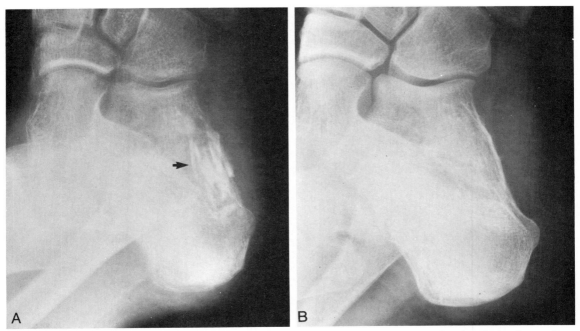

Figure 1–63. Healing of Cancellous Bone Graft. A simple cyst of the calcaneus was curetted and packed with cancellous bone graft. *A,* An oblique view at about 3 weeks shows strips of graft (arrow). *B,* Ten months later complete healing, with incorporation of the graft, has occurred.

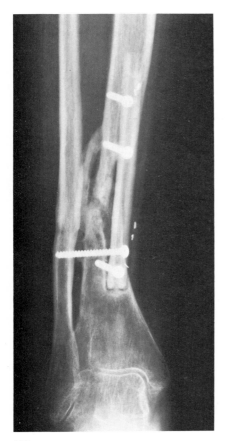

Figure 1–64. Nonunion of Vascularized Fibular Strut Graft. A fibular strut graft was used to bridge an area of nonunion. Examination several months later shows good incorporation of the graft proximally. Distally, however, the margins of the graft and adjacent host bone are smooth and sclerotic, suggesting nonunion.

The time to healing varies according to the site of bone graft. Tibial bone grafts for nonunion generally require 3 to 6 months to heal (Fig. 1–63).

Radiographic Evaluation

Donor Sites. Generally, the location and the sharp margins of the surgically created defects of donor sites help differentiate them from bone tumors or other lytic lesions. In these patients history provided to the radiologist is essential. Months after surgery, repair of the donor site occurs, making the margins slightly sclerotic and blurred.

Graft Sites. Bony union is documented by the presence of trabecular continuity between the graft and the host bone on standard views or on tomography. Fibrous union is suspected if a thin, radiolucent line persists at the graft-host interface.[242] In questionable cases stress views may be helpful to confirm solid union (the absence of motion) at the graft site.

Detection of Complications. Failure of incorporation of the graft is recognized on radiographs by the lack of trabecular continuity between the graft and the adjacent host bone (Fig. 1–64).[242] Stress views in these patients will show abnormal motion.

If the graft is not replaced by new bone, it will be resorbed and replaced by fibrous tissue. This is manifested on radiographs by a decrease in the size and density of the graft and, eventually, by its disappearance. In some cases, graft failure with eventual resorption is the result of infection, a situation that should be suspected when soft-tissue swelling and erosion and osteopenia of the adjacent host bone are present.

Graft *fracture,* leading to instability, may occur, or the graft may become *dislodged.* In anterior cervical spine fusions, anterior displacement of the graft may lead to dysphagia.

Reattachment of Severed Body Parts. Radiographic follow-up of reimplanted digits, metacarpals, wrists, and humeri shows some characteristic patterns of change (Table 1–21).[248] After digital reimplantation rapid decrease in the bone density of the distal fragment occurs for about 10 weeks, followed by improvement in bone density until it reaches that of the osteopenic proximal fragment (about 25 weeks). Callus increases progressively and usually becomes mature by 15 to 20 weeks. Soft-tissue swelling gradually decreases and disappears by 20 weeks.

Patients with osteomyelitis, nonunion, osteonecrosis, and soft-tissue infection may show radiographic patterns that differ from the usual. For example, osteosclerosis of the distal frag-

Table 1–21. Radiographic Findings After Surgical Replantation of Severed Digits

Radiographic Findings		Time
Bone density	Rapid osteopenia distally	—
	Improved density distally	10–25 weeks
	Improved density proximally and distally	25–40 weeks
Periosteal reaction at surgical site	Increases	10 weeks
Callus	Becomes mature	15–20 weeks
Soft-tissue swelling	Resolves by	20 weeks

After Kattapuram SV, Phillips WC: Radiology 149:59, 1983.

ment, rather than the usually noted osteopenia, suggests the presence of osteonecrosis.

Bone Scanning

Bone scanning has been used to study the viability of free vascularized bone grafts.[244, 249] Uptake of isotope by the graft indicates an intact vascular supply and the presence of metabolically active, viable bone. Conversely, absence of isotopic uptake on serial examinations suggests that the graft is not viable.

Osteotomy[250]

The term *osteotomy* refers to the surgical cutting of bone. These procedures are usually done to correct or lessen deformity. They may also be done to achieve limb shortening or lengthening.

A *closing wedge* osteotomy refers to the removal of a triangular wedge of bone from one side and approximation of the resected bony margins. An example is the intertrochanteric varus osteotomy.

An *opening wedge* osteotomy is performed by angulation of the bone causing one side of the osteotomy to open (Fig. 1–65). The defect is filled with bone graft.

In a *rotational* osteotomy the distal fragment is turned on its long axis.

Displacement osteotomy involves a shift in the position of the distal fragment in relation to the proximal fragment (e.g., McMurray intertrochanteric osteotomy).

"Shish kabob" osteotomies are used to correct severe bowing deformities of the long bones such as may occur in osteogenesis imperfecta. The shaft is cut in several places and the fragments threaded on an intramedullary rod.

Arthroplasty[251]

Arthroplasty refers to any operative procedure that attempts to reshape or realign the articular

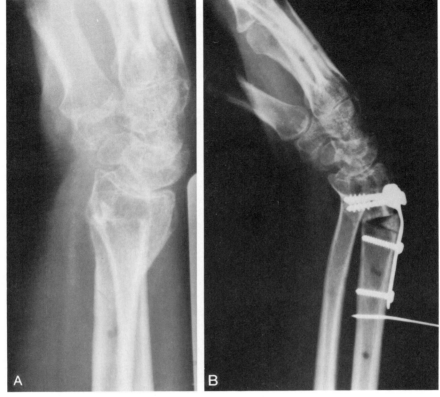

Figure 1–65. Opening Wedge Osteotomy. *A,* A lateral radiograph shows residual dorsal tilt of the distal radial articular surface caused by an old comminuted Colles' fracture. Marked limitation of pronation, flexion, and extension was noted clinically. *B,* An intraoperative lateral view shows a distal radial osteotomy with a wedge of bone inserted, redirecting the distal radial articular surface into a more normal volar tilt. Motion was improved.

surfaces of the joint using autogenous tissue or foreign materials. These procedures include partial or complete resection of the joint. *Hemiarthroplasty* involves resurfacing the more affected side of the joint with a metal or acrylic surface. The Neer humeral prosthesis and the McKeever knee prosthesis are examples.

Total-joint arthroplasty involves replacement of both sides of the joint. Most of the periarticular bone and soft tissue is preserved.

Types of Prostheses[251]

Total-joint prostheses are subclassified according to the degree of stability that the prosthesis itself provides. A *constrained* prosthesis is one that, in addition to resurfacing the joint, provides stability in patients in whom there is poor soft-tissue support because of marked bone loss or capsular and ligamentous laxity. Thus the prosthesis supplies the rigidity necessary for some function. In contrast, *unconstrained* prostheses are those that resurface the joint but provide little inherent stability. Stability must therefore be maintained by the patient's joint capsule and

ligaments. Between these two extremes *semiconstrained* prostheses provide some inherent stability by a built-in snap-lock fit or toggle effect.

Prosthetic Fixation

Fixation with Methylmethacrylate. The current era of total-joint replacement began with the introduction by Sir John Charnley of a total-hip prosthesis consisting of a nonreactive metallic femoral component and a polyethylene acetabular component secured to bone with methylmethacrylate. The methylmethacrylate has no adhesive properties when applied to wet bone but functions through a mechanical interlocking to distribute transmitted stresses evenly from the prosthesis to bone. Advantages to the use of cement fixation include the encasement of the components by cement, thus protecting them from corrosion; the potential for correction of incongruities between the implant and the surgical bed; the ability to orient prosthetic components independent of the shape of the surgically created bone bed; and the attainment of immediate stable fixation.[281] However, local and systemic reactions to methylmethacrylate may occur.

Local Reactions to Methylmethacrylate. Histological evaluation has shown three phases in the reaction of bone to methylmethacrylate: necrosis, repair, and a steady state.[262] Within the *first 3 weeks* after surgery, a zone of necrotic tissue and fibrin that may reach 3 mm in depth is formed. The cause of this necrosis is uncertain, but possibilities include a toxic effect from residual nonpolymerized monomer and thermal injury related to the polymerization of methylmethacrylate (an exothermic reaction).[259] From *3 weeks to 2 years* postoperatively, repair occurs and, in most cases, leads to the development of a fibrous layer along the cement-bone interface. The appearance is usually stable by *2 years,* with a 0.1 to 1.5 mm connective tissue membrane formed around the cement.

Radiological Correlates. Making the cement opaque (usually by the addition of barium sulfate) allows the interface between prosthesis and cement and cement and bone to be evaluated. Radiolucent zones present in the immediate postoperative period may represent unremoved cartilage, soft tissue, or blood within the prosthetic bed. Later, the connective tissue membrane between the cement and the bone is demonstrable by its relative lucency in comparison with the opaque cement on the one side and a thin zone of sclerotic bone that forms on the other side. With most cemented prostheses these zones of lucency are established by 6 months postoperatively, although they may occasionally begin later.

Lucencies of more than 2 mm suggest the possibility of loosening or infection. In cases of loosening the cement-bone lucent zones correlate, not to a fibrous layer (as described earlier), but to a synovium-like lining capable of producing substances that stimulate bone resorption.[255] In addition, reactions to methylmethacrylate, characterized by the presence of sheets of macrophages and the formation of large zones of resorption, have been noted.[257]

Systemic Reactions to Methylmethacrylate. Following the insertion of joint prostheses and methylmethacrylate into bone, a number of cardiovascular and pulmonary changes have been noted, including hypotension, cardiac irregularities, and hypoxemia. Of these, transient hypotension is the most frequent, occurring in many patients.[263] The fall in blood pressure occurs within minutes after the cement is applied and averages 3 to 5 minutes in duration.[267] A fall in arterial PO_2 is also noted. Both changes are more frequent and more pronounced after the femoral stem is pressed into the cement-

Table 1–22. Theories Suggested for the Production of Hypotension and Hypoxemia Following Joint Replacement Using Methylmethacrylate Cement

Effects of the Cement
  Bradycardia or myocardial depression
  Peripheral vasodilation
  Bronchoconstriction
  De-emulsification of fat
  Direct embolism effect
  Heat of polymerization
  Heat-produced emboli

Reflex Neurogenic Hypotension

Pulmonary Embolism
  Fat and marrow or air
  Secondary intravascular coagulation

Anesthesia
  Blocking of baroreceptor activity

Source: Weissman BN, Sosman JL, Braunstein E, et al.: J Bone Joint Surg (Am) 66:443, 1984, with permission.

filled marrow cavity than after the acetabular component is inserted.[267, 269] Several mechanisms have been implicated in the genesis of these reactions, including embolization of marrow contents and absorption of cement monomer into the blood (Table 1–22). Methylmethacrylate has been noted in a draining femoral vein after total hip replacement.[273] This occurrence provides a potential pathway for cement embolization to the lungs.

Other Methods of Fixation

Bony Ingrowth. Because of the relatively high incidence of loosening of total-hip prostheses (40 percent for the femoral component in one series), the idea that fixation with methylmethacrylate may not be the ultimate solution has been advanced, and a recently reborn alternative, bony ingrowth, has been suggested.[261] Unlike the large fenestrations of the Moore prosthesis, current attempts at achieving bony ingrowth make use of small surface recesses that produce porous layers into which bone gradually grows.[280]

Various factors affect the potential for bony ingrowth. One important one is the relative immobility of the prosthesis that must be achieved in order for bone ingrowth to occur. It is postulated that, for most of the width of the pore to be filled by bone, cyclic relative motion of an order of magnitude less than the pore size is tolerable. If the width of the pores for bony ingrowth is 100 μm, 10 μm of motion is tolerable, and this degree of relative immobility is apparently achievable in the hip.[280] If motion is excessive, fibrous tissue, rather than bone, may develop. Other considerations regarding fixation by bony ingrowth, summarized by Hedley and

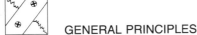
by Swanson and Freeman; include (1) the possibility that bony ingrowth will be replaced by fibrous tissue deposition after years of cyclic loading, (2) fatigue and corrosive changes may occur in implants not protected by methylmethacrylate; (3) atrophy of unloaded bone may occur; and (4) the possible difficulty in removing a failed implant.[276, 280] In contrast with fixation by cement, which may decrease with time, fixation by bony ingrowth should initially increase and then, it is hoped, remain stable.

Press (Interference) Fit.[280] Press fit is used, for example, in the Thompson femoral head prosthesis and in the Neer humeral head replacement. Fixation depends on the friction that is created between the prosthesis and the adjacent bone by making the implant bed smaller than the prosthesis. If the fit is imprecise or if bone remodeling occurs, loosening, particularly in weight-bearing areas, results. Thus if the stress transmitted to the underlying bone is too great, bone resorption with possible loss of fixation may occur. This type of fixation is therefore best

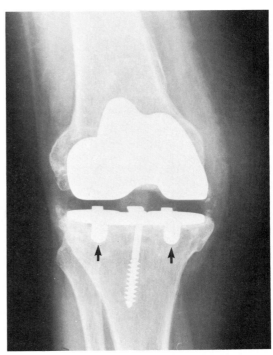

Figure 1–67. Screw Fixation for PCA Prosthesis. The screw maintains stability while bony ingrowth is occurring along the porous surfaces (arrows).

reserved for patients in whom functional demand is low and excessive stress is not achieved, or in whom temporary fixation is necessary until bony ingrowth occurs (Fig. 1–66).

Screw Fixation. Screw fixation alone is thought to be insufficient for the long-term. However, screws have been used to provide short-term fixation of prostheses in which gradual bony ingrowth is expected (Fig. 1–67).

References

X-Rays and Radiation Protection

1. Abrams HL: Sounding board. The "overutilization" of x-rays. N Engl J Med 300:1213–1216, 1979.
2. Antoku S, Russell WJ: Dose to the active bone marrow, gonads, and skin from roentgenography and fluoroscopy. Radiology 101:669–678, 1971.
3. Carmichael JHE, Warrick CK: Radiology now. The ten day rule—principles and practice. Br J Radiol 51:843–846, 1978.
4. Christensen EE, Curry TS III, Dowdey JE: An Introduction to the Physics of Diagnostic Radiology. Philadelphia, Lea & Febiger, 1978.
5. Doubilet PM, Judy PF: Dosimetry of radiological procedures and dose reduction in diagnostic radiology. Postgrad Radiol 1:309–323, 1981.
6. Drum DE: Personal communication, 1983.
7. Gregg EC: Radiation risks with diagnostic x-rays. Radiology 123:447–453, 1977.
8. Hall EJ: Radiobiology for the Radiologist. 2nd ed. New York, Harper & Row, 1978.

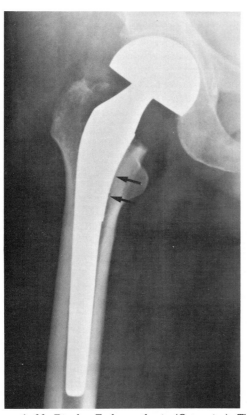

Figure 1–66. Bipolar Endoprosthesis (Osteonics). This prosthesis is press-fitted into the femoral canal. The press-fit maintains stability during bony ingrowth along the medial aspect (arrows) of the femoral component, which is covered with a porous metal surface.

9. Jacobson A, Conley JG: Estimation of fetal dose to patients undergoing diagnostic x-ray procedures. Radiology 120:683–685, 1976.
10. Kereiakes JG, Rosenstein M: Handbook of Radiation Doses in Nuclear Medicine and Diagnostic X-Ray. Boca Raton, Fla, CRC Press, 1980: 241–243.
11. Little JB: Environmental hazards. Ionizing radiation. N Engl J Med 275:929–938, 1966.
12. Little JB: Cellular effects of ionizing radiation. N Engl J Med 278:369–376, 1968.
13. Smith PG, Doll R: Mortality from cancer and all causes among British radiologists. Br J Radiol 54:187–194, 1981.
14. Zatz LM, Finston RA, Jones HH: Reduced radiation exposure in the operating room with video disc radiography. Radiology 110:475–477, 1974.

Magnification

15. De Smet AA, Templeton AW: Direct magnification radiography using conventional radiographic equipment. AJR 135:858–859, 1980.
16. Genant HK: Clinical applications of magnification in skeletal radiography. In Feldman F, ed. Radiology, Pathology and Immunology of Bones and Joints. A Review of Concepts. New York, Appleton-Century-Crofts, 1978: 133–138.
17. Genant HK, Doi K, Mall JC: Optical versus radiographic magnification for fine-detail skeletal radiography. Invest Radiol 10:160–172, 1975.
18. Griffiths HJ, Hunt R, Grindle T, Anderson M, Sandor T: The use of a primary magnification technic in metabolic bone disease. J Am Vet Radiol Society 18:12–18, 1977.
19. Mall JC, Genant HK, Rossmann K: Improved optical magnification for fine-detailed radiography. Radiology 108:707–708, 1973.
20. Mall JC, Genant HK, Silcox DC, McCarty DJ: The efficacy of fine-detail radiography in the evaluation of patients with rheumatoid arthritis. Radiology 112:37–42, 1974.
21. Meema HE, Rabinovich S, Meema S, Lloyd GJ, Oreopoulos DG: Improved radiological diagnosis of azotemic osteodystrophy. Radiology 102:1–10, 1972.
22. Weiss A: A technique for demonstrating fine detail in bones of the hands. Clin Radiol 23:185–187, 1972.

Tomography

23. Norman A: The value of tomography in the diagnosis of skeletal disorders. Radiol Clin North Am 8:251–258, 1970.

Computed Tomography

24. Abrams HL, McNeil BJ: Medical implications of computed tomography ("CAT scanning"). N Engl J Med 298:255–261, 310–328, 1978.
25. Alfidi RJ, MacIntyre WJ, Meaney TF, Chernak ES, Janicki P, Tarar R, Levin H: Experimental studies to determine application of CAT scanning to the human body. AJR 124:199–207, 1975.
26. Archer CR, Yeager V: Internal structures of the knee visualized by computed tomography. J Comput Assist Tomogr 2:181–183, 1978.
27. Berger PE, Kuhn JP: Computed tomography of tumors of the musculoskeletal system in children. Clinical applications. Radiology 127:171–175, 1978.
28. Bergstrom M, Sundman R: Picture processing in computed tomography. AJR 127:17–21, 1976.
29. Brooks RA, Di Chiro G: Theory of image reconstruction in computed tomography. Radiology 117:561–572, 1975.

30. Cann CE, Genant HK, Boyd DP: Precise measurement of vertebral mineral in serial studies using CT. In Proceedings of International Workshop on Bone and Soft Tissue Densitometry Using Computed Tomography. San Francisco, June 7–9. J Comput Assist Tomogr 3:847–862, 1979.
31. Carlson DH: CT evaluation of intra-articular fractures. South Med J 73:820–821, 1980.
32. Colley DP, Dunsker SB: Traumatic narrowing of the dorsolumbar spinal canal demonstrated by computed tomography. Radiology 129:95–98, 1978.
33. deSantos LA, Bernardino ME, Murray JA: Computed tomography in the evaluation of osteosarcoma: experience with 25 cases. AJR 132:535–540, 1979.
34. deSantos LA, Goldstein HM, Murray JA, Wallace S: Computed tomography in the evaluation of musculoskeletal neoplasms. Radiology 128:89–94, 1978.
35. Destouet JM, Gilula LA, Murphy WA: Computed tomography of long-bone osteosarcoma. Radiology 131:439–445, 1979.
36. Evens RG: New frontier for radiology: computed tomography. AJR 126:1117–1129, 1976.
37. Faerber EN, Wolpert SM, Scott RM, Belkin SC, Carter BL: Computed tomography of spinal fractures. J Comput Assist Tomogr 3:657–661, 1979.
38. Genant HK: Assessment of musculoskeletal disorders by computed tomography. In Feldman F, ed. Radiology, Pathology and Immunology of Bones and Joints. A Review of Concepts. New York, Appleton-Century-Crofts, 1978.
39. Genant HK: Computed tomography in diagnosis of bone and joint disorders. In Resnick D, Niwayama G, eds. Diagnosis of Bone and Joint Disorders. Philadelphia, WB Saunders, 1981.
40. Genant HK, Boyd D: Quantitative bone mineral analysis using dual energy computed tomography. Invest Radiol 12:545–551, 1977.
41. Genant HK, Wilson JS, Bovill EG, Brunelle FO, Murray WR, Rodrigo JJ: Computed tomography of the musculoskeletal system. J Bone Joint Surg (Am) 60:1088–1101, 1980.
42. Gilula LA, Murphy WA, Tailor CC, Patel RB: Computed tomography of the osseous pelvis. Radiology 132:107–114, 1979.
43. Ginaldi S, deSantos LA: Computed tomography in the evaluation of small round cell tumors of bone. Radiology 134:441–446, 1980.
44. Goldberg RP, Genant HK: Case report 67: Bone cyst of right ilium. Skeletal Radiol 3:118–121, 1978.
45. Gordon R: Dose reduction in computerized tomography. Invest Radiol 11:508–517, 1976.
46. Haaga JR: New techniques for CT-guided biopsies. AJR 133:633–641, 1979.
47. Handelberg F, Bellemans MA, Opdecam P, Casteleyn PP: The use of computerized tomographs in the diagnosis of thoracolumbar injury. J Bone Joint Surg (Br) 63:337–341, 1981.
48. Hardy DC, Murphy WA, Gilula LA: Computed tomography in planning percutaneous bone biopsy. Radiology 134:447–450, 1980.
49. Haughton VM, Syvertsen A, Williams AL: Soft tissue anatomy within the spinal cord as seen on computed tomography. Radiology 134:649–655, 1980.
50. Heiken JP, Lee JKT, Smathers RL, Totty WG, Murphy WA: CT of benign soft-tissue masses of the extremities. AJR 142:575–580, 1984.
51. Helms CA, Cann CE, Brunelle FO, Gilula LA, Chafetz N, Genant HK: Detection of bone-marrow metastases using quantitative computed tomography. Radiology 140:745–750, 1981.

52. Hinderling TH, Ruegsegger P, Anliker M, Dietschi C: Computed tomography reconstruction from hollow projections: an application to in vivo evaluation of artificial hip joints. J Comput Assist Tomogr 3:52–57, 1979.
53. Hounsfield GN: Picture quality of computed tomography. AJR 127:3–9, 1976.
54. Hunter JC, Johnston WH, Genant HK: Computed tomography evaluation of fatty tumors of the somatic soft tissues: Clinical utility and radiologic-pathologic correlation. Skeletal Radiol 4:79–91, 1979.
55. Jakob RP, Haertel M, Stussi E: Tibial torsion calculated by computerised tomography and compared to other methods of measurement. J Bone Joint Surg (Br) 62:238–242, 1980.
56. Koehler PR, Anderson RE, Baxter B: The effect of computed tomography viewer controls on anatomical measurements. Radiology 130:189–194, 1979.
57. Kuhn JP, Berger PE: Computed tomographic diagnosis of osteomyelitis. Radiology 130:503–506, 1979.
58. Kuhns LR, Borlaza GS, Seigel RS, Paramagul C, Berger PE: An in vitro comparison of computed tomography, xeroradiography, and radiography in the detection of soft-tissue foreign bodies. Radiology 132:218–219, 1979.
59. Levine E, Lee KR, Neff JR, Maklad NF, Robinson RG, Preston DF: Comparison of computed tomography and other imaging modalities in the evaluation of musculoskeletal tumors. Radiology 131:431–437, 1979.
60. McCullough EC, Payne JT: Patient dosage in computed tomography. Radiology 129:457–463, 1978.
61. McDavid WD, Waggener RG, Sank VJ, Dennis MJ, Payne WH: Correlating computed tomographic numbers with physical properties and operating kilovoltage. Radiology 123:761–762, 1977.
62. McLeod RA, Stephens DH, Beabout JW, Sheedy PF II, Hattery RR: Computed tomography of the skeletal system. Semin Roentgenol 13:235–247, 1978.
63. Miraldi F: Imaging principles in computed tomography. In Haaga JR, Alfidi RJ, eds. Computed Tomography of the Whole Body. St. Louis, CV Mosby, 1983.
64. O'Callaghan JP, Ullrich CG, Yuan HA, Kieffer SA: CT of facet distraction in flexion injuries of the thoracolumbar spine: The "naked" facet. AJR 134:563–568, 1980.
65. Rosenthal DI: Computed tomography in bone and soft tissue neoplasm: Application and pathologic correlation. Crit Rev Radiol 18:243–278, 1982.
66. Rosenthal DI, Aronow S, Murray WT: Iron content of pigmented villonodular synovitis detected by computed tomography. Radiology 133:409–411, 1979.
67. Roub LW, Drayer BP: Spinal computed tomography: Limitations and applications. AJR 133:267–273, 1979.
68. Seltzer S: CT of the musculoskeletal system. In Harvard Medical School. Syllabus of the Departments of Radiology and Continuing Education, Orthopedic Radiology Postgraduate Course, 1983.
69. Wall BF, Green DAC, Veerappan R: The radiation dose to patients from EMI brain and body scanners. Br J Radiol 52:189–196, 1979.
70. Weissberger MA, Zamenhof RG, Aronow S, Neer RM: Computed tomography scanning for the measurement of bone mineral in the human spine. J Comput Assist Tomogr 2:253–262, 1978.
71. White RR, Newberg A, Seligson D: Computerized tomographic assessment of the traumatized dorsolumbar spine before and after Harrington instrumentation. Clin Orthop 146:150–156, 1980.
72. Wittenberg J, Fineberg HV, Ferrucci JT Jr, Simeone JF, Mueller PR, vanSonnenberg E, Kirkpatrick RH: Clinical efficacy of computed body tomography, II. AJR 134:1111–1120, 1980.

Xeroradiography

73. Osterman FA Jr, Zeman GH, Rao GUV, Gayler B, Kirk BG, James AE Jr: Negative-mode soft-tissue xeroradiography. Radiology 124:689–694, 1977.
74. Otto RC, Pouliadis GP, Kumpe DA: The evaluation of pathologic alterations of juxtaosseous soft tissue by xeroradiography. Radiology 120:297–302, 1976.
75. Smith FW, Junor BJR: Xeroradiography of the hand in patients with renal osteodystrophy. Br J Radiol 50:261–263, 1977.
76. Verow PW, Dippy J: Soft tissue changes in early rheumatoid arthritis as seen on xeroradiography and non-screen radiographs. Clin Radiol 29:585–590, 1978.
77. Wolfe JN: Xeroradiography of the Breast. Springfield, Ill, CC Thomas, 1972.
78. Wolfe JN: Xeroradiography of the bones, joints, and soft tissues. Radiology 93:583–587, 1969.
79. Wolfe JN, Kapdi CC, Murphy HS: Atlas of Xeroradiographic Anatomy of Normal Skeletal Systems. Springfield, Ill, CC Thomas, 1978.

Bone Scanning

80. Bassett LW, Gold RH, Webber MM: Radionuclide bone imaging. Radiol Clin North Am 19:675–702, 1981.
81. Charkes ND: Bone scanning: Principles, technique, and interpretation. Radiol Clin North Am 8:259–270, 1970.
82. Desai A, Eymontt M, Alavi A, Schaeffer B, Dalinka MK: 99mTc-MDP uptake in nonosseous lesions. Radiology 135:181–184, 1980.
83. Dibos PE, Wagner HN Jr: Atlas of Nuclear Medicine, Vol. 4, Bone. Philadelphia, WB Saunders, 1978.
84. Genant HK, Bautovich GJ, Singh M, Lathrop KA, Harper PV: Bone-seeking radionuclides: An in vivo study of factors affecting skeletal uptake. Radiology 113:373–382, 1974.
85. Kirchner PT, Simon MA: Radioisotopic evaluation of skeletal disease. J Bone Joint Surg (Am) 63:673–681, 1981.
86. Krishnamurthy GT, Huebotter RJ, Tubis M, Blahd WH: Pharmacokinetics of current skeletal-seeking radiopharmaceuticals. AJR 126:293–301, 1976.
87. Lentle BC, Russell AS, Percy JS, Scott JR, Jackson FI: Bone scintiscanning updated. Ann Intern Med 84:297–303, 1976.
88. McNeil BJ: Rationale for the use of bone scans in selected metastatic and primary bone tumors. Semin Nucl Med 8:336–345, 1978.
89. Pendergrass HP, Potsaid MS, Castronovo FP: The clinical use of 99mTc-diphosphonate (HEDSPA). A new agent for skeletal imaging. Radiology 107:557–562, 1973.
90. Rosenthal DI, Chandler HL, Azizi F, Schneider PB: Uptake of bone imaging agents by diffuse pulmonary metastatic calcification. AJR 129:871–874, 1977.
91. Rosenthall L, Kaye M: Observations on the mechanism of 99mTc-labeled phosphate complex uptake in metabolic bone disease. Semin Nucl Med 6:59–67, 1976.
92. Sy WM, Mittal AK: Bone scan in chronic dialysis patients with evidence of secondary hyperparathyroidism and renal osteodystrophy. Br J Radiol 48:878–884, 1975.
93. Tilden RL, Jackson J, Enneking WF, DeLand FH,

McVey JT: 99mTc-polyphosphate: histological localization in human femurs by autoradiography. J. Nucl Med 14:576–578, 1973.

94. Weber DA, Keyes JW, Wilson GA, Landman S: Kinetics and imaging characteristics of 99mTc-labeled complexes used for bone imaging. Radiology 120:615–621, 1976.

Bone Scanning in Malignant Disease

95. Chew FS, Hudson TM: Radionuclide bone scanning of osteosarcoma: falsely extended uptake patterns. AJR 139:49–54, 1982.
96. Citrin DL: The role of the bone scan in the investigation and treatment of breast cancer. CRC Crit Rev Diagn Imaging, 13:39–55, 1980.
97. Corcoran RJ, Thrall JH, Kyle RW, Kaminski RJ, Johnson MC: Solitary abnormalities in bone scans of patients with extraosseous malignancies. Radiology 121:663–667, 1976.
98. Goldman AB, Becker MH, Braunstein P, Francis KC, Genieser NB, Firoonzia H: Bone scanning—osteogenic sarcoma. Correlation with surgical pathology. AJR 124:83–90, 1975.
99. Goldstein H, McNeil BJ, Zufall E, Treves S: Is there still a place for bone scanning in Ewing's sarcoma? Concise communication. J Nucl Med 21:10–12, 1980.
100. Goldstein H, McNeil BJ, Zufall E, Jaffe N, Treves S: Changing indications for bone scintigraphy in patients with osteosarcoma. Radiology 135:177–180, 1980.
101. Harbert JC: Efficacy of bone and liver scanning in malignant disease: facts and opinions. In Freeman LM, Weissman HS, eds. Nuclear Medicine Manual. New York, Raven Press, 1982: 373–401.
102. Huben RP, Schellhammer PF: The role of routine follow-up bone scans after definitive therapy of localized prostatic cancer. J Urol 128:510–512, 1979.
103. Katz RD, Alderson PO, Rosenshein NB, Bowerman JW, Wagner HN: Utility of bone scanning in detecting occult skeletal metastases from cervical carcinoma. Radiology 133:469–472, 1979.
104. Kaufman RA, Thrall JH, Keyes JW, Brown ML, Zakem JF: False negative bone scans in neuroblastoma metastatic to the ends of long bones. AJR 130:131–135, 1978.
105. McNeil BJ, Polak JF: An update on the rationale for the use of bone scans in selected metastatic and primary bone tumors. In Pauwels EKJ, Schutte HE, Taconis WK, eds. Bone Scintigraphy. The Hague, Martinus Nijhoff, 1981: 187–207.
106. McNeil BJ, Hanley J: Analysis of serial radionuclide bone images in osteosarcoma and breast carcinoma. Radiology 135:171–176, 1980.
107. Robbins GF, Knapper WH, Barrie J, Kripalani I, Lawrence J: Metastatic bone disease developing in patients with potentially curable breast cancer. Cancer 29:1702–1704, 1972.
108. Shafer RB, Reinke DB: Contribution of the bone scan, serum acid and alkaline phosphatase, and the radiographic bone survey to the management of newly-diagnosed carcinoma of the prostate. Clin Nucl Med 2:200–203, 1977.
109. Silberstein EB, Saenger EL, Tofe AJ, Alexander GW, Parke H-M: Imaging of bone metastases with 99mTc-Sn-EHDP (diphosphonate), 18 F, and skeletal radiography. A comparison of sensitivity. Radiology 107:551–555, 1973.
110. Sklaroff DM, Charkes ND: Bone metastases from breast cancer at the time of radical mastectomy. Surg Gynecol Obstet 127:763–768, 1978.

Joint Scanning

111. Aprill CN, Schuler SE, Weiss TE: Peripheral joint imaging: variations in normal children. J Nucl Med 13:367–372, 1972.
112. Desaulniers M, Fuks A, Hawkins D, Lacourciere Y, Rosenthall L: Radiotechnetium polyphosphate joint imaging. J Nucl Med 15:417–423, 1974.
113. O'Duffy JD, Wahner HW, Hunder GG: Joint imaging in polymyalgia rheumatica. Mayo Clin Proc 51:519–524, 1976.
114. Gomez E, Green FA, Hays MT: Joint imaging as a clinical aid in diagnosis and therapy of arthritic and related diseases. II. Bull Rheum Dis 25:791–793, 1974–1975.
115. Hoffer PB, Gerant HK: Radionuclide joint imaging. Semin Nucl Med 6:121–137, 1976.
116. Maxfield WS, Weiss TE, Shuler SE: Synovial membrane scanning in arthritic disease. Semin Nucl Med 2:50–70, 1972.
117. McCarty DJ, Polcyn RE, Collins PA, Gottschalk A: 99m-Technetium scintiphotography in arthritis. I. Technic and interpretation. Arthritis Rheum 13:11–32, 1970.
118. Wahner HW, O'Duffy JD: Peripheral joint scanning with technetium pertechnetate. Application in clinical practice. Mayo Clin Proc 51:525–531, 1976.
119. Weiss TE, Shuler SE: New techniques for identification of synovitis and evaluation of joint disease. I. Bull Rheum Dis 25:786–790, 1974–1975.

Scanning in Other Conditions

120. D'Ambrosia RD, Shoji H, Riggins RS, Stadalnik RC, Denardo GL: Scintigraphy in the diagnosis of osteonecrosis. Clin Orthop 130:139–143, 1978.
121. Geslien GE, Thrall JH, Espinosa JL, Older RA: Early detection of stress fractures using 99mTc-polyphosphate. Radiology 121:683–687, 1976.
122. Matin P: Bone scanning of trauma and benign conditions. In Freeman LM, Weissman HS, eds. Nuclear Medicine Annual. New York, Raven Press, 1982: 81–110.

Gallium Scanning and Osteomyelitis

123. Deysine M, Rafkin H, Russell R, Teicher I, Aufses AH: The detection of acute experimental osteomyelitis with 67Ga citrate scannings. Surg Gynecol Obstet 141: 40–42, 1975.
124. Deysine M, Rafkin H, Teicher I, Silver L, Robinson R, Manly J, Aufses AH: Diagnosis of chronic and postoperative osteomyelitis with gallium 67 citrate scans. Am J Surg 129:632–635, 1975.
125. Duszynski DO, Kuhn JP, Afshani E, Riddlesberger MM Jr: Early radionuclide diagnosis of acute osteomyelitis. Radiology 117:337–340, 1975.
126. Fanning A, Dierich H, Lentle B: Bone scanning with technetium 99mTc-polyphosphate in tuberculosis osteomyelitis. Tubercle 55:227–230, 1974.
127. Garnett ES, Cockshott WP, Jacobs J: Classical acute osteomyelitis with a negative bone scan. Br J Radiol 50:757–760, 1977.
128. Gelfand MJ, Silberstein EB: Radionuclide imaging. Use in diagnosis of osteomyelitis in children. JAMA 237:245–247, 1977.
129. Gilday DL, Eng B, Paul DJ, Paterson J: Diagnosis of osteomyelitis in children by combined blood pool and bone imaging. Radiology 117:331–335, 1975.
130. Handmaker H, Leonards R: The bone scan in inflammatory osseous disease. Semin Nucl Med 6:95–105, 1976.

131. Hoffer P: Gallium: mechanisms. J Nucl Med 21:282–285, 1980.

132. Lisbona R, Rosenthall L: Review article. An update on radionuclide imaging in benign bone disorders. J Can Assoc Radiol 29:188–192, 1978.

133. Letts RM, Afifi A, Sutherland JB: Technetium bone scanning as an aid in the diagnosis of atypical acute osteomyelitis in children. Surg Gynecol Obstet 140:899–902, 1975.

134. Majd M, Frankel RS: Radionuclide imaging in skeletal inflammatory and ischemic disease in children. AJR 126:832–841, 1976.

135. Russin LD, Staab EV: Unusual bone-scan findings in acute osteomyelitis: case report. J Nucl Med 17:617–619, 1976.

136. Seto H, Tonami N, Hisada K: Utility of combined 99m Tc-phosphate and 67Ga imaging in diagnosis of septic arthritis. Clin Nucl Med 3:1–3, 1978.

137. Teates CD, Williamson BRJ: "Hot and cold" bone lesion in acute osteomyelitis. AJR 129:517–518, 1977.

138. Treves S, Khettry J, Broker FH, Wilkinson RH, Watts H: Osteomyelitis: early scintigraphic detection in children. Pediatrics 57:173–185, 1976.

139. Tsan M-F: Studies on gallium accumulation in inflammatory lesions: III. Roles of polymorphonuclear leukocytes and bacteria. J Nucl Med 19:492–495, 1978.

Indium Scanning

140. Dewanjee MK, Chowdhury S, Jenkins D, Brown ML, Wagner HW: Identification of abscesses and thrombi by imaging of 111 In-labeled blood cells. Mayo Clin Proc 59:49–50, 1984.

141. Mountford PJ, Hall FM, Coakley AJ, Wells CP: Assessment of the painful hip prosthesis with 111 In-labelled leucocyte scans. Br J Radiol 55:378, 1982.

142. Propst-Proctor SL, Dillingham MF, McDougall IR, Goodwin D: The white blood cell scan in orthopedics. Clin Orthop 168:157–165, 1982.

Ultrasonography

143. Ambanelli U, Manganelli P, Nervetti A, Ugolotti V: Demonstration of articular effusions and popliteal cysts with ultrasound. J Rheumatol 3:134–139, 1976.

144. Baker ML, Dalrymple GV: Biological effects of diagnostic ultrasound: A review. Radiology 129:479–483, 1978.

145. Behan M, Kazam E: The echographic characteristics of fatty tissues and tumors. Radiology 129:143–151, 1978.

146. Braunstein E, Silver T, Martel W, Jaffe M: Ultrasonographic diagnosis of extremity masses. Skeletal Radiol 6:157–164, 1981.

147. Carpenter JR, Hattery RR, Hunder GG, Bryan RS, McLeod RA: Ultrasound evaluation of the popliteal space: comparison with arthrography and physical examination. Mayo Clin Proc 51:498–503, 1976.

148. deSantos LA, Goldstein HM: Ultrasonography in tumors arising from the spine and bony pelvis. AJR 129:1061–1064, 1977.

149. Forbes CD, Moule B, Grant M, Greig WR, Prentice CRM: Bilateral pseudotumors of the pelvis in a patient with Christmas disease with notes on localization by radioactive scanning and ultrasonography. AJR 121:173–176, 1974.

150. Goldberg BB: Ultrasonic evaluation of superficial masses. J Clin Ultrasound 3:91–94, 1975.

151. Hamilton JV, Flinn G, Haynie CC, Cefalo RC: Diagnosis of rectus sheath hematoma by B-mode ultrasound: A case report. Am J Obstet Gynecol 125:562–565, 1976.

152. Kaftori JK, Rosenberger A, Pollack S, Fish JH: Rectus sheath hematoma: ultrasonographic diagnosis. AJR 128:283–285, 1977.

153. Lawson TL, Mittler S: Ultrasonic evaluation of extremity soft-tissue lesions with arthrographic correlation. J Can Assoc Radiol 29:58–61, 1978.

154. Levine E, Lee KR, Neff JR, Maklad NF, Robinson RG, Preston DF: Comparison of computed tomography and other imaging modalities in the evaluation of musculoskeletal tumors. Radiology 131:431–437, 1979.

155. Meire HB, Lindsay DJ, Swinson DR, Hamilton EBD: Comparison of ultrasound and positive contrast arthrography in the diagnosis of popliteal and calf swellings. Ann Rheum Dis 33:221–224, 1974.

156. McDonald DG, Leopold GR: Ultrasound B-scanning in the differentiation of Baker's cyst and thrombophlebitis. Br J Radiol 45:729–732, 1972.

157. Moore CP, Sarti DA, Louie JS: Ultrasonographic demonstration of popliteal cysts in rheumatoid arthritis: A non-invasive technique. Arthritis Rheum 18:577–580, 1975.

158. Neiman HL, Yao JST, Silver TM: Gray-scale ultrasound diagnosis of peripheral arterial aneurysms. Radiology 130:413–416, 1979.

159. Nowotny C, Niessner H, Thaler E, Lechner K: Sonography: A method for localization of hematomas in hemophiliacs. Haemostasis 5:129–135, 1976.

160. Sarti DA, Louie JS, Lindstrom RR, Nies K, London J: Ultrasonic diagnosis of a popliteal artery aneurysm. Radiology 121:707–708, 1976.

161. Seltzer SE, Finberg HJ, Weissman BN: Arthrosonography—technique, sonographic anatomy, and pathology. Invest Radiol 15:19–28, 1980.

162. Seltzer SE, Finberg HJ, Weissman BN, Kido DK, Collier BD: Arthrosonography: gray-scale ultrasound evaluation of the shoulder. Radiology 132:467–468, 1979.

163. Silver TM, Washburn RL, Stanley JC, Gross WS: Gray scale ultrasound evaluation of popliteal artery aneurysms. AJR 129:1003–1006, 1977.

164. Smith EH, Bartrum RJ: Ultrasonically guided percutaneous aspiration of abscesses. AJR 122:308–312, 1974.

165. Wicks JD, Silver TM, Bree RL: Gray scale features of hematomas: an ultrasonic spectrum. AJR 131:977–980, 1978.

166. Wyatt GM, Spitz HB: Ultrasound in the diagnosis of rectus sheath hematoma. JAMA 241:1499–1500, 1979.

Nuclear Magnetic Resonance

167. Brady TJ, Rosen BR, Pykett IL, McGuire MH, Mankin HJ, Rosenthal DI: NMR imaging of leg tumors. Radiology 149:181–187, 1983.

168. Hull RG, Rennie JA, Eastmond CJ, Hutchison JM, Smith FW: Nuclear magnetic resonance (NMR) tomographic imaging for popliteal cysts in rheumatoid arthritis. Ann Rheum Dis 43:56–59, 1984.

169. Moon KL, Genant HK, Helms CA, Chafetz NI, Crooks LE, Kaufman L: Musculoskeletal applications of nuclear magnetic resonance. Radiology 147:161–171, 1983.

Fractures: When to X-Ray

170. Brand DA, Frazier WH, Kohlhepp WC, Shea KM, Hoefer AM, Ecker MD, Kornguth PJ, Pais MJ, Light TR: A protocol for selecting patients with injured extremities who need x-rays. N Engl J Med 306:333–339, 1982.

171. Cockshott WP, Jenkin JK, Pui M: Limiting the use of routine radiography for acute ankle injuries. Can Med Assoc J 129:129–131, 1983.

172. Kim H-R, Thrall JH, Keyes JW Jr: Skeletal scintigraphy following incidental trauma. Radiology 130:447–451, 1979.

173. Rosenthall L, Hill RO, Chuang S: Observation on the use of 99mTc-phosphate imaging in peripheral bone trauma. Radiology 119:637–641, 1976.

174. Nixon GW: Emergency room radiology. Refresher Course in Diagnostic Radiology. Sacred Heart Medical Center, Spokane, Washington, 1975.

Fracture Reporting

175. Cimmino CV: The radiologist and the orthopedist. Radiology 97:690–691, 1970.

176. Kaye JJ: The terminology and reportage of skeletal trauma. In American Roentgen Ray Society. Syllabus for the Categorical Course on Musculoskeletal Trauma, Atlanta, 1983.

177. Pitt MJ, Speer DP: Radiologic reporting of orthopedic trauma. Med Radiogr Photogr 58:14–18, 1982.

Fracture Healing

178. Aegerter E, Kirkpatrick JA Jr: The repair of fractures (Chap 8). In Orthopedic Disease. Physiology, Pathology, Radiology. Philadelphia, WB Saunders, 1975.

179. Basset CAL: Biophysical principles affecting bone structures. In Bourne GH, ed. The Biochemistry and Physiology of Bone, 3 vols., 2nd ed. New York, Academic Pr, 1972: 1–76.

180. Cave EF, Boyd RJ: Delayed union, nonunion and malunion of long bones. In Cave EF, Burke JF, Boyd RJ, eds. Trauma Management. Chicago, Year Book Medical Pub, 1974.

181. Cruess RL, Dumont J: Healing of bone, tendon, and ligament. In Rockwood CA Jr, Green DP, eds. Fractures. Philadelphia, JB Lippincott, 1975: 97–118.

182. Esterhai JL Jr, Brighton CT, Heppenstall RB, Alavi A, Desai AG: Detection of synovial pseudarthrosis by 99mTc scintigraphy: application to treatment of traumatic nonunion with constant direct current. Clin Orthop 161:15–23, 1981.

183. Harkess JW: Principles of fractures and dislocations. In Rockwood CA Jr, Green DP, eds. Fractures, Philadelphia, JB Lippincott, 1975.

184. Heppenstall RB: Fracture Treatment and Healing. Philadelphia, WB Saunders, 1980.

185. Houston CS, Swischuk LE: Occasional notes. Varus and valgus, no wonder they are confused. N Engl J Med 302:471–472, 1980.

186. Hulth A: Fracture healing: a concept of competing healing factors. Acta Orthop Scand 51:5–8, 1980.

187. Juhl JH: Traumatic lesions of bones and joints. In Juhl JH. Paul and Juhl's Essentials of Roentgen Interpretation, 4th ed, New York, Harper & Row, 1981: 127–143.

188. Kenzora JE: Repair of bone and fracture healing. In Cave EF, Burke JF, Boyd RJ, eds. Trauma Management. Chicago, Year Book Medical Pub, 1974.

189. Marty R, Denney JD, McKamey MR, Rowley MJ: Bone trauma and related benign disease: assessment by bone scanning. Semin Nucl Med 6:107–120, 1976.

190. Matin P: The appearance of bone scans following fractures, including immediate and long term studies. J Nucl Med 20:1227–1231, 1979.

191. Matin P: Bone scintigraphy in the diagnosis and management of traumatic injury. Semin Nucl Med 13:104–122, 1983.

192. McKibbin B: The biology of fracture healing in long bones. J Bone Joint Surg (Br) 60:150–162, 1978.

193. Muheim G: Assessment of fracture healing in man by serial 87mstrontium-scintimetry. Acta Orthop Scand 44:621–627, 1973.

194. Naimark A, Kossoff J, Leach RE: The disparate diameter. A sign of rotational deformity in fractures. J Can Assoc Radiol 34:8–11, 1983.

195. Naimark A, Miller K, Segal D, Kossoff J: Nonunion. Skeletal Radiol 6:21–25, 1981.

196. Nicholls PJ, Berg E, Bliven FE Jr, Kling JM: X-ray diagnosis of healing fractures in rabbits. Clin Orthop 142:234–236, 1979.

197. Renner RR, Mauler GG, Ambrose JL: The radiologist, the orthopedist, the lawyer, and the fracture. In Felson B. Roentgenology of Fractures and Dislocations. A Seminar in Roentgenology Reprints. New York, Grune & Stratton, 1978: 7–18.

198. Schultz RJ: The Language of Fractures. Baltimore, Williams & Wilkins, 1972.

199. Sevitt S: The healing of fractures of the lower end of the radius: a histological and angiographic study. J Bone Joint Surg (Br) 53:519–531, 1971.

200. Sevitt S: Healing of fractures in man. In Owen R, Goodfellow J, Bullough P, eds. Scientific Foundations of Orthopaedics and Traumatology. Philadelphia, WB Saunders, 1980: 258–273.

201. Sutton D: A Textbook of Radiology and Imaging. New York, Churchill Livingstone, 1980.

202. Urist MR, Mazet R Jr, McLean FC: The pathogenesis and treatment of delayed union and non-union: a survey of eighty-five ununited fractures of the shaft of the tibia and one hundred control cases with similar injuries. J Bone Joint Surg (Am) 36:931–966, 1954.

203. Wilson JN, ed. Watson-Jones Fractures and Joint Injuries, 5th ed, vol. 1. New York, Churchill Livingstone, 1976: 16–50.

Compression Plates

204. Bagby GW: Compression bone-plating. Historical considerations. J Bone Joint Surg (Am) 59:625–631, 1977.

205. Greiff J: Bone healing in rabbits after compression osteosynthesis: a comparative study between the radiological and histological findings. Injury 10:257–267, 1979.

206. Hicks JH: Rigid fixation as a treatment for hypertrophic non-union. Injury 8:199–205, 1976.

207. Kondo S. A bio-mechanical study on determining the indications of compression plating, with special reference to the friction coefficient of the fracture surface of human bone. Bull Osaka Med Sch 20:115–125, 1974.

208. Muller ME, Allgower M, Schneider R, Willenegger H: Manual of Internal Fixation: Technique Recommended by the AO-Group. Schatzker J, et al., trans. New York, Springer-Verlag, 1979.

209. Paavolainen P, Slatis P, Karaharju E, Holmstrom T. The healing of experimental fractures by compression osteosynthesis. I. Torsional strength. Acta Orthop Scand 50:369–374, 1979.

210. Paavolainen P, Penttinen R, Slatis P, Karaharju E. The healing of experimental fractures by compression osteosynthesis. II. Morphometric and chemical analysis. Acta Orthop Scand 50:375–383, 1979.

211. Paavolainen P, Karaharju E, Slatis P. Radiographic abnormalities in tubular bone after rigid plate fixation in rabbits. Acta Radiologica [Diagn] 19:119–126, 1978.

212. Ryan J. Compression in bone healing. Am J Nurs 74:1998–1999, 1974.
213. Sisk TD. Fractures. *In* Edmonson AS, Crenshaw AH, eds. Campbell's Operative Orthopedics. St. Louis, CV Mosby, 1980.

Intramedullary Fixation

214. Rush LV, Rush HL. Evolution of medullary fixation of fractures by the longitudinal pin. Am J Surg 78:324–333, 1949.
215. Rush LV, Rush HL. Intramedullary fixation of fractures of the humerus by the longitudinal pin. Surgery 27:268–275, 1950.
216. Küntscher GBG. The Küntscher method of intramedullary fixation. J Bone Joint Surg (Am) 40:17–26, 1958.

External Skeletal Fixation

217. Mears DC. External Skeletal Fixation. Baltimore, Williams & Wilkins, 1983.
218. Seligson D, Pope M. Concepts in External Fixation. New York, Grune & Stratton, 1982.

Electrical Stimulation

219. Brighton CT, Black J, Friedenberg ZB, Esterhai JL, Day LJ, Connolly JF. A multicenter study of the treatment of non-union with constant direct current. J Bone Joint Surg (Am) 63:2–13, 1981.
220. Compere CL. Electromagnetic fields and bones. JAMA 247:669, 1982.
221. Day L. Electrical stimulation in the treatment of ununited fractures. Clin Orthop 161:54–57, 1981.
222. Paterson DC, Lewis GN, Cass CA. Treatment of delayed union and nonunion with an implanted direct current stimulator. Clin Orthop 148:117–128, 1980.
223. Paterson DC, Lewis GN, Cass CA. Treatment of congenital pseudarthrosis of the tibia with direct current stimulation. Clin Orthop 148:129–135, 1980.
224. Peltier LF. A brief historical note on the use of electricity in the treatment of fractures. Clin Orthop 161:4–7, 1981.
225. Weber BG, Brunner C. The treatment of nonunions without electrical stimulation. Clin Orthop 161:24–32, 1981.

Stress Fractures

226. Baugher WH, Balady GJ, Warren RF, Marshall JL: Injuries of the musculoskeletal system in runners. Contemp Orthop 1:46–54, 1979.
227. Brower AC, Neff JR, Tillema DA: An unusual scapular stress fracture. AJR 129:519–520, 1977.
228. Daffner RH: Stress fractures: current concepts. Skeletal Radiol 2:221–229, 1978.
229. Daffner RH, Martinez S, Gehweiler JA Jr, Harrelson JM: Stress fractures of the proximal tibia in runners. Radiology 142:63–65, 1982.
230. El-Khoury GY, Wehbe MA, Bonfiglio M, Chow KC: Stress fractures of the femoral neck: a scintigraphic sign for early diagnosis. Skeletal Radiol 6:271–273, 1981.
231. Geslien GE, Thrall H, Espinosa JL, Older RA: Early detection of stress fractures using 99mTc-polyphosphate. Radiology 121:683–687, 1976.
232. Greaney RB, Gerber FH, Laughlin RL, Kmet JP, Metz CD, Kilcheski TS, Rao BR, Silverman ED: Distribution and natural history of stress fractures in U.S. Marine recruits. Radiology 146:339–346, 1983.
233. Meurman KOA: Less common stress fractures in the foot. Br J Radiol 54:1–7, 1981.

234. Pavlov H, Nelson TL, Warren RF, Torg JS, Burstein AH: Stress fractures of the pubic ramus. A report of twelve cases. J Bone Joint Surg (Am) 64:1020–1025, 1982.
235. Rosen PR, Micheli LJ, Treves S: Early scintigraphic diagnosis of bone stress and fractures in athletic adolescents. Pediatrics 70:11–15, 1982.
236. Roub LW, Gumerman LW, Hanley EN Jr, Clark MW, Goodman M, Herbert DL: Bone stress: a radionuclide imaging perspective. Radiology 132:431–438, 1979.
237. Sandrock AR: Another sports fatigue fracture. Stress fracture of the coracoid process of the scapula. Radiology 117:274, 1975.
238. Savoca CJ: Stress fractures: a classification of the earliest radiographic signs. Radiology 100:519–524, 1971.
239. Schneider HJ, King AY, Bronson JL, Miller EH: Stress injuries and developmental change of lower extremities in ballet dancers. Radiology 113:627–632, 1974.
240. Sweet DE, Allman RM: Stress fracture. RPC of the month from the AFIP. Radiology 99:687–693, 1971.
241. Wilcox JR Jr, Moniot AL, Green JP: Bone scanning in the evaluation of exercise-related stress injuries. Radiology 123:699–703, 1977.

Bone Graft

242. Bowerman JW, Hughes JL: Radiology of bone grafts. Radiol Clin North Am 13:67–77, 1975.
243. Cruess RL, Dumont J: Healing of bone, tendon and ligament. *In* Rockwood CA Jr, Green DP, eds. Fractures. Philadelphia, JB Lippincott, 1975.
244. Dee P, Lambruschi PG, Hiebert JM: The use of Tc-99m MDP bone scanning in the study of vascularized bone implants: concise communication. J Nucl Med 22:522–525, 1981.
245. Edmonson AS: Surgical techniques. *In* Edmonson AS, Crenshaw AH, eds. Campbell's Operative Orthopedics. St. Louis, CV Mosby, 1980: 20–22.
246. Enneking WF, Burchardt H, Puhl JJ, Piotrowski G: Physical and biological aspects of repair in dog cortical-bone transplants. J Bone Joint Surg (Am) 57:237–251, 1975.
247. Heppenstall RB: Bone grafting. *In* Heppenstall RB, ed. Fracture Treatment and Healing. Philadelphia, WB Saunders, 1980.
248. Kattapuram SV, Phillips WC: Severed body parts: radiologic evaluation following replantation. Radiology 149:59–63, 1983.
249. Lisbona R, Rennie WRJ, Daniel RK: Radionuclide evaluation of free vascularized bone graft viability. AJR 134:387–388, 1980.

Osteotomy

250. Ford LT: Osteotomies. Nomenclature and uses. Radiol Clin North Am 13:79–92, 1975.

Arthroplasty

251. Cooney WP III: Total joint arthroplasty: introduction to the upper extremity. Mayo Clin Proc 54:495–499, 1979.

Methylmethacrylate: Local Reaction, the Cement-Bone Interface

252. Charnley J, Follacci FM, Hammond BT: The long-term reaction of bone to self-curing acrylic cement. J Bone Joint Surg (B) 50:822–829, 1968.
253. Charnley J: The reaction of bone to self-curing acrylic cement. A long-term histological study in man. J Bone Joint Surg (Br) 52:340–353, 1970.

254. DeLee JG, Charnley J: Radiological demarcation of cemented sockets in total hip replacement. Clin Orthop 121:20–32, 1976.

255. Goldring SR, Schiller AL, Roelke M, Rourke CM, O'Neill DA, Harris WH: The synovial-like membrane at the bone-cement interface in loose total hip replacements and its proposed role in bone lysis. J Bone Joint Surg (Am) 65:575–584, 1983.

256. Harris WH, McCarthy JC Jr, O'Neill DA: Femoral component loosening using contemporary techniques of femoral cement fixation. J Bone Joint Surg (Am) 64:1063–1067, 1982.

257. Harris WH, Schiller AL, Scholler JM, Freiberg RA, Scott R: Extensive localized bone resorption in the femur following total hip replacement. J Bone Joint Surg (Am) 58:612–618, 1976.

258. Heilmann K, Diezel PB, Rossner JA, Brinkmann KA: Morphological studies in tissues surrounding alloarthroplastic joints. Virchows Arch [Pathol Anat] 366:93–106, 1975.

259. Reckling FW, Dillon WL: The bone-cement interface temperature during total joint replacement. J Bone Joint Surg (Am) 59:80–82, 1977.

260. Stauffer RN: Ten-year follow-up study of total hip replacement. With particular reference to roentgenographic loosening of the components. J Bone Joint Surg (Am) 64:983–990, 1982.

261. Sutherland CJ, Wilde AH, Borden LS, Marks KE: A ten-year follow-up of one hundred consecutive Muller curved-stem total hip-replacement arthroplasties. J Bone Joint Surg (Am) 64:970–982, 1982.

262. Willert H-G, Ludwig J, Semlitsch M: Reaction of bone to methacrylate after hip arthroplasty. A long-term gross, light microscopic, and scanning electron microscopic study. J Bone Joint Surg (Am) 56:1368–1382, 1974.

Methylmethacrylate: Systemic Reactions

263. Alexander JP, Barron DW: Biochemical disturbances associated with total hip replacement. J Bone Joint Surg (Br) 61:101–106, 1979.

264. Breed AL: Experimental production of vascular hypotension, and bone marrow and fat embolism with methylmethacrylate cement. Traumatic hypertension of bone. Clin Orthop 102:227–244, 1974.

265. Daniel WW, Coventry MB, Miller WE: Pulmonary complications after total hip arthroplasty with Charnley prosthesis as revealed by chest roentgenograms. J Bone Joint Surg (Am) 54:282–283, 1972.

266. Gooding JM, Weng J-T, Kirby RR, Smith RA: Methylmethacrylate seeks an appeal. South Med J 74:1209–1212, 1981.

267. Keret D, Reis DR: Intraoperative cardiac arrest and mortality in hip surgery. Possible relationship to acrylic bone cement. Orthop Rev 9:51–56, 1980.

268. Mallory TH, Kolodzik S: Fat embolization after total knee replacement. JAMA 236:1451, 1976.

269. Modig J, Busch C, Olerud S, Saldeen T, Waernbaum G: Arterial hypotension and hypoxaemia during total hip replacement: the importance of thromboplastic products, fat embolism and acrylic monomers. Acta Anesthesiol Scand 19:28–43, 1975.

270. Pedley RB, Meachim G, Gray T: Identification of acrylic cement particles in tissues. Ann Biomed Eng 7:319–328, 1979.

271. Petty W: Methylmethacrylate concentrations in tissues adjacent to bone cement. J Biomed Mater Res 14:427–434, 1980.

272. Rinecker H: New clinico-pathophysiological studies on the bone cement implantation syndrome. Arch Orthop Trauma Surg 97:263–274, 1980.

273. Weissman BN, Sosman JL, Braunstein EM, Dadkhahipoor H, Kandarpa K, Thornhill TJ, Lowell JD, Sledge CB: Intravenous methylmethacrylate after total hip replacement. J Bone Joint Surg (Am) 66:443–450, 1984.

274. Wong KC, Martin WE, Kennedy WF, Akamatsu TJ, Convery RF, Shaw CL: Cardiovascular effects of total hip placement in man: with observations on the effects of methylmethacrylate on the isolated rabbit heart. Clin Pharmacol Ther 21:709–714, 1977.

Prosthetic Fixation, Bony Ingrowth

275. Draenert K, Draenert Y: Possibilities and limitations of the cementless fixation of endoprosthetic components. *In* Morscher E, ed. The Cementless Fixation of Hip Endoprostheses. New York, Springer-Verlag, 1984: 46–51.

276. Hedley AK: Present state, problems, and future implications of porous-coated implants. *In* Riley LH, Jr, ed. Proceedings of the Eighth Open Scientific Meeting of the Hip Society, 1980. St. Louis, CV Mosby, 1980.

277. Ling RSM: The bonding of internal implants of bone. *In* Scientific Foundations of Orthopaedics and Traumatology. Owen R, Goodfellow J, Bullough P., eds. Philadelphia, WB Saunders, 1980: 472–481.

278. Salzer M, Knahr K, Frank P: Radiologic and clinical follow-ups of uncemented femoral endoprostheses with and without collars. *In* Morscher E, ed. The Cementless Fixation of Hip Endoprostheses. New York, Springer-Verlag, 1984: 161–167.

279. Schenk RK, Herrmann W: Histologic studies on the incorporation of uncemented implants. *In* Morscher E, ed. The Cementless Fixation of Hip Endoprostheses. New York, Springer-Verlag, 1984: 52–58.

280. Swanson SAV, Freeman MAR: The Scientific Basis of Joint Replacement. New York, Wiley, 1977.

281. Willert H-G, Buchhorn GH: Biocompatibility of endoprosthetic materials. *In* Morscher E, ed. The Cementless Fixation of Hip Endoprostheses. New York, Springer-Verlag, 1984: 29–38.

Chapter 2

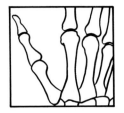

The
HAND

NORMAL STRUCTURE AND FUNCTION

Essential Anatomy

The remarkable strength and dexterity of the hand are reflected in its complex anatomy. Its structure has been viewed as a series of arches that are necessary to maintain the cupped shape of the palm and allow the thumb to oppose the other fingertips. These three essential arches are a fixed transverse arch through the distal carpal row, a mobile transverse arch through the metacarpal heads, and a linking longitudinal arch consisting of each ray (finger and metacarpal) with the apex at the metacarpophalangeal joint (Fig. 2–1).[2, 49] The inclusion of the wrist in this description is noteworthy because wrist structure and function are intimately related to hand function. Another functionally important concept is that of mobility around a central stable unit.

Thus the hand can be regarded as having a *fixed stable unit* composed of the second and third metacarpals and the distal carpal row and a *mobile unit* consisting of the thumb on the

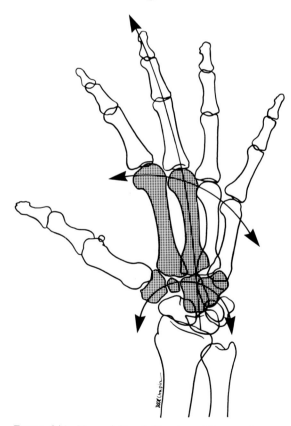

Figure 2–1. Normal Hand Structure. Three arches are present: a fixed transverse arch through the distal carpal row, a mobile transverse arch through the metacarpal heads, and linking longitudinal arches consisting of each finger and metacarpal. The fixed, stable unit of the hand (stippled) is shown. (After Tubiana R: The Hand, vol. 1. Philadelphia, WB Saunders, 1985, by permission.)

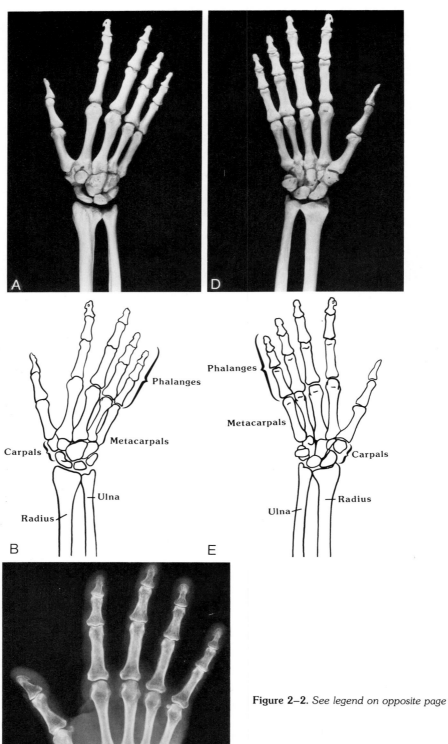

Figure 2–2. *See legend on opposite page*

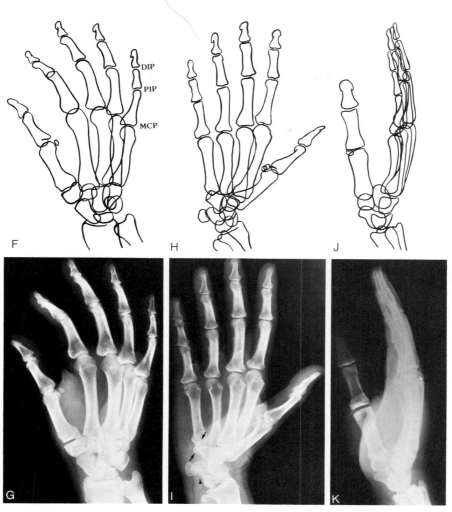

Figure 2–2. Normal Examination. Photographic, diagrammatic, and radiographic anatomy is shown in PA *(A to C)*, AP *(D, E)*, PA oblique *(F, G)*, AP oblique *(H, I)*, and lateral *(J, K)* views. On the PA oblique projection, note the excellent view of metacarpal heads, scaphoid-trapezium, and trapezium–first metacarpal joints. The AP oblique (ball-catcher's view) shows the fourth and fifth metacarpals and carpometacarpal joints, the hook of the hamate (arrows), and the pisiform triquetral joint (arrowhead) to advantage.

radial side and the fourth and fifth metacarpals on the ulnar side.[13, 14] The stability of the second and third carpometacarpal articulation is due largely to the geometry of the bony components.[13] The ring and fifth finger metacarpals are more mobile with about 15 degrees of dorsovolar motion possible at the ring finger and 25 degrees at the fifth finger carpometacarpal joints.[49]

The bony structures of the hand are shown in Figure 2–2. Each metacarpal has a head that includes the distal articular surface, a shaft, and a base. Two tubercles are noted on the dorsal aspect of the metacarpal at the sites of insertion of the collateral ligaments.

The phalanges of each digit also have a head distally, a shaft, and a base. The terminal tuft of each distal phalanx receives connective tissue strands that attach to the soft tissues of the fingertip. Numerous tendons also attach to the phalanges (Fig. 2–3), and knowledge of their insertions is especially important for evaluating avulsion fractures and understanding finger deformities.

The sesamoid bones are small ossicles located within tendons. The tendons are incorporated in the joint capsule to some extent, and the surface of the sesamoid that faces the joint is covered with articular cartilage. Sesamoid bones are almost always present at the thumb metacarpophalangeal joint, lying within the substance of the volar plate and at the sites of insertion of the flexor pollicis brevis (the radial sesamoid) and the adductor pollicis (ulnar sesamoid). Ses-

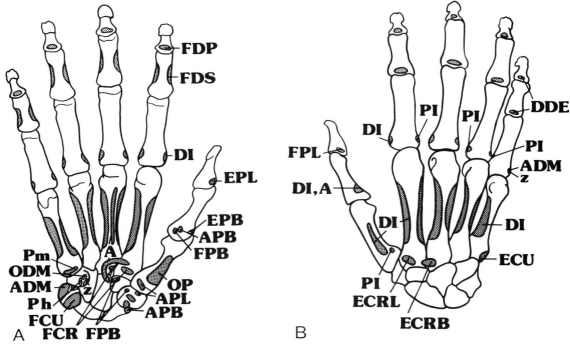

Figure 2–3. Sites of Tendon Insertion on Phalages and Metacarpals. *A,* Anterior view; *B,* posterior view. A = Adductor pollicis; ADM = abductor digiti minimi; APB = abductor pollicis brevis; APL = abductor pollicis longus; DDE = dorsal digital expansion (terminal and middle extensor tendons); DI = dorsal interossei; ECRB = extensor carpi radialis brevis; ECRL = extensor carpi radialis longus; ECU = extensor carpi ulnaris; EPB = extensor pollicis brevis; EPL = extensor pollicis longus; FCR = flexor carpi radialis; FCU = flexor carpi ulnaris; FDP = flexor digitorum profundus; FDS = flexor digitorum superficialis; FPB = flexor pollicis brevis; FPL = flexor pollicis longus; OP = opponens pollicis; ODM = opponens digiti minimi; PI = palmar interossei; Ph = pisohamate ligament; Pm = pisometacarpal ligament; Z = flexor digiti minimi brevis. (After McMinn RMH, Hutchings RT. The Color Atlas of Human Anatomy. Chicago, Year Book Med, 1977.)

amoid bones occur in other sites as well, as shown in Figure 2–4. They are involved in arthritis and may be fractured or dislocated as a consequence of trauma.[11]

Muscular control of the hand is derived from two major muscle groups: the extrinsics and the intrinsics.[5] The *extrinsic* muscles originate in the elbow and forearm and insert on the hand. They provide the power and endurance necessary for normal hand function. This group of muscles includes the forearm flexor-pronator and extensor-supinator muscles, each of which in general exerts its main action across a single joint. The *intrinsic* muscles originate and insert in the hand. They exert their action on more than one joint and help position the fingers to achieve dexterity by cupping the palm or spreading the hand. The muscles of the thenar and hypothenar eminences, the interosseous muscles, the lumbricals, the adductor pollicis, the short flexor of the thumb, and the palmaris brevis muscles are in this group (Figs. 2–3 and 2–5).

The metacarpophalangeal (MCP) joints of the index through fifth fingers are ball-and-socket

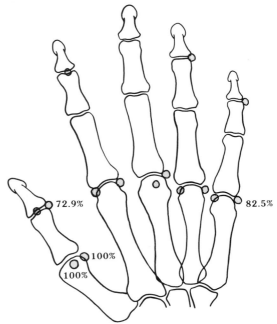

Figure 2–4. Sesamoids. The usual locations of the sesamoid bones of the hand are shown.

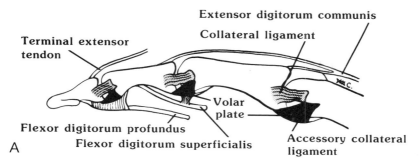

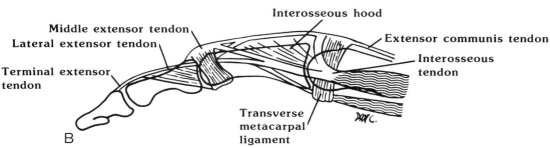

Figure 2–5. Flexors and Extensors of the Fingers.

joints that allow motion in flexion and extension (90 degrees flexion to 15 degrees extension), abduction-adduction (50 to 60 degrees), and rotation (15 to 20 degrees).[10] The stability of the MCP joints is due to muscular forces and the passive stability provided by the joint capsule, volar plate, and collateral ligaments (Figs. 2–6 and 2–7). Anteriorly the volar plate is an area of thickening of the joint capsule that prevents

hyperextension. Distally, it has a strong attachment to the base of the proximal phalanx and proximally, a looser attachment to the metacarpal neck. The volar plates of the index through fifth finger metacarpophalangeal joints are joined

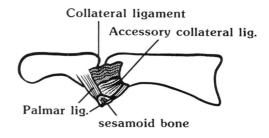

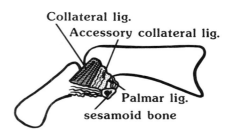

Figure 2–7. Collateral Ligaments. Diagrammatic view of the MCP collateral ligaments in extension and flexion. Collateral ligaments of the MCPs are more lax in extension than in flexion, whereas PIP collateral ligaments are taut in both positions.

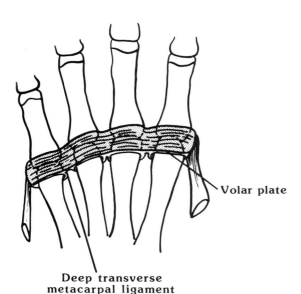

Figure 2–6. Normal MCP. Deep transverse metacarpal ligaments are seen connecting the volar plates.

by deep transverse metacarpal ligaments. The collateral ligament consists of two parts, a dorsal metacarpophalangeal ligament and a volar accessory collateral ligament that attaches to the volar plate. The collateral ligaments of the MCPs are looser in extension than in flexion. Thus there is more abduction-adduction motion possible when the fingers are held in extension. This also means that immobilization of the MCP joints in extension may lead to shortening of the collateral ligaments and subsequent restriction of joint motion.

The extensor mechanism of the MCP joint consists of a dorsal hood that contains centrally the extensor tendon of the extrinsic group and, more peripherally and volarly, the interosseous and lumbrical tendons of the intrinsic group (Fig. 2–5). The extensor hood slips back and forth over the MCP joint.[10] Flexion of the MCP joint results primarily from the intrinsic muscles and secondarily from the flexor digitorum muscles.[49]

The metacarpal articular surface extends farther anteriorly than posteriorly and is enclosed by the joint capsule that attaches close to but not on the articular cartilage margins of the metacarpal and the proximal phalanx. A small area of bone between the capsular insertion and the articular cartilage surface is particularly vulnerable to early erosion in rheumatoid arthritis. The proximal interphalangeal (PIP) joints are essentially hinge joints that allow motion from 5 degrees of hyperextension to 115 degrees of flexion.[10, 13] No motion other than flexion-extension occurs. This stability is crucial for function and results from the geometric configuration of the joint and presence of the joint capsule, the volar plate, the collateral ligaments, and the fibrous flexor sheaths that insert on or just proximal and distal to the volar plate. The joint capsule is thin dorsally but is reinforced by the central slip of the extensor tendon, which continues on to insert into the dorsal tubercle at the base of the middle phalanx. As in the MCP joints, the collateral ligament on either side of the PIP joint consists of two parts. In contrast to the relative laxity of the collateral ligaments in the extended MCP, the collateral ligaments at the PIP joints are taut in both flexion and extension and therefore provide stability in both positions.[51] The PIP joints are flexed by the flexor digitorum sublimis, which inserts on the middle phalanx, and are extended by a dual system consisting of the extensor digitorum and the dorsal expansion of the intrinsic muscles.[49]

The distal interphalangeal (DIP) joints are structurally similar to the PIP joints. Flexion of about 80 degrees is produced by the flexor digitorum profundus, which inserts on the volar

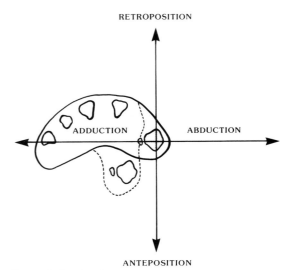

Figure 2–8. Thumb Motions. (Redrawn from Tubiana R: The Hand, Vol 1. WB Saunders, 1981.)

surface of the base of the distal phalanx. Extension is produced by action of the terminal extensor tendon, which inserts on the dorsal aspect of the distal phalanx.[12]

The motions of the thumb are complex (Fig. 2–8). Apposition of the thumb actually includes a series of motions at the MCP and interphalangeal joints.

Normal Radiographic Anatomy

Routine examination of the hand includes the wrist and consists of posteroanterior (PA), oblique, and lateral views. All of the carpals and fingers must be included on each film. In the PA view, fingers and forearms should be flat on the film with the fingers separated to permit the soft tissues of each digit to be seen. Three (frontal, oblique, and lateral) coned, well-positioned views of individual digits should be done in cases of localized injury. Radiographic factors are adjusted to permit both bony structures and soft tissues to be seen on one examination.

In order to avoid confusion, the fingers should be named (thumb, index, middle or long, ring, and little or fifth) rather than numbered. The terms *radial* and *ulnar* are preferred to *lateral* and *medial*; *volar* (palmar) and *dorsal* (extensor), to *anterior* and *posterior*.

Normal Bony Anatomy

Normal bony anatomy is shown in Figure 2–2. The axis of the second metacarpal is normally in line with the long axis of the radius and forms an angle of 115 degrees with the distal radial articular surface.[65] The proximal phalanges of the index, middle, and fifth fingers are normally ulnar deviated in relation to the metacarpal shafts.[13]

Normal Soft Tissue Anatomy

The normal soft tissues of the hand can be studied on routine examination or with special techniques such as low kV radiography or xerography, which display them to advantage. The soft tissue density around the DIP and PIP joints is composed of joint capsules and contents and collateral ligaments. At the level of the MCPs, fat is noted around the soft tissue density that includes the capsules and adjacent interosseous and lumbrical muscles (see Fig. 2–14). Fischer attempted to quantify the amount of periarticular soft tissue present.[16] In normal subjects the width of the base of the adjacent phalanx was subtracted from the width of the periarticular soft tissue. At the DIP joints the periarticular soft tissues may normally measure only 1 mm more than the width of the base of the distal phalanx. Larger differences were noted at the PIP and MCP joints.

Metacarpophalangeal, Proximal Interphalangeal, and Distal Interphalangeal Joint Arthrography

Technique. As described by Rosenthal and co-workers, injection of each of these joints is done in a similar manner.[19] The patient is positioned prone on the fluoroscopic table with the palm of the affected hand down. After antiseptic skin preparation, an injection site is localized fluoroscopically over the midline or paramedian joint space. The skin is infiltrated with 1 percent lidocaine, and a 25-gauge needle is advanced into the selected site. If there are signs or symptoms suggesting abnormality in a particular location, the injection is made away from that site. Contrast material is injected until there is increased resistance or complete filling of the joint on fluoroscopy. This requires less than 1 ml of contrast agent. A double contrast study using 0.1 to 0.3 ml of contrast material and air to make a total volume of 1 ml can be done, particularly if the articular cartilage is the primary area of interest. Posteroanterior, oblique, and lateral fluoroscopic spot films are obtained and may be followed by magnification radiographs, traction radiographs, tomography, or a combination of these.

Normal Arthrographic Findings. The joint capsule of the MCP attaches proximally near the articular margins of the metacarpal head and distally near the base of the proximal phalanx

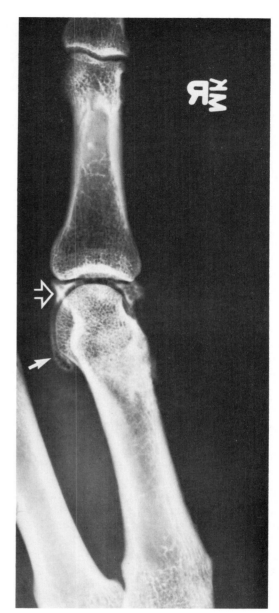

Figure 2–9. Normal Metacarpophalangeal Joint Arthrogram (Fifth Finger). The prominent volar recess (arrow) and smooth articular cartilage surfaces are well seen in this magnification view from a double contrast study. Lateral (open arrow) and medial indentations are caused by the adjacent collateral ligaments. (Courtesy of Dr. Daniel Rosenthal, Massachusetts General Hospital, Boston, Mass.)

(Fig. 2–9). Recesses projecting from the volar aspect of the capsule can be noted, and, on the posteroanterior view, medial and lateral indentations in the capsule due to the proximity of the collateral ligaments can be seen. The artic-

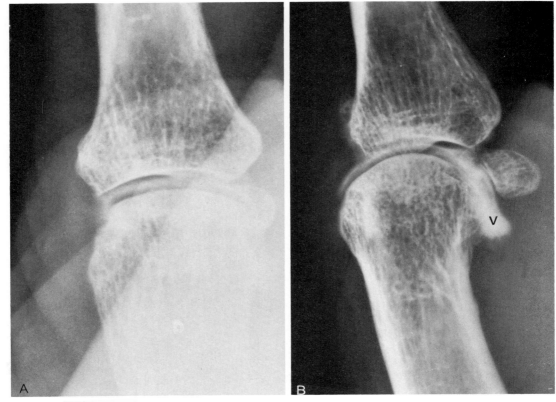

Figure 2–10. Normal Thumb Metacarpophalangeal Joint Arthrogram. AP *(A)* and oblique *(B)* views. The prominent volar recess (V) and its relation to the sesamoids are well shown.

ular cartilage surfaces appear smooth, with the metacarpal cartilage appearing somewhat thicker than the proximal phalangeal cartilage.

The normal thumb MCP joint exhibits dorsal and volar recesses around the metacarpal head and a small dorsal recess around the base of the proximal phalanx (Fig. 2–10). A very small recess is present radially at the volar margin of the proximal phalanx.[39]

The contour of the proximal interphalangeal joint capsule is similar to that of the metacarpophalangeal joint. Impressions due to the intact collateral ligaments will be noted on either side on posteroanterior radiographs (Fig. 2–11). Recesses will be noted along the dorsal and volar aspects of the proximal phalangeal head and neck. Arthrograms of the distal interphalangeal joints show similar findings.

Abnormal Findings. Arthrography of these joints can confirm collateral ligament laxity (the affected side of the capsule appears to bulge), volar plate injury (contrast agent extravasation from that region of the volar plate), fibrous ankylosis of the joint,[19] and synovial disease, including rheumatoid arthritis and synovial osteochondromatosis (Fig. 2–12).

ABNORMAL CONDITIONS

Soft Tissue Abnormalities: Arthritis

Rheumatoid Arthritis

In evaluating soft tissue changes in the hands, both the character and the distribution of the swelling are important. Fusiform soft tissue swelling at the proximal interphalangeal joints, metacarpophalangeal joints, and ulnar styloids makes a diagnosis of rheumatoid arthritis very likely, even when there are no bony abnormalities (Fig. 2–13).[24]

On the PA view the soft tissues over the normal proximal interphalangeal joints and marginal metacarpophalangeal joints are slightly convex, and the space between the index and middle finger metacarpophalangeal joints is greater than that between the middle, ring, and fifth MCP joints. The soft tissues around the joints can be measured and compared with the normal values described by Fischer.[16]

Fusiform swelling of the joints due to capsular distension by effusion and pannus is characteristic of rheumatoid arthritis. In the proximal

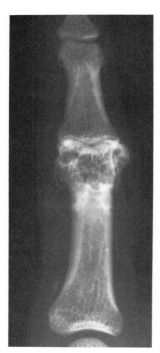

Figure 2–11. Normal PIP Arthrogram. The articular cartilage is better seen on the ulnar side of the joint in this example. Bubbles of gas account for observed filling defects. (Courtesy of Dr. Daniel Rosenthal, Massachusetts General Hospital, Boston, Mass.)

interphalangeal joints, moderate swelling is readily appreciated in posteroanterior views, but mild swelling should be confirmed by obliteration of the normal knuckle creases on the oblique view (Fig. 2–13).

Metacarpophalangeal swelling is more difficult to detect, and comparison with other fingers is necessary. The index and middle finger metacarpophalangeal joints are the earliest and most often to be affected.[25] Capsular distension can be detected by separation of the metacarpal heads, bulging of the web spaces, and increased convexity of the marginal soft tissues of the metacarpophalangeal joints of the thumb and index and fifth fingers (Fig. 2–14).

Psoriatic Arthritis and Reiter's Syndrome

In contrast to the fusiform soft tissue swelling around joints that occurs in rheumatoid arthritis, the swelling that occurs in psoriatic arthritis or in Reiter's syndrome may involve the entire digit, producing a "sausage" appearance (Fig. 2–15). This diffuse swelling is attributed to simultaneous involvement of the interphalangeal joints, tendon sheaths, and surrounding tissues.[23] In Reiter's syndrome the feet are typically more severely involved than the hands (Fig. 2–16).[25]

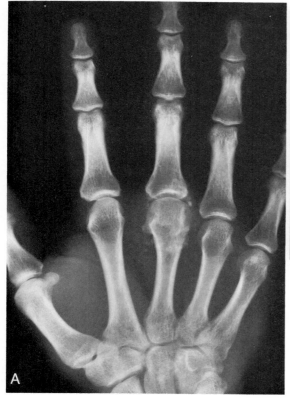

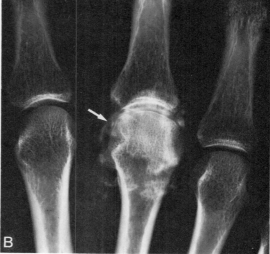

Figure 2–12. Synovial Osteochondromatosis. A, PA view prior to contrast agent injection shows multiple calcified densities in the region of the third MCP joint capsule. B, Arthrography shows contrast around some of these densities (arrow), confirming their intraarticular location.

79

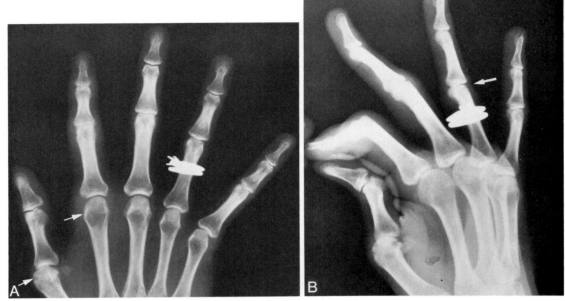

Figure 2–13. Proximal Interphalangeal Joint Swelling in Rheumatoid Arthritis. *A,* PA view shows fusiform swelling of the index finger PIP and MCP and the middle finger PIP. There is early erosion of the thumb and index MCPs (arrows) and the index PIP. *B,* Oblique view confirms swelling of the middle finger PIP by showing displacement and smoothing of the knuckle creases in comparison with those of the normal ring finger (arrow).

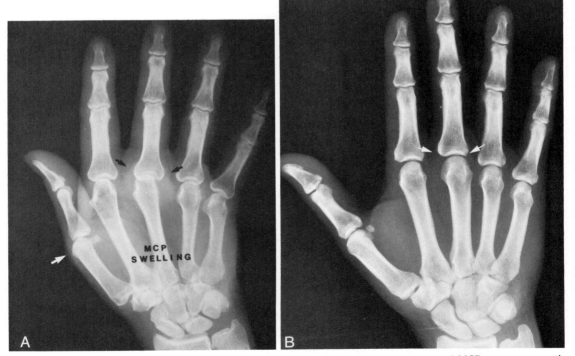

Figure 2–14. MCP Swelling. *A,* Several of the findings of MCP capsular distention in a central MCP are present at the middle finger, including separation of the metacarpal heads, increased soft tissue density, flattening of the concavities of the web spaces, and displacement of fat around the intrinsic muscles and capsules (arrows). There is slight swelling of the thumb MCP as indicated by the bulge in the overlying soft tissue contour (white arrow). *B,* Normal appearances for comparison with A. Arrows indicate the third MCP pericapsular fat.

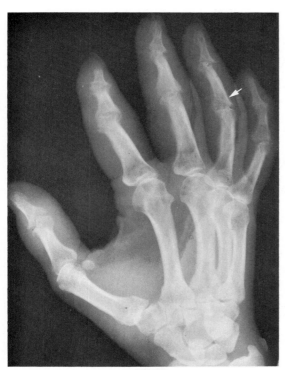

Figure 2–15. Psoriatic Arthritis with Diffuse Swelling. There is a diffuse swelling of all of the fingers owing to IP and tendon sheath involvement, producing "sausage" digits. Thin periosteal reaction is noted along several middle phalanges (arrow).

Pigmented Villonodular Synovitis

(PVNS, or Giant Cell Tumor of Tendon Sheath)

PVNS occurs in diffuse and localized, intraarticular, and extraarticular forms. The localized extraarticular form is the most frequent and usually involves the tendon sheaths or joint capsules of the hands, especially the fingers. According to Phalen and associates, this lesion is the second most frequent subcutaneous tumor of the hand, only ganglia being more common.[37]

Typically, a solitary, slowly enlarging, painless mass is noted. It is not fixed to the overlying skin and is nontender. The flexor tendon sheaths are most often involved.[35] Characteristic radiographic findings include the presence of a solitary, lobulated, uncalcified soft tissue mass; normal bony mineralization; and normal cartilage spaces (Fig. 2–17).[33] The mass may produce pressure erosion of the adjacent bone.

Differential diagnostic possibilities include ganglia (distinguished clinically by their cystic feel, aspiration of mucinous material, or transillumination), xanthomas, other benign tendon sheath tumors, and synovial sarcoma.[37]

Soft Tissue Abnormalities: Injuries

Gamekeeper's Thumb

This term was originally applied to a disability noted in Scottish gamekeepers, who killed wounded rabbits by stretching and hyperextending their necks. The rabbit's head was held between the gamekeeper's thumb and index finger, and if a loose grip was applied, the chronic stress due to the impact of the animal's neck against the ulnar side of the gamekeeper's thumb resulted in collateral ligamentous damage.[40] This condition is now recognized to result from a number of traumatic incidents, including abduction and extension of the thumb against the strap of a ski pole.[45, 46] Disabling instability of pinch, chronic pain, or both may result.[41]

Anatomy.[39, 48] The fibrous capsule of the thumb MCP is reinforced anteriorly by the volar plate, dorsally by the extensor pollicis brevis,[39] and on the radial and ulnar sides by the collateral ligaments (Fig. 2–18). There are actually two parts to the ulnar collateral ligament, a "proper" ulnar collateral ligament that limits abduction of the thumb MCP when the joint is flexed beyond 20 degrees and an accessory collateral ligament that serves the same function when the joint is extended. Under normal circumstances no more than 20 degrees of abduction is possible when the thumb is in either the extended or the slightly flexed position.

The two most common disruptions that are known to produce gamekeeper's thumb are avulsion of the proper collateral ligament from its phalangeal attachment and disruption of both collateral ligaments. The torn ligament may be folded back with its torn edge protruding under the proximal edge of the adductor aponeurosis. Thus the adductor aponeurosis blocks the return of the ligament to its normal position. This condition, described by Stener, requires surgical treatment.

Plain Film Findings.[41, 46] Avulsion fractures of the ulnar or ulnar–volar border of the proximal phalanx occur in many cases, and in most, such a fracture indicates that the joint is unstable. Significant displacement or rotation of the avulsed fragment may mean that healing without surgery would be inadequate or associated with lengthening of the ligament and chronic instability (Fig. 2–19). Involvement of more than 10 percent of the articular surface also suggests the need for surgical repair. Volar subluxation of the proximal phalanx may be noted on lateral radiographs.

Stress Views. Abduction stress views of the normal as well as the injured thumb are neces-

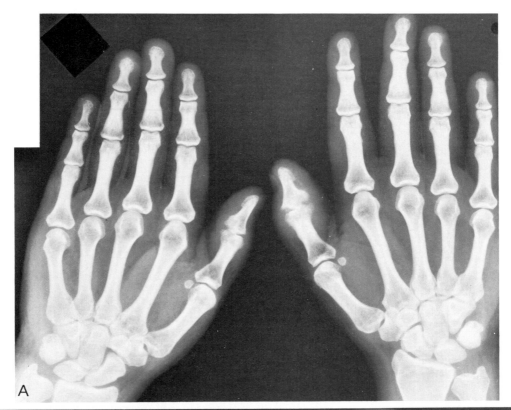

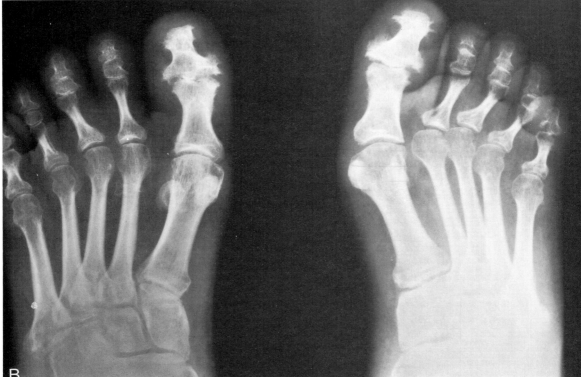

Figure 2–16. Reiter's Syndrome. *A,* Initial hand radiographs show diffuse swelling of the right thumb and more focal swelling of the left. There is periosteal reaction and erosion of the right thumb IP. Some nail changes are present. The patient clinically showed classic features of Reiter's syndrome. *B,* Views of the feet 2 years later show erosion and sclerosis of the great toe IP joints. There is periosteal reaction along several of the left phalanges, erosion of several PIPs, and swelling of several toes, particularly the right great toe. The findings are identical to those seen in psoriatic arthritis. *C,* There is bilateral sacroiliitis.

Illustration continued on opposite page

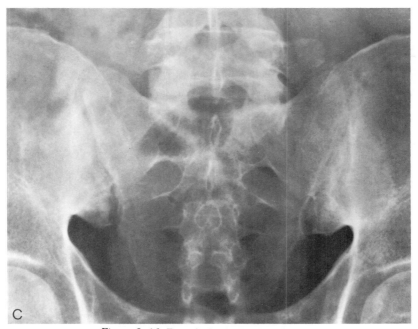

Figure 2–16. Reiter's Syndrome *Continued*

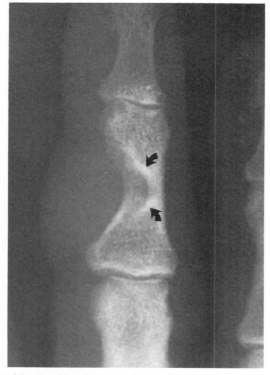

Figure 2–17. Giant Cell Tumor of Tendon Sheath. A coned view of the middle finger shows a noncalcified soft tissue mass producing smooth erosion (arrows) of the middle phalanx.

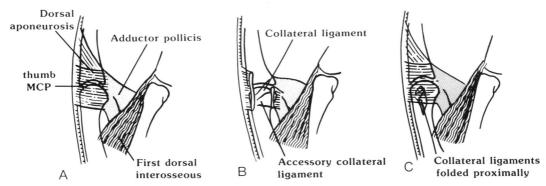

Figure 2–18. The Thumb MCP. *A*, The aponeurosis. *B*, Collateral ligaments. *C*, Gamekeeper's thumb with folding back of the collateral ligaments.

sary. Local anesthesia may be required to allow demonstration of instability. Bowers and Hurst noted normal thumb abduction to be about 15 ± 5 degrees, although higher normal values have been reported.[39] Abduction to 30 degrees or more or 10 degrees or more than the unaffected side is considered abnormal. Widening of the ulnar aspect of the joint and radial subluxa-

tion of the proximal phalanx on the metacarpal may be noted.

Arthrography.[39, 42, 45] After contrast agent injection posteroanterior, lateral, and abduction stress views in the flexed position are done. Abnormal findings include (1) leakage of contrast material through the capsule along the abductor muscle or along the tendons of the

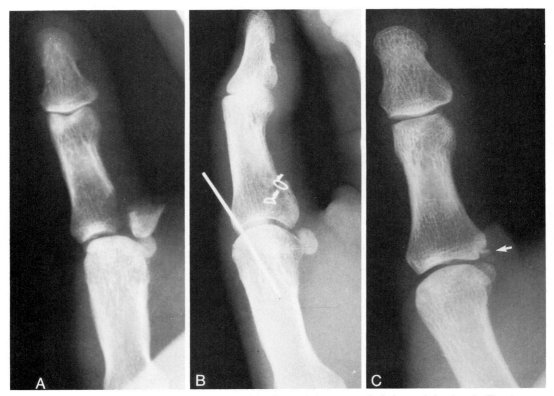

Figure 2–19. Gamekeeper's Thumb. *A*, A fracture of the base of the proximal phalanx of the thumb. The fragment is rotated 90 degrees. There is mild radial subluxation of the thumb proximal phalanx. *B*, The postoperative radiograph confirms almost anatomic reduction of the fracture fragments. The pin through the MCP provides stability during healing. *C*, Another patient with an old injury documented by small avulsion fracture fragments (arrow) at the thumb base.

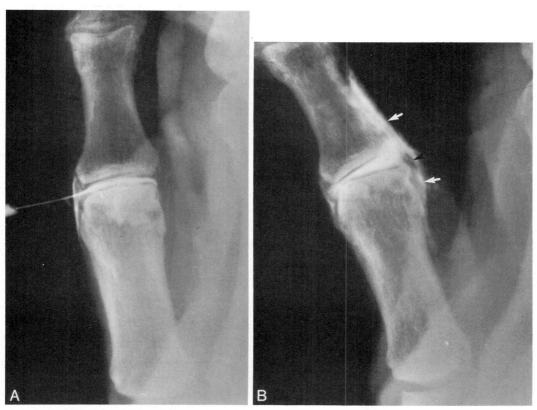

Figure 2–20. Gamekeeper's Thumb Confirmed by Arthrography. *A,* Normal PA view after contrast injection shows extravasation laterally at the puncture site but no extravasation medially. *B,* The same view, of a cadaver, after production of a gamekeeper's lesion shows marked widening of the joint space medially and contrast extravasation (arrows). The filling defect (arrowhead) is the torn collateral ligament.

THE HAND

extensor pollicis brevis and longus muscles (Fig. 2–20); (2) leakage of contrast around the edge of an everted collateral ligament.

The presence of a capsular tear differentiates patients with strains from those with true capsular injuries. The diagnosis of a trapped, everted collateral ligament suggests the need for surgical intervention.

Mallet Finger

Mallet finger (baseball finger, or dropped finger) refers to flexion deformity at the DIP joint that results from extensor tendon damage or avulsion. The injury results from forced flexion of the end of an extended finger. These injuries are classified as being of either tendinous or bony origin, since the type of injury influences treatment (Fig. 2–21). The mallet finger of *tendon origin* may result from stretching of the extensor tendon fibers over the DIP joint, complete rupture of the extensor tendon, or avulsion of a small fragment of the distal phalanx by the extensor tendon. Such a small avulsion fracture

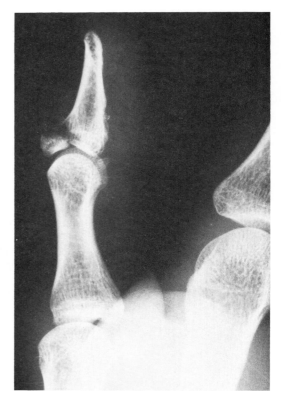

Figure 2–22. Mallet Finger. An avulsion fracture of the base of the thumb distal phalanx involving more than one third of the articular surface. Surgical reduction was performed.

was noted in almost one quarter of cases reviewed by Stark and colleagues.[47] Treatment of the mallet deformity of tendinous origin usually involves hyperextending the distal joint and flexing the proximal joint to allow apposition of torn edges of the extensor tendon or shortening of an attenuated extensor tendon.[51] Mallet finger of *bony origin* results from fractures involving one third or more of the dorsal articular surface of the distal phalanx (Figs. 2–22 and 2–23). These injuries are differentiated from those grouped as tendon injuries because the bony lesion may require open reduction and internal fixation, particularly when there is subluxation of the DIP joint.

Radiographic Findings. Lesions limited to the extensor tendon will show flexion deformity at the DIP joint without visible fracture. Small avulsion fractures of the dorsal margin of the distal phalanx should be looked for carefully, although these fractures are treated in the same way as tendon injuries.[51] Secondary hyperextension of the PIP joint may occur because of imbalance of the extensor mechanism.

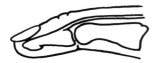

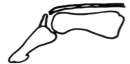

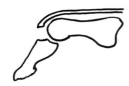

Tendon origin

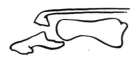

Bone origin

Figure 2–21. Classification of Mallet Finger.

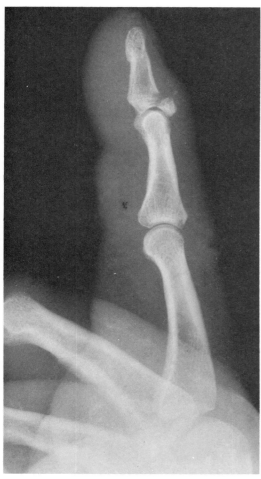

Figure 2–23. Mallet Finger. An avulsion fracture of the dorsal aspect of the base of the distal phalanx. More than one third of the articular surface is involved. Such lesions may require open reduction and internal fixation, particularly if there is subluxation of the DIP joint.

Mallet finger of bony origin is identified radiographically by the presence of a distal phalangeal fracture that involves one third or more of the dorsal articular surface (Figs. 2–22 and 2–23). The proximal fragment is often tilted or rotated and the remainder of the phalanx subluxed volarly. With treatment radiographic evidence of bony union can be seen at 8 to 10 weeks.[51]

Other Soft Tissue Injuries

Proximal Interphalangeal Joints. Proximal interphalangeal joint injuries include damage to the collateral ligaments from excessive abduction or adduction stress. Complete ligamentous rupture is identified by noting a displaced avulsion fracture or abnormal widening of the joint on abduction or adduction stress films.[51]

Volar plate injuries result from forced hyperextension of the PIP joint. Usually, the volar plate is pulled from its firm distal attachment to the base of the middle phalanx rather than from its weaker proximal attachments. Bony avulsion fracture may be noted on radiographic examination, particularly on lateral or oblique views (Fig. 2–24).[43] Hyperextension deformity of the proximal interphalangeal joint may be present and is sometimes associated with compensatory flexion of the distal interphalangeal joint.[51] Surgical treatment is suggested for fractures that involve more than 30 percent of the articular surface.[43]

Metacarpophalangeal Joints. Metacarpophalangeal joint dislocations are evident clinically. Radiographic examination allows identification of irreducible lesions if the joint space is wide or if a sesamoid is noted within the joint space, documenting the fact that the volar plate has been torn and its free end displaced into the joint.

Fractures

Phalangeal Fractures[49, 51, 53, 56]

Distal Phalanx. Distal phalangeal fractures account for more than half of all hand fractures. Fractures that do not involve the proximal articular surface have been divided into three types: longitudinal fractures, transverse fractures, and crushed-eggshell comminuted fractures of the distal tuft (Fig. 2–25). Crush injuries resulting in comminuted fractures are the most common, but, in general, significant displacement does not occur because of the presence of fibrous tissue septa that radiate from the bone into the soft tissues (Fig. 2–26). Displaced and angulated fractures of the distal phalanx are considered unstable and may require internal fixation.[49]

Distal phalangeal fractures may heal by fibrous rather than bony union, and complete bony union may not be demonstrable on radiographs for many months. Protective splinting is usually discontinued, however, after 3 to 4 weeks. Smith and Rider note that absence of bony union cannot be assumed until 1 year has elapsed.[56]

Proximal and Middle Phalangeal Fractures. Fractures of the shafts of the phalanges may be classified as stable, unstable, or intraarticular. Stable fractures are nondisplaced or impacted, and there is neither angular deformity in any plane nor any rotational deformity. Rotational

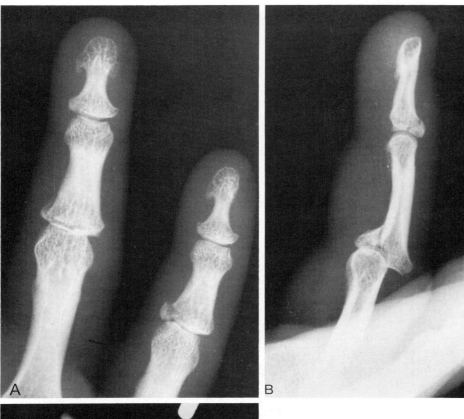

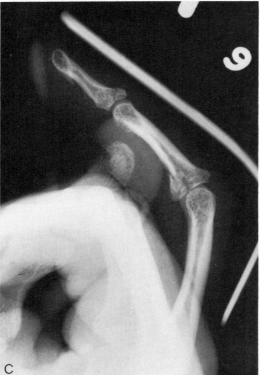

Figure 2–24. PIP Fracture Dislocation.
A, PA view immediately after injury shows swelling around the ring and fifth finger PIP joints. Avulsion fractures of the radial corners of the middle phalanges (at the sites of collateral ligament insertion) are shown. The overlap of the phalanges at the ring finger PIP joint (in the absence of PIP flexion) suggests dislocation. *B,* Coned lateral view of the ring finger confirms dislocation at the PIP joint. There is also a fracture of the base of the distal phalanx at the site of attachment of the terminal extensor tendon. *C,* Repeat lateral examination after attempted reduction of the PIP joint shows that reduction is inadequate; the articular surfaces are not parallel, and a gap remains at the fracture site. Open reduction and internal fixation were done. The distal reduction was adequate.

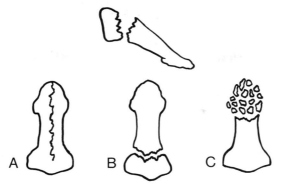

Figure 2–25. Distal Phalangeal Fractures. Longitudinal *(A)*, transverse *(B)*, and crush *(C)* fractures are shown.

deformity is better evaluated on clinical than on radiological examination, however. Green and Rowland suggest that stable fractures be treated by taping the injured finger to the adjacent finger.[51] Range-of-motion exercises are encouraged to prevent joint stiffness. Follow-up radiographs are obtained to detect any displacement or angular deformity that may develop.

Unstable fractures usually show displacement on initial examination (Figs. 2–27 to 29). They are reduced by closed manipulation and immobilized with external devices to prevent displacement. Fractures that are unstable after closed reduction, particularly long oblique fractures of the proximal phalanx, require internal fixation.

Fractures involving the articular surface may require open reduction and internal fixation to restore anatomical alignment to the joint surface (Fig. 2–30). Intraarticular fractures are grouped by type and location:

1. Fractures of the base of the proximal phalanx are usually avulsion fractures at the distal insertion of the collateral ligament (Fig. 2–31). Open reduction and internal fixation are required if the fragment is large.
2. Fractures of the base of the middle phalanx.
   A. Avulsion of bone from the dorsal aspect by the central tendon of the extensor apparatus produces a boutonnière deformity.
   B. Volar chip fractures are usually accompanied by dorsal subluxation or dislocation of the middle phalanx (Fig. 2–32). (See volar plate injuries.)
   C. Lateral fractures result from avulsion of

Text continued on page 94

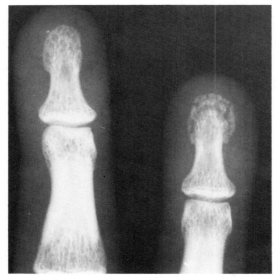

Figure 2–26. Tuft Fracture. A comminuted fracture of the ring finger distal tuft; minimal displacement of fracture fragments is characteristic.

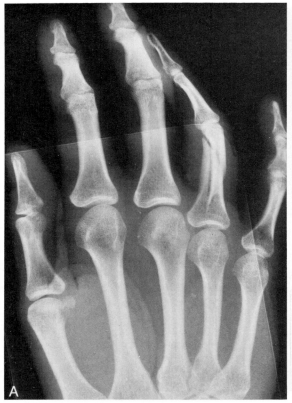

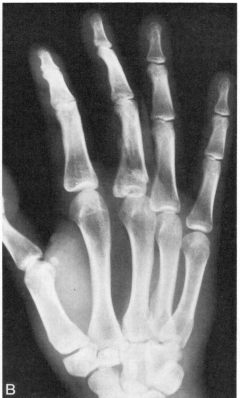

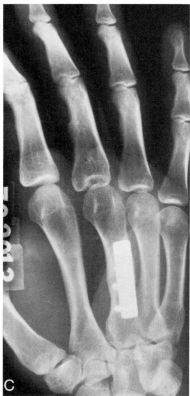

Figure 2–27. Proximal Phalangeal Fractures with Rotational Deformity. *A,* PA view through aluminum splint of an oblique fracture through the fourth proximal phalangeal shaft of the ring finger. Although rotational deformity is usually best identified clinically, it is confirmed in this case by noting the lateral projection of the ring finger in comparison with the oblique view of the other fingers. *B,* Another patient with a healed third proximal phalangeal fracture had residual rotational malalignment that was more obvious clinically than radiologically. *C,* A derotational metacarpal osteotomy was required.

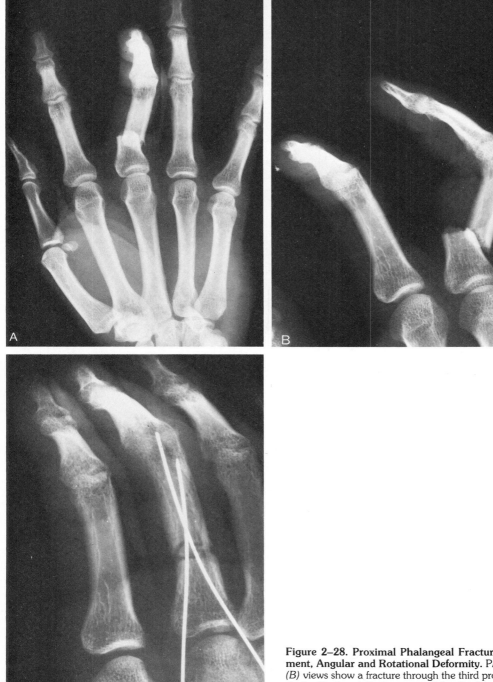

Figure 2–28. Proximal Phalangeal Fracture with Displacement, Angular and Rotational Deformity. PA *(A)* and oblique *(B)* views show a fracture through the third proximal phalangeal shaft with dorsal displacement of the distal fragment. The distal fragment is seen in an almost lateral projection in comparison with the oblique view of the proximal fragment and the other fingers. *C,* Reduction and fixation with two pins sufficed to restore alignment and allow healing to occur.

91

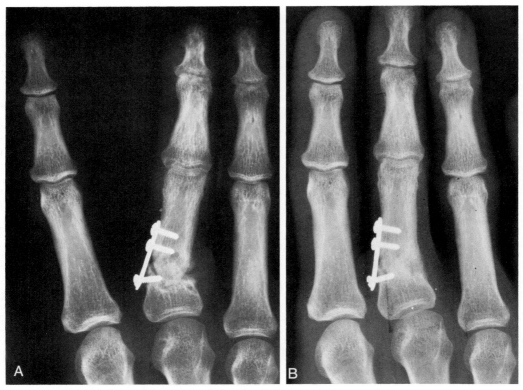

Figure 2–29. Proximal Phalangeal Fracture with Angular Deformity. *A,* PA view 4 months after internal fixation of an angulated proximal phalangeal fracture shows incomplete healing with residual angular deformity and displacement of the proximal portion of the screw and plate. *B,* Healing occurred with less deformity after K wires were inserted.

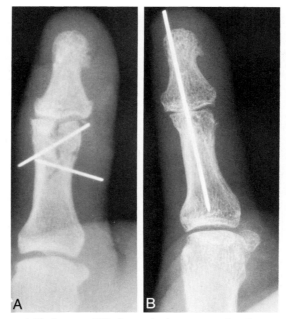

Figure 2–30. Fracture of Proximal Phalanx at PIP Joint. *A,* An attempted reduction of this comminuted proximal phalangeal fracture was unsuccessful in reestablishing a smooth articular surface. *B,* IP fusion was eventually necessary to relieve pain.

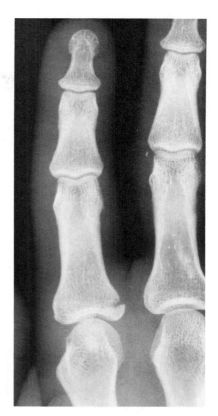

Figure 2–31. Intraarticular (MCP) Fracture. An avulsion fracture at the site of insertion of the ulnar collateral ligaments. Internal fixation was necessary to ensure healing without deformity of the articular surface.

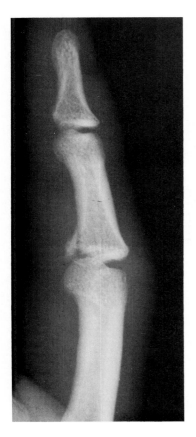

Figure 2–32. Avulsion Fracture. There is a fracture of the anterior aspect of the base of the middle phalanx caused by avulsion by the volar plate.

bone by a collateral ligament. Treatment depends on the size of the fracture fragment, with internal fixation used for large fracture fragments.

3. Condylar fractures may involve one or both condyles. Open reduction and internal fixation are often required to achieve and maintain anatomical reduction.

4. Comminuted intraarticular fractures. Anatomical restoration is usually not possible in these cases, and they therefore are treated by traction rather than by internal fixation.

Metacarpal Fractures[49, 51]

The Thumb. Fractures of the thumb metacarpal are divided into intraarticular and extraarticular types. *Bennett's fracture* is an intraarticular fracture dislocation that occurs following an axial blow to the partially flexed metacarpal. The metacarpal base dislocates, but strong ligamentous connections (the deep ulnar ligament) between the anterior portion of the metacarpal base (the volar lip) and the trapezium restrain this portion of the metacarpal, producing an avulsion fracture (Fig. 2–33). *Rolando's fracture*

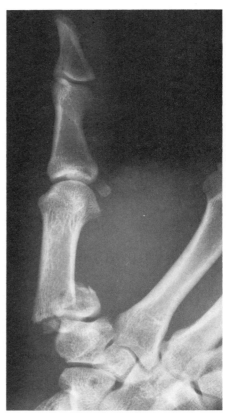

Figure 2–34. Rolando's Fracture. This is a comminuted fracture of the thumb metacarpal with dislocation of the carpometatacarpal joint. The comminution makes this a Rolando's rather than a Bennett's fracture.

is also an intraarticular fracture, but, in addition to the anterior fragment seen in Bennett's fracture, a dorsal fragment is present (Figs. 2–34 and 2–35). Bennett's fracture should be anatomically reduced, but because of the comminution present in Rolando's fracture, anatomical reduction may be impossible.

Extraarticular fractures may be transverse or oblique in orientation. Residual angular deformity of up to 30 degrees may be present with no detectable limitation of motion.[51]

Other Metacarpal Fractures.[49, 51] These fractures have been classified according to location into ones involving the metacarpal head (distal to the insertion of the collateral ligaments), neck, shaft, and base. Fractures of the metacarpal neck, including the "boxer's" fracture of the fifth metacarpal, are quite common. Angular deformity with the apex of the angle directed dorsally and comminution of the anterior cortex is frequent (Fig. 2–36). This comminution predisposes to recurrent deformity after the angulation has been reduced. Angular deformity is of less

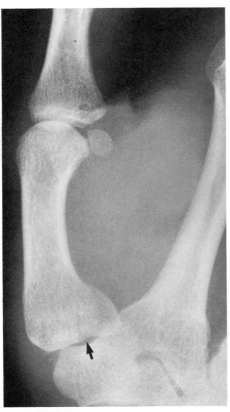

Figure 2–33. Bennett's Fracture. There is a fracture of the anterior lip of the base of the thumb metacarpal (arrow).

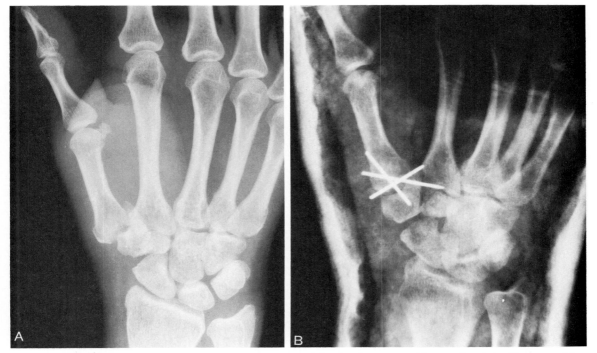

Figure 2–35. Rolando's Fracture. *A,* A comminuted fracture of the thumb metacarpal base with radial subluxation of the metacarpal. *B,* Open reduction and pinning resulted in improved positions of the fracture fragments and reduction of the subluxation.

serious consequence in the ring and fifth fingers, in which there is some mobility at the carpo-metacarpal joints, than in the index and middle fingers, where there is no mobility of these joints and where residual angular deformity results in protrusion of the metacarpal head into the palm and a painful grip. For these reasons no residual angular deformity is acceptable in the index and middle finger metacarpals (Fig. 2–37). The degree of angular deformity acceptable in the fourth and fifth metacarpals has been debated. Green and Rowland suggest reduction of acute fourth and fifth metacarpal neck fractures if more than 10 degrees of angular deformity is present,[51] but other authors accept considerably more deformity (Fig. 2–38).[57] Significant rotatory abnormalities should be corrected.

Metacarpal shaft fractures may be subdivided according to the type of fracture into transverse, oblique, and comminuted types. Transverse fractures are usually angulated dorsally owing to the distal pull of the interosseous muscles. As with angular deformity of metacarpal neck fractures, some degree of angulation may be acceptable in the fourth and fifth metacarpals, but any degree of angular deformity in the second or third metacarpal is unacceptable. The more proximal the fracture site in the metacarpal, the

more apparent will be the angular deformity; therefore, less angulation can be accepted in proximal fractures than in more distal ones.

Oblique fractures of the metacarpals tend to result in shortening and rotation rather than in angular deformity (Fig. 2–39). This is especially true in the second and fifth metacarpals, in which the deep transverse metacarpal ligament attaches to only one side of the volar plate. According to Green and Rowland, 2 or 3 mm of shortening is unassociated with functional loss so long as no angular deformity is present.[51]

Fractures of the bases of the index, middle, and ring metacarpals usually result from crush injuries. Severely angulated metacarpal fractures, fractures of the metacarpal bases, and distal carpal fractures suggest the possibility of accompanying carpometacarpal dislocation.

Fischer notes that the PA view is especially valuable in establishing a diagnosis of carpometacarpal dislocation (Fig. 2–40).[16] The carpal and metacarpal articular cortices are normally parallel with a 1 to 2 mm cartilage space between them. The ulnar margins of the hamate and fifth metacarpal base should be aligned when films are properly taken with the forearm flat on the table. Alterations in these findings suggest dislocation, which may then be con-
Text continued on page 100

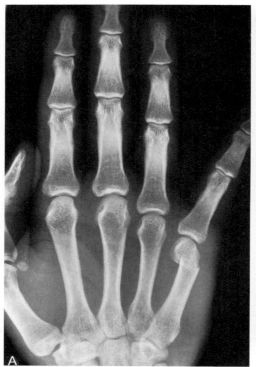

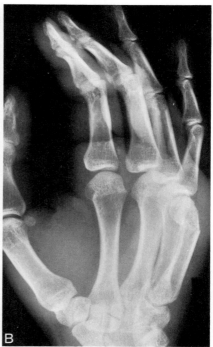

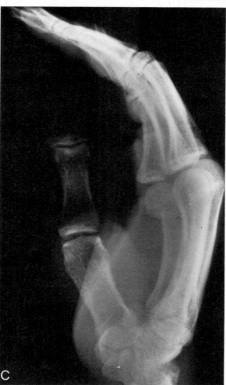

Figure 2–36. Boxer's Fracture. The fracture of the fifth metacarpal neck with angular deformity, apex dorsal, is characteristic. The metacarpal head is rotated radially. PA *(A)*, oblique *(B)*, lateral *(C)*.

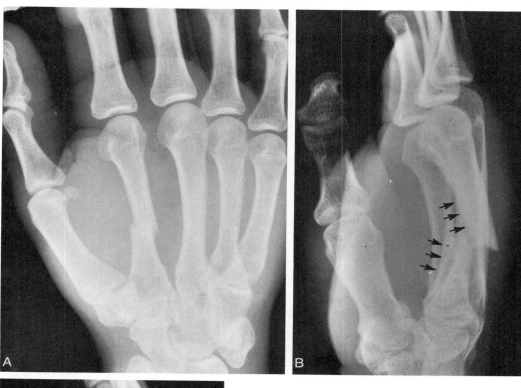

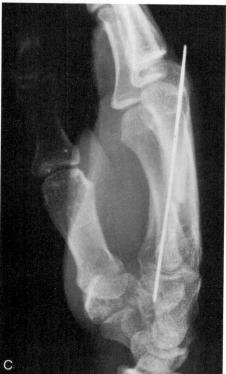

Figure 2–37. Second Metacarpal Fracture. A, PA view of a mildly displaced transverse fracture of the second metacarpal. B, The lateral view shows angular deformity (arrows on anterior cortex of second metacarpal). Because of the limited mobility of the index and middle carpometacarpal joints, residual angular deformity may result in protrusion of the metacarpal head into the palm and a painful grip. C, Internal fixation was done to correct the angular deformity.

THE HAND

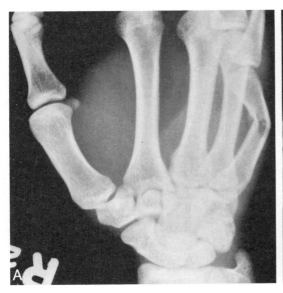

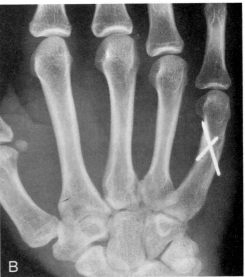

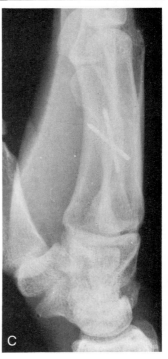

Figure 2–38. Fifth Metacarpal Fracture. *A*, Oblique view shows a fracture of the fifth metacarpal shaft with moderate angular deformity. Healing occurred with the fracture in this position. *B* and *C*, Osteotomy was required to correct the deformity.

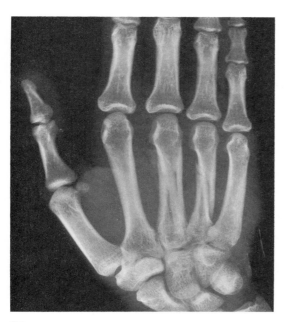

Figure 2–39. Oblique Metacarpal Fractures. Oblique fractures of the third and fourth metacarpal shafts have resulted in some shortening but no rotational deformity.

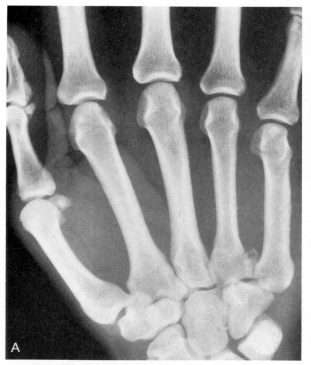

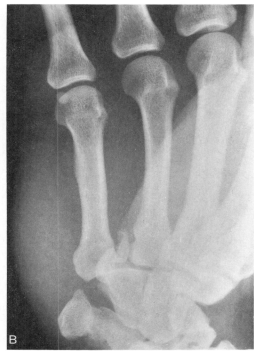

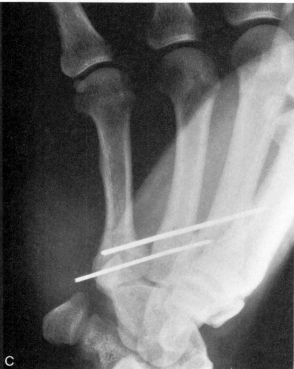

Figure 2–40. Fracture-Dislocation, Fifth Carpo-metacarpal Joint. *A*, The PA view shows ulnar deviation of the base of the fifth metacarpal and a bony fragment between the fourth and fifth metacarpals. *B*, The ball-catcher's view better demonstrates the ulnar subluxation of the metacarpal and the origin of the fracture fragment. *C*, Internal fixation and pinning were required to reduce and maintain this fracture-dislocation.

firmed on other views. Carpometacarpal fracture dislocations usually require open reduction and internal fixation.

Basal Joint Arthritis of the Thumb[58–61]

The large amount of motion possible at the thumb carpometacarpal joint is the result of motion at the trapezium–first metacarpal, trapezium–second metacarpal, trapezium–trapezoid, and trapezium–scaphoid joints. These basal joints are critical to hand function because they allow the thumb to be positioned appropriately.

Burton classified arthritic involvement of the thumb base into three clinical groups:

Group 1 is the most common group and includes middle-aged patients with no history of major trauma.

Group 2 consists of younger patients with underlying injuries such as Bennett's fracture, with secondary instability or osteoarthritis.

Group 3 patients have underlying rheumatoid arthritis. (About 35 percent of patients with rheumatoid arthritis will develop basal joint involvement.)[58]

Symptoms and signs related to arthritic involvement of the thumb base include pain and

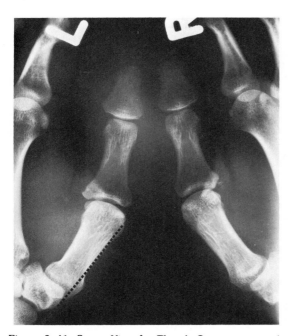

Figure 2–41. Stress View for Thumb Carpometacarpal Joint. The tips of the thumbs are pressed together. No subluxation of the trapezium–first metacarpal joints is present. A line drawn along the radial aspect of the thumb metacarpal falls near (not lateral to) the trapezium.

swelling, instability, crepitation, deformity, loss of motion, and decreased strength.

Radiographic Findings

Radiographic features depend on the demonstration of instability at the thumb base, the presence of osteoarthritis at the thumb carpometacarpal joint or at adjacent joints, and the documentation of secondary deformities of the thumb MCP and interphalangeal (IP) joints.

Normally, the radial cortex of the thumb metacarpal is nearly in line with the lateral side of the trapezium (Fig. 2–41). Subluxation of the thumb metacarpal is documented by displacement of this line lateral to the trapezium. This is brought out on stress views obtained by pressing the tips of the thumbs together or pinching the index finger and thumb together. The film is centered over the carpometacarpal joint. Osteoarthritis is demonstrable, as in other joints, by the presence of osteophytes, cartilage space narrowing, subchondral sclerosis, and cysts (Figs. 2–42 and 2–43). Abnormalities at the thumb carpometacarpal joint may result in secondary distal joint imbalance. The distal portion of the thumb metacarpal shaft becomes adducted, and eventual hyperextension deformity occurs at either the metacarpophalangeal or the interphalangeal joint (Fig. 2–44).

The severity of basal joint damage may be graded according to radiographic and clinical features as:

Stage 1–ligamentous laxity. The hypermobility of the thumb carpometacarpal, with the metacarpal base subluxing dorsally and laterally, may be demonstrated on stress views. Routine radiographs may be normal or may show mild hypertrophic lipping.

Stage 2–definite osteoarthritis. Chronic subluxation and osteoarthritis are present, with cartilage space narrowing, subchondral sclerosis, and osteophyte formation.

Stage 3–pantrapezial osteoarthritis. In these cases, osteoarthritis involves not only the trapezium–first metacarpal joint but also the adjacent joints, including the trapezium–second metacarpal (86.2 percent), the trapezioscaphoid joint (48.3 percent), and the trapezium–trapezoid joint (34.6 percent).

Stage 4–involvement of the thumb metacarpophalangeal joint is present.

Treatment

Several methods of treatment are proposed and depend largely on the degree of involvement. In localized disease (stage 2), treatment has been by fusion of the carpometacarpal joint or by joint replacement. In pantrapezial disease (stage

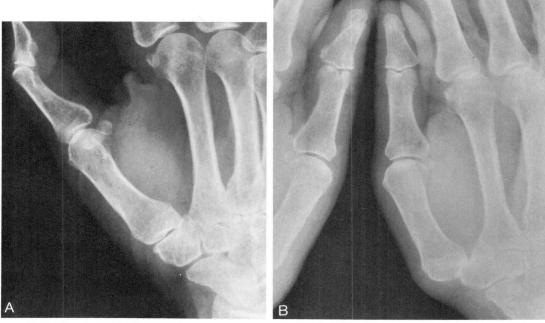

Figure 2–42. Osteoarthritis Thumb Carpometacarpal. *A,* Moderate cartilage loss at the metacarpal-trapezial joint with mild hypertrophic lipping. No subluxation is seen. *B,* The stress view shows marked radial displacement of the thumb metacarpal with the lateral cortex of the metacarpal laterally displaced in comparison with the trapezium.

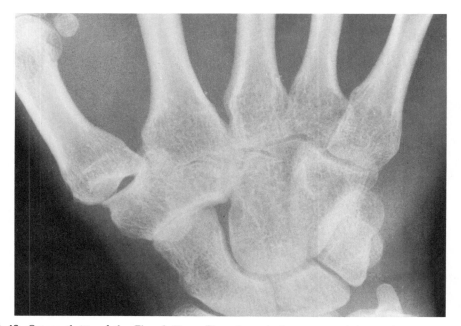

Figure 2–43. Osteoarthritis of the Thumb Base. There is marked narrowing of the scaphoid-trapezial and scaphoid-trapezoid articulations. Mild osteoarthritis in the thumb carpometacarpal joint is documented by the presence of osteophytes but little cartilage narrowing.

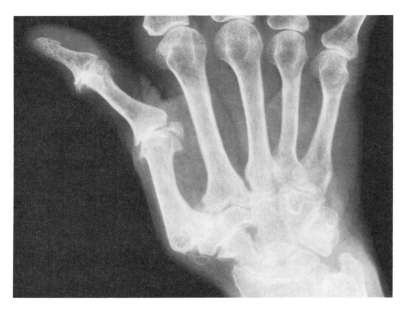

Figure 2–44. Osteoarthritis of the Thumb Base, Severe. There is severe osteoarthritis at the thumb metacarpal-trapezial joint with complete cartilage loss, sclerosis, osteophytic lipping, radial subluxation of the metacarpal, and several separate ossicles suggesting loose bodies. There is also severe involvement of the scaphoid-trapezial and scaphoid-trapezoid joints. The adduction of the thumb metacarpal has resulted in secondary MCP hyperextension. Osteoarthritic changes are noted at the thumb MCP and IP.

3), it is postulated that carpometacarpal fusion will produce increased stress on the other involved articulations, and therefore arthroplasty rather than carpometacarpal fusion is suggested.

Finger Deformities

Finger deformities are caused by arthritic and traumatic damage that upset the normal balance of forces in the hand. These deformities are complex. Brief explanations are provided here; the interested reader is referred to published reports for further details.[62, 67]

Boutonnière Deformity

This deformity is characterized by flexion at the proximal interphalangeal (PIP) joint and hyper-

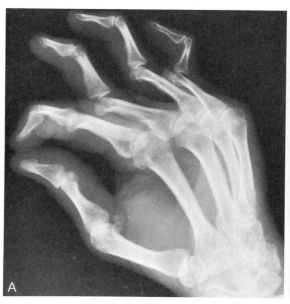
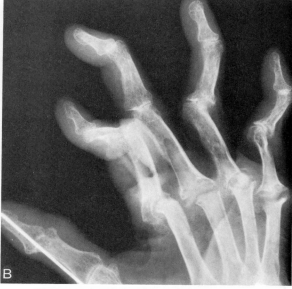

Figure 2–45. Finger Deformities. *A,* Swan neck deformity. There is hyperextension at the PIP joints and flexion at the DIP joints of most of the fingers. Despite these striking deformities and the dislocation at the thumb carpometacarpal joint, there is no erosion. This combination of deformity without erosion or cartilage space narrowing is characteristic of systemic lupus erythematosus. *B,* Boutonnière deformity. The flexion of the PIP and hyperextension of the DIP of the index finger are characteristic of a boutonnière deformity. There are swan neck deformities of the other fingers. Also noted is disruption of the index and middle finger Silastic MCP prostheses.

extension at the distal interphalangeal (DIP) joint (Fig. 2–45). It is most often a consequence of rheumatoid arthritis, in which capsular distension at the PIP joint produces weakening and relative lengthening of the central tendon, resulting in ineffective PIP extension. The lateral bands are displaced toward the palm, anterior to the axis of joint motion, so that they act as flexors rather than extensors of this joint. The pull of these lateral bands at their insertions on the distal phalanx also produces hyperextension of the DIP joint.[67]

Boutonnière deformities may also result from traumatic avulsion of the insertion of the central extensor tendon from the dorsal aspect of the base of the middle phalanx. This produces flexion deformity of the PIP joint. Tearing of soft tissue connections to the lateral bands of extensor tendons allows these tendons to slip below the axis of motion of the PIP joint, further increasing flexion. The displaced lateral bands limit flexion of the DIP joint and eventually produce hyperextension of this joint.[51]

Swan Neck Deformity

Swan neck deformity consists of hyperextension at the PIP joint and flexion at the DIP joint (Fig. 2–45). In patients with rheumatoid arthritis, the deformity results from limited PIP flexion caused by synovitis of the flexor tendon sheath.[67] Hyperextension occurs because of the relative increase in intrinsic muscle pull on the central tendon and inflammatory changes producing laxity of the anterior joint capsule. Eventually, the lateral bands become displaced dorsally, further increasing PIP extension. The flexor digitorum profundus tendon flexes the DIP joint.

Thumb Deformities[64, 67]

Thumb deformities occur in both rheumatoid arthritis and osteoarthritis. Nalebuff described three types of deformity in patients with rheumatoid arthritis (Fig. 2–46). The Nalebuff type I deformity consists of flexion at the MCP joint and hyperextension at the IP joint and is the most common thumb deformity in rheumatoid arthritis. Deformity results from synovitis at the MCP joint with stretching of the capsule and extensor apparatus and ulnar displacement of the extensor pollicis longus. Extension of the MCP joint is therefore reduced, and flexion deformity results. Hyperextension of the IP joint occurs because of the pull of the extensor pollicis longus and extensor insertions of the intrinsic muscles.

Nalebuff types II and III deformities result from damage at the thumb carpometacarpal joint. In type II deformity there is carpometacarpal dislocation, adduction of the thumb metacarpal, and secondary hyperextension of the thumb IP. Flexion deformity of the MCP may follow. In type III deformity hyperextension at the thumb MCP follows the adduction contracture at the carpometacarpal joint. Flexion at the IP joint follows, producing a swan neck deformity. Treatment depends on the severity and location of the abnormality and includes joint fusion and tendon transfer surgery.

Metacarpophalangeal Subluxation

In rheumatoid arthritis ulnar deviation of the fingers at the MCP joints, extensor tendon subluxation, and palmar subluxation of the proximal phalanges may occur (Fig. 2–47). Rheumatoid involvement of the MCP joints allows the occur-

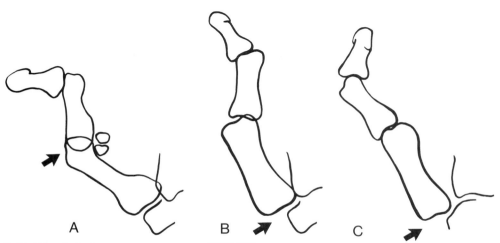

Figure 2–46. Thumb Deformities. A, Diagram of Nalebuff type I deformity. The arrow indicates the site of primary involvement. B, Nalebuff type II deformity. C, Nalebuff type III deformity.

Illustration continued on following page

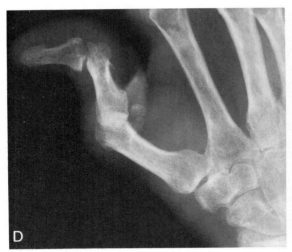
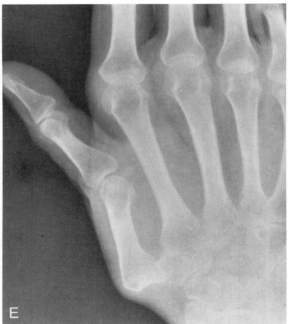

Figure 2–46. Thumb Deformities *Continued. D,* Nalebuff type I deformity: Rheumatoid arthritis has resulted in damage to the thumb MCP with flexion deformity. There is secondary hyperextension of the IP joint. *E,* Nalebuff type III deformity: Damage of the thumb carpometacarpal has resulted in lateral dislocation of the proximal thumb metacarpal. Hyperextension at the thumb MCP and flexion at the IP are secondary findings. (Same patient as in Figure 2–45A.)

rence of the normally resisted tendency toward ulnar deviation and palmar subluxation that the common flexor tendons produce.[66, 67]

Metacarpophalangeal (MCP) Prostheses

Although metal to plastic prostheses are available, the most frequently used prostheses for the MCP joints are the silicone rubber prostheses of the Swanson and Niebauer types.[69–71, 80–82] The Swanson prosthesis consists of a single silicone rubber (Silastic) piece with a central curved section and a stem on each end (Fig. 2–48). Motion results both from the hinge action of the central portion of the prosthesis and from pistoning of the stem within the bone.[71, 76, 81] In contrast, the stems of the Niebauer prosthesis are coated with Dacron mesh to allow bony ingrowth.[80] Since these stems then become fixed within the medullary canal, finger motion will result only from the hinge action of the midportion of the prosthesis. In general, relief of pain originating at the MCPs, correction of deformity, and between 30 and 75 degrees of motion can be obtained postoperatively.[79]

Postoperative radiographs allow demonstration of the degree of correction of deformity, the positions of the components, and the detection of most complications. On the posteroanterior view, the hinge portion of the prosthesis is seen as a rectangular area of slight increased density with the long axis of the rectangle parallel to the resection margin of the metacarpal (Fig. 2–49). The dense band is located proximally. The lateral view shows the concavity of the hinge to be directed anteriorly. The proximal portions of the stem may protrude 1 to 2 mm from the cut surface of the bone. A thin layer of periosteal new bone may develop along the adjacent shafts close to the resection margin without any other evidence to suggest infection.

Radiographically identifiable complications include recurrence of deformity, development of rotational deformity, fracture of the prosthesis, dislocation of the stems of the prosthesis, and infection.[69-71, 79] Prosthetic fracture is not uncommon, occurring in 26.6 percent of early types of Swanson and 38.2 percent of Niebauer prostheses in one series (Fig. 2–50).[69] Fracture usually involves the base of the distal stem and may be associated with instability and subluxation or dislocation of the joint. Fracture of a Swanson prosthesis may not correlate with clinical deterioration and may be noted incidentally on follow-up radiographs. In the series of Beckenbaugh and associates satisfactory function was

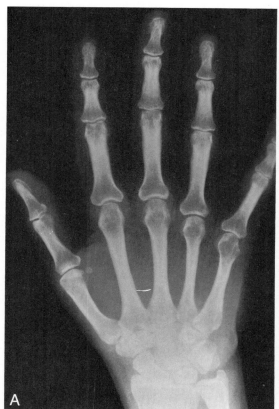

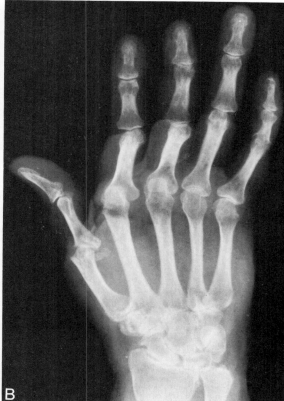

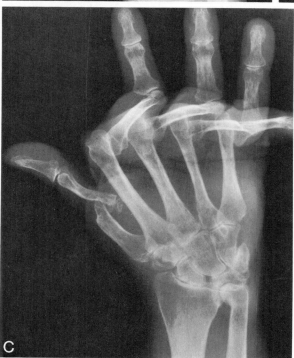

Figure 2–47. Rheumatoid Arthritis with Progressive Deformity. *A,* 1962. Normal examination. *B,* 1970. There is now severe deformity of the thumb, index, and middle fingers. Hyperextension of the index, middle, and ring finger PIPs is present but is better demonstrated on oblique views. There is erosion of the fifth PIP and DIP, the thumb, index, and fifth MCPs, and ulnar styloid and cartilage narrowing of several PIPs, MCPs, and the intercarpal and radiocarpal joints. *C,* 1977. The ulnar deviation and MCP subluxation are now severe, and there is striking PIP hyperextension at the index, middle, and ring fingers and at the thumb MCP. Ulnar carpal subluxation and mild widening of the scapholunate distance are also present.

105

THE HAND

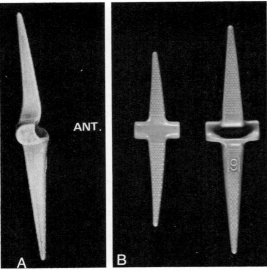

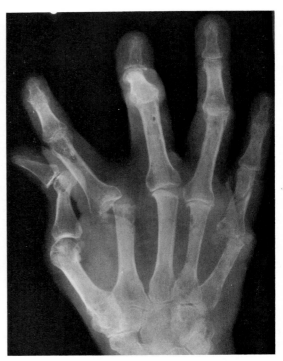

Figure 2–48. Silastic (Swanson) MCP Prosthesis. *A,* Lateral view. *B,* The dorsal and volar aspects are shown. Flexion-extension motion is a combination of bending of the midportion and pistoning of the stems of the prosthesis within the bone.

Figure 2–50. Fractured MCP Prostheses. This patient with systemic lupus erythematosus and severe hand deformity underwent multiple surgical procedures and insertion of Swanson MCP prostheses at the index through fifth fingers 12 years previously. There has been fracture of the index and fifth finger prostheses with fragmentation of the prostheses and displacement of the bone ends. The bony apposition at the third and fourth MCPs raises the possibility of prosthetic fracture here as well. An oblique fracture of the fifth finger proximal phalanx is noted.

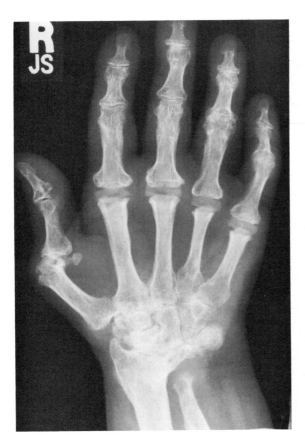

Figure 2–49. Silastic Prostheses. PA radiograph. The bases of the prostheses are parallel and flush with the resected ends of the metacarpals.

preserved in about 50 percent of joints with fractured Swanson prostheses. Mechanical failure is more likely to result from fracture of a Niebauer prosthesis, which functions as a fixed hinge rather than as a dynamic spacer. Synovitis or lymphadenopathy may follow prosthetic fracture and release of silicone particles (Fig. 2–51).[74]

Infection is uncommon, occurring in less than 1 percent of cases and usually remaining confined to one MCP.[69, 71, 77] Radiographic evidence of infection includes increasing soft tissue swelling, osteoporosis, bone destruction, and periosteal reaction (Fig. 2–52). Removal of the prosthesis and treatment with antibiotics is curative.

Interphalangeal Joint Fusion

Indications. Fusion of the small joints of the hand has been used to correct instability or deformity resulting from arthritis, injury, or paralysis and to alleviate pain resulting from these disorders when conservative therapy has failed.

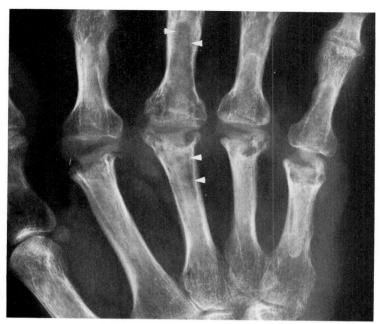

Figure 2–51. Foreign Body Reaction after Silicone Prosthesis. There is bone resorption (arrowheads) about the stems of the middle finger MCP prosthesis. At surgery a marked foreign body reaction to material consistent with Silastic was found. The radiographic appearance suggests infection, but this was never documented.

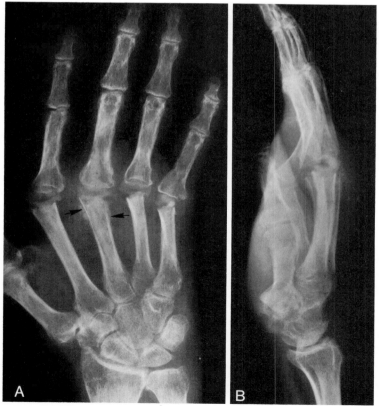

Figure 2–52. Infected MCP Prosthesis. *A* and *B,* This patient with severe rheumatoid arthritis and ulnar deviation underwent Swanson MCP arthroplasty at the index, middle, ring, and fifth fingers. Infection about the middle finger prosthesis is suggested by the marked soft tissue swelling and periosteal reaction (arrows) present. The prosthesis was removed.

Arthrodesis is also used in conjunction with certain tendon transfer operations. Generally, if two adjacent joints of a digit are involved, fusion of one will accelerate degenerative changes in the other so that if one of the involved joints is to be fused, the other should be replaced.

Position of Fusion. The position at which the joint is fused varies with the digit and the joint. Since the index finger is used mainly for pinch, some surgeons prefer fusion in an almost straight position, but because the ulnar digits are more involved with grasp, surgeons often fuse them in a somewhat flexed position. Kilgore and Graham recommend fusion in 10 to 25 degrees of flexion at the DIP, 25 to 45 degrees at the PIP, 25 to 45 degrees at the MCP, 10 degrees of flexion and 10 degrees of pronation at the thumb IP, and 10 to 15 degrees of flexion and 10 to 15 degrees of pronation at the thumb MCP.[5]

Although the details of the suggested operative procedures vary, in general bone is removed from the joint margins, and the resected bone ends are perfectly apposed. The position is maintained by Kirschner wires and external immobilization.

Healing and Complications. Healing is primarily judged radiologically by the appearance of trabecular continuity across the fusion site. This usually requires 7 to 10 weeks. Complications include nonunion (5 percent overall in one series),[83] which is especially frequent in patients with neurological disturbances. Malalignment of the digit may also occur.

References

Essential Anatomy

1. Eyler DL, Markee JE: The anatomy and function of the intrinsic musculature of the fingers. J Bone Joint Surg (Am) 36:1–9, 1954.
2. Flatt AF: Kinesiology of the hand. AAOS Instructional Course Lectures 18:266–281, 1961.
3. Harris C Jr, Rutledge GL: The functional anatomy of the extensor mechanism of the finger. J Bone Joint Surg (Am) 54:713–726, 1972.
4. Kaplan EB: Functional and Surgical Anatomy of the Hand. 2nd ed. Philadelphia, JB Lippincott, 1965.
5. Kilgore ES Jr, Graham WP III: The Hand. Surgical and Non-Surgical Management. Philadelphia, Lea & Febiger, 1977.
6. Kuczynski K: The proximal interphalangeal joint. J Bone Joint Surg (Br) 50:656–663, 1963.
7. Landsmeer JMF: Anatomical and functional investigations on the articulations of human fingers. Acta Anat (Suppl 24) 25:1–69, 1955.
8. Landsmeer JMF: Power grip and precision handling. Ann Rheum Dis 21:164–170, 1962.
9. Landsmeer JMF: Atlas of Anatomy of the Hand. Edinburgh, Churchill Livingstone, 1976.
10. Linscheid RL, Dobyns JH: Total joint arthroplasty, the hand. Mayo Clin Proc 54:516–526, 1979.
11. Resnick D, Niwayama C, Feingold ML: The sesamoid bones of the hands and feet. Radiology 123:57–62, 1977.
12. Tubiana R, Valentin P: Anatomy of the extensor apparatus. The physiology of finger extension. Surg Clin North Am 44:897–918, 1964.
13. Tubiana R: The Hand. vol. 1. Philadelphia, WB Saunders, 1981.
14. Wood-Jones F: The Principles of Anatomy as Seen in the Hand. 2nd ed. Baltimore, Williams & Wilkins, 1942.
15. Zancolli E: Structural and Dynamic Basis of Hand Surgery. 3rd ed. Philadelphia, JB Lippincott, 1979.

Normal Radiographic Anatomy

16. Fischer E: Low kilovolt radiography. In Resnick D, Niwayama G, eds. Diagnosis of Bone and Joint Disorders. Philadelphia, WB Saunders, 1981.
17. Lewis RW: The Joints of the Extremities. A Radiographic Study. Springfield, Ill., CC Thomas, 1955.
18. Linscheid RL: Arthrography of the metacarpophalangeal joint. Clin Orthop 103:91, 1974.
19. Rosenthal DI, Murray WT, Smith RJ: Finger arthrography. Radiology 137:647–651, 1980.
20. Weston WJ: The normal arthrogram of the metacarpophalangeal, metatarsophalangeal and interphalangeal joints. Australas Radiol 13:211–218, 1969.
21. Yeh H-C, Wolf BS: Radiographic anatomical landmarks of the metacarpo-phalangeal joints. Radiology 122:353–355, 1977.

Rheumatoid Arthritis, Psoriatic Arthritis, and Reiter's Syndrome

22. Avila R, Pugh DG, Slocumb CH, Winkelmann RK: Psoriatic arthritis: A roentgenologic study. Radiology 75:691–701, 1960.
23. Baker H, Golding DN, Thompson M: Psoriasis and arthritis. Ann Intern Med 58:909–925, 1963.
24. Berens DL, Lockie LM, Lin R, Norcross BM: Roentgen changes in early rheumatoid arthritis. Wrists—hands—feet. Radiology 82:645–654, 1964.
25. Martel W, Braunstein EM, Borlaza G, Good AE, Griffin PE Jr: Radiologic features of Reiter's disease. Radiology 132:1–10, 1979.
26. Mason RM, Murray RS, Oates JK, Young AC: A comparative radiological study of Reiter's disease. J Bone Joint Surg (Br) 41:137–148, 1959.
27. Peterson CC Jr, Silbiger ML: Reiter's syndrome and psoriatic arthritis. Their roentgen spectra and some interesting similarities. AJR 101:860–871, 1967.
28. Reiter H: Uber ein bisher unerkannte spirochaetinfektion (spirochaetosis arthritica). Dtsch Med Wochenschr 42:1535–1536, 1916.
29. Sholkoff SD, Glickman MG, Steinbach HL: Roentgenology of Reiter's syndrome. Radiology 97:497–503, 1970.
30. Weinberger HJ: Reiter's syndrome re-evaluated. Arthritis Rheum 5:202–210, 1962.
31. Weissman BNW, Sosman JL: The radiology of rheumatoid arthritis. Orthop Clin North Am 6:653–674, 1975.
32. Weldon WV, Scalettar R: Roentgen changes in Reiter's syndrome. AJR 86:344–350, 1961.

Pigmented Villonodular Synovitis

33. Breimer CW, Freiberger RH: Bone lesions associated with villonodular synovitis. AJR 79:618–629, 1958.
34. Docken WP: Pigmented villonodular synovitis: A review with illustrative case reports. Semin Arthritis Rheum 9:1–22, 1979.
35. Jaffe HL, Lichtenstein L, Sutro CJ: Pigmented villonodular synovitis, bursitis and tenosynovitis: A discus-

sion of the synovial and bursal equivalents of the tenosynovial lesion commonly denoted as xanthoma, xanthogranuloma, giant cell tumor or myeloplaxoma of the tendon sheath, with some consideration of this tendon sheath lesion itself. Arch Pathol 31:731–765, 1941.

36. Jones FE, Soule EH, Coventry MB: Fibrous xanthoma of synovium (giant-cell tumor of tendon sheath, pigmented nodular synovitis). J Bone Joint Surg (Am) 51:76–86, 1969.

37. Phalen GS, McCormack LJ, Gazale WJ: Giant-cell tumor of tendon sheath (benign synovioma) in the hand: Evaluation of 56 cases. Clin Orthop 15:140–151, 1959.

38. Wagner ML, Spjut HJ, Dutton RV, Glassman AL, Askew JB: Polyarticular pigmented villonodular synovitis. AJR 136:821–823, 1981.

Soft Tissue Injuries

39. Bowers WH, Hurst LC: Gamekeeper's thumb. J Bone Joint Surg (Am) 59:519–524, 1977.

40. Campbell CS: Gamekeeper's thumb. J Bone Joint Surg (Br) 37:148–149, 1955.

41. Frank WE, Dobyns J: Surgical pathology of collateral ligamentous injuries of the thumb. Clin Orthop 83:102–114, 1972.

42. Linscheid RL: Arthrography of the metacarpophalangeal joint. Clin Orthop 103:91, 1974.

43. Nance EP Jr, Kaye JJ, Milek MA: Volar plate fracture. Radiology 133:61–64, 1979.

44. Neviaser RJ, Wilson JN, Lievano A: Rupture of the ulnar collateral ligament of the thumb (gamekeeper's thumb). Correction by dynamic repair. J Bone Joint Surg (Am) 53:1357–1364, 1971.

45. Resnick D, Danzig LA: Arthrographic evaluation of injuries of the first metacarpophalangeal joint: Gamekeeper's thumb. AJR 126:1046–1052, 1976.

46. Smith RJ: Post-traumatic instability of the metacarpophalangeal joint of the thumb. J Bone Joint Surg (Am) 59:14–21, 1977.

47. Stark HH, Boyes JH, Wilson JN: Mallet finger. J Bone Joint Surg (Am) 44:1061–1068, 1962.

48. Stener B: Displacement of the ruptured ulnar collateral ligament of the metacarpo-phalangeal joint of the thumb. J Bone Joint Surg (Br) 44:869–879, 1962.

Fractures

49. Bora EW Jr, Osterman AL: Injuries of the hand. In Heppenstall RB, ed. Fracture Treatment and Healing. Philadelphia, WB Saunders, 1980.

50. Eaton RG: Joint Injuries of the Hand. CC Thomas, Springfield, Ill., 1971.

51. Green DP, Rowland SA: Fractures and dislocations in the hand. In Rockwood CA, Green DP, eds. Fractures. Philadelphia, JB Lippincott, 1975.

52. Hunter JM, Cowen NJ: Fifth metacarpal fractures in a compensation clinic population. A report on one hundred and thirty-three cases. J Bone Joint Surg (Am) 52:1159–1165, 1970.

53. Kaplan L: The treatment of fractures and dislocations of the hand and fingers. Surg Clin North Am 20:1695–1720, 1940.

54. Kaye JJ: Hand and wrist. In Felson B, ed. Roentgenology of Fractures and Dislocations. New York, Grune & Stratton, 1978.

55. Pritsch M, Engel J, Farin I: Manipulation and external fixation of metacarpal fractures. J Bone Joint Surg (Am) 63:1289–1291, 1981.

56. Smith FL, Rider DL: A study of the healing of one hundred consecutive phalangeal fractures. J Bone Joint Surg 17:91–109, 1935.

57. Stark HH: Troublesome fractures and dislocations of the hand. AAOS Instructional Course Lectures 19:130–149, 1970.

Basal Joint Arthritis of the Thumb

58. Burton RI: Basal joint arthrosis of the thumb. Orthop Clin North Am 4:331–348, 1973.

59. Dickson RA, Morrison JD: The pattern of joint involvement in hands with arthritis at the base of the thumb. Hand 2:249–255, 1979.

60. Swanson AB: Disabling arthritis at the base of the thumb: Treatment by resection of the trapezium and flexible (silicone) implant arthroplasty. J Bone Joint Surg (Am) 54:456–471, 1972.

61. Swanson AB, Swanson GG, Watermeier JJ: Trapezium implant arthroplasty: Long-term evaluation of 150 cases. J Hand Surg 6:125–141, 1981.

Finger Deformities

62. Heywood AWB: The pathogenesis of the rheumatoid swan neck deformity. Hand 2:176–183, 1979.

63. Kleinert HE, Frykman G: The wrist and thumb in rheumatoid arthritis. Orthop Clin North Am 4:1085–1096, 1973.

64. Nalebuff EA: Diagnosis, classification and management of rheumatoid thumb deformities. Bull Hosp J Dis Orthop Inst 29:119–137, 1968.

65. Shapiro JS: The etiology of ulnar drift: A new factor. J Bone Joint Surg (Am) 50:634, 1968.

66. Smith EM, Juvinall RC, Bender LF, Pearson JR: Role of the finger flexors in rheumatoid deformities of the metacarpophalangeal joints. Arthritis Rheum 7:467–480, 1964.

67. Swanson AB, Swanson GG: Pathogenesis and pathomechanics of rheumatoid deformities in the hand and wrist. Orthop Clin North Am 4:1039–1056, 1973.

MCP Prostheses

68. Aptekar RG, Davie JM, Cattell HS: Foreign body reaction to silicone rubber. Complication of a finger joint implant. Clin Orthop 98:231–232, 1974.

69. Beckenbaugh RD, Dobyns JH, Linscheid RL, Bryan RS: Review and analysis of silicone-rubber metacarpophalangeal implants. J Bone Joint Surg (Am) 58:483–487, 1976.

70. Beckenbaugh RD: New concepts in arthroplasty of the hand and wrist. Arch Surg 112:1094–1098, 1977.

71. Calenoff L, Stromberg WB: Silicone rubber arthroplasties of the hand. Radiology 107:29–34, 1973.

72. Christie AJ, Weinberger KA, Dietrich M: Silicone lymphadenopathy and synovitis. Complications of silicone elastomer finger joint prostheses. JAMA 237:1463–1464, 1977.

73. Gillespie TE, Flatt AE, Youm Y, Sprague BL: Biomechanical evaluation of metacarpophalangeal joint prosthesis designs. J Hand Surg 4:508–521, 1979.

74. Groff GD, Schned AR, Taylor TH: Silicone-induced adenopathy eight years after metacarpophalangeal arthroplasty. Arthritis Rheum 24:1578–1581, 1981.

75. Kircher T: Silicone lymphadenopathy. A complication of silicone elastomer finger joint prostheses. Hum Pathol 2:240–244, 1980.

76. Millender LH, Nalebuff EA: Metacarpophalangeal joint arthroplasty utilizing the silicone rubber prosthesis. Orthop Clin North Am 4:349–371, 1973.

77. Millender LH, Nalebuff EA, Hawkins RB, Ennis R: Infection after silicone prosthetic arthroplasty in the hand. J Bone Joint Surg (Am) 57:825–829, 1975.

78. Millender LH, Nalebuff EA: Reconstructive surgery in the rheumatoid hand. Orthop Clin North Am 6:709–732, 1975.

79. Nalebuff EA, Millender LH: Reconstructive surgery and rehabilitation of the hand. *In* Kelley WN, Harris ED Jr, Ruddy S, Sledge CB, eds Textbook of Rheumatology. Philadelphia, WB Saunders, 1981: pp 1900–1920.

80. Niebauer JJ, Shaw JL, Doren WW: Silcone-dacron hinge prosthesis design, evaluation, and application. Ann Rheum Dis 28 Suppl., 56–59, 1969.

81. Swanson AB: Flexible implant resection arthroplasty. Hand 4:119–134, 1972.

82. Swanson AB, Swanson GG: Flexible implant resection arthroplasty: A method for reconstruction of small joints in the extremities. AAOS Instructional Course Lectures 27:27–60, 1978.

IP Fusion

83. Carroll RE, Hill NA: Small joint arthrodesis in hand reconstruction. J Bone Joint Surg (Am) 51:1219–1221, 1969.

Chapter 3

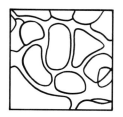

The
WRIST

NORMAL STRUCTURE AND FUNCTION

Essential Anatomy

Bony Anatomy

The carpal bones may be thought of as being divided into two rows: a proximal row consisting of the lunate and triquetrum and a distal row, including the trapezium, trapezoid, capitate, and hamate (Fig. 3–1).[44] The proximal carpal row is termed an *intercalated segment* because its position is determined by forces acting on its proximal and distal articulations.[18] When such a

system is compressed, a zigzag pattern of collapse, analogous to the positions of cars in a train if the first car stops short, occurs (Fig. 3–2). Collapse deformity is normally prevented by linkage of the proximal and the distal carpal rows by the scaphoid and its connecting ligaments.

Compartmental Anatomy

Anatomically, the wrist joint is separated into a number of compartments by the many ligaments that attach to the carpal bones. These compartments, shown in Figure 3–3, are of considerable significance for the interpretation of arthrograms and for identifying various patterns of arthritic involvement. The compartments are as follows:

1. Radiocarpal compartment
2. Midcarpal compartment
3. Pisiform–triquetral compartment
4. Carpometacarpal compartments (two)
5. Intermetacarpal compartments (three)
6. Inferior radioulnar compartment

The *radiocarpal* compartment lies between the proximal carpal row and the distal radius and triangular fibrocartilage complex. On its ulnar side two projections are noted from the joint space, a proximal prestyloid recess between the meniscus homologue and the triangular fibrocartilage and a distal recess that extends to the triquetrum. The prestyloid recess abuts on the ulnar styloid, a relationship important in the development of ulnar styloid erosion in rheumatoid arthritis. On its radial aspect the radiocarpal compartment contacts the "bare areas" (areas unprotected by articular cartilage) of the scaphoid and the radial styloid.[5]

The *midcarpal* compartment includes articulations between the proximal and the distal carpal rows. The *pisiform–triquetral* compart-

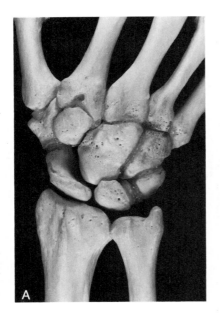

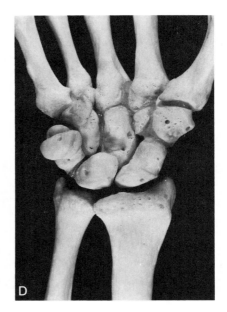

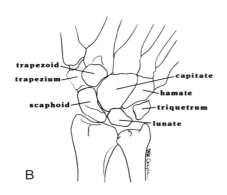

trapezoid

trapezium

scaphoid

capitate

hamate

triquetrum

lunate

B

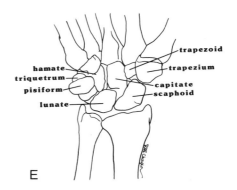

hamate

triquetrum

pisiform

lunate

trapezoid

trapezium

capitate

scaphoid

E

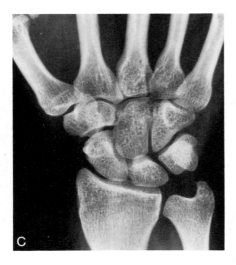

C

Figure 3–1. Photographic, Diagrammatic, and Radiographic Anatomy of the Wrist. *A, B, C,* Dorsal aspect; *D, E,* volar aspect.

Illustration continued on opposite page

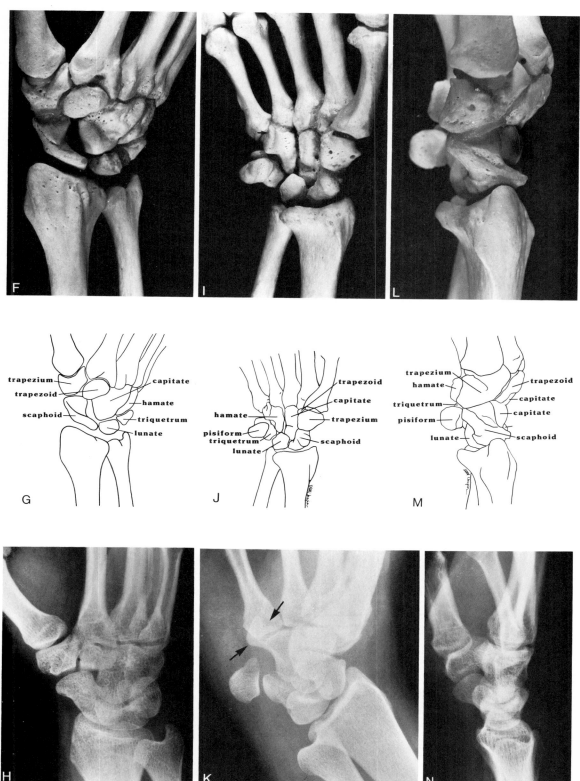

Figure 3–1. Photographic, Diagrammatic, and Radiographic Anatomy of the Wrist *Continued. F, G, H,* Oblique view (partial pronation); *I, J, K,* oblique ("ball-catcher's") view (partial supination); the hook of the hamate (arrows) is well seen; *L, M, N,* lateral view from the radial side.

113

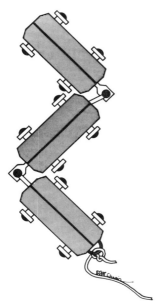

Figure 3–2. Zigzag Collapse. The proximal carpal row is an *intercalated segment* because its position is determined by forces acting on its proximal and distal articulations. Compression of such a system results in a zigzag pattern of collapse, analogous to the position of cars in a train when the first car stops short.

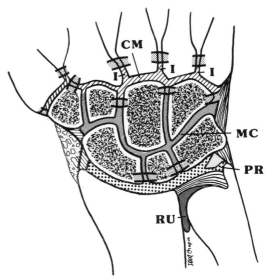

Figure 3–3. Carpal Compartments. The wrist joint is separated into various compartments by ligaments that attach to carpal bones. Radiocarpal (dotted), midcarpal (MC), carpometacarpal (CM), intermetacarpal (I), inferior radioulnar (RU) compartments, and prestyloid recess (PR) are shown. The anterior pisiform-triquetral compartment is not shown.

ment is a small synovial cavity between the volar aspect of the triquetrum and the dorsal aspect of the pisiform. This compartment is separated from the radiocarpal joint by the meniscus–homologue attachment to the triquetrum.

The two *carpometacarpal* compartments consist of a separate thumb compartment with its own joint capsule and a common compartment for the other metacarpals.[27]

The *inferior radioulnar* compartment lies between the cartilage-covered surfaces of the radius and the ulna and is separated from the radiocarpal joint by the triangular fibrocartilage complex (Fig. 3–4). The triangular fibrocartilage complex functions as a cushion that prevents articulation between the ulna and the carpus and is a major stabilizer of the distal radioulnar joint. When viewed end-on, the triangular configuration of the fibrocartilage, with its base attached to the radius and its apex inserted into the fossa at the base of the ulnar styloid and intertwined with the ulnar collateral ligament, is apparent. In 31 to 53 percent of anatomic specimens there are perforations in this structure that allow communication between compartments.[3, 7]

Ligamentous Anatomy (Fig. 3–5)

The ligaments of the wrist have been classified by Taleisnik into an *extrinsic* group that connects

the carpals to the radius or metacarpals and an *intrinsic* group that originates and inserts on the carpal bones.[8] Ligamentous support is considerably greater on the volar aspect of the wrist than on the dorsum. The volar radiocarpal ligaments (of the extrinsic group) are the most important and consist of radiolunate, radioscaphoid–capitate and radioscaphoid–lunate segments. The latter two ligaments attach the proximal pole of the scaphoid to the volar aspect of the radius and prevent rotatory subluxation of the scaphoid.[8] Among the intrinsic group of ligaments are those that loosely connect the scaphoid to the trapezium (distally) and to the lunate (proximally) and allow the scaphoid to rotate as the wrist is flexed or extended. An area on the volar aspect of the wrist, adjacent to the lunate and capitate (the "space of Poirier"), is devoid of ligaments and thus is a site of potential weakness.[6]

Function

Functionally, the wrist articulations consist of a radiocarpal joint with radioscaphoid and radiolunate components and a midcarpal joint between the proximal and distal carpal rows. Wrist motion is complex, with an average of 70 degrees of dorsiflexion (extension), 75 degrees of volar flexion, 15 to 25 degrees of radial abduction (deviation), and 30 to 60 degrees of ulnar

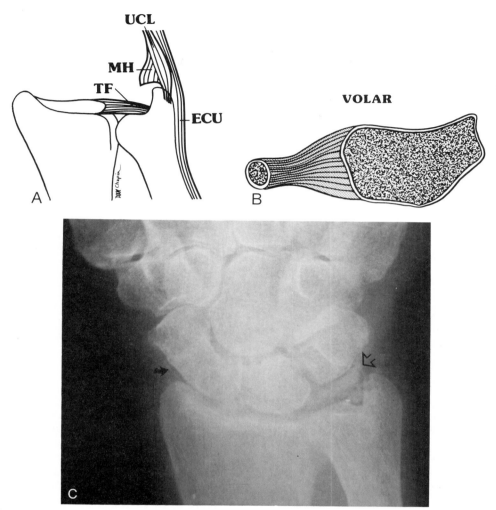

Figure 3–4. Triangular Fibrocartilage Complex. *A,* This complex includes the triangular fibrocartilage (articular disc, TF), the meniscus homologue (MH), the ulnar collateral ligament (UCL), and the dorsal and volar radioulnar ligaments (not shown). The extensor carpi ulnaris tendon (ECU) is shown. *B,* The triangular fibrocartilage (dotted) attaches to the ulnar border of the radius and the distal ulna. The triangular shape is evident on this transverse section through the radius and ulnar styloid. The volar aspect of the wrist is labeled. *C,* Chondrocalcinosis. There is heavy calcification of the articular cartilage (curved arrow) and the area of the triangular fibrocartilage complex (open arrow).

abduction possible because of a combination of radiocarpal and midcarpal motion (Fig. 3–6). Both the radiocarpal and the midcarpal joints participate in radial deviation but not in equal amounts, 60 to 65 percent of motion occurring at the midcarpal joint.[9] As radial deviation proceeds, the distal pole of the scaphoid tips toward the palm to clear the radial styloid.[11] During ulnar deviation motion also occurs at both midcarpal and radiocarpal joints, but relatively more motion occurs at the radiocarpal joint. Pronation-supination motion of the hand takes place at both the proximal (elbow) and the distal radioulnar joints.

Normal Radiographic Examination

Standard radiographic examination of the wrist includes posteroanterior, oblique, and lateral views (Fig. 3–1). This examination may be supplemented by views in radial or ulnar deviation, in flexion or extension, in compression or traction, or by fluoroscopy.

Bony Structures

Posteroanterior View. Views of the wrist are usually taken in the posteroanterior projection with the forearm pronated. When this is the case, the ulnar styloid is seen in profile, in

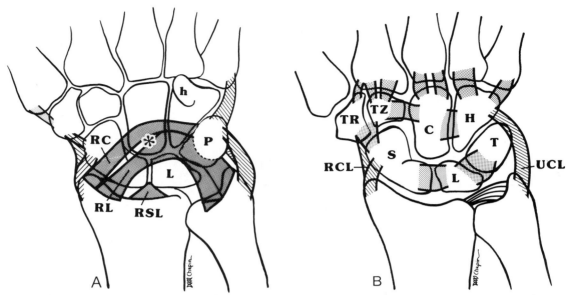

Figure 3–5. Carpal Ligaments. *A,* Volar ligaments. Volar radiocarpal ligaments (of the extrinsic group) are the most important and include radiolunate (RL), radioscaphoid capitate (RC), and radioscaphoid lunate (RSL) portions. The last two connect the proximal pole of the scaphoid to the volar aspect of the radius and prevent rotatory subluxation of the scaphoid. The space of Poirier(*) is a gap in the volar ligaments and a site of potential weakness. *B,* Intercarpal, carpometacarpal, and collateral ligaments, dorsal view. S = scaphoid; L = lunate; T = triquetrum; P = pisiform; TR = trapezium (greater multangulum); TZ = trapezoid (lesser multangulum); C = capitate; H = hamate; h = hook of hamate; RCL = radial collateral ligament; UCL = ulnar collateral ligament.

contrast to views taken in supination, in which the ulnar styloid overlaps the central portion of the distal ulna (Fig. 3–7). Three smooth arcuate lines can normally be constructed along the carpal articular surfaces (Fig. 3–8). One runs along the proximal margins of the scaphoid, the lunate, and the triquetrum; a second along the distal concave aspects of these bones; and a third along the proximal margins of the capitate and hamate.[14] With the wrist in the neutral position, one half or more of the lunate should contact the distal radial articular surface.[14]

The shapes of the carpals on the PA view vary with wrist flexion. The profile of the lunate is somewhat triangular in shape with dorsiflexion or palmar flexion and tends toward the rectangular in the neutral position. As radial deviation or palmar flexion takes place, the distal pole of the scaphoid tilts toward the palm, producing a foreshortened appearance. The contour of the scaphoid elongates as the wrist is ulnar deviated or extended.

Ulnar Variance. The length of the ulna relative to the radius, the ulnar variance, may be

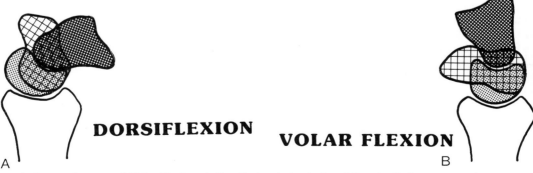

Figure 3–6. Dorsiflexion and Volar Flexion. *A,* Dorsiflexion (extension) and *B,* volar flexion movements are caused by motion at both the radiocarpal and the midcarpal joints. The rotation of the distal pole of the scaphoid (crosshatched) toward the palm in volar flexion is evident.

116

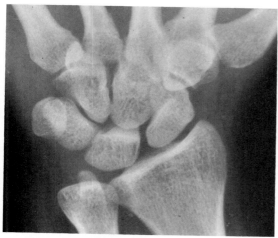

Figure 3–7. Supination. A view taken with the hand in supination shows the ulnar styloid projected over the central portion of the distal ulna. In pronation the ulnar styloid is border forming and seen in profile.

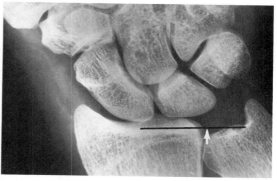

Figure 3–9. Ulnar Variance. The relationship between the length of the ulna and that of the radius at the wrist, termed ulnar variance, is shown. A line is extended from the distal radial articular surface (anteriorly) toward the ulna, and the distance from this line to the distal ulna (arrow) is measured in millimeters.

found by extending a line along the distal articular surface of the radius toward the ulna and measuring the distance from this line to the distal ulna (Fig. 3–9).[13] Normally, the radius and ulna are almost the same length (the measured difference in distance being $+0.27 \pm 1.69$ mm for whites),[13] although wrist and forearm position and centering of the x-ray tube have been noted to influence the measurements obtained.[1a]

When the ulna is shorter than the radius, the term *negative ulnar variance* is used. *Positive*

ulnar variance indicates that the ulna projects farther distally than does the radius. An abnormally short ulna has been implicated in the genesis of avascular necrosis of the lunate; a relatively long ulna is associated with perforation of the triangular fibrocartilage.[7]

Radial and Ulnar Deviation Views (Fig. 3–10). As the wrist is radially deviated, the distal pole of the scaphoid rotates toward the palm to clear the radial styloid. This produces a foreshortened appearance of the scaphoid and, often, a ring-like contour to its distal pole since the distal scaphoid is projected end-on. The scapholunate distance remains normal (less than 2 mm). As the wrist is moved in to ulnar deviation, the scaphoid rotates (its distal pole moving dorsally and toward the ulna) and appears to elongate. This change in contour of the scaphoid attests to its normal linkage to the proximal and the distal carpal rows and excludes the presence of scapholunate dissociation.

As the hand is radially deviated, the lunate moves toward the ulna and may no longer contact the radial articular surface. However, with ulnar deviation contact is restored.

Oblique Views. The standard oblique view is taken in the PA position, with the hand in partial pronation. Scaphoid, trapezium, and thumb base are seen to advantage. The AP view in partial supination (ball-catcher's view) shows the pisiform and the hamate well and profiles the intervening joint.

Lateral View

Longitudinal Axes of Radius, Lunate, and Capitate.[15, 18] Lateral views in any degree of palmar flexion or dorsiflexion should show the cup of the distal radial articular surface to contain the lunate and the cup of the lunate to contain

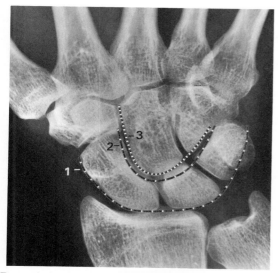

Figure 3–8. Wrist Arcs. Three arcuate lines can normally be constructed along the carpal articular surfaces: one along the proximal margins of the scaphoid, lunate, and triquetrum (1); another along the distal aspects of these bones (2); and a third along the proximal margins of the capitate and hamate (3).

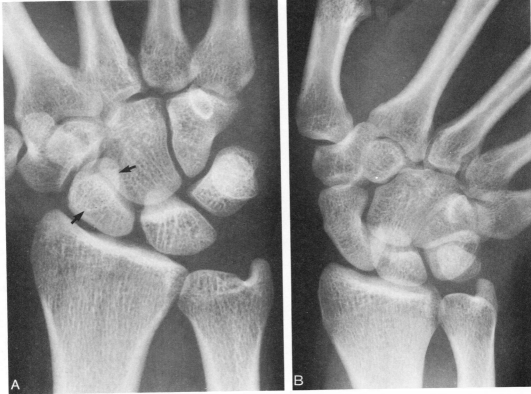

Figure 3–10. Radial and Ulnar Deviation. *A,* In radial deviation the scaphoid rotates toward the palm and assumes a foreshortened appearance. The circular density (arrows) represents the distal pole of the scaphoid on end. *B,* In ulnar deviation the full length of the scaphoid is seen. Note the change in the position of the lunate with respect to the distal radius.

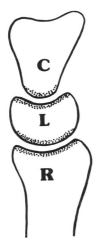

Figure 3–11. Normal Radial–Lunate–Capitate Relationships. The cup of the distal radial (R) articular surface (dotted) normally contains the lunate (L), and the cup of the distal lunate articular surface contains the capitate (C). These relationships are true in any degree of volar flexion or dorsiflexion.

the capitate (Fig. 3–11). In neutral position, longitudinal axes through the third metacarpal, the capitate, the lunate, and the radius all fall on the same line. This ideal situation is actually uncommon, but in most cases the axes are within 10 degrees of this line (Fig. 3–12).[14] The axis of the radius is constructed as a line parallel to the center of the radial shaft. The axis of the lunate can be drawn through the midpoints of its proximal and distal articular surfaces. The axis of the capitate is drawn through the centers of its head and its distal articular surface.

Longitudinal Axis of the Scaphoid. The long axis of the scaphoid is represented by a line drawn through the midpoints of its proximal and distal poles.[18] Another method, more easily seen on lateral views, is that proposed by Gilula and Weeks, consisting of connecting the ventral convexities of the scaphoid that are visible on the lateral view (Fig. 3–13).[15]

Normally, the angle formed between the long axis of the radius, the lunate, and the capitate

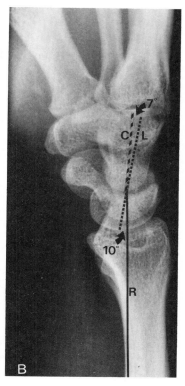

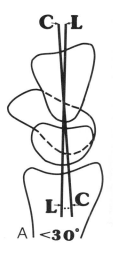

Figure 3–12. Radio–Lunate–Capitate Axis. Diagram *(A).* Normal lateral radiograph *(B).* The capitate axis (C) is drawn from the midpoint of its head to the center of its distal articular surface or the center of the base of the third metacarpal. The lunate axis (L) may be constructed as the perpendicular to a line through the distal poles of the lunate or, more accurately, through the center of its proximal and distal poles. The axis of the radius (R) is drawn as a line parallel to the center of the radial shaft. Although theoretically these lines should superimpose, angles between them of up to 30 degrees may be found in normal subjects. (Redrawn from Gilula LA, Weeks PM: Radiology 129:641, 1978.)

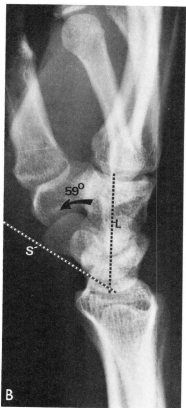

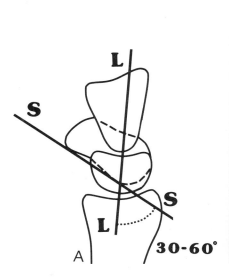

Figure 3–13. Scapholunate Axis. *A,* Diagram. The axis of the scaphoid (S) can be drawn as a line down its center or as a line connecting its proximal and distal volar convexities (used in this example). The lunate axis (L) is drawn as a perpendicuar to a line through its distal poles or as a line through the center of its proximal and distal poles (as shown). *B,* Normal scapholunate axis. (*A* is redrawn from Gilula LA, Weeks PM: Radiology 129:641, 1978.)

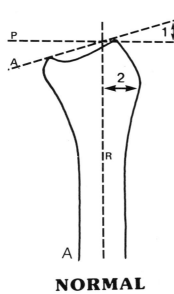

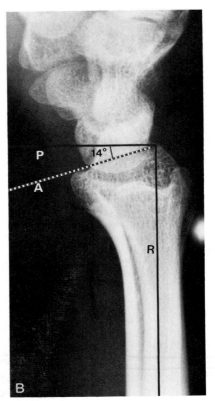

NORMAL

Figure 3–14. Tilt of Distal Radial Articular Surface. *A,* Tilt of the distal radial articular surface (1) is measured as the angle of intersection between a line drawn across the most distal points of the radial articular surface (A) and a perpendicular (P) to the axis of the radial shaft (R). Normally, a volar tilt of about 5 degrees is noted. The distal shift (useful in evaluating fracture deformities) is the distance between the midshaft of the radius and its most dorsal prominence (2). *B,* Normal example. (Redrawn from van der Linden W, Ericson R: J Bone Joint Surg (Am) 63:1285, 1981.)

and that of the scaphoid (termed the *scapholunate angle*) ranges between 30 and 60 degrees and averages 47 degrees.[18] This angle is abnormal in patients with carpal instability.

Distal Radial Articular Surface. The normal volar tilt of the radius can be measured on lateral views by noting the angle of intersection between a line drawn tangentially across the most distal points of the radial articular surface and a perpendicular to the midshaft of the radius (Fig. 3–14). This normally ranges from 11 degrees of volar tilt to 4 degrees of dorsal tilt and averages about 5 degrees of volar tilt.[16]

Carpal Tunnel Views. Views taken with the hand hyperextended and the beam angled along the volar aspect of the wrist show the bony margins of the carpal tunnel (Fig. 3–15). The axial orientation of computed tomography shows this area to advantage.

Soft Tissues

Posteroanterior View

The Cartilage Spaces. The distances between the carpal bones are normally equal throughout and are unchanged by radial or ulnar deviation. Widening of the scapholunate distance to between 2 and 4 mm may be abnormal, and more than 4 mm is definitely abnormal.[15]

The Scaphoid Fat Stripe. A triangular or linear collection of fat is normally present along the radial aspect of the scaphoid, bounded by tendons of the abductor pollicis longus and the extensor pollicis brevis and by the radial collateral ligament (Fig. 3–16). Fractures of the scaphoid, the radial styloid, and the first metacarpal often result in displacement or obliteration of this fat stripe. This result is a useful indicator of adjacent fracture, since an abnormal fat stripe was noted in 13 of 15 (87 percent) patients with scaphoid fractures but in only 14 of 400 (3.5 percent) control subjects.[58]

The Tendon Sheaths. On the radial aspect of the wrist, linear collections of fat are noted along tendons of the abductor pollicis longus and extensor pollicis brevis (Fig. 3–17). When these tendons run in a single sheath, their combined density is outlined by fat. Localized edema of the soft tissues, such as occurs in de Quer-

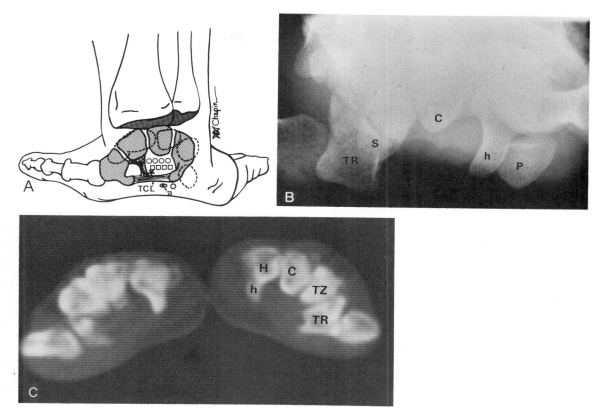

Figure 3–15. Carpal Tunnel. *A*, Diagram of the carpal tunnel, which is bounded dorsally by the carpal bones and volarly by the transvese carpal ligament (TCL) that inserts on the trapezium, scaphoid, and occasionally the radial styloid and extends to the pisiform and hook of the hamate. Flexor tendons and median nerve (asterisk) are located within the tunnel. Ulnar nerve and artery (a) are outside the tunnel. *B*, Standard carpal tunnel projection, and *C*, computed tomogram of the carpal tunnel. The trapezium (TR), trapezoid (TZ), capitate (C), and hamate (H) form the base of the carpal tunnel. P = pisiform, h = hook of hamate, and S = scaphoid.

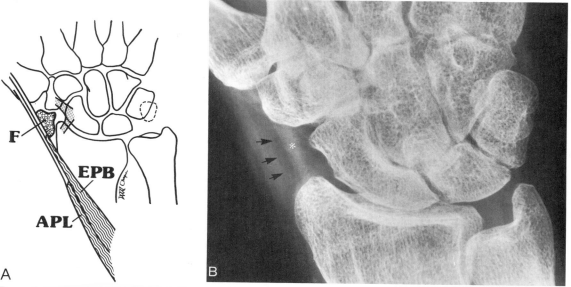

Figure 3–16. Scaphoid Fat Stripe. *A*, The normal linear (or triangular) collection of fat (F) between tendons of the abductor pollicis longus (APL) and extensor pollicis brevis (EPB) and the radial collateral ligament. *B*, Normal scaphoid fat stripe (arrows). The linear density (asterisk) is an overlying vein. (After Terry DW Jr, Ramin JE: AJR 124:25, 1975.)

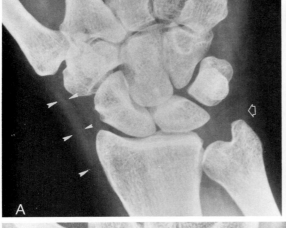

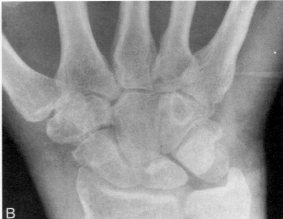

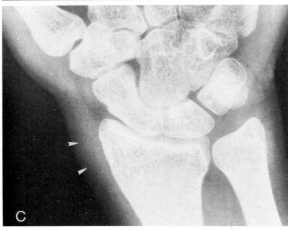

Figure 3–17. Radial Tendon Sheaths. *A,* PA view of a normal wrist shows fat lines around the extensor pollicis brevis and the abductor pollicis longus (arrowheads). The scaphoid fat stripe is along the ulnar aspect of these tendons. On the ulnar side of the wrist, subcutaneous fat adjacent to the extensor carpi ulnaris tendon is seen (open arrow). *B,* Rheumatoid involvement of these tendon sheaths has resulted in obliteration of normally present fat lines. *C,* De Quervain's tenosynovitis. Combined soft tissue densities of the abductor pollicis longus and the extensor pollicis brevis (arrowheads) are abnormally widened and cause the usually almost straight soft tissue contour to bulge.

vain's tenosynovitis, will obliterate these fat lines. Residual thickening of the tendon sheath can be appreciated by separation of the fat lines and displacement of the subcutaneous fat.[17, 20]

On the ulnar aspect of the wrist, fat along the extensor carpi ulnaris tendon is often visible. Inflammatory processes such as rheumatoid arthritis may obliterate these fat stripes and thicken the tendon shadow, increasing the amount of soft tissue density along the ulnar styloid.[19]

Lateral View

The Pronator Quadratus Line. In virtually all normal individuals, lateral views of the wrist demonstrate a linear fat collection just anterior to the distal radius and ulna (Fig. 3–18). Anatomical studies show this fat plane to lie anterior to the pronator quadratus muscle.

Fractures involving the distal radius or ulna often show volar displacement, blurring, irregularity, or obliteration of this fat collection, and these findings should initiate a careful search for an otherwise occult fracture.[53] Volar to the pronator quadratus line, another fat line separates the flexor digitorum profundus and the flexor digitorum sublimis muscles.

Wrist Arthrography

Technique. Wrist arthrography is commonly limited to injection of the radiocarpal joint. Preliminary films are obtained, with additional stress views taken before contrast medium injection if ligamentous integrity is the clinical concern. Two approaches to the radiocarpal joint are commonly used. In one, injection is made through a *dorsal* approach into the area between the radius and the scaphoid or between the radius and the lunate. Care is taken to avoid contrast agent extravasation into the scapholunate area or inadvertent injection of the midcarpal joint, since either of these errors may result in a nondiagnostic examination. The patient is positioned prone on the fluoroscopic table, with the palm down on the table and the wrist slightly flexed over a triangular sponge. After the area is washed and draped, the puncture site is selected under fluoroscopic guidance. The skin

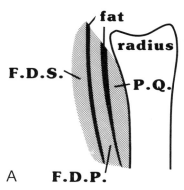

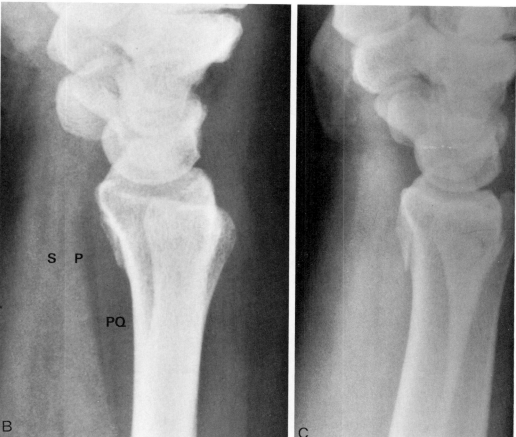

Figure 3–18. Pronator Quadratus Line. *A,* Diagrammatic representation of the volar fat lines that may normally be seen. PQ = pronator quadratus; FDP = flexor digitorum profundus; FDS = flexor digitorum sublimis. *B,* Normal radiograph several weeks after a distal radial fracture. PQ = pronator quadratus; P = flexor digitorum profundus; S = flexor digitorum sublimis. *C,* Lateral radiograph immediately after injury shows poor definition of fat lines due to hemorrhage and edema (same patient as in *B*).

is infiltrated with 1 percent lidocaine, and a 22-gauge, 1½-inch needle is introduced perpendicular to the skin. The flexed position of the wrist should open the joint dorsally and lessen the possibility that the dorsal lip of the radius will obstruct needle entry into the joint.

The second approach is a *lateral* one. The hand is positioned with the thumb up and the ulnar side of the wrist slightly flexed over an angled sponge. The site of injection is identified by palpating the tip of the radial styloid; the needle enters just distal to that site and is directed downward at an angle of about 45 degrees into the joint space between the radial styloid and the scaphoid.

With either approach, correct needle placement is confirmed by injecting a small amount of contrast medium (e.g., Reno–M–60) and noting its flow away from the needle tip and along the radiocarpal joint. The pattern of filling is then observed fluoroscopically until the injection is complete; 1.0 to 1.5 ml of contrast agent usually is adequate. The needle is then withdrawn, and PA, oblique, and lateral radiographs are obtained before and after exercise.

Normal Arthrogram. The cavity of the radiocarpal joint is smooth in contour and separate from the other wrist compartments (Fig. 3–19). It is bounded distally by the articular surfaces of the scaphoid, the lunate, and the triquetrum and proximally by the distal radius and the triangular fibrocartilage. On the radial side, contrast medium extends to the area of the radial collateral ligament. Two diverticula project from the ulnar aspect of the joint, a proximal prestyloid recess and a distal recess adjacent to the triquetrum. Anterior recesses of variable size and number extend proximally.[27]

Although the radiocarpal compartment is

Table 3–1. **Communication Between RC***
Compartment and Other Sites

Site of Communication	Dissection (%)	Arthrography (%)
RC compartment and flexor tendon sheaths	—	0
RC compartment and extensor tendon sheaths	—	0
RC and midcarpal compartments	—	13
lunate-triquetrum	36	—
lunate-scaphoid	40	
RC and radioulnar compartments	30–60	7–16
RC and pisiform-triquetral compartments	35.6	—

Sources: Leibolt FL: Surg Gynecol Obstet 66:1008, 1938; Harrison MO, Freiberger RH, Ranawat CS: AJR 112:480, 1971; Trentham DE, Hamm RL, Masi AT: Semin Arthritis Rheum 5:105, 1975. *RC = radiocarpal.

thought to be separate from the other wrist compartments, anatomic communications between compartments have been noted in more than one third of dissections (Table 3–1). These communications appear to be much less commonly demonstrated by arthrography than by dissection. For example, arthrographic exami-

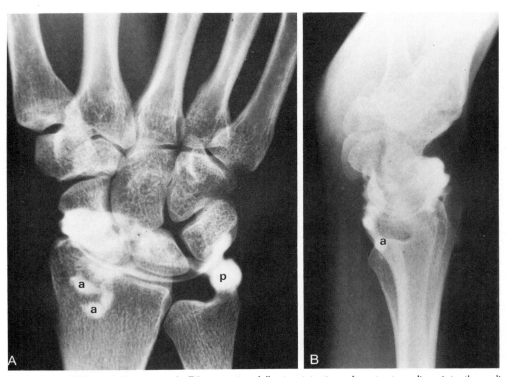

Figure 3–19. Normal Wrist Arthrogram. A, PA projection following injection of contrast medium into the radiocarpal compartment. There is no filling of the midcarpal or radioulnar compartments. Prominent anterior (a) and prestyloid (p) recesses are noted. B, Lateral view. The anterior recesses (a) are well seen.

nation of cadaver wrists by Harrison and associates disclosed communication between the radiocarpal and radioulnar joints in only 16 percent and between the radiocarpal and midcarpal joints in only 13 percent.[22]

ABNORMAL CONDITIONS

Fractures and Dislocations

Colles' Fracture

In 1814 Abraham Colles described the clinical features of the fracture that now bears his name. The fracture was noted to occur about 1½ inches proximal to the end of the radius and to result in characteristic deformity due to the dorsal angulation of the distal radial fragment and the wrist.[29] Radiologic examination has since revealed the presence of comminution, impaction, or extension of the fracture into the radiocarpal joint in some cases and the presence of an ulnar styloid fracture (due to avulsion by the triangular fibrocartilage) in more than half (53.2 percent).[30, 33]

The Colles' fracture usually occurs in older persons after a fall on an outstretched hand.

The resulting "dinner fork" deformity is characteristic.[33]

Radiographic Examination. On the lateral view in a normal wrist, the articular surface of the radius will be noted to be tipped volarly about 10 degrees. In Colles' fracture the articular surface of the radius is displaced or angled dorsally (Figs. 3–20 to 3–22). The deformity may resemble dislocation, but this can be excluded by noting the preservation of contacts between the radial articular surface and the lunate and between the distal lunate surface and the capitate. Colles' fractures result in shortening of the radius. This can be measured by noting the millimeters of overlap at the fracture site, and the decrease in distance that the radial styloid projects distal to the ulna or the radial angle (Fig. 3–21).[32, 34] According to van der Linden and Ericson, only two measurements are necessary, dorsal displacement (i.e., the dorsal angle) and radial displacement.[34]

Postreduction Films. Postreduction radiographs should show that the length of the radius is restored and dorsal displacement of the distal fragment corrected. The volar tilt of the distal radial articular surface should be reestablished if possible. If not, the radial articular surface should

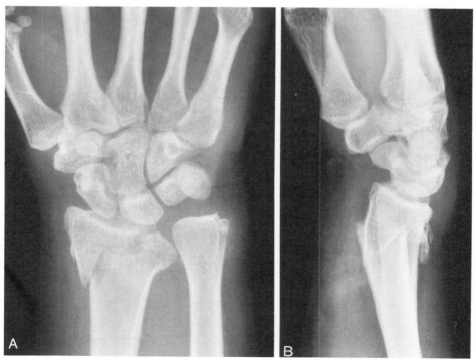

Figure 3–20. Colles' Fracture. *A*, PA view shows a comminuted distal radial fracture that extends into the radial articular surface. Despite articular involvement, the term *Colles' fracture* is still applicable. Irregularity of the distal ulna suggests an avulsion fracture. *B*, Lateral view confirms the "dinner fork" deformity.

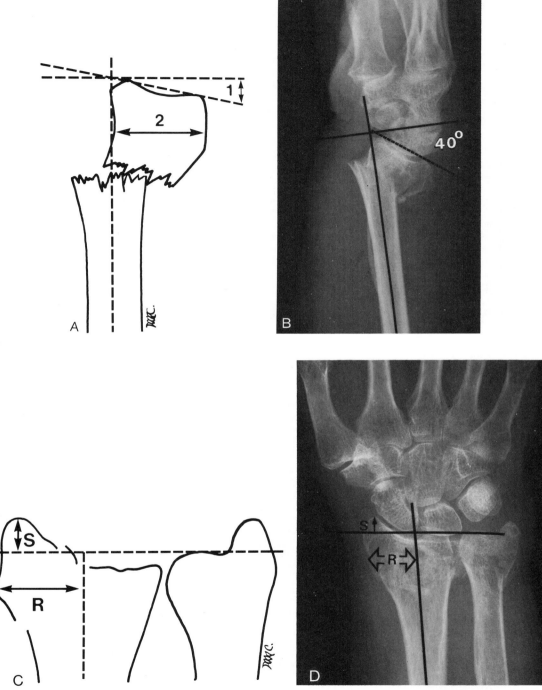

Figure 3–21. Measurement of Postfracture Radial Deformity. *A,* Lateral views allow angle of inclination of radial articular surface (dorsal angle 1) to be measured. This is the angle between a perpendicular to the long axis of the radial shaft and a line connecting the poles of the articular surface. The dorsal shift (2) is the distance from the long axis of the radius to its most dorsal point. *B,* Example of Colles' fracture with 40 degree of dorsal angulation of the articular surface. *C,* PA radiograph allows degree of shortening (S) to be assessed by comparison with normal side. Degree of shortening is the decrease in distance that the radial styloid projects distal to the ulna. Measurement is from a perpendicular to the long axis of the radius drawn through the articular surface of the ulna. Radial shift (R) is the increase in distance from the long axis of the radius to the most radial part of the styloid process. *D,* Example of shortening (S) and radial shift (R). (Redrawn from van der Linden W, Ericson R: J Bone Joint Surg (Am) 63:1285–88, 1981.)

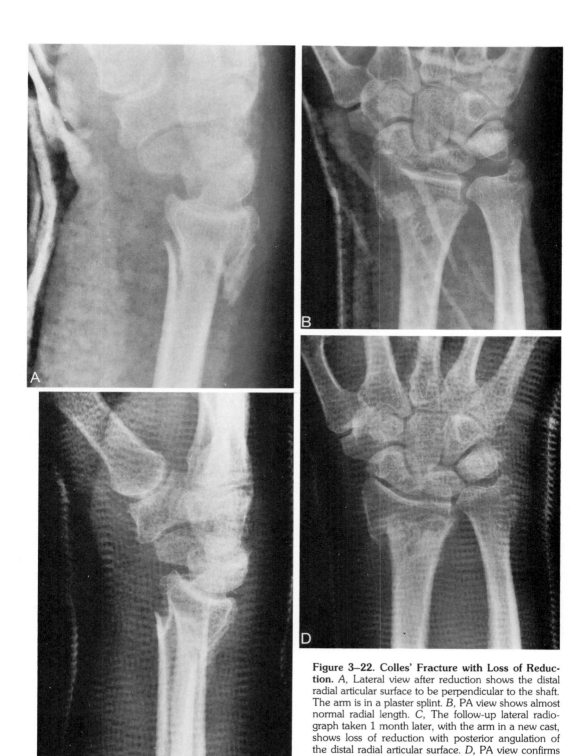

Figure 3–22. Colles' Fracture with Loss of Reduction. *A,* Lateral view after reduction shows the distal radial articular surface to be perpendicular to the shaft. The arm is in a plaster splint. *B,* PA view shows almost normal radial length. *C,* The follow-up lateral radiograph taken 1 month later, with the arm in a new cast, shows loss of reduction with posterior angulation of the distal radial articular surface. *D,* PA view confirms marked shortening of the radius as compared with the ulna.

be at least in neutral alignment (90 degrees to the radial shaft).[32, 33]

Inadequate reduction or overreduction may occur. Even with immobilization, recurrence of deformity (Fig. 3–22) or development of a reverse deformity (due to slipping of the distal radial fragment anteriorly) may occur.[33] Remanipulation is possible for up to 4 to 6 weeks; therefore, prompt recognition of positional changes is important.

Results. Although Colles noted that even with inadequate reduction "the limb will at some remote period again enjoy perfect freedom in all its motions, and be completely exempt from pain,"[29] subsequent studies have not been as optimistic. Bacorn and Kurtzke noted postfracture disability to occur more frequently with increasing age and increasing residual deformity.[30] Cooney, Dobyns, and Linscheid noted complications in 19 percent of nonreferred patients.[31] Complications include neuropathies (medial, ulnar, or radial nerve), radiocarpal or radioulnar osteoarthritis, malposition and malunion at the fracture site, and the shoulder–hand syndrome (Figs. 3–23 and 3–24).

A number of injuries have been noted to occur in association with Colles' fractures, and these may go unnoticed unless carefully sought. These injuries include scaphoid, radial head, and Bennett's fractures and intercarpal ligament injuries.

Barton's and Smith's Fractures

In 1838, John Rhea Barton described "a subluxation of the wrist, consequent to a fracture through the articular surface of the carpal extremity of the radius". The carpus and the fragment could be displaced dorsally or volarly, although currently only the volarly displaced variety is termed a Barton's fracture.[38] In 1847 Robert William Smith described an "exceedingly rare" injury consisting of fracture of the distal radius with displacement of the distal fragment and carpus volarly, the deformity opposite to the Colles' fracture. Since the fracture does not involve the articular surface of the radius, it should not be confused with Barton's fracture.[39]

Despite the difference between Smith's and Barton's fractures noted previously, the most frequently cited classification of Smith's fractures is that of Thomas, which actually includes both fractures (Fig. 3–25).[40] Classification was based on the obliquity of the fracture line and the presence of articular involvement:

Type I fractures extend across the distal cancellous bone of the radius, and there is volar displacement of the distal fragment, often with an ulnar styloid process fracture.

Type II fractures are really Barton's fractures involving the volar margin of the distal articular surface of the radius and with volar and proximal displacement of the fragment and carpus.

Type III fractures extend through the distal

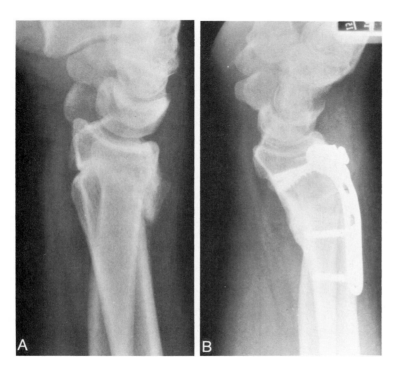

Figure 3–23. Malposition after Colles' Fracture. *A,* Lateral view shows residual dorsal tilt of the radial articular surface. *B,* Osteotomy was necessary owing to loss of grip strength associated with the malposition.

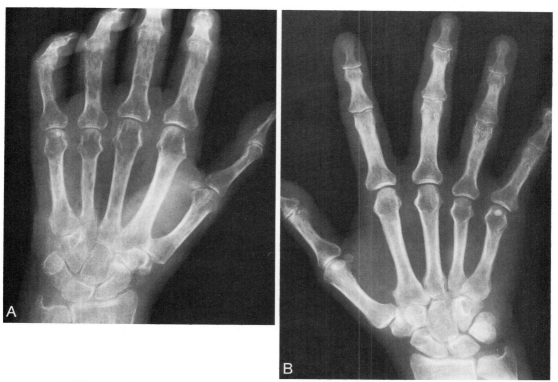

Figure 3–24. Sudeck's Atrophy. *A,* PA view of the left hand and wrist after a Colles' fracture shows fingers held in flexion and marked osteopenia. No residual radial deformity was present. Burning pain and diffuse soft tissue swelling were noted. *B,* Comparison view of normal right side.

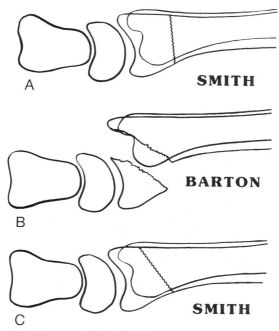

Figure 3–25. The Thomas Classification of Smith's Fractures. *A,* Type I. Fracture line extends through the distal cancellous bone of the radius. There is volar displacement of the distal fragment. *B,* Type II are really Barton's fractures and involve the anterior margin of the distal radial articular surface. There is volar and proximal displacement of the distal fragment and the wrist. *C,* Type III are distal radial fractures in which the fracture line is slightly oblique on lateral radiographs. (After de Oliveira JC: J Bone Joint Surg (Am) 55:586, 1973.)

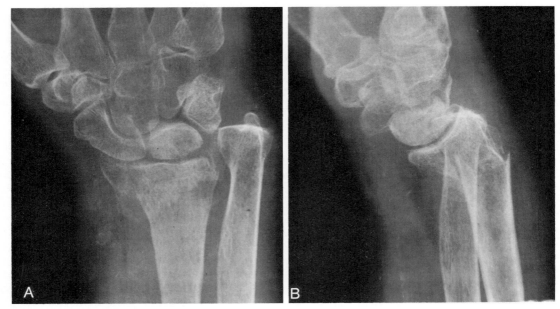

Figure 3–26. Smith's Fracture. There is a comminuted fracture of the distal radius (Thomas type I) with volar angulation and displacement. A nondisplaced fracture line extends to the articular surface. *A*, PA view. *B*, Lateral view.

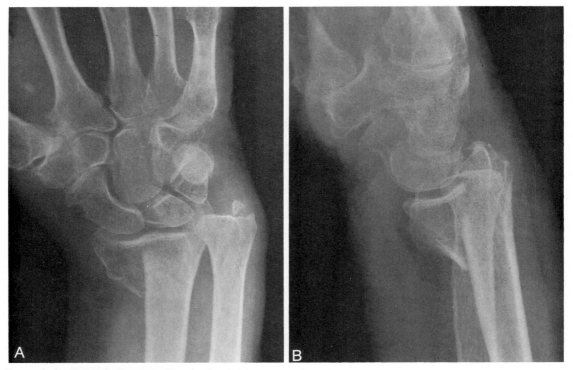

Figure 3–27. Barton's Fracture. The distal radial fracture involves the articular surface, and there is proximal and radial displacement of the volar fragment. An ulnar styloid fracture is present. This fracture would correspond to type II of the Thomas classification. *A*, PA view. *B*, Lateral view.

radius and are slightly oblique on lateral radiographs.

Although Smith noted that the fracture results from a fall on the back of the hand, current theory suggests a fall with the wrist in dorsiflexion and the forearm supinated.[32] However, direct injury to the dorsum of the hand in motorcycle crashes has been noted to produce a Smith's fracture.[40]

Radiographic Findings. In Smith's fracture lateral views show a fracture of the distal radial metaphysis with the distal articular surface angled volarly (Fig. 3–26). Differentiation from carpal dislocation is made by noting the preservation of articulation between the distal radius and the lunate. In Barton's fracture the fracture line extends through the articular surface of the radius, and the distal fragment is angled volarly (Fig. 3–27).

Treatment. Differentiation between Smith's and Barton's fractures is not purely academic; Smith's fractures may be treated by manipulation and immobilization, but Barton's fractures are usually unstable, and open reduction and internal fixation are often necessary (Fig. 3–28).[32, 35-37, 40] Smith's fractures, in which the fracture line is oblique (type III), also tend to be unstable. Healing occurs 5 to 6 weeks after reduction.[32]

Radioulnar Dislocations

Damage to the distal radioulnar joint may be seen in a large number of congenital and acquired abnormalities.[47] Madelung's deformity, in which the radius is abnormally short, is associated with radioulnar dislocation (Fig. 3–29).[46] Fractures of the distal radius (Colles', Smith's), fractures of the shafts of both radius and ulna, and isolated fractures of the ulnar shaft may be accompanied by dislocations of the radioulnar joint. In rheumatoid arthritis damage to the triangular fibrocartilage complex and the joint capsule may result in radioulnar dislocation, with weakness and pain.

Traumatic dislocations of the radioulnar joint are usually the result of hyperpronation or hypersupination injuries. In the former the ulna will be dorsal to the carpals and the radius, while in the latter the ulna will be volar. Cadaver studies have shown that dislocation cannot occur

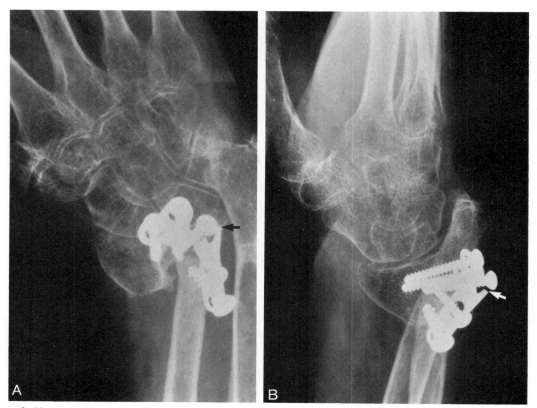

Figure 3–28. Barton's Fracture with Nonunion. Despite an attempt at internal fixation, the distal radial fracture remains unhealed and has collapsed, with marked shortening and radial deviation. The plate has fractured (arrow). *A,* PA view. *B,* Oblique view.

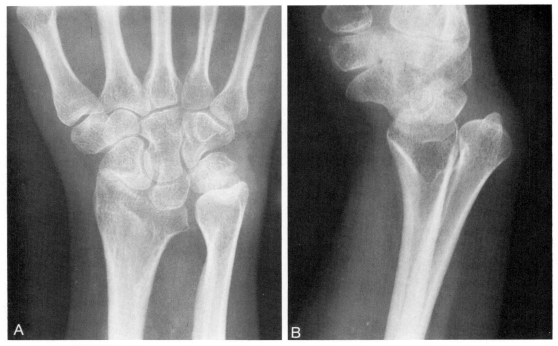

Figure 3–29. Madelung's Deformity. *A,* PA view. The ulnar aspect of the radius is abnormally short. *B,* Lateral view. The ulna is positioned dorsally with respect to the radius.

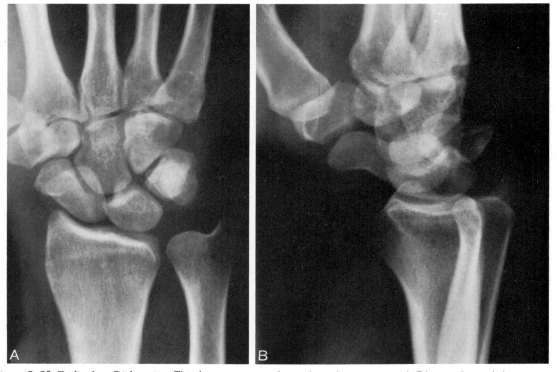

Figure 3–30. Radioulnar Dislocation. This diagnosis was made on physical examination. *A,* PA view shows slight separation between the radius and the ulna. *B,* Dorsal position of the distal ulna with relation to the radius is shown on this slightly off-lateral view.

without the presence of a tear in the triangular fibrocartilage complex.[42] Dislocations at the distal radioulnar joint are apparently due to displacement of the radius rather than the ulna, and therefore the phrase *dislocation of the distal ulna* is inaccurate. Dameron suggests the terms *distal radioulnar dislocation—ulna volar* and *distal radioulnar dislocation—ulna dorsal* to describe the resulting deformity.[42]

The diagnosis of dislocation at the radioulnar joint may be difficult clinically with characteristic deformities obscured by soft tissue swelling. Dorsal position of the distal ulna produces a prominence in this area while volar position of the distal ulna results in a wrist that is narrower than normal in anteroposterior dimension.

Radiographic Examination. Radiographic findings associated with radioulnar dislocation include the following (Fig. 3–30):[42]

1. Abnormal rotation of the ulna with the ulnar styloid overlying the central portion of the distal ulna may be seen despite the usual PA pronation radiograph.

2. Widening of the radioulnar distance on the PA view may be seen in ulna dorsal dislocations.

3. Superimposition of the radius and ulna on the frontal view is present in ulna ventral dislocations.

4. True lateral views (with the radial styloid overlying the center of the distal radius) will confirm the relative anterior or posterior position of the ulna. Less than optimal positioning, however, makes diagnosis inaccurate. To obviate this problem, Mino and colleagues recommend computed tomography (CT) through the distal radioulnar joint (Fig. 3–31).

Arthrography. Injection of contrast agent into the radiocarpal compartment should fill only that

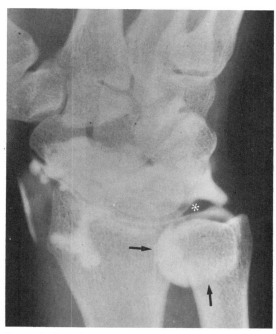

Figure 3–32. Filling of the Radioulnar Compartment. PA view after injection of contrast material into the radiocarpal joint shows contrast in the radioulnar compartment (arrows). The triangular fibrocartilage is well seen (asterisk), outlined by contrast on its proximal and distal surfaces.

compartment. Filling of the inferior radioulnar compartment suggests a tear in the triangular fibrocartilage complex if the clinical setting is appropriate (Fig. 3–32). However, anatomical studies have shown perforation (said to be caused by degenerative changes) in the triangular fibrocartilage complex in one third to one half of cadaver specimens,[3] although arthrograms have demonstrated communications between these compartments considerably less often.[22] The significance of such communication must be interpreted with caution.[72a]

Scaphoid Fractures[54, 55, 59]

Scaphoid fractures make up more than 60 percent of all carpal injuries. Seventy percent of these fractures occur through the middle third of the scaphoid, 10 percent through the distal third, and 20 percent through the proximal third (Fig. 3–33). The location and orientation of the fracture line influence the rate of healing. Since the blood supply to the scaphoid enters distally, fractures of the distal and middle thirds of the bone tend to heal more quickly than do fractures of the proximal pole. Thus Osterman and Bora suggest that longer immobilization may be necessary for proximal pole fractures (12 to 16 weeks) than for distal and midthird fractures (8

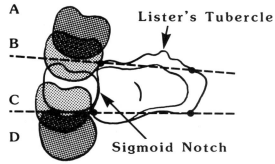

Figure 3–31. CT for the Diagnosis of Radioulnar Dislocation. The ulna is normally located within the sigmoid notch, between axes (dashed) drawn along the dorsal and the volar surfaces of the radius. Subluxation (ulnar positions B and C) and dislocation (ulnar positions A and D) can be detected by the position of the ulna relative to these axes. (After Mino DE, Palmer AK, Levinsohn EM: J Hand Surg 8:23, 1983.)

Lister's Tubercle

Sigmoid Notch

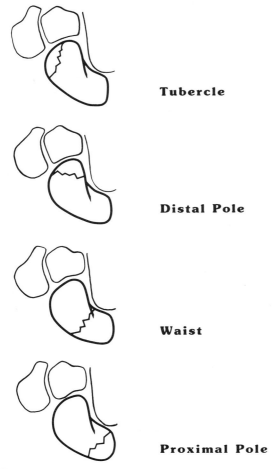

Tubercle

Distal Pole

Waist

Proximal Pole

Figure 3–33. Scaphoid Fracture Locations. Most fractures involve the middle third (waist) of the scaphoid.

to 12 weeks).[54] Fractures that are directed along the longitudinal axis of the scaphoid are subjected to greater shearing forces and therefore may require longer periods of immobilization than are necessary for the healing of transversely oriented fractures.

The major factor leading to nonunion of scaphoid fractures is delayed or inadequate immobilization; treatment therefore is often begun even when radiographic confirmation is lacking. Thus, according to Osterman and Bora, individuals without radiographically demonstrable fractures who are clinically suspected of having nondisplaced scaphoid fractures should be immobilized in a cast for several weeks and then reexamined.[54] If radiographs remain normal and clinical examination has returned to normal, immobilization is discontinued. Usually, if a fracture is present, sufficient resorption has occurred along the fracture line to make it apparent on repeat radiographs. However, if tenderness per-

sists and the radiographs remain normal, another period of immobilization followed by repeat radiographs is advocated (Fig. 3–34).

An alternative course has been suggested by Ganel and co-workers, who noted that a negative bone scan 24 to 72 hours after injury excludes fracture at this site.[49] Therefore, in clinically suspicious cases with negative or inconclusive radiographs, a cast is applied and a bone scan (with the cast on) is performed; if this is negative, immobilization is discontinued.

Radiographic Examination. Multiple views of the wrist are indicated in patients with suspected scaphoid fractures. In addition to PA lateral and oblique projections, angled and magnification views (Fig. 3–35) and views with the wrist in ulnar deviation may be helpful in demonstrating subtle fracture lines.

Early radiographic diagnosis requires a high index of suspicion and careful attention to detail. Soft tissue changes may be helpful since obliteration or displacement of the scaphoid fat stripe has been noted to occur in most patients with scaphoid fractures (Fig. 3–36).[58] This fat stripe is normally seen paralleling the lateral aspect of the scaphoid. Within an hour after injury the fat stripe is displaced or obliterated by local hemorrhage; therefore the presence of a normal fat stripe after injury essentially excludes a scaphoid fracture.[51] Days to months later when edema and hemorrhage resolve, the normal fat line returns.[58]

Radiographic Evidence of Healing. Immobilization is often continued until there is radiographic evidence of union. When trabecular continuity is not complete, increased density along the fracture site or on each side of the fracture site (in a recent fracture) provides evidence that healing is occurring. Inadequate healing is documented by motion at the fracture site or bone resorption along the fracture margins with the formation of cyst-like areas of lucency (Figs. 3–34 and 3–38).

Complications

Avascular Necrosis (AVN). The blood supply to the scaphoid is derived primarily from the radial artery. A volar branch enters the scaphoid tubercle to supply blood to the distal 20 to 30 percent of the bone. The proximal 70 to 80 percent of the scaphoid is supplied by an artery that enters distally along the dorsal ridge. Thus the entire blood supply to the scaphoid enters through its distal pole.[50] AVN may occur following fractures through the waist of the scaphoid and is an expected sequel of proximal pole fractures. Increased density of the proximal fragment, indicating avascular necrosis, has been noted on radiographs in about 30 percent of

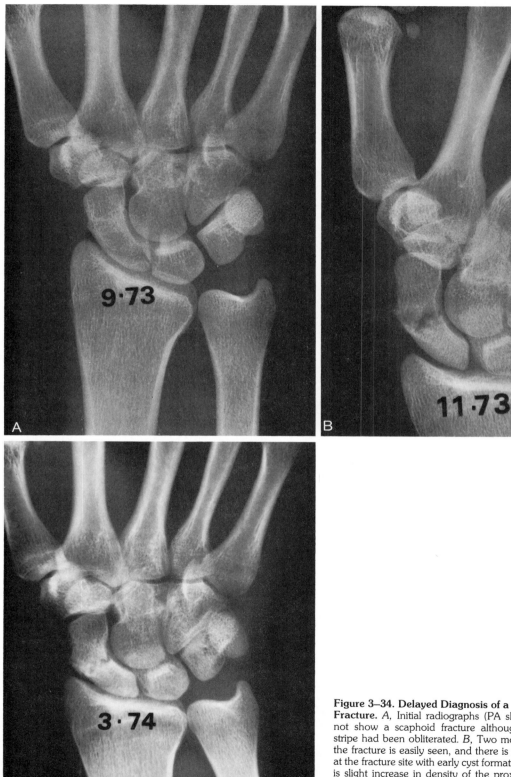

Figure 3–34. Delayed Diagnosis of a Scaphoid Fracture. *A,* Initial radiographs (PA shown) did not show a scaphoid fracture although the fat stripe had been obliterated. *B,* Two months later the fracture is easily seen, and there is resorption at the fracture site with early cyst formation. There is slight increase in density of the proximal pole of the scaphoid, indicative of avascular necrosis. *C,* Four months later, after immobilization, healing is occurring.

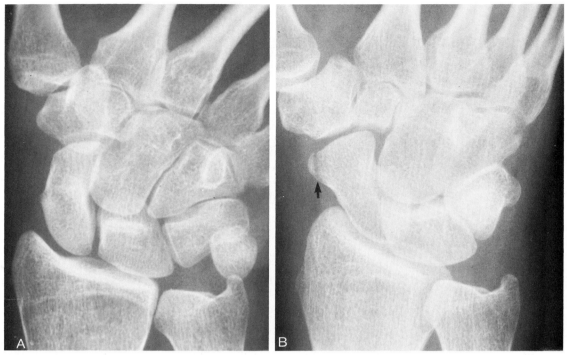

Figure 3–35. Scaphoid Tubercle Fracture. *A*, Routine scaphoid view with the wrist in ulnar deviation shows no fracture. *B*, A standard oblique view, however, shows a nondisplaced fracture of the scaphoid tubercle (arrow).

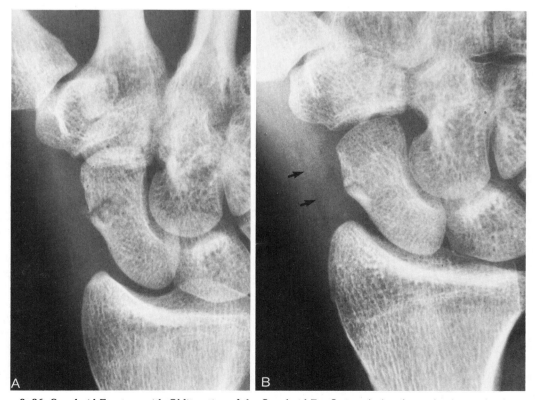

Figure 3–36. Scaphoid Fracture with Obliteration of the Scaphoid Fat Stripe. *A*, A radiograph taken within hours after injury shows the scaphoid fracture and the absence of the normal scaphoid fat stripe. *B*, Follow-up radiograph 1½ months later shows healing of the fracture and a normal scaphoid fat stripe (arrows).

136

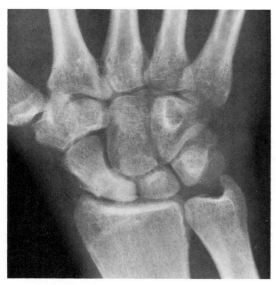

Figure 3–37. Avascular Necrosis of the Proximal Pole of the Scaphoid after Scaphoid Fracture. The PA view demonstrates striking increase in density of the proximal pole. The fracture (between the waist and proximal pole) did not heal.

patients (Fig. 3–37).[55, 56] It does not indicate inevitable nonunion, and both the fracture and the avascular area may go on to heal.

Nonunion. Nonunion of scaphoid fractures is due primarily to delay in diagnosis, or lack of adequate immobilization, or both.[59] Contributing factors include anatomical features such as the presence of articular cartilage covering five of the six scaphoid surfaces, healing by endosteal reaction only,[59] failure to achieve anatomical reduction,[54] and a tenuous blood supply in some cases.[54]

Radiographic Findings Indicating Nonunion. Fractures that have not been immobilized develop bone resorption along the fracture margins within a few weeks and further resorption producing "cavities," or cyst-like lucencies, by 2 to 3 months (Figs. 3–38 and 3–40). Sclerotic edges of the fracture site (typical of nonunion) appear only after several months or years (Fig. 3–39).[56] Osterman and Bora suggest that nonunion is present when there is no evidence of healing on three sets of radiographs taken at 1-month intervals.[54]

Bipartite Scaphoid. The presence of a congenitally bipartite scaphoid has been mentioned. However, Louis and associates conclude that this appearance is actually a post-traumatic one because no example of a bipartite scaphoid was found in a review of hand radiographs of more than 17,000 children or in fetal hand specimens (Fig. 3–38).[52]

Treatment of Nonunion and AVN. A number of surgical techniques have been developed for the treatment of complications following scaphoid fracture. Appropriate treatment requires identification of delayed union or nonunion alone or with the presence of associated AVN, superimposed osteoarthritis, or both.

Bone grafting and electrical stimulation have been used when secondary osteoarthritis has not developed. The *Matte-Russe graft* procedure includes removal of fibrotic tissue and sclerotic bone from the nonunion site and insertion of autogenous cancellous and corticocancellous graft (Figs. 3–39 and 3–40).[54, 56] The time to union averages more than 16 weeks.[59] Electrical stimulation may be done after the percutaneous insertion of electrodes under local anesthesia or transcutaneously. For union to occur 8 to 12 weeks are necessary.[54]

Nonunion associated with AVN but without secondary osteoarthritis has been treated with a variety of methods, including immobilization, Matte-Russe fusion, limited carpal fusion, prosthetic replacement of the scaphoid, and excision of the proximal pole of the scaphoid (Fig. 3–40).[54, 55]

Excision of the radial styloid, radiocarpal fusion, and proximal row carpectomy have been used after radiocarpal arthritis has developed (Figs. 3–41 and 3–42).[54, 55]

Carpal Dislocations

Most wrist injuries, including dislocations, result from forced dorsiflexion of the wrist. Dislocation occurs first at the midcarpal joint, with the capitate dislocating dorsally on the lunate (a perilunate dislocation).[62, 65] This dislocation is followed by scaphoid injury: either fracture, allowing the distal fragment to dislocate dorsally with the capitate, or ligamentous rupture at the proximal pole, allowing the scaphoid to rotate dorsally. The progression of injury involves the triquetrolunate area, with tearing of the radial triquetral ligaments.[63] As spontaneous reduction of the perilunate dislocation occurs, the lunate is displaced volarly by the capitate, and a lunate dislocation results. Thus, lunate dislocation is thought to be the end stage of a perilunate dislocation.[60, 62, 65] The classification of wrist dislocations by Green and O'Brien is of interest because it places dorsal perilunate dislocation in the same group as volar dislocation of the lunate, emphasizing the concept that these lesions are different stages of the same basic injury (Table 3–2).[62]

Dorsal Perilunate and Volar Lunate Dislocations. The designation *dorsal perilunate dislocation* is applied when the lateral view shows

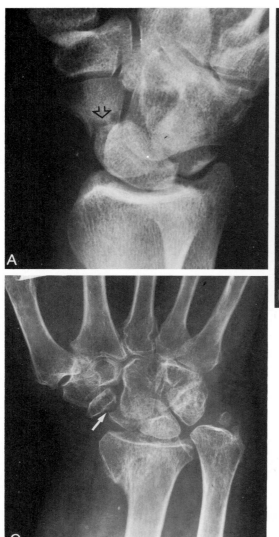

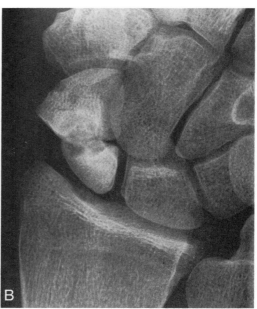

Figure 3–38. Nonunion of Scaphoid Fractures. *A,* Months after injury there is cystic resorption (arrow) along the fracture margins, suggesting nonunion. *B,* Another patient shows more striking cystic resorption, and there is sclerosis around the fracture site. *C,* This patient has residual deformity from a prior Colles' fracture. The apparent "bipartite" scaphoid is the result of an old fracture with nonunion (arrow).

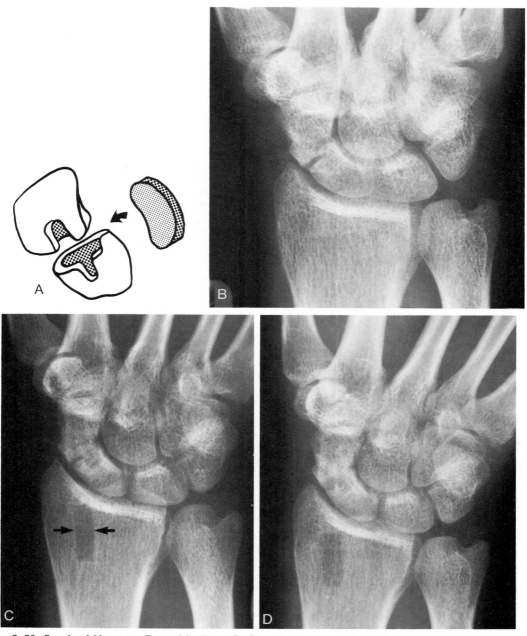

Figure 3–39. Scaphoid Nonunion Treated by Bone Grafting. *A,* Diagram of the Matte-Russe bone graft procedure. *B,* Smooth fracture lines and a gap at the fracture site more than 6 months after injury attest to nonunion. *C,* A Matte-Russe bone graft has been done with bone taken from the distal radius (arrows). *D,* Healing has occurred. (Redrawn from Osterman AL, Bora FW, Jr: Injuries of the wrist. *In* Heppenstall, R.B. Fracture Treatment and Healing. WB Saunders, 1980.)

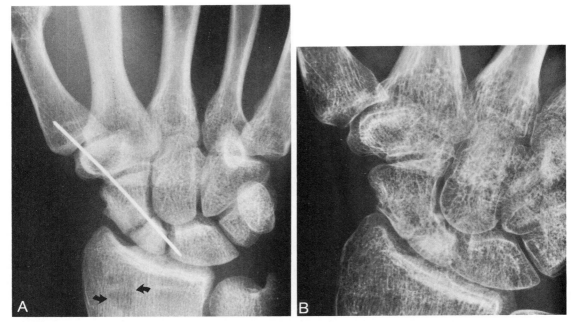

Figure 3–40. Scaphoid Nonunion Treated by Bone Grafting. *A,* Postoperative view documents avascular necrosis of the proximal pole. Bone graft taken from the distal radius has been placed at the fracture site. A pin holds the fracture fragments in position and fixes the scaphoid to the trapezium. Arrows indicate donor graft site. *B,* Seven months later there is healing across the fracture site. There is marked osteopenia (due to immobilization) with the exception of a small area of the proximal scaphoid that remains sclerotic.

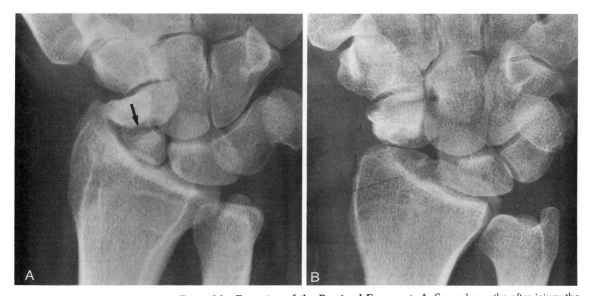

Figure 3–41. Scaphoid Nonunion Treated by Resection of the Proximal Fragment. *A,* Several months after injury the scaphoid fracture (arrow) has not healed. There is bone resorption at the fracture site and some sclerosis but no narrowing of the cartilage space. *B,* The proximal pole of the scaphoid has been removed.

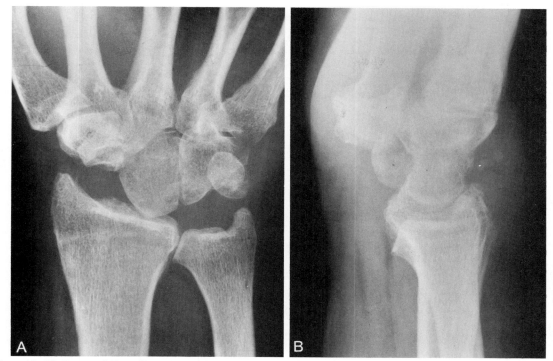

Figure 3–42. Proximal Row Carpectomy. The patient had a scaphoid fracture complicated by avascular necrosis and radiocarpal osteoarthritis. He underwent a proximal row carpectomy. *A,* PA view. The absence of the scaphoid, lunate, and triquetrum is shown. There is articulation between the capitate and the radius. *B,* The lateral view shows the radiocapitate articulation.

displacement of the capitate dorsally in relation to the lunate and the relationship of the lunate to the distal radial articular surface is maintained (Fig. 3–43; Table 3–3). The proximal pole of the scaphoid is rotated dorsally, making it more horizontal in orientation than is normal. On the PA view densities of the capitate and the lunate overlap, and the carpus appears foreshortened. Damage to the volar radiocarpal ligament complex results in a gap between the scaphoid and the lunate.

Table 3–2. Classification of Carpal Dislocations

I. Dorsal perilunate/volar lunate dislocation*
II. Dorsal transscaphoid perilunate dislocation*
III. Volar perilunate/dorsal lunate dislocation
IV. Variants
    Transradial styloid perilunate dislocation*
    Naviculocapitate syndrome
    Transtriquetral fracture-dislocation
    Miscellaneous
V. Isolated rotary scaphoid subluxation
    Acute subluxation
    Recurrent subluxation
VI. Total dislocation of the scaphoid

Source: Green DP, O'Brien ET: Clin Orthop 149:55, 1980.
*The most common patterns of injury.

Volar lunate dislocation is identified on the lateral radiograph by the displacement of the lunate volar to the lip of the radius (Fig. 3–44). The distal articular surface of the lunate is tipped volarly (the "spilled teacup" sign).[62] Spontaneous reduction of a transient perilunate dislocation is suggested by partial contact between the capitate and the distal radial articular surface. On the PA view abnormal rotation of the lunate results in its appearing triangular or wedge shaped, rather than normally trapezoidal. Intermediate patterns, between the classic dorsal perilunate and the volar lunate dislocation, may be seen.

Damage to the median nerve is a frequent clinical complication. Closed reduction may be successful early after injury, and postreduction radiographs should confirm complete reduction. Residual scapholunate dissociation (identified on the frontal view by widening of the scapholunate space), a foreshortened appearance to the scaphoid with a circular (or ring) appearance to its distal pole, a more horizontal orientation of the scaphoid than normal, and a scapholunate angle of more than 80 degrees may occur (see section on scapholunate dissociation). Usually, this is an indication for surgery, since secondary osteoar-

Table 3–3. **Radiographic Findings in Carpal Dislocations**

Projection	Dorsal Perilunate Dislocation	Lunate Dislocation
Lateral	Lunate seated in concave distal radius*	Lunate tilted and displaced anteriorly†
	Capitate displaced dorsally	Capitate partially seated in distal radial articular surface
	Rotation of scaphoid with proximal pole dorsal	
PA	Overlap of proximal and distal carpals Scapholunate gap Foreshortening of scaphoid	Lunate triangular in configuration

*See Figure T3–3A.
†See Figure T3–3B.

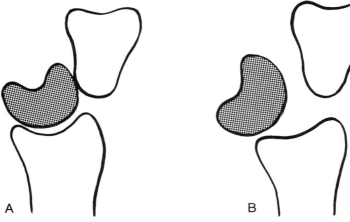

Figure T3–3

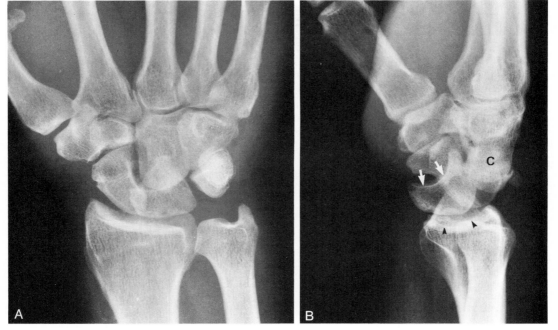

Figure 3–43. Dorsal Perilunate Dislocation. *A,* The PA view shows apparent loss of the capitate-lunate cartilage space and, owing to its volar rotation, a triangular-shaped lunate. *B,* The lateral view confirms the posterior position of the capitate (C) in relation to the lunate. The distal articular surface of the lunate is well seen (arrows) now that it no longer contains the capitate. The proximal articular surface of the lunate maintains contact with the radius (arrowheads).

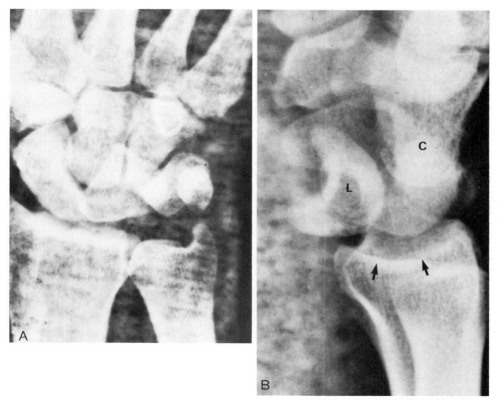

Figure 3–44. Lunate Dislocation. *A,* In the PA view through plaster the lunate, because of its abnormal rotation, shows a triangular shape. There is loss of the normal arcuate line along the proximal carpal row. *B,* The lateral view confirms the loss of contact between the capitate (C) and the lunate (LL) and between the lunate and the radial articular surface (arrows).

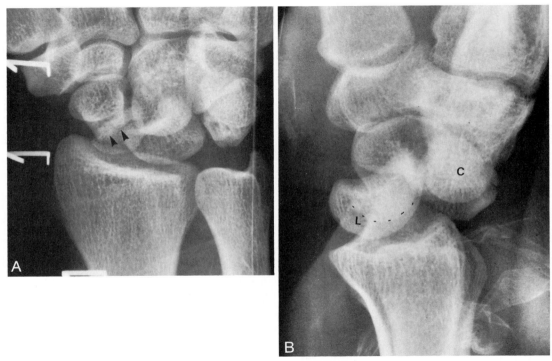

Figure 3–45. Transscaphoid Perilunate Dislocation. *A,* There is a fracture through the scaphoid (arrowheads). The lunate is somewhat triangular in appearance as a result of its abnormal rotation. *B,* The lateral view confirms the integrity of the radiolunate articulation and the abnormal posterior position of the capitate (C) in relation to the lunate (L). The proximal pole of the scaphoid (dotted) has shifted anteriorly with the lunate and is superimposed on it.

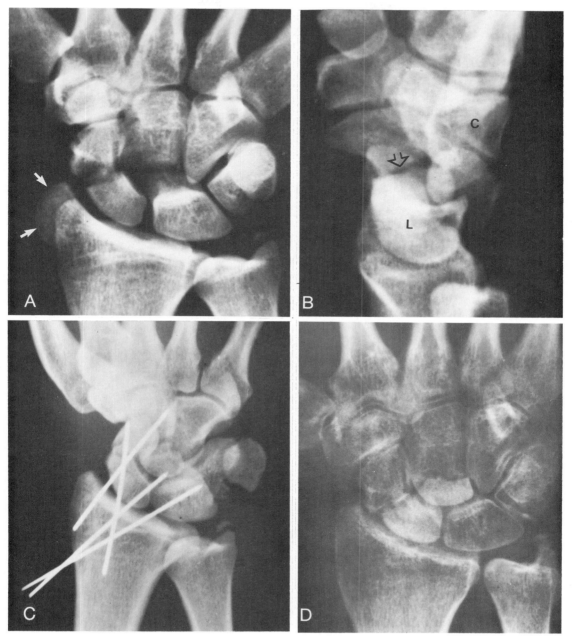

Figure 3–46. Naviculocapitate Syndrome. *A,* There is a scaphoid waist fracture, an ulnar styloid fracture, and a fracture of the proximal pole of the capitate, with the fragment (arrows) displaced so that it overlies the radial styloid. *B,* The lateral view shows the empty lunate (L) articular surface. The capitate (C) is displaced slightly posteriorly. The scaphoid fracture can be seen (arrow). *C,* After open reduction and internal fixation has been performed, an oblique view shows the fracture fragments repositioned. *D,* A follow-up radiograph 4 months after injury shows increased density of the proximal poles of the scaphoid and capitate, indicating avascular necrosis. The fractures have not yet healed.

Table 3–4. Carpal Instability Patterns

	Normal	Dorsiflexion Instability	Palmar Flexion Instability	Ulnar Translocation	Dorsal Subluxation	Palmar Subluxation
Scapholunate angle	30°–60°	60–80° = borderline; > 80° = abnormal	< 30°	Normal	Normal	Normal
Capitate–lunate angle	0–30°	Normal	> 30°	Normal	Normal	Normal
Comments		Lunate tipped dorsally; scaphoid tipped toward palm	Lunate and scaphoid tipped toward palm	> 50% lunate medial to radius on PA view with hand in neutral	Shift of carpals dorsal to midplane of radius on lateral view	Shift of carpals anterior to midplane of radius on lateral view

Source: Gilula LA, Weeks PM: Radiology 129:641, 1978.

thritis may result if the scapholunate dissociation remains untreated.

Residual tilting of the lunate dorsally (dorsiflexion instability) should also be looked for on the immediate postreduction and follow-up radiographs. Identification of this tilting suggests the need for open reduction.

Dorsal Trans-Scaphoid Perilunate Dislocation. The findings in this injury are similar to those of the dorsal perilunate dislocation except that there is in addition a fracture through the waist of the scaphoid (Fig. 3–45). The distal pole of the scaphoid is displaced dorsally in relation to the capitate, and the proximal pole remains with the lunate.

After closed reduction, restoration of the normal radiolunate-capitate relationships should be demonstrated on the lateral view, and the scaphoid fracture should be anatomically positioned. Failure to reduce or loss of reduction of the scaphoid fracture may lead to nonunion, post-traumatic dorsiflexion instability, or both. Therefore, open reduction and internal fixation are often indicated if anatomical reduction of the scaphoid fracture is not obtained or is not maintained.

Transradial Styloid Perilunate Dislocation. Perilunate or lunate dislocation may be associated with radial styloid, rather than scaphoid, fracture. As emphasized by Green and O'Brien, one should suspect this combination when evaluating a patient with an apparently isolated radial styloid fracture.[62]

Naviculocapitate Syndrome. This designation refers to the association of a midcarpal dislocation with a fracture of the proximal pole of the capitate and rotation of the fracture fragment 90 or 180 degrees (Fig. 3–46). Residual displacement of the capitate fragment after closed reduction may be an indication for operative intervention.

Carpal Instability

Disruption of normal alignment between carpals and between the carpals and the radius is termed *carpal instability.*[68] It may be due to fracture, to ligamentous damage as a consequence of trauma, or to inflammatory conditions such as rheumatoid arthritis. (Although fractures produce instability similar to that from other causes, they are discussed separately, earlier in the chapter.)

Classification. Linscheid and co-workers classify carpal instability into two major types, dorsal and volar, depending on whether the distal lunate articular surface is directed dorsally (dorsiflexed) or volarly (palmar-flexed) relative to the long axes of the radius and capitate.[73] The terms used are *dorsiflexion instability,* or *dorsiflexed intercalated segment instability* (abbreviated DISI), and *volar flexion instability,* or *volar-flexed* (palmar-flexed) *intercalated segment instability* (VISI). In addition ulnar translocation of the carpals and dorsal and volar subluxation of the carpals have been recognized.

Radiographic Examination (Table 3–4). Although characteristic abnormalities may be identified on routine radiographic examination, patients with persistent unexplained pain or limitation of wrist motion who are suspected of having ligamentous instability may require additional views. The full series includes (1) posteroanterior views in neutral as well as in ulnar and radial deviation; (2) anteroposterior views with the fist tightly clenched (compression); (3) routine oblique view; (4) lateral views with the wrist in neutral, flexion, and extension; and (5) lateral view in neutral position with the fist clenched.[69]

The views in flexion and extension and in radial and ulnar deviation help to demonstrate the dynamics of wrist motion. The clenched-fist views compress the wrist, tending to force the capitate into the space between the scaphoid and the lunate and to rotate the scaphoid toward the palm, thus revealing any tendency for abnormal scaphoid rotation or scapholunate separation.[69] Transient subluxation may be demonstrated during fluoroscopic examination.[74]

Scapholunate Dissociation. Scapholunate dissociation may accompany any of the four collapse patterns previously mentioned, but it is

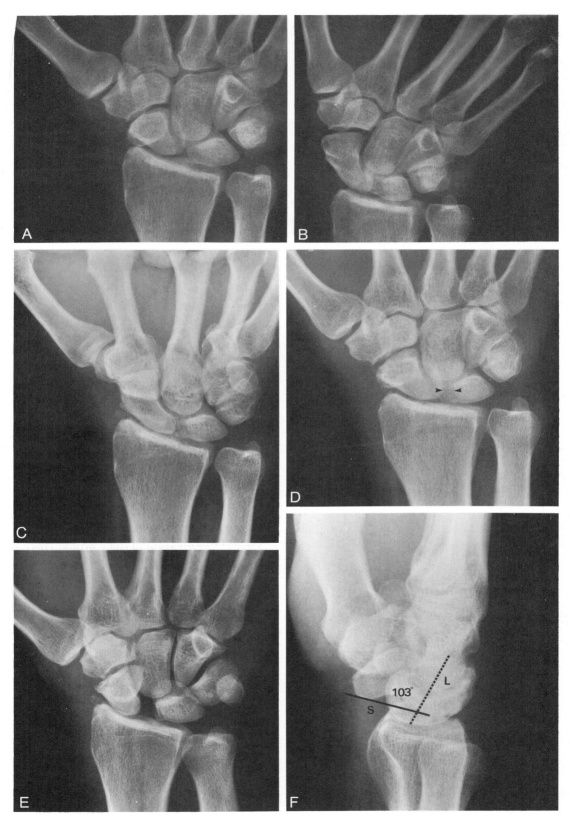

Figure 3–47. *See legend on opposite page*

almost always an accompanying finding in cases of dorsiflexion instability.[68] Characteristically, the scaphoid rotates in such a way that its proximal pole is directed more dorsally and its distal pole more volarly than is normal, thus producing rotatory subluxation of the scaphoid.[69] The condition usually results from ligamentous disruption due to trauma or to rheumatoid arthritis. Experimental sectioning of the interosseous scapholunate ligament produces minimal separation between these bones.[6] When the radioscaphoid ligament (between the radius and the dorsal aspect of the scaphoid) is also divided, scapholunate dissociation is produced.

The condition may be associated with pain, decreased grip strength, and clicking or snapping and may lead to secondary degenerative arthritis.[72, 73]

Findings may be normal on standard radiographic views, and the additional views described previously may be necessary. Abnormal findings (Figs. 3–47 and 3–48) include the following:[72]

1. *A wide scapholunate distance* (the "Terry Thomas sign," from British actor Terry Thomas's wide space between his front teeth). Normally the scapholunate distance is less than 2 mm.[73] Ligamentous disruption is suspected when a measurement of 2 to 4 mm is present and is certain if the measured distance is 4 mm or more.[69] Widening of the scapholunate space may be demonstrated at the time of fluoroscopy, when the wrist is observed during a range of motion. Linscheid and associates noted widening of this distance in dorsiflexion and ulnar or forced radial deviation.[73]

2. *Foreshortened appearance of the scaphoid.* This appearance is due to rotation of the distal pole of the scaphoid toward the palm. In contrast to the normal wrist, this foreshortening does not disappear on ulnar deviation.

3. *Ring sign.* This sign refers to the density produced by the cortex of the distal pole of the scaphoid seen end-on because of the abnormal scaphoid rotation. Normal individuals may exhibit this finding on frontal views taken with the hand in radial deviation; however, this appearance should not persist when the hand is ulnar deviated.

4. Arthrography can confirm disruption of the scapholunate ligament by demonstrating *extension of contrast medium* into the midcarpal cartilage space after the radiocarpal joint has been injected (Fig. 3–49).

Dorsiflexion Instability (DISI). In dorsiflexion instability the distal articular surface of the lunate faces dorsally. The scaphoid remains in normal position, or its distal pole tips toward the palm. Thus, the carpal rows are no longer linked normally.[69]

Radiographic findings of dorsiflexion instability include (1) overlap of the lunate and capitate on a PA view with the hand and forearm flat against the film and (2) an increased scapholunate angle (greater than 80 degrees) on lateral view.[68, 69]

Volar Flexion Instability (VISI). In volar flexion instability the distal articular surface of the lunate is tilted volarly (Fig. 3–50). The distal portion of the capitate is directed dorsally, increasing the capitolunate angle to greater than 30 degrees.[68] The scapholunate angle is less than 30 degrees. Frontal views show that the lunate overlaps the capitate.

Ulnar Translocation. In this condition the carpals are shifted toward the ulna, leaving an abnormally wide space between the radial styloid and the scaphoid.[68] On the frontal view in neutral position the trapezium is closer than normal to the radial styloid, and 50 percent or more of the lunate does not contact the distal radial articular surface.[69] On ulnar deviation the lunate does not return to its normal position above the radius. This is a fairly common deformity in patients with rheumatoid arthritis (Fig. 3–51).[67]

Dorsal Subluxation of the Carpus. This condition is characterized by shift of the entire carpus dorsal to the midpoint of the distal radial articular surface. Normally, the distal radial articular surface tilts volarly, and the dorsal lip of the radius presents a barrier to dorsal displacement of the carpals. Loss of this barrier may result from an impacted Colles' fracture, allowing subsequent dorsal subluxation of the carpals to occur.

Anterior Displacement of the Carpus. This abnormality is most frequent in patients with

---

Figure 3–47. Scapholunate Dissociation. All views show an abnormally wide separation between the proximal scaphoid and the lunate, although in several the gap (arrowheads, in traction view) is obscured by the superimposed lunate. In this figure, the supination view most clearly shows the separation. The lateral view shows the dorsal tilt of the lunate, indicating dorsal intercalated segmental instability (DISI), and the scapholunate angle is increased. The scaphoid (S) and lunate (L) axes and the scapholunate angle are indicated.

A, PA; *B*, ulnar deviation; *C*, compression; *D*, traction; *E*, supination; and *F*, lateral views.

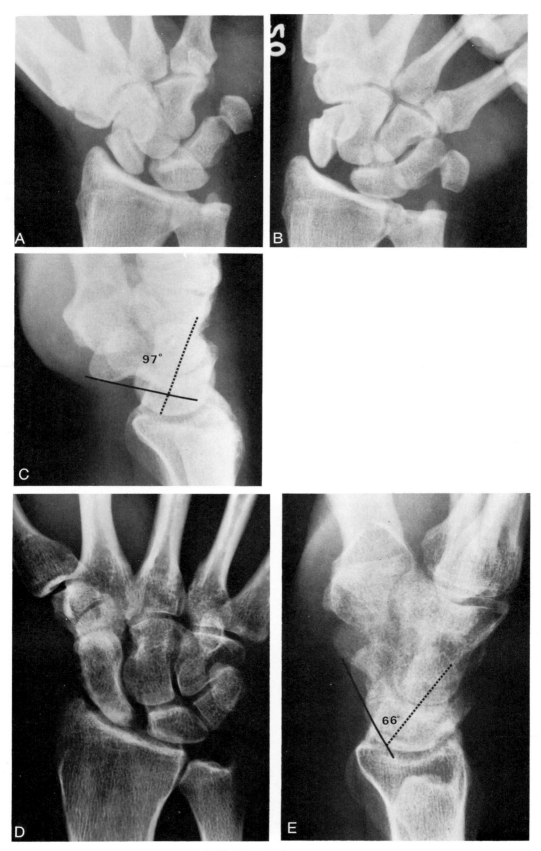

Figure 3–48. *See legend on opposite page*

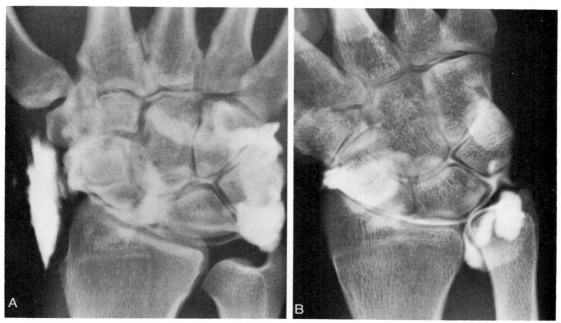

Figure 3–49. Scapholunate Dissociation Arthrogram. *A,* Injection of the radiocarpal joint showed filling of the scapholunate articulation and extension of contrast into the midcarpal and the carpometacarpal compartments. The lunate-triquetral space is also filled but was noted on fluoroscopy to fill from the midcarpal joint (retrograde), indicating that the proximal ligaments were intact. The contrast agent along the radial aspect of the wrist was extravasated during injection. The radial injection site insures that any extravasation will not obscure the scapholunate area. *B,* In another patient the lunate-triquetral space fills with contrast material injected into the radiocarpal joint. The slight offset of the lunate and triquetrum attests to the instability at this level (lunate-triquetral instability). The radioulnar joint has also filled, indicating a perforation in the triangular fibrocartilage.

Figure 3–48. Scapholunate Dissociation. *A,* An AP view with the hand in radial deviation shows the normally foreshortened appearance of the scaphoid in this position. The scapholunate distance is slightly wide. *B,* The ulnar deviation view shows that the scaphoid has not rotated normally and therefore continues to show a foreshortened appearance. The marked widening of the scapholunate distance is brought out in this view. *C,* The lateral view shows the scaphoid to be more horizontal in position than normal, with increase in the scapholunate angle. The scaphoid axis (solid line) and the lunate axis (dashed line) are marked. Postoperative PA view *(D)* and lateral view *(E)* show that the scaphoid has been rotated so that its distal pole is more dorsal than on preoperative views, and the scaphoid no longer has a foreshortened appearance. The distal pole of the scaphoid has been fused to the trapezium and the trapezoid. The scapholunate distance continues to be abnormally wide, but the scapholunate angle is decreased.

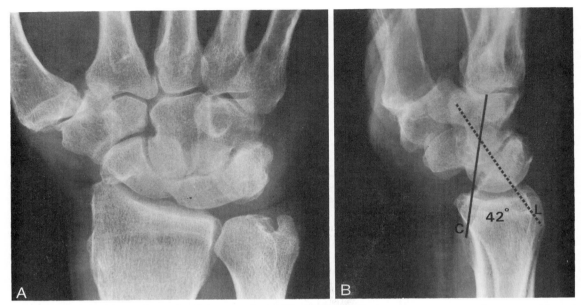

Figure 3–50. Volar Flexion Intercalated Segment Instability (VISI). *A,* PA view shows an apparently narrow midcarpal cartilage space and overlap of proximal and distal carpal rows. The lunate appears triangular in shape because of its abnormal tilt. *B,* Lateral view confirms anterior tilt of the lunate and dorsal tilt of the distal capitate, with an increased (more than 30 degrees) capitolunate angle.

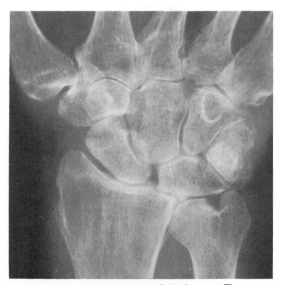

Figure 3–51. Rheumatoid Arthritis with Ulnar Translocation of the Lunate. The proximal carpal row has shifted toward the ulna, documented by the failure of the radial articular surface to contact at least 50 per cent of the lunate articular surface. Also noted are narrowing of the radiocarpal cartilage space, slight widening of the scapholunate distance, and small osteophytes from the lunate. The ulna is now articulating with the lunate.

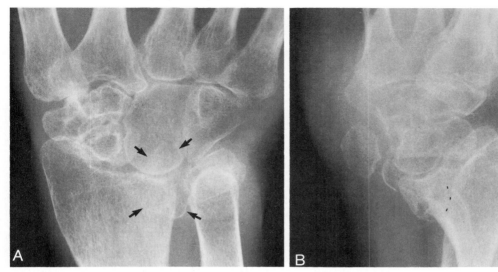

Figure 3–52. Anterior and Ulnar Subluxation of the Wrist in Rheumatoid Arthritis. *A,* PA view shows the lunate (arrows) overlying the distal radius and radioulnar joint. The scaphoid has rotated, giving it a foreshortened appearance. *B,* An oblique view confirms anterior (as well as ulnar) subluxation of the lunate (dashed line) owing to extensive erosion of the anterior aspect of the radius. Erosion of the pisiform is incidentally noted.

rheumatoid arthritis.[67] The carpals are displaced anterior to the midline of the radius (Fig. 3–52).

Kienböck's Disease

Robert Kienböck described the radiographic and clinical features of the disorder that he called traumatic malacia of the lunate.[80] It is believed that this condition represents post-traumatic avascular necrosis occurring in a susceptible population.[76] Individuals thought to be prone to the development of this disorder include those with variations in blood supply and those with relatively short ulnae.[81] Such short ulnae (negative ulnar variance) have been noted more frequently in patients with Kienböck's disease than in a normal population, and this variation is thought to lead to a concentration of forces on the lunate.[54, 76, 78]

Kienböck's disease is more frequently seen in males and is usually unilateral, with a tendency for involvement of the dominant hand.[54, 76, 80] A history of prior injury is often obtained, and radiographically identifiable fractures have been noted in 72 percent of patients in one series.[76]

Radiographic Findings. Radiographic findings have been classified by Lichtman and coworkers into the following stages (Figs. 3–53 and 3–54):[82]

Stage 1–Linear or compression fracture of the lunate with normal bone density is noted.

Stage 2–Density of the lunate appears in-

creased in relation to that of the other carpal bones. Later in this stage there is loss of height of the radial aspect of the lunate.

Stage 3–Collapse of the lunate associated with proximal migration of the capitate and spreading of the proximal carpal row is evident. Collapse can be quantified by noting the ratio between the length of the carpus and the length of the third metacarpal (Fig. 3–55). Normally, this ratio is 0.54 ± 0.03.[83, 84] Rotatory subluxation of the scaphoid may occur.

Stage 4–There is secondary osteoarthritis. Early diagnosis may be facilitated by the use of tomography to demonstrate lunate fracture.[76, 82] Bone scanning may be of help.[77a]

Treatment. Several modes of treatment have been suggested, depending on the deformity and the presence of secondary osteoarthritis. Immobilization alone may be accompanied by collapse of the lunate, resulting in carpal instability. Before lunate collapse occurs ulnar lengthening to correct negative ulnar variance has been suggested (Fig. 3–56).[54, 76] Silastic replacement of the lunate has been thought to be most satisfactory in early stages, before marked collapse has occurred, although Stark and colleagues recommend this procedure only after collapse.[84] Lunate excision, removal of the proximal carpal row, and radiocarpal fusion have been suggested when secondary osteoarthritis has occurred.[54, 76, 77, 79, 82]

153

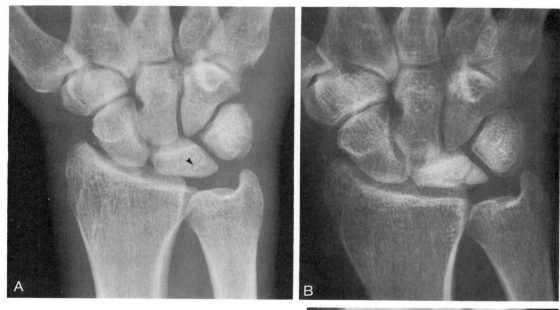

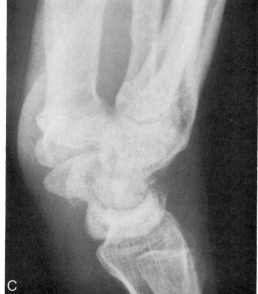

Figure 3–53. Kienböck's Disease (Stages 1 and 2). *A*, PA radiograph shows slightly increased density of the lunate. A faint fracture line is seen (arrowhead). The cartilage spaces remain normal. PA *(B)* and lateral *(C)* views 8 months later show flattening of the lunate in addition to a more marked increase in its density. Increased density in these cases is due to a combination of factors: osteoporosis of the adjacent bones, compression of trabeculae, and the laying down of new bone on dead trabeculae.

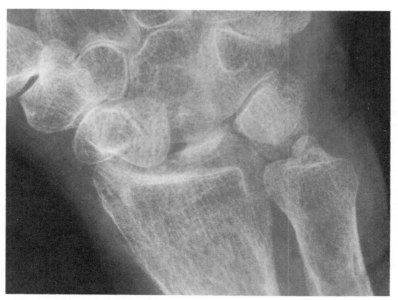

Figure 3–54. Kienböck's Disease (Stage 3). There is marked flattening of the lunate, apparently representing the end stage of Kienböck's disease. This was an incidental finding.

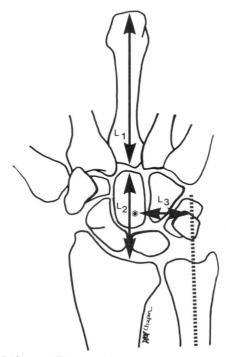

Figure 3–55. Measuring Carpal Deformity. The *carpal height* (L_2) is the distance from the base of the third metacarpal to the distal radius. When L_2 is divided by the third metacarpal length (L_1), the result is normally 0.54 ± 0.03. Collapse of the wrist is indicated by a decrease in this ratio. The *carpal–ulnar distance* (L_3) is measured as the perpendicular distance from the center of the head of the capitate to a line through the long axis of the ulna. The ratio of this distance to the third metacarpal length (L_3:L_1) is normally 0.3 ± 0.03. A decrease in this ratio indicates shift of the carpals in an ulnar direction. (Redrawn from McMurtry RY, et al. J Bone Joint Surg (Am) 59:899, 1977.)

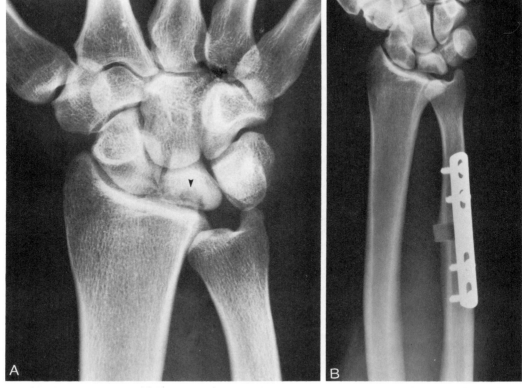

Figure 3–56. Avascular Necrosis of the Lunate. *A,* PA view shows increased density of the lunate with a proximal lucent area (arrowhead) characteristic of avascular necrosis. The subchondral cortex of the proximal lunate is flattened, but the radiocarpal cartilage space remains normal. The ulna is abnormally short (negative ulnar variance). *B,* A bone graft has been inserted in the ulna to correct the negative ulnar variance.

Wrist Fusion

Severe wrist damage, particularly in patients with advanced rheumatoid arthritis, may be treated by wrist fusion or by arthroplasty. The fusion technique of Millender and Nalebuff includes excision of the distal ulna and the articular cartilage, fibrous tissue, and sclerotic bone of the radiocarpal joint (Fig. 3–57).[90] A Steinmann pin is placed through the carpus, the distal end exiting between the second and third metacarpals and the proximal end positioned in the radial shaft. Additional staples are placed across the dorsal aspect of the radiocarpal joint. Currently, it is felt that the wrist should be positioned in the neutral or slightly flexed position.[92] Alternative techniques of wrist fusion include the insertion of bone graft[85] and the technique of Mannerfelt and Malmsten, in which a Rush rod is inserted into the shaft of the third metacarpal and is driven into the medullary canal of the radius.[88]

Following successful fusion stability, strength, and dexterity are increased and relief of pain originating in the radiocarpal joint is noted.[85, 90, 91] Flexion–extension motion is eliminated, but supination and pronation are preserved. Complications are uncommon but include infection, pseudarthrosis, and distal migration of the pin (Fig. 3–58).

Wrist Prostheses

Wrist fusion may result in functional disability in patients with bilateral disease or severe proximal joint disease, such as frequently occurs in those with rheumatoid arthritis. Patients in whom pain is the predominant symptom but in whom significant range of motion is preserved may be reluctant to undergo fusion. In these cases arthroplasty rather than fusion is considered. Nalebuff and Millender favor wrist arthroplasty over fusion when there are good bone stock, an adequate third metacarpal intramedullary canal, functioning extensor tendons, and involvement of the opposite wrist. Contraindications to arthroplasty include marked deformity or instability, excessive bone loss, and the presence of multiple tendon ruptures.[87, 92]

Several types of wrist replacement are available (Figs. 3–59 and 3–62). The Swanson sili-

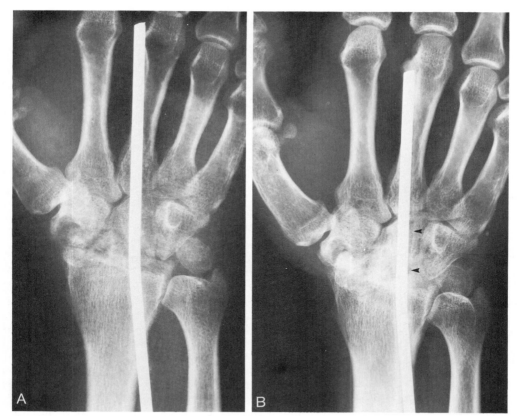

Figure 3–57. Carpal Fusion. The patient had a scaphoid fracture with nonunion and avascular necrosis for which he underwent bone grafting, eventual Silastic replacement of the scaphoid, and finally wrist fusion. PA views immediately after surgery *(A)* and 1 year later *(B)* show that much of the proximal carpal row has been excised. The rod protrudes from the radius and has migrated proximally and loosened distally (arrowheads), but the fusion is solid, with trabecular continuity across the radiocarpal joint at 1 year.

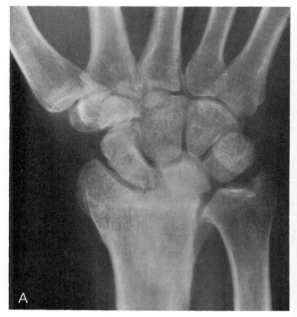

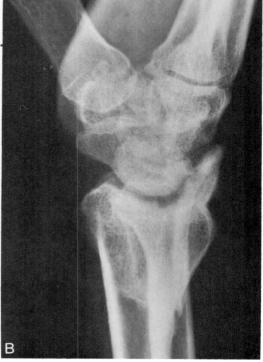

Figure 3–58. Failed Wrist Fusion. *A,* PA view suggests trabecular continuity across the radiocarpal joint. *B,* Lateral view, however, shows a shelf of bone posteriorly but no fusion across the joint.

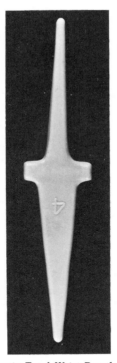

cone rubber prosthesis is similar in shape to the silicone rubber finger prosthesis (Figs. 3–59 and 3–60). The lunate, the proximal scaphoid, the radial half of the triquetrum, and the radial styloid are resected so that the resection margins are perpendicular to the long axis of the radius. The distal ulna is usually resected, and an ulnar prosthesis may or may not be inserted. The wrist prosthesis is placed so that the distal stem is in the capitate and the third metacarpal and the proximal stem is in the radius. The central portion of the prosthesis should be flush against the radius and the capitate, and the alignment of the hand on the wrist should be correct. The capsule is closed with sutures that pass through drill holes in the dorsal and radial aspects of the radial cortex.

Radiographically identifiable complications include osteomyelitis (although no such case was reported in 37 wrist prostheses reviewed by Goodman and associates), failure to seat the distal stem of the prosthesis within the medullary canal of the third metacarpal, recurrence of or failure to correct the deformity, collapse of the carpus around the prosthesis, and prosthetic fracture. Fracture of the prosthesis was noted in 8 percent of cases reviewed by Goodman and

Figure 3–59. Silastic Total Wrist Prosthesis. View from the dorsal surface shows the broad proximal and thin distal stems of the prosthesis.

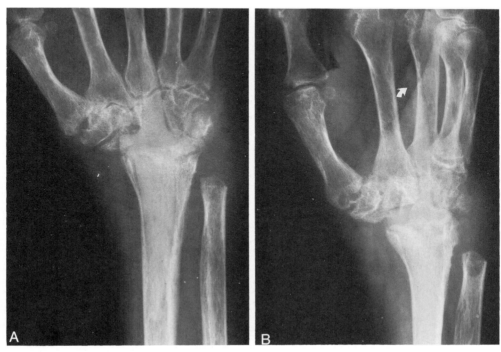

Figure 3–60. Silastic Wrist Prosthesis. This patient with severe rheumatoid arthritis underwent radiocarpal replacement with a Silastic prosthesis. *A,* PA view shows that the ulnar portion of the scaphoid and the proximal capitate have been removed. The lunate is subluxed toward the ulna. A Silastic prosthesis with the proximal stem in the radius and the distal stem overlying the third metacarpal is seen. The distal ulna has been resected. *B,* Oblique view shows the distal stem (arrow) to lie at least partially outside the metacarpal.

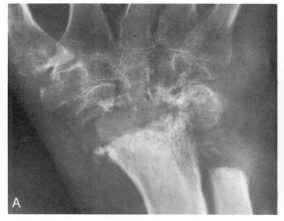

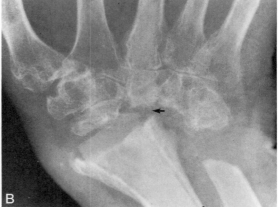

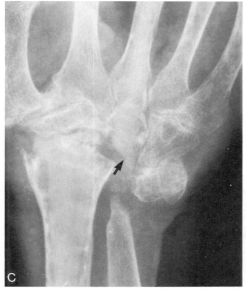

Figure 3–61. Fracture of Silastic Total Wrist Prosthesis. *A,* A total wrist prosthesis is in place. *B,* Radiographs 2 years later show disruption of the prosthesis at the base of the distal stem (arrow) and marked ulnar subluxation of the carpals. *C,* Another case in which the prosthesis has broken between the barrel and distal stem (arrow) and the carpus has shifted toward the ulna. (Courtesy of Dr. Lewis Millender, Brookline, Mass.)

colleagues. In all cases fracture occurred between the distal stem and the barrel of the prosthesis, and in two of the three prosthetic fractures in this series, failure to correct ulnar deviation was noted prior to component fracture (Fig. 3–61).

In addition to the silicone rubber prosthesis, metal-to-plastic prostheses in which the components are secured with methylmethacrylate cement have been developed (Fig. 3–62).[86, 89, 94] The Meuli prosthesis consists of two metal components separated by a freely movable polyethylene ball. The distal metallic component has a cupped articular surface and two stems, which are cemented into the carpus and second and third metacarpals. The proximal metal trunnion component is cemented into the radius. Complications have included infection, difficulties in technical insertion, dislocation, and stem breakage.

Carpal Prostheses

Silicone rubber implants are available for replacement of the scaphoid or lunate. The prostheses developed by Swanson and Swanson have the shape of the normal bone but more prominent concavities and a projecting stem that fits into an adjacent carpal bone in order to facilitate placement of the prosthesis at surgery and provide early postoperative stability (Figs. 3–63 to 3–65). The stem of the scaphoid prosthesis fits into the trapezium and that of the lunate into the triquetrum. These implants act as space fillers that prevent migration of the other carpal bones. Such prostheses are usually considered for patients with avascular necrosis of the lunate, long-standing carpal dislocation, localized osteoarthritis, or severe or complicated scaphoid fractures. In appropriate cases carpal stability and motion are said to be improved, and pain is relieved. Soft tissue support and

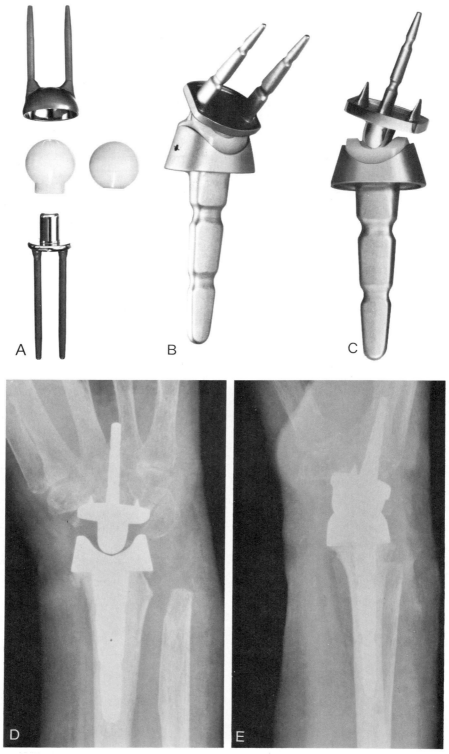

A   B   C

D   E

Figure 3–62. *See legend on opposite page*

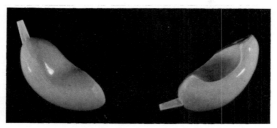

Figure 3–63. Swanson Silastic Scaphoid Prosthesis. The stem of the prosthesis is inserted into the trapezium to help provide stability.

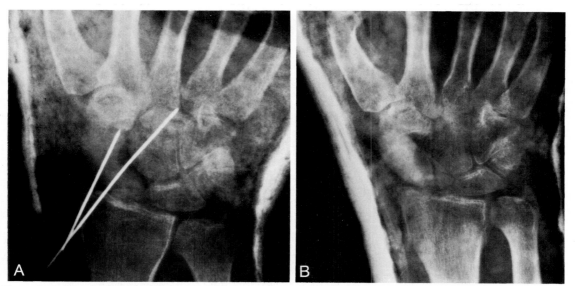

Figure 3–64. Scaphoid Prosthesis. *A*, Immediate postoperative view through plaster shows the scaphoid prosthesis held by two pins. *B*, After removal of the pins the scaphoid has rotated. There is dislocation at the scaphotrapezial joint.

Figure 3–62. Cemented Total Wrist Prostheses. *A*, Meuli total wrist prosthesis. The Meuli prosthesis consists of two separate, stemmed, metal components with a freely movable polyethylene piece between them. The stems of the proximal component are cemented into the radius, and those of the cupped distal component are cemented into the second and third metacarpals. The stems may be bent to achieve proper position. Other models of this prosthesis are available with changes in the distal fixation stems. The distal ulna and radius, scaphoid, lunate, and triquetrum and the proximal capitate are excised. *B* and *C*, Volz (AMC) total wrist prostheses (Howmedica). These prostheses allow motion in two planes (radioulnar deviation and flexion-extension). The components are cemented into the radius and second and third metacarpals. *D*, PA and *E*, lateral views of a Volz prosthesis in place. The tip of the distal stem is incorrectly placed outside the metacarpal shaft.

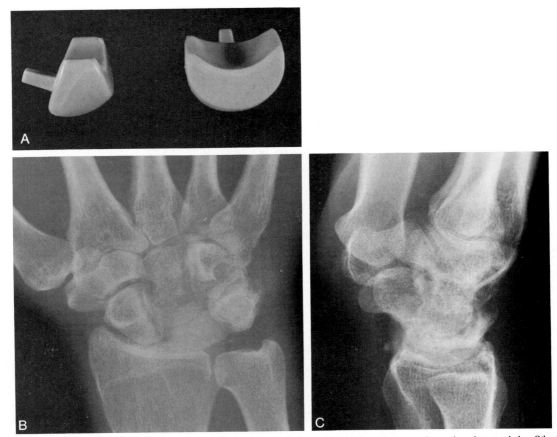

Figure 3–65. Lunate Prosthesis (Swanson and Swanson). *A,* Lateral and frontal views show the shape of the Silastic prosthesis. The stem is inserted into the triquetrum for stability. *B,* PA view, and *C,* lateral view, show a Silastic lunate replacement done because of avascular necrosis (Kienböck's disease).

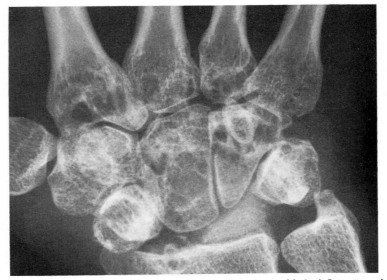

Figure 3–66. Synovitis Following Insertion of a Silastic Lunate Prosthesis. Marked flattening of the prosthesis and development of soft tissue swelling, bone erosion, and cyst-like areas have occurred. (Courtesy of Dr. Daniel I. Rosenthal, Boston, Mass.)

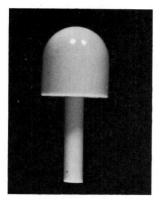

Figure 3–67. Distal Ulnar Silastic Prosthesis.

foreign body reaction may occur in response to silicone particles (Fig. 3–66).[97, 102]

A silicone rubber implant to cap the distal ulna after the ulnar head has been resected has been developed. This implant is used in patients with rheumatoid arthritis in particular because in these cases resection of the distal ulna (the Darrach procedure) may be complicated by instability of the distal ulna due to poor ligamentous support. In addition progressive shift of the carpals toward the ulna, bony overgrowth at the resected bone margin, rupture of the extensor tendons where they contact an irregular edge of resected bone, and loss of function of the extensor carpi ulnaris tendon have been noted. Apparently, capping of the distal ulna by a stemmed implant preserves the anatomical relationships and the function of the distal radioulnar joint. The Swanson prosthesis has an intramedullary stem and a cuffed, dome-shaped head (Fig. 3–67). The prosthesis is placed so that its stem fits snugly into the canal and its cuff covers the bone end loosely. For stability sutures may be passed through both the implant and the drill holes in the ulna. Postoperative complications include malposition or distal migration of the implant. Bone resorption at the resection margins has been noted and is thought to be due to vascular impairment from too tight a fit of the cuff of the prosthesis on the distal ulna (Fig. 3–68).

continuity must be present or established around the prostheses; therefore their use is contraindicated in cases in which this support is inadequate.

Generalized cartilage loss in the wrist and markedly decreased space for insertion of the prosthesis are other contraindications. The size of the prosthesis selected must be appropriate. Small Kirschner wires may be inserted for the immediate postoperative period in order to transfix the prosthesis and hold it in proper alignment to the other carpal bones. Radiologically detectable complications include dislocation, malposition and fragmentation of the prosthesis, and infection (Fig. 3–64). In addition a

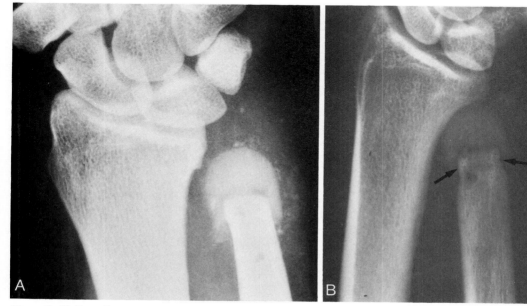

Figure 3–68. Bone Resorption Under Silastic Ulnar Prosthesis. *A,* Immediate postoperative, and *B,* follow-up, radiographs. Tapering of the cortical margins (arrows) and bone loss from the distal ulna have occurred since the immediate postoperative examination.

Carpal Tunnel Syndrome

This entrapment syndrome is due to compression of the median nerve as it passes (with the flexor tendons of the fingers) through the carpal tunnel. The carpal tunnel is bounded dorsally by the bones of the carpus and anteriorly by the transverse carpal ligament, which inserts on the trapezium, the scaphoid, and occasionally the radial styloid and extends to the pisiform and the hook of the hamate (see Fig. 3–15). Within this tunnel the median nerve may be compressed, usually by tenosynovitis of the flexor tendons. This condition is usually localized and is unassociated with systemic disease. However, rheumatoid arthritis; hypothyroidism; amyloidosis; gout; acromegaly; and a variety of local disorders, including an adjacent osteoid osteoma, may occur in association with this syndrome.[103, 104]

The median nerve is a mixed sensory-motor nerve, but sensory changes usually occur first, with numbness or paresthesias of the thumb, the index, the middle and one half of the ring finger, usually worse at night and often bilateral, noted.[104] Pain may extend proximally into the forearm, shoulder, or neck.

Radiographic examination may be of some help in assessing the presence of systemic disorders or localized abnormalities such as an osteoid osteoma. The carpal tunnel view may show evidence of rheumatoid erosion. Injection of contrast material into the synovial sheaths of the flexor tendons allows demonstration of tenosynovitis.[105]

Calcific Tendinitis

Calcific tendinitis, comparable in all respects to the more frequent variety in the shoulder, may occur in tendons of the wrist and the fingers.[107, 109, 111–113] The flexor carpi ulnaris tendon is the most commonly reported site. This tendon inserts on the pisiform and then continues distally, as the pisohamate and pisometacarpal ligaments, to insert on the hamate and the fifth metacarpal.[110] Calcification in this tendon or in the adjacent ulnar styloid recess is therefore projected on radiographs proximal or distal, lateral, medial, or volar to the pisiform (Fig. 3–69).

Acute symptoms are associated with focal inflammation resulting in severe localized pain, tenderness, swelling, erythema and warmth, and painful limitation of motion. Prior trauma related to occupational and recreational activities such as golf, typing, violin playing, and bowling may precipitate acute symptoms. The treatment is similar to that for calcific tendinitis elsewhere. Calcification may disappear as symptoms subside.

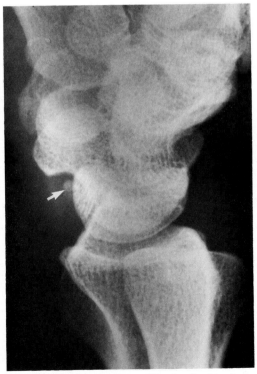

Figure 3–69. Calcific Tendinitis. Pain, localized tenderness, and soft tissue swelling were noted after an evening of bowling. The lateral radiograph of the wrist confirms calcification in the area of the flexor carpi ulnaris tendon (arrow).

References

Normal Anatomy and Function

1. International Federation of Societies for Surgery of the Hand: Terminology for Hand Surgery. Brentwood, Essex, Westbury, 1970.

1a. Epner RA, Bowers WH, Guilford WB: Ulnar variance—The effect of wrist positioning and roentgen film technique. J Hand Surg 7:298–305, 1982.

2. Kauer JMG: Functional anatomy of the wrist. Clin Orthop 149:9–20, 1980.

3. Leibolt FL: Surgical fusion of wrist joint. Surg Gynecol Obstet 66:1008–1023, 1938.

4. MacConaill MA: The mechanical anatomy of the carpus and its bearings on some surgical problems. J Anat 75:166–175, 1941.

5. Martel W, Hayes JT, Duff IF: The pattern of bone erosion in the hand and wrist in rheumatoid arthritis. Radiology 84:204–214, 1965.

6. Mayfield JK, Johnson RP, Kilcoyne RF: The ligaments of the human wrist and their functional significance. Anat Rec 186:417–428, 1976.

7. Palmer AK, Werner FW: The triangular fibrocartilage complex of the wrist—anatomy and function. J Hand Surg 61:153–171, 1981.

8. Taleisnik J: The ligaments of the wrist. J Hand Surg 1:110–118, 1976.
9. Tubiana R: The Hand. Vol. 1. Philadelphia, WB Saunders, 1981.
10. Warwick R, Williams PL: Gray's Anatomy. 36th Br. ed. Philadelphia, WB Saunders, 1982.
11. Youm Y, Flatt AE: Kinematics of the wrist. Clin Orthop 149:21–32, 1980.

Normal Radiographic Examination

12. Arkless R: Cineradiography in normal and abnormal wrists. AJR 96:837–844, 1966.
13. Gelberman RH, Salamon PB, Jurist JM, Posch JL: Ulnar variance in Kienböck's disease. J Bone Joint Surg (Am) 57:674–676, 1975.
14. Gilula LA: Carpal injuries: analytic approach and case exercises. AJR 133:503–517, 1979.
15. Gilula LA, Weeks PM: Post-traumatic ligamentous instabilities of the wrist. Radiology 129:641–651, 1978.
16. Keats TE, Teeslink R, Diamond AE, Williams JH: Normal axial relationships of the major joints. Radiology 87:904–907, 1966.
17. Lewis RW: The Joints of the Extremities, A Radiographic Study. Springfield, Ill. CC Thomas, 1955.
18. Linscheid RL, Dobyns JH, Beabout JW, Bryan RS: Traumatic instability of the wrist: Diagnosis, classification and pathomechanics. J Bone Joint Surg (Am) 54:1612–1632, 1972.
19. Resnick D: Rheumatoid arthritis of the wrist: Why the ulnar styloid? Radiology 112:29–35, 1974.
20. Weston WJ: De Quervain's disease. Br J Radiol 40:446–448, 1967.

Wrist Arthrography

21. Dalinka MK, Turner ML, Osterman AL, Batra P: Wrist arthrography. Radiol Clin North Am 19:217–226, 1981.
22. Harrison MO, Freiberger RH, Ranawat CS: Arthrography of the rheumatoid wrist joint. AJR 112:480–486, 1971.
23. Iveson JMI, Hill AGS, Wright V: Wrist cysts and fistulae: An arthrographic study of the rheumatoid wrist. Ann Rheum Dis 34:388–394, 1975.
23a. Palmer AK, Levinsohn EM, Kuzma GR: Arthrography of the wrist. J Hand Surg 8:15–23, 1983.
24. Ranawat CS, Harrison MO, Jordan LR: Arthrography of the wrist joint. Clin Orthop 83:6–12, 1972.
25. Resnick D: Arthrography in the evaluation of arthritic disorders of the wrist. Radiology 113:331–340, 1974.
26. Resnick D: Rheumatoid arthritis of the wrist: the compartmental approach. Med Radiogr Photogr 52:50–87, 1976.
27. Trentham DE, Hamm RL, Masi AT: Wrist arthrography: Review and comparison of normals, rheumatoid arthritis and gout patients. Semin Arthritis Rheum 5:105–120, 1975.
28. Weissman BN: Arthrography in arthritis. Radiol Clin North Am 19:379–392, 1981.

Colles' Fracture

29. Colles A: On the fracture of the carpal extremity of the radius. Abr. transl. Clin Orthop 83:3–5, 1972. Original, Edinb Med Surg J 10:181, 1814.
30. Bacorn RW, Kurtzke JF: Colles' fracture: A study of two thousand cases from the New York State Workman's Compensation Board. J Bone Joint Surg (Am) 35:643–658, 1953.
31. Cooney WP III, Dobyns JH, Linscheid RL: Compli-

cations of Colles' fracture. J Bone Joint Surg (Am) 62:613–619, 1980.
32. Dobyns JH, Linscheid RL: Fractures and dislocations of the wrist. In Rockwood CA Jr, Green DP, eds. Fractures. Philadelphia, JB Lippincott, 1975.
33. Fahey JH: Fracture and dislocations about the wrist. Surg Clin North Am 37:19–40, 1957.
34. van der Linden W, Ericson R: Colles' fracture. How should its displacement be measured and how should it be immobilized? J Bone Joint Surg (Am) 63:1285–1288, 1981.

Barton's and Smith's Fractures

35. De Oliveira JC: Barton's fractures. J Bone Joint Surg (Am) 55:586–594, 1973.
36. Ellis J: Smith's and Barton's fractures. J Bone Joint Surg (Br) 47:724–727, 1965.
37. Mills TJ: Smith's fracture and anterior marginal fracture of radius. Br Med J [Clin Res] 2:603–605, 1957.
38. Peltier LF: Eponymic fractures: John Rhea Barton and Barton's fractures. Surgery 34:960–970, 1953.
39. Peltier LF: Eponymic fractures: Robert William Smith and Smith's fractures. Surgery 45:1035–1042, 1959.
40. Thomas FB: Reduction of Smith's fracture. J Bone Joint Surg (Br) 39:463–470, 1957.

Radioulnar Dislocations

41. Coleman HM: Injuries of the articular disc at the wrist. J Bone Joint Surg (Br) 42:522–529, 1960.
42. Dameron TB Jr: Traumatic dislocation of the distal radio-ulnar joint. Clin Orthop 83:55–63, 1972.
43. Darrach W: Partial excision of lower shaft of ulna for deformity following Colle's fracture. Ann Surg 57:764–765, 1913.
44. Dobyns JH, Linscheid RL: Fractures and dislocations of the wrist. In Rockwood CA Jr, Green DP, eds. Fractures. Philadelphia, JB Lippincott, 1975.
45. Frykman G: Fracture of the distal radius including sequelae—shoulder–hand–finger syndrome, disturbance in the distal radio-ulnar joint and impairment of nerve function. A clinical and experimental study. Acta Orthop Scand [Suppl] 108:3–155, 1967.
46. Kessler I, Hecht O: Present application of the Darrach procedure. Clin Orthop 72:254–260, 1970.
46a. Mino DE, Palmer AK, Levinsohn EM: The role of radiography and computerized tomography in the diagnosis of subluxation and dislocation of the distal radioulnar joint. J Hand Surg 8:23–31, 1983.
47. Vesely DG: The distal radio-ulnar joint. Clin Orthop 51:75–91, 1967.

Scaphoid Fractures

48. Barr JS, Elliston WA, Musnick H, Delorme TL, Hanelin J, Thibodeau AA: Fracture of the carpal navicular (scaphoid) bone. An end-result study in military personnel. J Bone Joint Surg (Am) 35:609–625, 1953.
49. Ganel A, Engel J, Oster Z, Farine I: Bone scanning in the assessment of fractures of the scaphoid. J Hand Surg 4:540–543, 1979.
50. Gelberman RH, Menon J: The vascularity of the scaphoid bone. J Hand Surg 5:508–513, 1980.
51. Haverling M, Sylven M: Soft tissue abnormalities at fracture of the scaphoid. Acta Radiol [Diagn] (Stockh) 19:497–501, 1978.
52. Louis DS, Calhoun TP, Garn SM, Carroll RE, Burdi AR: Congenital bipartite scaphoid—fact or fiction? J Bone Joint Surg (Am) 58:1108–1112, 1976.
53. MacEwan DW: Changes due to trauma in the fat plane overlying the pronator quadratus muscle: A radiologic sign. Radiology 82:879–886, 1964.

54. Osterman AL, Bora FW: Injuries of the wrist. *In* Heppenstall RB, ed. Fracture Treatment and Healing. WB Saunders, Philadelphia, 1980.

55. Pennsylvania Orthopedic Society: Evaluation of treatment for non-union of the carpal navicular. J Bone Joint Surg (Am) 44:169–174, 1962.

56. Russe O: Fracture of the carpal navicular. Diagnosis, non-operative treatment and operative treatment. J Bone Joint Surg (Am) 42:759–768, 1960.

57. Taleisnik J, Kelly PJ: The extraosseous and intraosseous blood supply of the scaphoid bone. J Bone Joint Surg (Am) 48:1125–1137, 1966.

58. Terry DW, Remain JE: The navicular fat stripe. A useful roentgen feature for evaluating wrist trauma. AJR 124:25–28, 1975.

59. Verdan C, Narakas A: Fractures and pseudarthrosis of the scaphoid. Surg Clin North Am 48:1083–1095, 1968.

Carpal Dislocations

60. Campbell RD Jr, Lance EM, Yeoh CB: Lunate and perilunar dislocations. J Bone Joint Surg (Br) 46:55–72, 1964.

61. Dunn AW: Fractures and dislocations of the carpus. Surg Clin North Am 52:1513–1538, 1972.

62. Green DP, O'Brien ET: Classification and management of carpal dislocations. Clin Orthop 149:55–72, 1980.

63. Johnson RP: The acutely injured wrist and its residuals. Clin Orthop 149:33–44, 1980.

64. Taleisnik J: Post-traumatic carpal instability. Clin Orthop 149:73–82, 1980.

65. Wagner CJ: Fracture-dislocations of the wrist. Clin Orthop 15:181–196, 1959.

66. Wiot JF, Dorst JP: Less common fractures and dislocations of the wrist. Radiol Clin North Am 4:261–276, 1955.

Carpal Instability

67. Collins LC, Lidsky MD, Sharp JT, Moreland J: Malposition of carpal bones in rheumatoid arthritis. Radiology 103:95–98, 1972.

68. Dobyns JH, Linscheid RL, Chao EYS, Weber ER, Swanson GE: Traumatic instability of the wrist. AAOS Instructional Course Lectures 11:182–199, 1975.

69. Gilula LA, Weeks PM: Post-traumatic ligamentous instabilities of the wrist. Radiology 129:641–651, 1978.

70. Gilula LA: Carpal injuries: Analytic approach and case exercises. AJR 133:503–517, 1979.

71. Howard FM, Fahey T, Wojcik E: Rotatory subluxation of the navicular. Clin Orthop 104:134–139, 1974.

72. Hudson TM, Caragol WJ, Kaye JJ: Isolated rotatory subluxation of the carpal navicular. AJR 126:601–611, 1976.

72a. Levinsohn EM, Palmer AK: Arthrography of the traumatized wrist. Correlation with radiography and the carpal instability series. Radiology 146:647–651, 1983.

73. Linscheid RL, Dobyns JH, Beabout JW, Bryan RS: Traumatic instability of the wrist: Diagnosis, classification and pathomechanics. J Bone Joint Surg (Am) 54:1612–1632, 1972.

74. Protas JM, Jackson WT: Evaluating carpal instabilities with fluoroscopy. AJR 135:137–140, 1980.

Kienböck's Disease

75. Armistead RB, Linscheid RL, Dobyns JD, Beckenbaugh RD: Ulnar lengthening in the treatment of Kienböck's disease. J Bone Joint Surg (Am) 64:170–178, 1982.

76. Beckenbaugh RD, Shives TC, Dobyns JH, Linscheid RL: Kienböck's disease. The natural history of Kienböck's disease and consideration of lunate fractures. Clin Orthop 149:98–106, 1980.

77. Dornan A: The results of treatment in Kienböck's disease. J Bone Joint Surg (Br) 31:518–520, 1949.

77a. Duong RB, Nishiyama H, Mantil JC, Bever JD, Duong SL, Weinberg S: Kienböck's disease: Scintigraphic demonstration in correlation with clinical, radiographic, and pathologic findings. A case report. Clin Nucl Med 7:418–420, 1982.

78. Gelberman RH, Salamon PB, Jurist JM, Posch JL: Ulnar variance in Kienböck's disease. J Bone Joint Surg (Am) 57:674–676, 1975.

79. Gillespie, HS: Excision of the lunate bone in Kienböck's disease. J Bone Joint Surg (Br) 43:245–249, 1961.

80. Kienböck R: Concerning traumatic malacia of the lunate and its consequences: degeneration and compression fractures. Abr. transl. Clin Orthop 149:4–8, 1980.

81. Lee MLH: Intra-osseous arterial pattern of the carpal lunate bone and its relationship to avascular necrosis. Acta Orthop Scand 33:43–55, 1963.

82. Lichtman DM, Mack GR, MacDonald RI, Gunther SF, Wilson JN: Kienböck's disease: The role of silicone replacement arthroplasty. J Bone Joint Surg (Am) 59:899–908, 1977.

83. McMurtry RY, Youm Y, Flatt AE, Gillespie TE: Kinematics of the wrist. II. Clinical applications. J Bone Joint Surg (Am) 60:955–961, 1978.

84. Stark HH, Zemel NP, Ashworth CR: Use of a hand-carved silicone-rubber spacer for advanced Kienböck's disease. J Bone Joint Surg (Am) 63:1359–1370, 1981.

Wrist Fusion and Total-Wrist Prostheses

85. Allende BT: Wrist arthrodesis. Clin Orthop 142:164–167, 1979.

86. Beckenbaugh RD: Total joint arthroplasty: The wrist. Mayo Clin Proc 54:513–515, 1979.

87. Goodman MJ, Millender LH, Nalebuff EA, Philips CA: Arthroplasty of the rheumatoid wrist with silicone rubber: an early evaluation. J Hand Surg 5:114–121, 1980.

88. Mannerfelt L, Malmsten M: Arthrodesis of the wrist in rheumatoid arthritis: A technique without external fixation. Scand J Plast Reconstr Surg 5:124–130, 1971.

89. Meuli HC: Arthroplasty of the wrist. Clin Orthop 149:118–125, 1980.

90. Millender LH, Nalebuff EA: Reconstructive surgery in the rheumatoid hand. Orthop Clin North Am 6:709–732, 1975.

91. Millender LH, Nalebuff EA: Arthrodesis of the rheumatoid wrist: an evaluation of sixty patients and a description of a different surgical technique. J Bone Joint Surg (Am) 55:1026–1034, 1973.

92. Nalebuff EA, Millender LH: Reconstructive surgery and rehabilitation of the hand. *In* Kelley WN, Harris ED Jr, Ruddy S, Sledge CB, eds. Textbook of Rheumatology. Philadelphia, WB Saunders 1981: 1900–1920.

93. Swanson AB: Flexible implant arthroplasty for arthritic disabilities of the radiocarpal joint: A silicone rubber intramedullary stemmed flexible hinge implant for the wrist joint. Orthop Clin North Am 4:383–393, 1973.

94. Volz RG: The development of a total wrist arthroplasty. Clin Orthop 116:209–214, 1976.

Carpal Prostheses

95. Barber H, Goodfellow J: Acrylic lunate prostheses: A long-term follow-up. J Bone Joint Surg (Br) 56:706–711, 1974.
96. Lichtman DM, Mack GR, MacDonald RI, Gunther SF, Wilson JN: Kienböck's disease: The role of silicone replacement arthroplasty. J Bone Joint Surg (Am) 59:899–908, 1977.
97. Rosenthal DI, Rosenberg AE, Schiller AL, et al. Destructive arthritis due to silicone: a foreign body reaction. Radiology 149:69–72, 1983.
98. Stark HH, Zemel NP, Ashworth CR: Use of a hand-carved silicone-rubber spacer for advanced Kienböck's disease. J Bone Joint Surg (Am) 63:1359–1370, 1981.
99. Swanson AB: Silicone rubber implants for the replacement of the carpal scaphoid and lunate bones. Orthop Clin North Am 1:299–309, 1970.
100. Swanson AB: Implant arthroplasty for disabilities of the distal radioulnar joint. Orth Clin North Am 4:373–382, 1973.
101. Swanson AB, Swanson GG: Flexible implant resection arthroplasty: A method for reconstruction of small joints in the extremities. AAOS Instructional Course Lectures 27:27–60, 1978.
102. Telaranta T, Solonen KA, Tallroth K, et al.: Bone cysts containing silicone particles in bones adjacent to carpal Silastic implant. Skeletal Radiol 10:247–249, 1983.

Carpal Tunnel Syndrome

103. Christian CL: Diseases of the joints. In Beeson PB, McDermott W, Wyngaarden JB, eds. Cecil Textbook of Medicine. Philadelphia, WB Saunders, 1979.
104. Nakano KK: Entrapment neuropathies. In Kelley WN, Harris ED Jr, Ruddy S, Sledge CB, eds. Textbook of Rheumatology. Philadelphia, WB Saunders, 1981.
105. Resnick D: Roentgenographic anatomy of the tendon sheaths of the hand and wrist: Tenography. AJR 124:44–51, 1975.
106. Tanzer RC: The carpal tunnel syndrome. Clin Orthop 15:171–179, 1959.

Calcific Tendinitis

107. Cooper W: Calcareous tendinitis in metacarpophalangeal region. J Bone Joint Surg (Am) 24:114–122, 1942.
108. Cowan IJ, Stone JR: Painful periarticular calcifications at wrist and elbow: Diagnosis and treatment. JAMA 149:530–533, 1952.
109. De Palma AF: Calcareous deposits in soft tissues about the proximal interphalangeal joint of the index finger. J Bone Joint Surg (Am) 29:808–809, 1947.
110. Gandee RW, Harrison RB, Dee PM: Peritendinitis calcarea of flexor carpi ulnaris. AJR 133:1139–1141, 1979.
111. Gondos B: Calcification about wrist associated with acute pain (periarthritis calcarea). Radiology 60:244–251, 1953.
112. Martin JF, Brogdon BG: Peritendinitis calcarea of the hand and wrist. AJR 78:74–85, 1957.
113. Medl WT: Tendinitis, Tenosynovitis, "trigger finger," and de Quervain's disease. Orthop Clin North Am 1:375–382, 1970.

Chapter 4

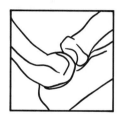

The

ELBOW

NORMAL STRUCTURE AND FUNCTION

Essential Anatomy

The elbow joint consists of three articulations: a lateral articulation between the capitellum (little head; also spelled *capitelum*) and the radius, a medial articulation between the trochlea and the trochlear notch of the ulna, and the radioulnar articulation. The bony structures are shown in Figure 4–1. Medial and lateral epicondyles project from the distal humerus proximal to its articular surface. The larger medial epicondyle is the site of origin of the flexor muscles of the forearm and the ulnar collateral ligament. The lateral epicondyle is the site of origin of the superficial extensor muscles of the forearm and the deeper radial collateral ligament.

The coronoid and radial fossae are indentations on the anterior aspect of the distal humerus that receive the coronoid process of the ulna and the radial head when the elbow is flexed. The posterior olecranon fossa receives the olecranon process of the ulna when the elbow is fully extended. Loose bodies, fracture fragments, or hardware within the olecranon fossa will block proper seating of the olecranon and, as a consequence, will impede full elbow extension. The bone between these anterior and posterior fossae is thin and in some cases absent, forming the supratrochlear fossa. In 1 percent of the white population and less often in blacks a bony outgrowth protrudes from the anteromedial aspect of the humerus (Fig. 4–2). This supracondyloid process may be connected to

169

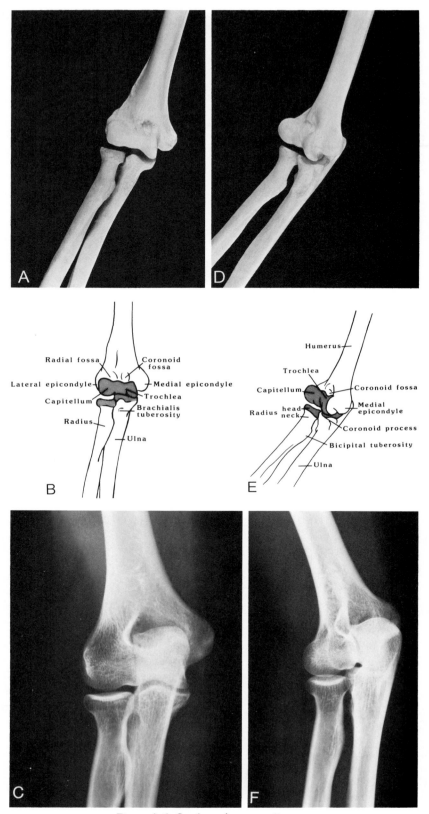

Figure 4–1. *See legend on opposite page*

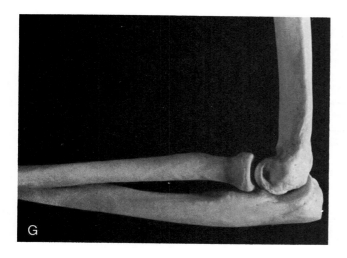

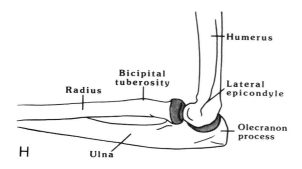

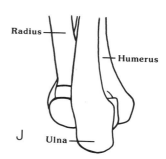

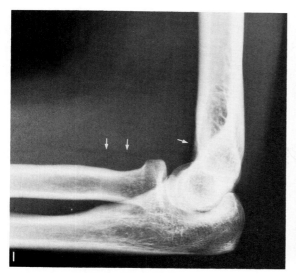

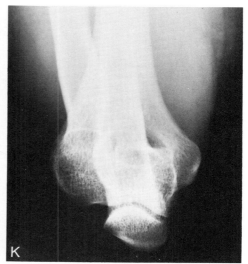

Figure 4–1. Normal Bony Structures. Photographic, diagrammatic, and radiographic anatomy of the normal elbow in the *A-C*, anterior; *D-F*, external oblique; *G-I*, lateral; and *J, K*, tangential olecranon, projections. The supinator line (two arrows) and the anterior fat pad (single arrow) are seen.

171

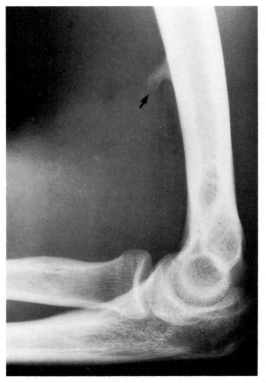

Figure 4–2. Supracondyloid Process. This well-defined bony excrescence (arrow) arises from the anterior, medial aspect of the humerus. It may rarely be associated with symptomatic median nerve compression.

the medial epicondyle by an abnormal ligament, and this connection sometimes results in compression of the median nerve against the spur.[1, 2, 4, 6, 7]

The olecranon process of the ulna has a trochlear notch containing a longitudinal ridge and adjacent concavities that articulate with the

trochlea, which is contoured to fit them. The coronoid process forms the distal margin of the trochlear notch.

The proximal radius consists of a head, neck, and tuberosity. The radial head articulates with both the capitellum and the radial notch of the ulna. The bicipital tuberosity is the site of insertion of the biceps tendon. More distally the radius has a normally curved appearance, with a lateral bow of about 9 degrees and a dorsal bow of about 6 degrees.

Motion
The elbow essentially is a hinge joint with about 150 degrees of flexion possible from the neutral (completely extended) position (Fig. 4–3). The biceps brachii, brachioradialis, and brachialis muscles are the primary elbow flexors, while the triceps is the extensor of the elbow joint (Fig. 4–4).[5]

The radioulnar joint allows 80 degrees of pronation and supination of the forearm (Fig. 4–3).[6] In supination the radius and the ulna are almost parallel, but in pronation the radius swings around and crosses the ulna.

Soft Tissues
The articular surfaces of the elbow are enclosed by a joint capsule consisting of an inner synovial lining and an outer fibrous layer that is thickened medially and laterally to form the ulnar and radial collateral ligaments (Fig. 4–5).[3] The synovial membrane inserts peripheral to the margins of the articular cartilage and is increased in surface area by the presence of several recesses: an anterior recess with two superior projections over the radial and the coronoid fossae, a posterior recess over the posterior surface of the distal humerus, an annular recess extending under and bulging beyond the annular ligament,

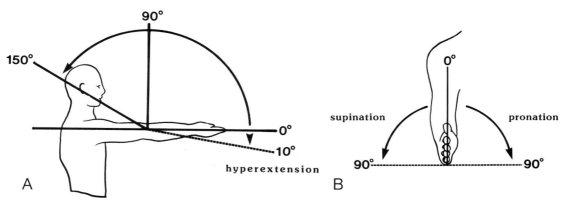

Figure 4–3. Elbow Motion. *A,* Range of flexion, extension motion. *B,* Proximal and distal radioulnar joints and interosseous membrane allow about 90 degrees of pronation and supination motion.

The annular (orbicular) ligament originates and inserts on the margins of the radial notch of the ulna and encircles the radial head, keeping it in contact with the ulna during elbow motion. The radial collateral ligament inserts into the annular ligament. More distally, the radius and ulna are joined by the obliquely oriented fibers of the strong interosseous membrane, which originates proximally on the radius 1 inch below the radial tuberosity and inserts distally on the ulna, merging with the capsule of the distal radioulnar joint. At the wrist the joint capsule and the triangular fibrocartilage complex unite these bones.

The cubital tunnel is a fibroosseous compartment through which the ulnar nerve and ulnar collateral artery pass as they proceed from the arm to the forearm (Fig. 4–7). The more superficial component of this tunnel is the arcuate ligament that extends from the medial epicondyle to the medial surface of the olecranon.[6] The deep components are the ulnar collateral ligament of the elbow and the underlying bony margins of the humeral groove between the inferior aspect of the medial epicondyle and the medial edge of the trochlea. The tunnel is widest when the arm is extended and narrows with arm flexion when the arcuate ligament becomes taut, the ulnar ligament, redundant, and the interval between the medial epicondyle and the olecranon process, increased.

Normal Radiographic Appearances

The usual radiographic examination includes a lateral view with the arm in 90 degrees of flexion, an anteroposterior (AP) view with the arm extended, and an AP view with the arm extended and externally rotated (Fig. 4–1). When full extension is not possible, views may be obtained with the forearm flat on the film, the humerus flat on the film, or the point of the elbow on the film and the humerus and forearm equally elevated from the film.

Bony Relationships

On the AP radiograph in supination a valgus carrying angle is noted between the ulna and the humerus (Fig. 4–8); this is functionally important because it allows objects to be carried in the hand without their impinging against the lateral aspect of the thigh. Usually the carrying angle is stated as being larger in women than in men. Beals, however, noted no significant sex difference.[8] Normal values for males range from 2 to 26 degrees (average 11 degrees) and for

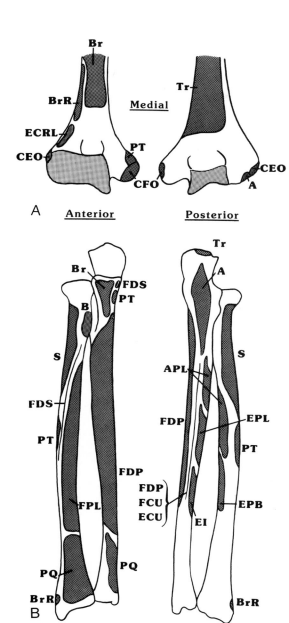

Figure 4–4. Muscular Insertions Near the Elbow. Anterior and posterior views of the distal humerus, radius, and ulna are shown. A = Anconeus; APL = abductor pollicis longus; B = biceps; Br = brachialis; BrR = brachioradialis; CEO = common extensor tendon origin; CFO = common flexor tendon origin; ECRL = extensor carpi radialis longus; ECU = extensor carpi ulnaris; EI = extensor indicis; EPB = extensor pollicis brevis; EPL = extensor pollicis longus; FCU = flexor carpi ulnaris; FDP = flexor digitorum profundus; FDS = flexor digitorum superficialis; FPL = flexor pollicis longus; PQ = pronator quadratus; PT = pronator teres; S = supinator; Tr = triceps.

and a radioulnar (sacciform) recess extending from the annular recess between the radius and the ulna (Fig. 4–6). These can be readily seen on arthrography (see Fig. 4–12).

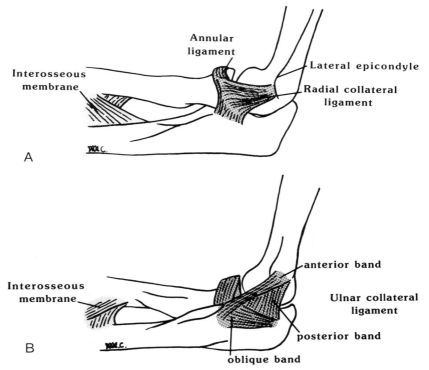

Figure 4–5. Collateral Ligaments. *A,* The radial collateral ligament and the annular ligament with which it merges. *B,* The ulnar collateral ligament with its anterior, posterior, and oblique portions.

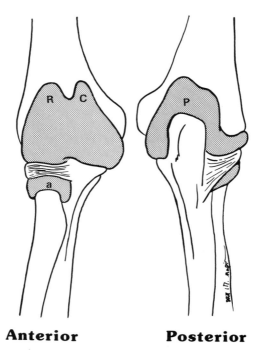

Anterior   **Posterior**

Figure 4–6. Joint Capsule. Anterior and posterior views show the anterior recess, with superior radial (R) and coronoid (C) extensions, a posterior recess (P), and an annular recess (a) extending under the annular ligament.

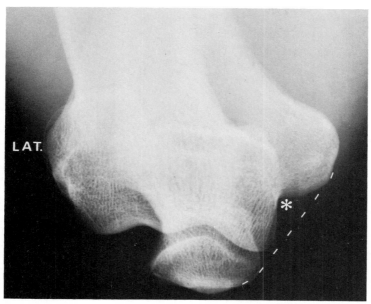

Figure 4–7. Cubital Tunnel. The ulnar nerve (asterisk) lies in a tunnel bridged by the arcuate ligament (dashed line), which extends from the medial epicondyle to the olecranon process. (After Wadsworth TG: The Elbow. Edinburgh, Churchill Livingstone, 1982, by permission.)

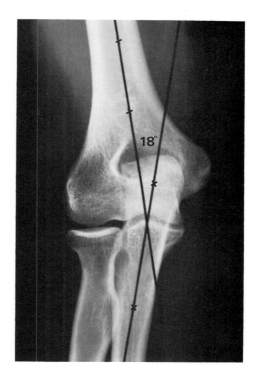

Figure 4–8. Carrying Angle. The carrying angle may be determined by noting the angle of intersection betwee a line connecting midpoints in the distal humerus and a line connecting midpoints in the proximal ulna. (*Method of* Beals RK: Clin Orthop 119:194, 1976.)

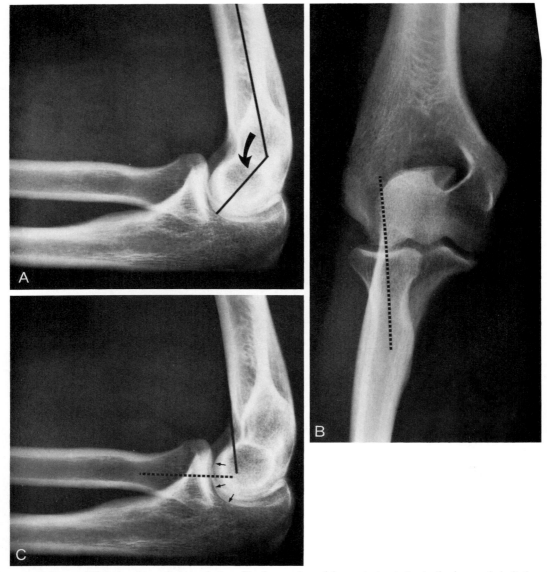

Figure 4–9. Normal Relationships. *A,* Lateral view. The humeral condyles project anterior to the humeral shaft, forming an angle of about 140 degrees (arrow) with the shaft. *B* and *C,* On the AP and lateral views, respectively, a line (dashed) bisecting the proximal radial shaft passes through the capitellum (arrows). A line drawn along the anterior surface of the humeral cortex (solid line) normally passes through the middle third of the capitellum.

females from 1 to 22 degrees (average 13 degrees).[9]

Several other normal angles and relationships are shown on standard radiographs (Fig. 4–9). These have particular value when subtle changes in contour or position are sought, particularly when distal humeral fractures are clinically suspected. On the AP radiograph the humeral articular surface is not quite perpendicular to the humeral shaft. This obliquity averages 85 degrees in males (range 77 to 95 degrees) and 83 degrees in females (range 72 to 91 degrees)

when measured on the ulnar side (Fig. 4–9).[9] On the lateral radiograph the articular surfaces of the humerus project anteriorly, forming an angle of about 140 degrees with the midshaft of the humerus.[10] Because of this anterior angulation, a line drawn along the anterior surface of the humeral cortex normally passes through the middle third of the capitellum.[10] Posterior displacement of the capitellum as a consequence of fracture will be readily apparent because the anterior humeral cortical line will then fall on the anterior one third of the capitellum or altogether

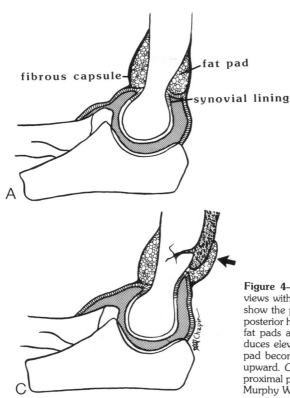

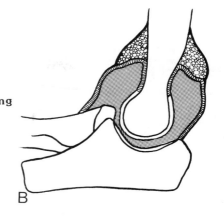

Figure 4–10. Elbow Fat Pads. *A,* Normal lateral views with the arm flexed to 90 degrees should not show the posterior fat pad, which is held against the posterior humerus by the triceps tendon. The anterior fat pads are normally visible. *B,* Joint effusion produces elevation of the fat pads so that the posterior pad becomes visible and the anterior pad is bowed upward. *C,* Extraarticular fractures may displace the proximal portion of a fat pad (arrow). (Redrawn from Murphy W, Siegel MJ: Radiology 124:659, 1977.)

anterior to it. The radial head normally articulates with the capitellum, and a line bisecting the proximal radial shaft should always pass through the capitellum on any radiographic view.[10] Absence of this relationship indicates dislocation.

Soft Tissues

Anterior and Posterior Fat Pads. These collections of fat are located between the fibrous capsule and the synovial membrane and are significant in that they allow evaluation of joint distension (Fig. 4–10). Two of these fat pads are anteriorly situated over the coronoid and radial fossae, but on lateral radiographs they are superimposed and appear as one triangular lucency with a straight anterior surface.[19] These anterior fat pads are routinely seen on lateral views with the elbow in flexion.[25] The single posterior fat pad overlies the olecranon fossa and is pressed into the fossa when the arm is flexed. It is therefore inapparent on routine lateral views obtained with the elbow in 90 degrees of flexion and, indeed, was not seen in 300 normal elbows studied by Norell or in 99 normal cases studied by Kohn.[22, 25] Nonetheless, Murphy and Siegel note that this fat line is occasionally seen in normal subjects as a 1 mm linear lucency and suggest that in these cases either the fat pad is of unusually large size or its positioning is slightly oblique.[22, 23] The posterior fat pad will routinely be seen if the elbow is examined in extension.

The Supinator Line. On the normal lateral radiograph with the elbow in flexion, a thin lucent line parallels the ventral aspect of the proximal third of the radius (Fig. 4–11).[26] This lucency, the supinator line, overlies the supinator muscle and is therefore separated by 1 to 1.3 cm from the anterior margin of the radius. Its importance lies in the fact that it is elevated, widened, or blurred in virtually all cases of acute radial head fracture,[26] and it may also be displaced in cases of septic or rheumatoid arthritis.[34]

Arthrography

Technique. The patient is positioned either sitting next to or lying prone on the fluoroscopic table with the elbow flexed to 90 degrees and the lateral side of the arm up. Our personal preference is to use the prone position since the seated patient occasionally feels faint. For single-contrast examinations a syringe with about 6 ml of contrast (e.g., Reno–M 60) and 2 ml of 1 percent Xylocaine is prepared and attached to a connector tube. After the preliminary films are evaluated fluoroscopy to determine the midpoint

THE ELBOW

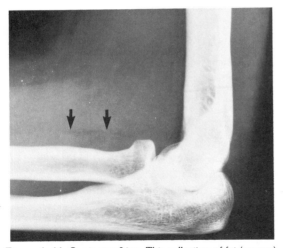

Figure 4–11. Supinator Line. This collection of fat (arrows) overlies the supinator muscle and parallels the proximal radius.

of the radiocapitellar joint is done. The skin over that site is prepared, and the skin and subcutaneous tissue anesthetized with 1 percent Xylocaine. A 22-gauge, 1½-inch needle is then inserted perpendicular to the radiocapitellar joint and advanced until a decrease in resistance is noted. As in arthrography of the knee, as much joint fluid as possible is aspirated and is sent for culture, or additional analysis, or both as the clinical situation warrants. If no fluid is obtained, intraarticular needle position is confirmed by the injection of a small amount of positive contrast. If the needle tip is intraarticular, the contrast mixture is seen to flow immediately away from the needle and to outline the articular surface. When positive contrast alone is used, the joint is filled until the patient feels some fullness in the elbow. This usually requires about 5 ml of contrast, but up to 10 ml may be necessary.[12]

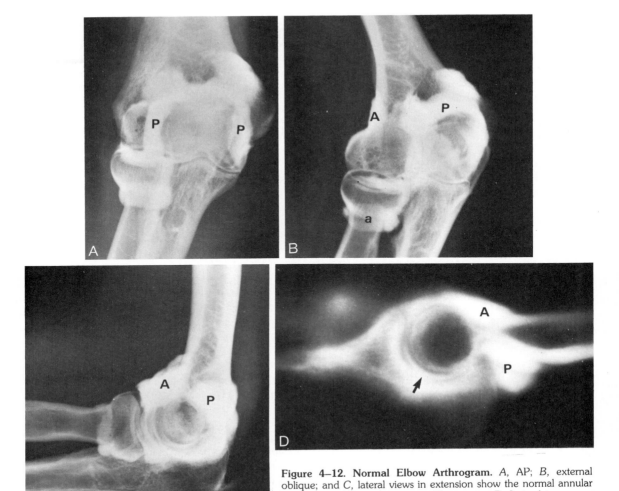

Figure 4–12. Normal Elbow Arthrogram. *A,* AP; *B,* external oblique; and *C,* lateral views in extension show the normal annular (a), anterior (A), and posterior (P) recesses. *D,* Lateral tomogram with the arm extended. The area of the trochlea that is devoid of cartilage (arrow) is seen.

A double-contrast technique requires the instillation of positive contrast (e.g., Reno–M 60), air, and usually epinephrine, but the exact amounts of each of these are somewhat controversial. Hudson suggests 0.5 to 1.5 ml of positive contrast, 8 to 12 ml of air, and 0.1 to 0.2 ml of a 1:1000 solution of epinephrine.[17] Hall suggests the use of smaller quantities of positive contrast material (0.3 to 0.5 ml), larger amounts of air (8 to 15 ml), and 0.1 ml of epinephrine.[16]

Single, positive contrast studies are usually done for evaluation of the synovial lining, synovial cysts, or capsular rupture, the last requiring examination within a few days of injury.[12, 17] The films obtained depend on the clinical situation but usually include lateral views in flexion and extension, internal and external oblique views, and an AP view. When a synovial cyst is suspected, films after exercise may fill an otherwise unrecognized cavity.

Double-contrast arthrography has been suggested as the method of choice for the demonstration of loose bodies or evaluation of articular cartilage. Fluoroscopy and spot filming are done and if necessary are supplemented by multidirectional tomography using the thinnest possible sections taken at 2 to 4 mm intervals.

Normal Arthrographic Anatomy. The distended joint capsule shows two anterior projections over the radial and coronoid fossae of the humerus, likened to rabbit ears (Fig. 4–12). The posterior recess of the capsule is particularly deep behind the olecranon fossa and behind the radial head. The joint space continues under the annular ligament and bulges distal to it, forming the annular recess. The radioulnar recess extends between the proximal portions of the radius and ulna.

Articular cartilage is present along the anterior and inferior surfaces of the capitellum and the anterior, inferior, and posterior surfaces of the trochlea.[14] Of note is a normal defect in the articular cartilage of the midportion of the trochlear notch (Fig. 4–12).[17]

ABNORMAL CONDITIONS

Soft Tissue Abnormalities

Elevation of Anterior and Posterior Fat Pads (Positive Fat Pad Sign)

Norell, in 1954, was the first to note the importance of visualization of the posterior fat pad in the diagnosis of elbow joint effusion (Fig. 4–13).[25] He noted that none of 300 normal

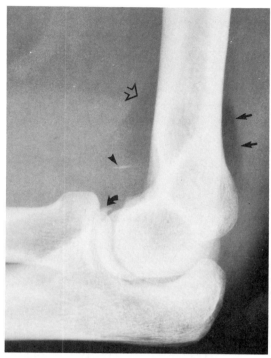

Figure 4–13. Coronoid Process Fracture with Hemarthrosis. The posterior fat pad (arrows) is clearly seen on this lateral view with the arm flexed to 90 degrees, indicating joint effusion. The anterior fat pad (open arrow) is well seen. There is a fracture of the coronoid process (curved arrow), and a loose body (arrowhead) is present.

elbows showed a fat line posteriorly, but 74 percent of children with elbow fractures demonstrated this abnormality on lateral radiographs. Failure to see the posterior fat pad in the other fracture patients was attributed to the presence of an overlying cast, severe fractures or dislocations in which the joint capsule was presumably ruptured, an extracapsular fracture location, or suboptimal radiographic technique.

Additional observations have been made regarding the appearance of the elbow fat pads including the following:[21, 23]

1. A 1 mm lucency, thought to be due to an unusually large fat pad or oblique positioning, is occasionally seen in apparently normal patients. It is prudent, however, to carefully examine each of these patients clinically and radiographically as though they had a truly positive fat pad sign.

2. When intraarticular fluid is present, the inferior aspect of the posterior fat pad is elevated, and the fat pad takes on a semilunar shape.

3. Elevation of the anterior fat pad may be recognized as definitely abnormal if its lower, inferior margin becomes concave, an appear-

Table 4–1. **Relationship Between Fat Pad Displacement and the Presence of an Elbow Fracture**

| | + Fat Pad Sign | | − Fat Pad Sign | |
Series	Fracture	No Fracture	Fracture	No Fracture
Smith and Lee	23 (82%)	5 (18%)	0	61 (100%)
Norell	118 (76%)	38 (24%)		
Kohn	120 (80%)	30 (20%)		
Bohrer (children)	5 (42%)	7 (58%)		

Sources: Smith DN, Lee JR: Injury 10:115, 1978; Norell HG: Acta Radiol [Diagn] (Stockh) 42:205, 1954; Kohn AM: AJR 82:867, 1959; Bohrer SP: Clin Radiol 21:90, 1970.

ance likened to a ship's sail. Elevation of the anterior fat pad is occasionally present when the posterior fat pad is not displaced.

4. A variety of other conditions may be associated with positive fat pad signs owing to the presence of intraarticular masses or fluid. These include hemophilia, rheumatoid arthritis, gout, pseudogout, neuropathic arthropathy, infection, pigmented villonodular synovitis, osteoid osteoma, osteochondromatosis, and osteochondritis dissecans.

Abnormal Supinator Line

Elevation, blurring, or widening of the supinator line (in addition to joint effusion) was noted to accompany all acute radial head fractures studied by Rogers and MacEwan.[26] In patients with trauma but without identifiable fracture, only 10 percent had abnormalities of this line. The presence of these abnormalities (or a positive fat pad sign, described previously) warrants careful clinical and radiologic examination, with additional oblique views to fully evaluate the possibility of an occult fracture, particularly one involving the radial head (Table 4–1).

Lipohemarthrosis

Lateral views with horizontal beam technique allow delineation of small amounts of fat within the fluid-filled joint. According to Yousefzadeh and Jackson this finding indicates the presence of an intraarticular fracture or capsular injury.[29]

Olecranon Bursitis and Nodules

The normal olecranon bursa caps the olecranon process and is separate from the elbow joint proper (Fig. 4–14). Distension of the bursa is most often associated with trauma or rheumatoid arthritis and produces a homogeneous soft tissue density on radiographs. Saccular protrusions that extend down the extensor surface of the forearm may develop.[34]

Rheumatoid nodules may also be located over the olecranon process and the extensor surface of the ulna. Typically, these have a reticular pattern on radiographs, with no associated calcification or bone erosion (Fig. 4–15).[33] Gouty tophi, in contrast, are not as discrete, are of increased density due to the deposition of calcium urate, and produce local bone erosion and new bone formation (Fig. 4–16).[33]

Loose Bodies

Cartilaginous or osteocartilaginous loose bodies may be found in the elbow, usually as a consequence of osteochondritis dissecans or osteoarthritis.[36] Less frequent causes include acute osteochondral fractures, synovial osteochondromatosis, and neuropathic joints. Loose bodies

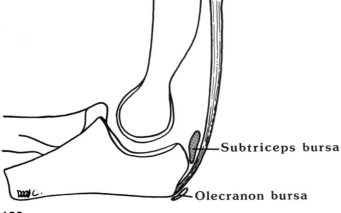

Figure 4–14. Bursae. The superficial olecranon bursa and the bursa between the triceps and the olecranon process are shown.

Subtriceps bursa

Olecranon bursa

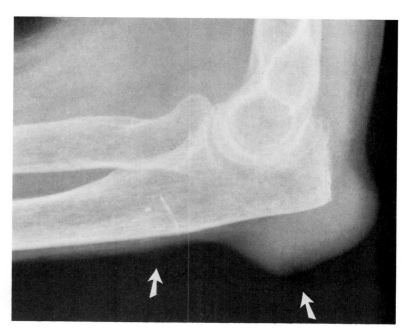

Figure 4–15. Rheumatoid Nodules. These nodules (arrows) typically do not calcify and do not erode adjacent bone.

are most often found in the anterior portions of the joint but may lodge posteriorly in the olecranon fossa, producing a radiographic appearance that may simulate osteoid osteoma or a supratrochlear foraminal bone (Figs. 4–17 to 4–19).[35] The diagnosis is suggested on standard radiographs if ossification or calcification overlying the expected area of the joint capsule is present, and it is confirmed on arthrography, often with tomography, if the fragment is completely surrounded by contrast material.

Rheumatoid Arthritis

Elbow joint involvement occurs in 40 to 50 percent of patients with long-standing rheumatoid arthritis.[30] The joint becomes distended owing to effusion, synovial hypertrophy, edema, and the presence of loose bodies.[34] The distension of the joint capsule is seen anteriorly as displacement of the anterior fat pad and supinator line, sometimes producing a "reverse 3" shape (Fig. 4–20); posteriorly, there is elevation of the fat pad. A subtriceps bursitis may be

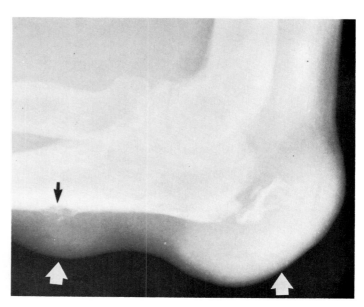

Figure 4–16. Gouty Tophi. A lateral view of the elbow shows soft tissue masses (tophi, white arrows). Ossification of the tophus over the olecranon process and erosion of the ulna (black arrow), findings not seen with rheumatoid nodules but typical of gout, are present.

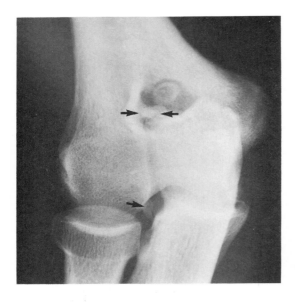

Figure 4–17. Loose Bodies. There is a large, well-corticated density overlying the olecranon fossa. The appearance could be confused with the osteoid osteoma shown in Figure 4–19 or with a supratrochlear foraminal bone. The presence of other, smaller densities (arrows) suggests the correct diagnosis.

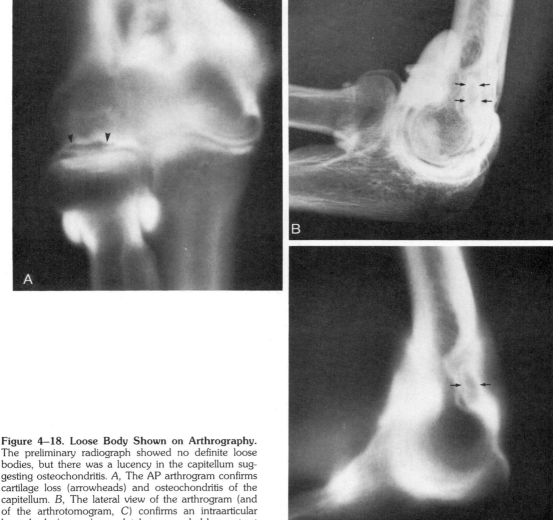

Figure 4–18. Loose Body Shown on Arthrography. The preliminary radiograph showed no definite loose bodies, but there was a lucency in the capitellum suggesting osteochondritis. *A,* The AP arthrogram confirms cartilage loss (arrowheads) and osteochondritis of the capitellum. *B,* The lateral view of the arthrogram (and of the arthrotomogram, *C*) confirms an intraarticular loose body (arrows) completely surrounded by contrast medium.

182

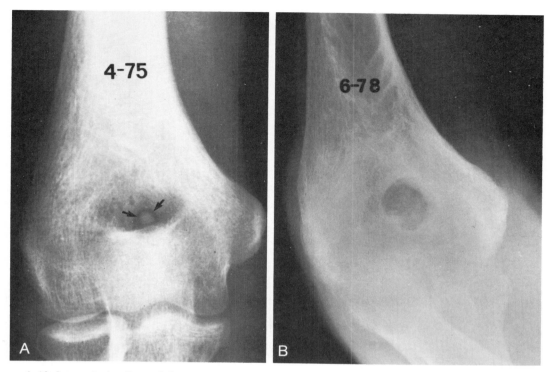

Figure 4–19. Intraarticular Osteoid Osteoma. *A,* An AP view taken in 1975 shows a small area of lucency with central calcification (arrows) in the distal humerus. This was misinterpreted as being a normal ossicle. *B,* Three years later the area of lucency has enlarged, and the calcifications are more irregular in appearance. Joint effusion, flexion contracture, and cartilage loss have occurred in the interim, apparently because of the synovitis that may accompany intraarticular osteoid osteomas.

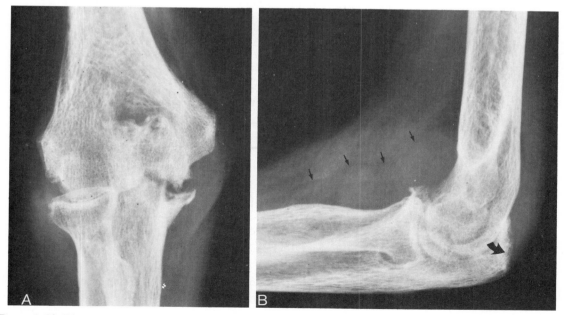

Figure 4–20. Rheumatoid Arthritis. *A,* The AP view shows erosion of the coronoid process and the distal humerus. There is radiocapitellar cartilage space narrowing. *B,* On the lateral view the anterior and posterior fat pads, the supinator line (arrows), and the joint capsule are elevated (producing a ''reverse 3'' appearance anteriorly), indicating joint distension. There is erosion of the olecranon process (curved arrow) and adjacent soft tissue swelling due to subtriceps bursitis.

183

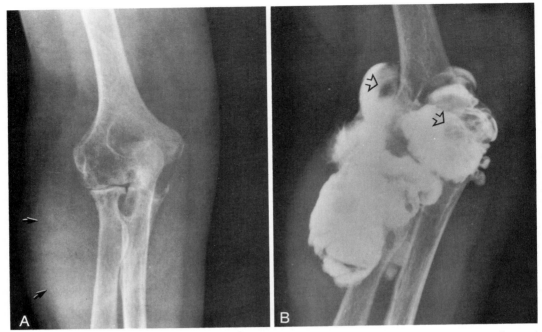

Figure 4–21. Rheumatoid Cyst. *A,* The AP view shows erosion of the distal humerus and ulna and radiocapitellar cartilage-space narrowing. There is a soft tissue mass laterally (arrows). *B,* An oblique view of the arthrogram shows the irregular sac-like extension of the joint that produced the soft tissue mass noted in *A.* Irregularity and enlargement of the joint capsule and the filling defects (open arrows) are typical features of rheumatoid arthritis. (From Weissman BN: Radiol Clin North Am 19:379, 1981.)

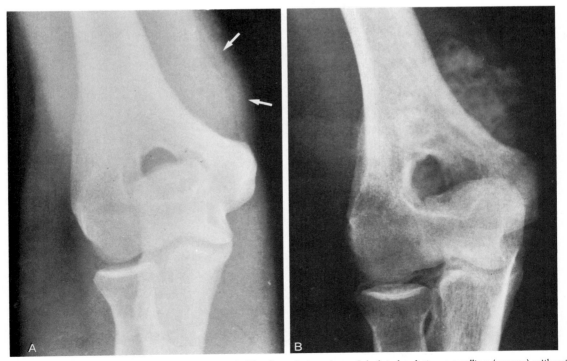

Figure 4–22. Pigmented Villonodular Synovitis. *A,* The frontal view shows lobulated soft tissue swelling (arrows) without calcification. The cartilage spaces are normal. *B,* The single positive contrast arthrogram shows numerous filling defects. (From Weissman BN: Radiol Clin North Am 19:379, 1981.)

present with swelling and adjacent bone erosion (Fig. 4–20).

Arthrography in patients with rheumatoid arthritis may show multiple filling defects, sacculation, lymphatic and supratrochlear lymph node filling, and filling of cysts (Fig. 4–21). The presence of nodular filling defects is a nonspecific finding that may also be seen in patients with pigmented villonodular synovitis (Fig. 4–22) or synovial (osteo)chondromatosis. Antecubital cysts, analogous to popliteal cysts, have been reported in the elbows of patients with rheumatoid arthritis.[31, 32] The cysts extend distally from the joint, medially or laterally, and occasionally rupture into the adjacent soft tissues, producing local induration, heat, swelling, and tenderness (Fig. 4–21). Involvement may be bilateral.

Elbow Fractures

For discussion, fractures of the elbow will be subdivided according to the bone involved.

Humeral Fractures

Humeral fractures are subdivided by location into (1) supracondylar; (2) transcondylar; (3) intercondylar (dicondylar T or Y); (4) condylar (medial or lateral); (5) articular surface; and (6) epicondylar. Types 2 through 6 are intracapsular.

In general, intracapsular fractures require the restoration of a smooth articular surface and the removal of fracture fragments, loose bodies, and deformed bone that impede normal motion. Extracapsular fractures and elbow dislocations are associated with different complications, particularly damage to neurovascular structures and myositis ossificans.[56]

Supracondylar Fractures. Supracondylar fractures are uncommon in adults. They are usually divided into two types: the *extension* type, in which the distal fragment is located posterior to the proximal humeral shaft, and the *flexion* type, in which the distal fragment is located anterior to the humeral shaft (Fig. 4–23). The extension fracture is more frequent,[45, 52] and it is more likely to be associated with damage to neurovascular structures in the antecubital region.

The AP radiograph usually reveals a transverse fracture line just above the origin of the joint capsule. The presence of angulation, displacement, and rotation of the distal fragment should be ascertained.

On the lateral radiograph in spite of the extracapsular location of these fractures, the posterior fat pad may be seen to be posteriorly displaced. Murphy and Siegel note that this displacement is due to hemorrhage associated with these fractures, which causes displacement of the *proximal* portion of the fat pad (Fig. 4–10).[23] With intraarticular fractures, in contrast, hemarthrosis elevates the distal aspect of the fat pad. In extension fractures the lateral view usually shows posterior angulation of the distal fragment

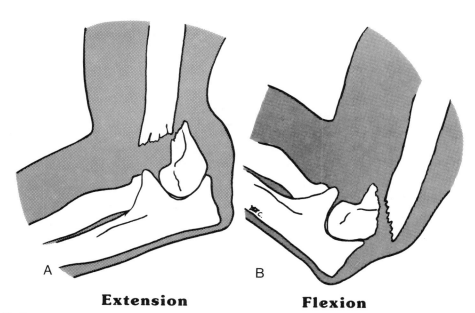

Extension   **Flexion**

Figure 4–23. Supracondylar Fractures. *A,* In the extension type of fracture the distal fragment is posterior to the proximal humeral shaft. *B,* In the flexion type of fracture the distal fragment is anterior to the proximal humeral shaft.

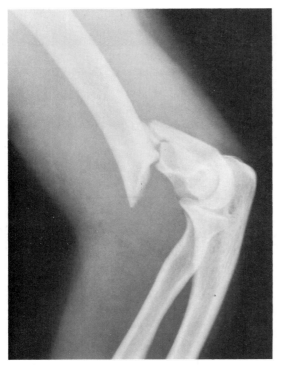

Figure 4–24. Supracondylar Fracture, Extension Type. The lateral view shows an oblique fracture of the distal humerus, with angular deformity. The distal fragment is displaced posteriorly.

(Fig. 4–24). When this angulation is mild, radiographic findings may be subtle. However, the lateral radiograph will show a decrease in the normal anterior tilt of the distal articular surface with respect to the humerus, and a line drawn along the anterior aspect of the humeral shaft will intersect the capitellum anterior to its middle third instead of at its normal intersection with the middle third.

Treatment consists of closed reduction and the application of a cast or splint,[45, 52] the fracture usually healing in 8 to 12 weeks. Alternatively, traction may be used, particularly if there is significant swelling in the antecubital area. Fixation by percutaneous pins or open reduction and internal fixation are alternatives; the latter is chosen when a satisfactory closed reduction cannot be obtained or when there is vascular damage.

The flexion type of supracondylar fracture is defined on the lateral view by the anterior displacement of the distal humeral fragment (Fig. 4–25). Closed reduction and immobilization, or open reduction and internal fixation (if reduction cannot otherwise be obtained), may be used for treatment. In contrast to the extension type of fracture, vascular injury is rare.

Transcondylar Fractures. These fractures involve the distal humerus at the level of the epicondyles and the olecranon fossa and are therefore within the joint capsule (Fig. 4–26). They are usually relatively nondisplaced and are treated by closed methods. Excess callus production in the coronoid or olecranon fossae may result in limitation of motion.

Intercondylar T or Y Fractures. These fractures are usually due to direct trauma, in which a force applied to the proximal ulna drives the wedge-shaped olecranon into the distal humeral articular surface.

Radiographic examination shows a T- or Y-shaped fracture with the vertical limb extending through the articular surface. These fractures have been subdivided according to their radiographic appearance into four types (Fig. 4–27): (1) nondisplaced fracture between the capitellum and the trochlea, (2) fracture with separation of the capitellum and the trochlea but no rotation of the fragments, (3) fracture with rotation of the fragments, and (4) fracture with severe comminution of the articular surfaces and widespread separation of the humeral condyles.[66]

Treatment is directed toward realigning the condyles with respect to the proximal humerus and to each other in order to establish a smooth joint surface.[45, 52] Type I fractures are usually treated conservatively. Treatment of Type II

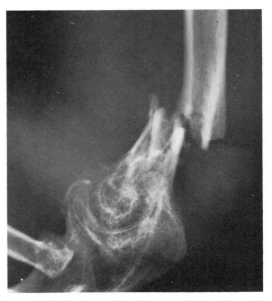

Figure 4–25. Supracondylar Fracture, Flexion Type. The lateral view of this patient with osteogenesis imperfecta shows anterior displacement of the distal humeral fragment, making this a fracture of the flexion type. There is marked osteopenia. The radial head is dislocated from an old injury and from surgery.

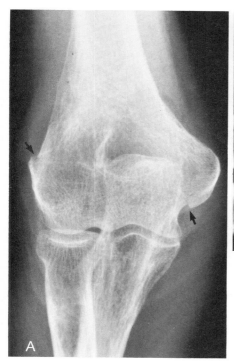

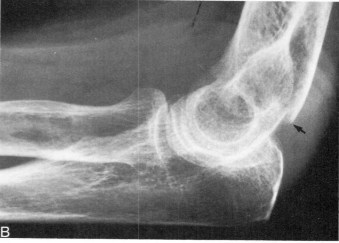

Figure 4–26. Transcondylar Fracture. *A*, AP and *B*, lateral views show cortical discontinuity medially, laterally, and posteriorly (arrows), but no fracture line is visible.

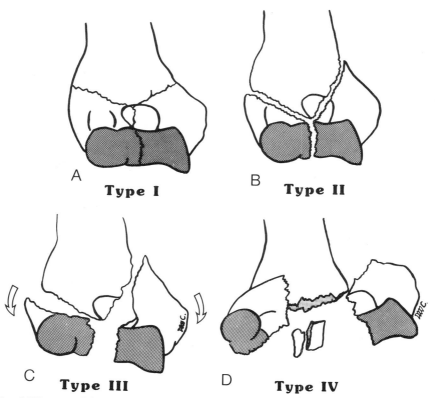

Figure 4–27. T and Y Intercondylar Fractures. *A*, In type I fractures the fracture fragments are not displaced. *B*, In type II injury there is separation of the capitellum and the trochlea but no rotation of fracture fragments. *C*, The fracture fragments are rotated. *D*, There is comminution of the articular surfaces and marked separation of the humeral condyles.

fractures ranges from conservative therapy (frequently used in the elderly) to more aggressive methods, including overhead traction, pins in plaster, and open reduction with internal fixation. Type III fractures usually require operative reduction and internal fixation. Type IV fractures, with marked comminution of the articular surface, have been treated with overhead olecranon traction, resection arthroplasty, or prosthetic joint replacement. Of importance is the observation that the final clinical result may not coincide with the final radiographic appearance, since excellent function may coexist with distorted anatomy, and poor function may be present in spite of optimal radiographic appearances.[45] Radiographically demonstrable complications include nonunion, limitation of motion due to bony deformity of the coronoid or olecranon fossae, and, rarely, avascular necrosis.

Condylar Fractures

Oblique Fractures of a Single Condyle. Lateral condylar fractures are more frequent than medial ones. Lateral condylar fractures are divided into two types based on the position of the fracture line in relation to the lateral ridge of the trochlea and the trochlear groove (Fig. 4–28).[60] Type I fractures involve only the lateral aspect of the joint. Since the lateral ridge is not separated, the elbow joint itself is stable in the medial-lateral plane (Figs. 4–29 and 4–30). In contrast type II fractures involve the midportion

of the joint, through or medial to the trochlear groove, and dislocation in the medial-lateral direction therefore usually occurs. There may be associated disruption of the ulnar collateral ligament, with an increase in the valgus carrying angle of the elbow.

Eppright and Wilkins stress the differentiation between lateral condylar fractures and fractures of the capitellum.[45] Condylar fractures have both articular and nonarticular (i.e., epicondyle) components, whereas a fracture of the capitellum involves only the articular surface and supporting bone.

Type I fractures may be treated nonoperatively or with internal fixation. Type II fractures are usually treated with open reduction and internal fixation.

Medial condylar fractures are treated conservatively if there is no displacement or with reduction and internal fixation if displacement is present.[52] The incidence of post-traumatic arthritis is higher than with lateral condylar fractures.

Fractures of the Distal Humeral Articular Surface

Fractures of the Capitellum. These fractures represent less than 1 percent of all elbow fractures. Radiographic findings may be subtle, depending upon the amount of subchondral bone included in the fracture fragment (Fig. 4–31). Some (type I) fractures include a significant bony

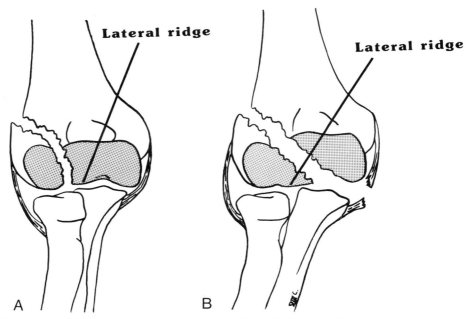

Figure 4–28. Milch Classification of Abduction Lateral Condylar Fractures. *A,* Type I fractures involve only the lateral side of the elbow, and the joint is stable in the medial–lateral plane. *B,* In type II fractures the fracture line is medial to the lateral ridge of the trochlea, and dislocation may occur. The ulnar collateral ligament may be torn.

188

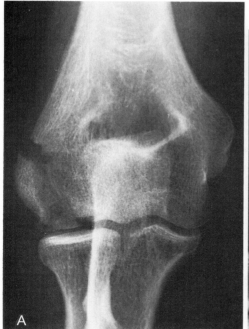
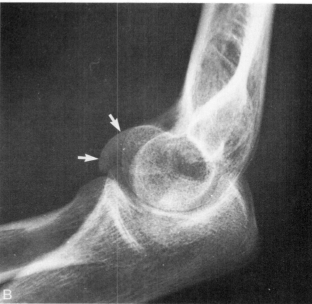

Figure 4–29. Lateral Condylar Fracture (Milch Type I). *A,* AP view. The fracture extends through the articular surface and the more proximal humerus. *B,* Lateral view. The condyle (arrows) is rotated anteriorly.

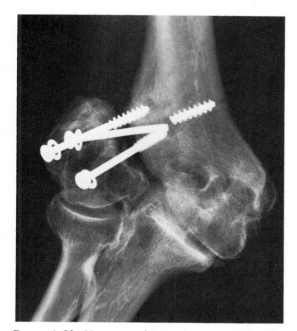

Figure 4–30. Nonunion of Lateral Humeral Condylar Fracture. The patient had a comminuted distal humeral fracture 15 years before the examination. This AP view shows three cancellous screws across the lateral condyle: One screw is broken, and the condyle remains separate from the humerus, with smooth fracture margins indicative of nonunion. There is deformity of the trochlea and some secondary osteoarthritis.

fragment, whereas others (type II fractures) include articular cartilage with only a small amount of attached bone.[45] Careful search for the bony fragment is necessary, and it is usually seen on the lateral view in an anterior location, proximal to the main body of the capitellum. Radial head fractures may coexist, and hemarthrosis, with elevation of the fat pads, is the rule. Treatment may be by closed or open reduction with excision or replacement of the fragment.

Fracture of the Trochlea. This is an extremely uncommon injury. The diagnosis should be considered when a fragment is seen on the medial side of the joint, just distal to the medial epicondyle.

Epicondylar Fractures. These are uncommon lesions in adults. Unlike avulsion injuries in children, lesions in adults are usually the result of direct trauma, and the more prominent medial epicondyle therefore is more likely to be involved. The fracture fragment is usually pulled anteriorly and distally by the attached forearm flexors, and, in rare cases associated with elbow dislocation, the medial epicondyle may become trapped within the joint (see Fig. 4–53). This possibility should be strongly considered if the fragment overlies the level of the joint, since simple avulsion of the epicondyle does not pull

189

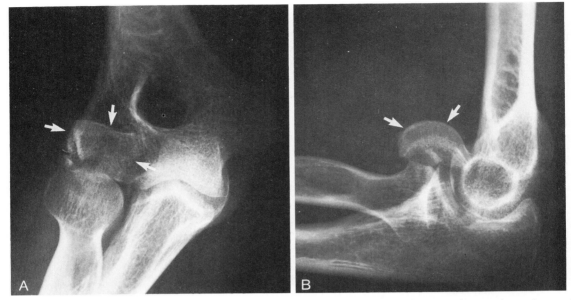

Figure 4–31. Capitellar Fracture. AP *(A)* and lateral *(B)* views. There is a fracture involving the articular surface and adjacent subchondral bone of the capitellum. The fracture fragment (arrows) is displaced and rotated anteriorly.

the involved fragment as far distally as the joint line.[63]

The ossification center of the medial epicondyle fuses within the distal humerus at about age 20, but in some adults fusion does not occur. This is usually a bilateral finding, and comparison views therefore may reassure the uncertain examiner as to the presence or absence of fracture.

Treatment is usually by conservative means with early resumption of motion.[52] Fibrous union may occur but apparently does not jeopardize the clinical outcome.

Radial Fractures

Radial Head Fracture. Radial head fracture is a common elbow injury in adults. The majority of cases result from a fall on the outstretched arm and the minority from a direct blow to the lateral aspect of the elbow.[52, 55] At the time of injury the joint is forced into valgus alignment, and damage to the medial soft tissues or capitellum may result.

Physical examination usually demonstrates painful pronation and supination and limited flexion and extension motion as well as tenderness to palpation of the radial head.

Radiologic Examination. The suspicion of a radial head fracture requires careful radiographic examination for confirmation. Besides the standard radiographic examination (AP, AP in supination, and lateral views), multiple additional

oblique views may be necessary to document a fracture line. Greenspan and Norman suggest a lateral view with the x-ray tube angled 45 degrees toward the head.[51] This position projects the radial head anterior to the ulna and, therefore, free of overlapping structures. Oblique and angled views are indicated in patients with strong clinical indications of radial head fracture and in those patients with an appropriate history of injury and with displacement of fat pads indicating joint effusion (see section on periarticular fat pads) (Fig. 4–32). Smith and Lee studied patients with minor elbow injuries who presented to an emergency room. Eighty-two percent of patients with displaced fat pads had fractures, but none of the patients with normal fat pad position had fractures.[28] Rogers, however, notes that the absence of fat pad displacement in adults does not reliably exclude a fracture.[67] Elevation or blurring of the supinator line helps focus attention on the radius, and in one series all patients with acute radial head fractures had abnormalities of this line along with joint effusion.[26]

Most radial head fractures involve the lateral aspect of the head and are vertically oriented.[67] The amount of the articular surface involved and the presence of comminution, displacement, or angulation should be noted, since these features are important in treatment planning (Figs. 4–33 and 4–34).[55, 57, 59] Capitellar fractures should be suspected and looked for if there are

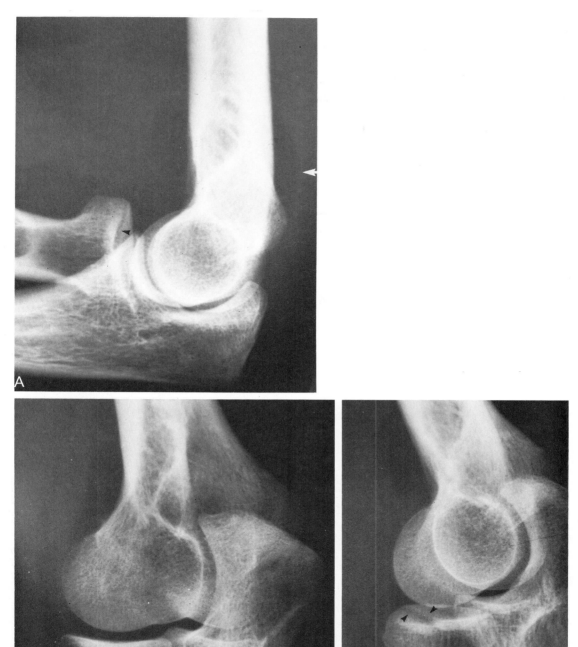

Figure 4–32. Radial Head Fracture. *A,* A lateral radiograph obtained shortly after injury shows displacement of the posterior fat pad (arrow), indicating joint effusion (hemarthrosis). No definite fracture is seen, although a questionable lucency (arrowhead) was noted overlying the radius. In this setting the presence of an effusion is strong evidence for an intracapsular fracture, and therefore multiple oblique views were done. *B,* An external rotation view failed to show a fracture. *C,* An off-lateral view confirmed the presence of the radial head fracture (arrowheads), with slight depression of the lateral articular surface.

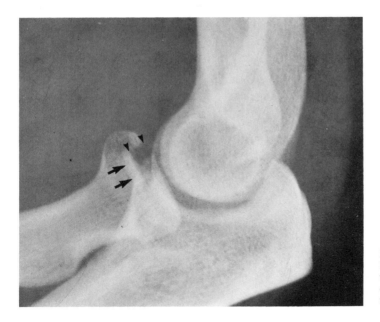

Figure 4–33. Depressed Fracture of the Radial Head. A focal area of depression of the articular surface is present (arrows). The degree of depression is indicated by the distance between the arrowheads.

free fragments within the joint proximal to the radial head, since radial head fractures are only rarely displaced proximally (Fig. 4–34).[45]

Classification. Mason has classified radial head fractures by their radiographic appearance (Fig. 4–35): *type I*—fissure fractures or marginal fractures without displacement, *type II*—marginal fractures with displacement (the involved segment being separated, depressed, impacted, or angulated), *type III*—comminuted fractures involving the whole radial head.[57]

Eppright and Wilkins noted that radial head fractures accompanying elbow dislocations are associated with a higher complication rate, especially the development of myositis ossificans. They therefore suggest adding another category

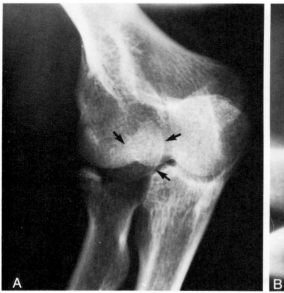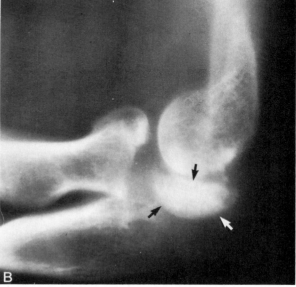

Figure 4–34. Displaced Radial Head Fracture. *A,* An external oblique view taken weeks after injury shows deformity of the radial head with absence of the medial two thirds of its articular surface. A bony fragment (arrows) overlies the capitellum. *B,* A lateral tomogram shows the defect in the radius and more clearly defines the bony fragment (arrows), which is apparently derived from the radial head because no large capitellar defect was identified. The patient underwent radial head excision and Silastic replacement.

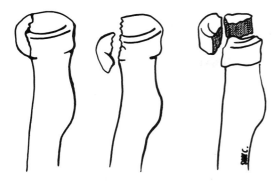

Type I   **Type II**   **Type III**

Figure 4–35. Mason Classification of Radial Head Fractures. Type I, nondisplaced marginal fractures. Type II, marginal fractures with depression, displacement, or angulation of the fragments. Type III, comminuted fractures involving the entire radial head.

to the above: (*type IV*)–radial head fractures associated with elbow dislocation.[45]

Treatment.[45, 52, 55, 57, 69] Type I (nondisplaced) fractures are usually treated nonoperatively. Type II (marginal fractures with displacement) lesions have been treated by both surgical and conservative measures. McLaughlin recommended primary radial head excision if the radial articular surface was depressed by more than 3 mm or if there was more than 30 degrees of angulation.[45] Mason suggested radial head resection if more than one fourth of the radial head was involved, observing that damage to more than one fourth of the radial head will interfere with forearm rotation.[57] Radin and Riseborough used involvement of two thirds of the head as the criterion for surgical excision.[65] Heppenstall advocates a regimen in which early motion is started and, at the end of a 2-week period of observation, radial head excision is performed if good functional recovery has not occurred.[52]

In type III (comminuted) fractures radial head excision is often performed shortly after injury. Interoperative radiographs are helpful in identifying any fragments of the radial head that remain, since the entire head should be excised at a level proximal to the annular ligament. Subluxation of the distal radioulnar joint due to the relative shortening of the radius may occur, but according to Heppenstall, this is usually of little clinical consequence (Fig. 4–36). Swanson and associates have used a Silastic radial head replacement to maintain radial length and radiocapitellar contact.

Type IV fractures are treated first by reducing the dislocation and then by early excision of the radial head if the chosen criteria for excision are met.

Radial Neck Fractures. Radial neck fractures are uncommon injuries in adults. When they

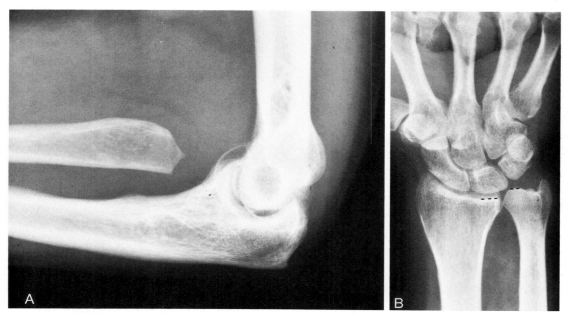

Figure 4–36. Radial Shortening at Wrist after Radial Head Excision. A, Following a comminuted radial head fracture, radial head excision was done. There is elevation of the proximal radius. B, Wrist pain developed postoperatively, and subsequent wrist films show the radius to be shorter than the ulna (dashed lines). Ulnar shortening was eventually performed after conservative therapy failed.

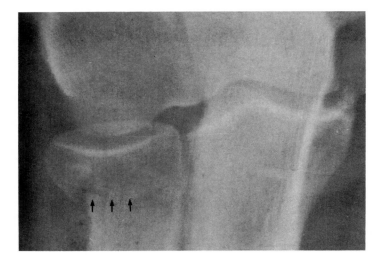

Figure 4–37. Radial Neck Fracture. There is a transverse, slightly impacted radial neck fracture (arrows).

occur, they are often associated with other injuries, including fractures of the olecranon process or posterior dislocations of the elbow.[55] These fractures are seen on the lateral view as an abrupt step-off between the radial head and neck and on the frontal views as a line of increased density (Fig. 4–37).[67]

Ulnar Fractures

Olecranon Fractures. The olecranon process proximally and the coronoid process farther distally form the trochlear notch of the ulna, which articulates with the trochlea of the humerus. This articulation allows motion in the AP plane and provides mediolateral stability. There-fore, all fractures of the olecranon that involve the articular surface potentially disrupt the stability of the elbow joint.[45]

The triceps tendon inserts on the olecranon process. The fascia overlying the triceps muscle extends medially and laterally to insert onto the deep fascia of the forearm and the periosteum of the olecranon and the proximal ulna. If these soft tissue structures remain intact, displacement of fracture fragments will be minimal; conversely, if they are torn, displacement can occur.[45]

Olecranon fractures usually result from a direct fall on the point of the elbow, and this mechanism frequently produces comminution

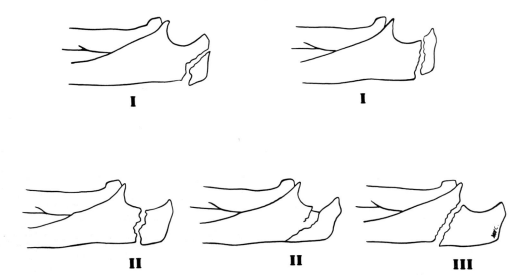

Figure 4–38. Classification of Olecranon Fractures. The classification of Horne and Tanzer divides fractures by their locations as seen on the lateral radiograph. Type I fractures involve the proximal third, type II the midthird, and type III the distal third. (Redrawn from Horne JG, Tanzer TL: J Trauma 21:469, 1981.)

with marked displacement of the major olecranon fragment. Indirect force, from a fall on the outstretched arm, for example, more often produces an oblique or transverse fracture with minimal displacement. Hyperextension, associated with dislocation, may also produce olecranon fractures. The diagnosis of olecranon fracture is usually apparent on physical examination, with limited elbow extension, localized swelling and tenderness, and, often, a palpable bony defect present.

Classification. A number of classification schemes are available. Wadsworth classified fractures as avulsion (type I), displacement of a large fragment (type II), and comminuted (type III) and recommended screw fixation in types II and III fractures when a large fragment was present.[72]

Horne and Tanzer classified these fractures by their location on lateral radiographs (Fig. 4–38): Type I fractures involve the proximal third of the olecranon, type II the middle third of the articular surface, and type III the distal third.[53] The majority of fractures involve the middle third.

Radiologic Examination. Radiologic examination defines the degree of displacement of the olecranon fragments and the degree of comminution (Figs. 4–39 and 4–40). Eppright and Wilkins note the importance of insisting on a true lateral view for accurate appraisal of the fracture and any associated dislocation.[45]

Treatment. Nondisplaced fractures are usu-ally treated nonoperatively, whereas displaced fractures are most often treated by open reduction and internal fixation. The criteria for considering the fracture nondisplaced are (1) separation of fracture fragments by less than 2 mm, (2) no increase in this separation with flexion to 90 degrees, and (3) the patient's ability to actively extend the elbow against gravity.[45, 55]

With conservative treatment, bony union is complete by 6 to 8 weeks.[45] Radiographs are taken at about 1 week to confirm the continued absence of displacement.

Several types of operative intervention are available, including the following:

1. *Tension-band wiring* involves the placement of two Kirschner wires longitudinally through the olecranon process across the fracture site. A wire figure-of-8 suture extends from the tip of the olecranon process over the subcutaneous border of the ulna. This wire is anchored proximally by the K-wires and distally through a drill hole in the ulna (Figs. 4–39 and 4–41).[44, 62]

2. Internal fixation is accomplished with a *wire loop* or a figure-of-8 wire.

3. An oblique *compression screw* traverses the fracture site and penetrates the anterior cortex of the ulna. The screw should not violate the articular surface.

4. The comminuted fragments are excised and the triceps tendon is reattached to the ulna.[47]

Complications. Radiographically identifiable

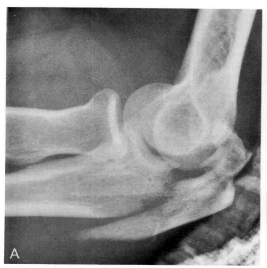
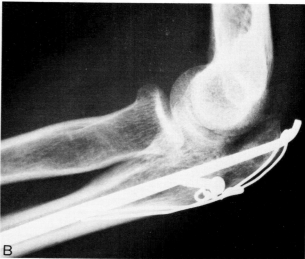

Figure 4–39. Olecranon Fracture. *A,* The lateral view shows a comminuted olecranon fracture. *B,* The postoperative lateral view shows an irregular trochlear surface posteriorly due to removal of comminuted fracture fragments that included a portion of the articular surface. The main distal fragment with its articular surface and the main proximal fragment with the attached triceps tendon were reduced and held by a cortical screw and a tension band. Pain and limitation of motion persisted postoperatively.

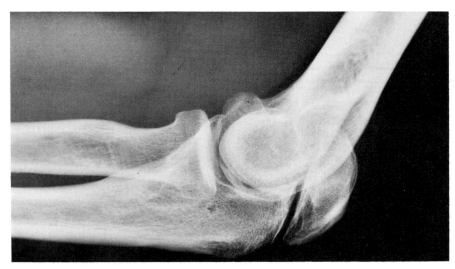

Figure 4–40. Patella Cubiti. The olecranon ossification center has remained separate from the remainder of the ulna. The appearance may be confused with an ununited fracture.

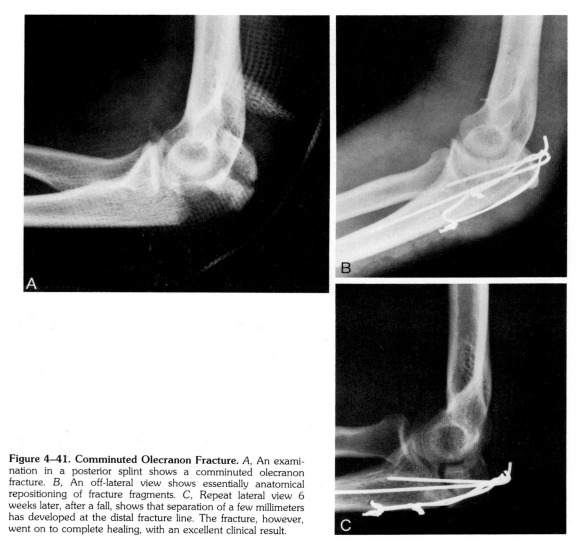

Figure 4–41. Comminuted Olecranon Fracture. *A,* An examination in a posterior splint shows a comminuted olecranon fracture. *B,* An off-lateral view shows essentially anatomical repositioning of fracture fragments. *C,* Repeat lateral view 6 weeks later, after a fall, shows that separation of a few millimeters has developed at the distal fracture line. The fracture, however, went on to complete healing, with an excellent clinical result.

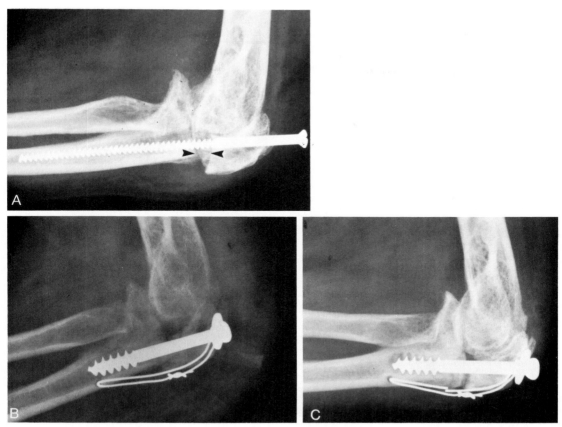

Figure 4–42. Nonunion of Olecranon Fracture. *A,* The lateral radiograph shows evidence of prior radial head excision and arthroplasty with olecranon osteotomy. The osteotomy is ununited (arrowheads). It appears that the screw across the olecranon fragments had not been completely advanced or had backed out so that the screw threads cross the fracture site, and compression of fracture fragments is not achieved. The protruding proximal end of the screw has resulted in localized soft tissue swelling. There is severe cartilage-space narrowing due to rheumatoid arthritis. *B,* The screw was removed and replaced by a cancellous screw and a tension band wire. There is incongruity of the articular surface. *C,* Months later there is motion at the osteotomy site, indicated by the wide fracture line, the bone resorption about the distal part of the screw, and the break in the wire.

complications include post-traumatic arthritis and nonunion, the latter occurring in approximately 5 percent of patients (Fig. 4–42).[45]

Coronoid Process Fractures. These fractures usually occur in association with posterior dislocations of the elbow as a result of avulsion by the brachialis muscle when the elbow is hyperextended. A part of the coronoid process may remain loose within the joint in which case surgical exploration is indicated (see Fig. 4–13).[45]

Sideswipe Fracture

This injury occurs when an elbow protruding from a car window (resting on the window ledge) is hit directly by a vehicle approaching in the opposite direction, by a fixed object, or by the car's overturning. Injuries vary from soft tissue trauma alone to one or more bone injuries, including olecranon fracture, radial and ulnar fractures, dislocation, and humeral fracture.

Sports-Related Injuries

The elbow may be the site of a number of changes due to the acute and chronic trauma sustained during sports activities. Gore and coworkers reviewed some of the radiographic changes in symptomatic athletes, the majority of whom were baseball players, and related the radiographic changes to the incurred stresses.[49] Most focal injuries resulted from the valgus position of the elbow that is achieved during the acceleration phase of pitching. This position results in compression of the lateral side of the joint and distraction of the medial side. In adults these medial distraction forces stress the ulnar collateral ligament and its attachments to the coronoid tubercle of the ulna and the medial

197

Table 4–2. **Sports-Related Elbow Injuries and Precipitating Stresses**

Types of Stress	Resulting Injuries (Adult)
Diffuse	Humeral hypertrophy; radial head and coronoid process hypertrophy; olecranon process hypertrophy
Humeral Shaft	Spiral fracture humeral shaft
Medial Tension	Acute: avulsion fracture medial epicondyle; fracture ulnar spur
	Chronic: ulnar traction spur; hyperostosis ulnar groove; loose bodies
Lateral Compression	Acute: osteochondral fracture;
	Chronic: loose bodies
Extension	Acute: avulsion olecranon process
	Chronic: osteochondral loose bodies

Source: Gore RM et al: AJR 134::971, 1980.

epicondyle. The changes associated with this and other stresses are shown in Table 4–2.

Forearm Fractures

Forearm fractures are usually the result of direct trauma, with severe injury generally associated with fractures of both bones and milder injury with single-bone fractures. These fractures are subdivided, depending on which bones are involved.

Fractures of Both Bones

These fractures of the forearm are often due to direct trauma but may result from indirect injury consequent to a fall on the outstretched arm. The clinical diagnosis is usually obvious, but radiographic examination allows documentation of the degree of deformity and comminution.

Radiographic Examination. Radiographs of the forearm must include the wrist and the elbow, since, as in the pelvis and other areas that have a ring-like configuration, one displaced fracture is often accompanied by another or by dislocation at the adjacent joint. Other fractures of the distal humerus or the wrist may occur simultaneously.

Evans described the tuberosity view, in which the position of the bicipital tuberosity can be assessed and correlated with the degree of rotation of the proximal radius (Fig. 4–43).[46] Such

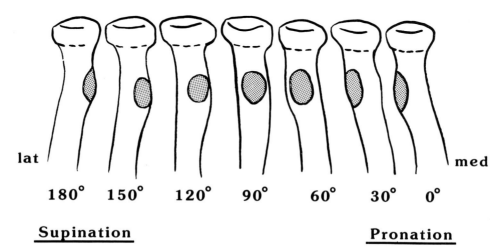

Figure 4–43. Rotation of the Radius Gauged by Appearance of the Biceps Tuberosity. The biceps tuberosity is seen in profile on the medial side of the radius when the proximal radius is in maximum (180 degrees) supination and is seen end-on at 90 degrees. With maximum pronation (0 degrees) the tuberosity is in profile on the lateral margin of the radius. (Redrawn from Evans EM: J Bone Joint Surg 27:373, 1945.)

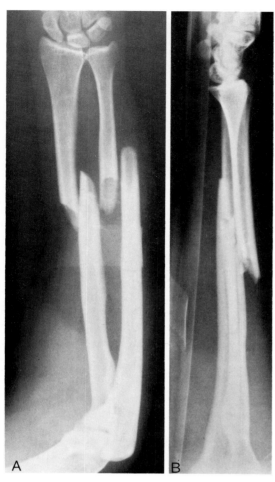

Figure 4–44. Fracture of Both Bones of the Forearm. *A,* PA and *B,* lateral views show the distal fracture fragments displaced laterally and dorsally. The supination of the proximal radius (on lateral view of the forearm, AP view of the elbow) is indicated by the medially directed profile of the biceps tuberosity.

evaluation is of importance because it allows the distal radial fragment to be rotated appropriately to align with the proximal fragment.

Treatment. Because of the severity of the injury necessary to fracture both bones of the forearm, most of these fractures are displaced (Fig. 4–44). Closed reduction has been suggested as appropriate in undisplaced fractures;[40] otherwise, open reduction is usually recommended. Correction of both angular deformity and rotational deformity is mandatory in order to regain normal supination and pronation motion. The bow of the radius and the interosseous space must be preserved. Matthews and colleagues noted experimentally that angular deformity of 20 degrees in one or both of the bones of the forearm resulted in limitation of

motion.[59] Rotation of the proximal radius can be judged by noting the contour of the bicipital tuberosity, and the forearm can then be aligned to the proximal fragment. Following closed reduction, frequent radiographs are necessary to document continued adequacy of position. Compression plating with a five- or six-hole plate is recommended,[52, 58] and additional bone grafting is done when the fractures are comminuted. Although intramedullary rods have been used, round rods may not control rotation of the fracture fragments and may be associated with nonunion. Grace and Eversmann noted better forearm range-of-motion in patients with fractures of both bones of the forearm if early active motion was instituted after plating.[50]

Healing and Complications. Usually, healing occurs within 6 months. Delayed healing refers to cases in which healing takes 6 to 10 months and nonunion to those in which the fracture has not solidly united by 10 months.[40] Complications include infection, delayed union, nonunion (1.8 percent with compression plating),[58] and radioulnar synostosis.[70]

Single-Bone Fractures

Radial Fractures. Isolated radial shaft fractures are relatively uncommon injuries. They are subdivided into those that involve the proximal two thirds and those that involve the distal one third.

Fractures of the proximal two thirds of the radial shaft are further subdivided into those that involve the proximal portion of the radius, between the supinator and the pronator teres muscles, and those that occur distal to the pronator teres (Fig. 4–45). In the more proximal group the unopposed pull of the biceps brachii and the supinator markedly supinate the proximal fragment.[38] Therefore, undisplaced fractures in this region are immobilized with the forearm in full or almost full supination. If the fracture occurs at the distal site, the supination of the proximal fragment is balanced by the pull of the pronator teres, and the proximal fragment assumes a neutral position. The forearm does not, therefore, have to be significantly supinated in order to be aligned with the proximal fragment. Displaced fractures are usually treated with open reduction and internal fixation, often with the use of compression plates.[38, 52]

Distal Third Radial Fractures. The term *Galeazzi fracture* refers to a fracture at the junction of the middle and distal thirds of the radius with dislocation or subluxation of the distal radioulnar joint. If the triangular fibrocartilage complex is not torn, an avulsion fracture of the

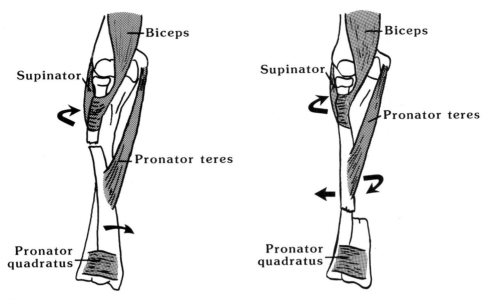

Figure 4–45. Rotation of Radial Fracture Fragments. *A,* Fractures that occur proximal to the pronator teres insertion are characterized by marked supination of the proximal fragment, caused by the unopposed pull of the biceps brachii and the supinator. *B,* When the fracture is distal to the pronator teres insertion, the proximal fragment is less supinated because the pull of the supinator is balanced by that of the pronator teres. (Redrawn from Wilson JN, ed.: Watson-Jones Fractures and Joint Injuries. 5th ed., 2 vols. Edinburgh, Churchill Livingstone, 1976, by permission.)

ulnar styloid occurs. This injury has also been called a reverse Monteggia fracture, Piedmont fracture, and fracture of necessity,[38] signifying that open reduction and internal fixation are mandatory. Hughston, of the Piedmont Orthopaedic Society, noted several factors that tend to displace these fractures and make internal fixation necessary.[54] Thus the weight of the hand (even in a cast) tends to displace the distal fragment volarly, the pull of the pronator quadratus and brachioradialis tends to rotate the distal fragment toward the ulna and draw it proximally, and the pull of the thumb abductors and extensors shorten the radial side of the wrist and relax the radial collateral ligament.[54]

Radiographs confirm the presence of a fracture between the mid- and distal portions of the radial shaft, which is usually transverse or short oblique in type (Fig. 4–46). Dislocation of the radioulnar joint is manifested by widening of the

radioulnar distance and the relatively dorsal position of the distal ulna.

Open reduction and internal fixation, usually with a plate and screws, is necessary in order to maintain good pronation and supination motion and to avoid arthritic changes in the distal radioulnar joint.

Ulnar Fractures. Isolated ulnar shaft fractures are fairly common and are usually due to direct trauma (hence the term *nightstick fracture*). Nondisplaced fractures are treated conservatively and take about 3 months to unite.[38] Proximal fractures are more likely to become displaced following conservative therapy, and careful radiographic follow-up for loss of position is required (Fig. 4–47). Displaced fractures are treated with open reduction and internal fixation, usually by a compression plate and screws.

Isolated fractures of the ulna have a reputation for nonunion, with a reported incidence of up

Table 4–3. **Classification of Monteggia Fractures**

Type	Radial Head Dislocation	Ulnar Fracture	Radial Fracture
Type I (60%)	Anterior	Any level, anterior angulation	—
Type II (15%)	Posterior or posterolateral	Shaft fracture, posterior angulation	—
Type III (20%)	Lateral or anterolateral	Metaphysis	—
Type IV (5%)	Anterior	At level of radial fracture	Proximal one-third

Source: Bado JL: Clin Orthop 50:71, 1967.

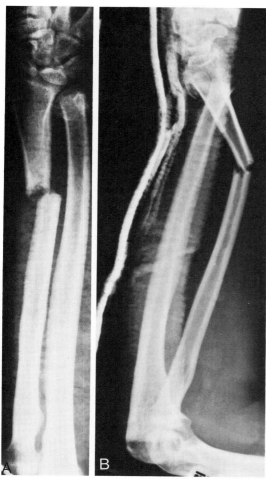

Figure 4–46. Galeazzi Fracture. The term Galeazzi fracture applies to fractures of the radial shaft at the junction of the mid- and the distal thirds and disruption (dislocation or avulsion fracture) of the radioulnar joint. *A,* The PA view shows a radial shaft fracture at the junction of the mid- and the distal thirds. Increased density overlies the distal ulna, suggesting superimposition of ulnar fracture fragments. No radial head dislocation is present. *B,* The lateral view shows striking angular deformity (apex anterior) of the radial fracture. There is a fracture of the distal ulna, with 1 shafts width dorsal displacement of the distal fragment, angular deformity (apex anterior), and overriding.

to 20 percent for this complication.[42] Nonunion has been defined as absence of healing by 1 year.[42] The middle third and the junction of the mid- and distal thirds of the ulna are particularly susceptible to this complication since these areas have a poor blood supply because of the termination of branches of the nutrient artery at the junction of the middle and distal thirds of the bone.

The Monteggia Fracture. In 1814 Giovanni Battista Monteggia described the combination of a fracture of the proximal third of the ulna and an anterior or a posterior dislocation of the radial head.[64] This concept was expanded in 1959 by Bado, who coined the term *Monteggia lesion* to include injuries in which anterior, posterior, or lateral dislocation of the radius was associated with fracture of the ulna or of both the radius and the ulna (Table 4–3).[39]

The mechanism of production of the Monteggia lesion is still debated, with either forced pronation at the time of a fall on the outstretched arm or a direct blow to the ulna suggested as the cause.[41] On physical examination the fracture deformity is usually apparent, but the radial head displacement can be recognized only by an astute clinician. Similarly, the ulnar fracture is usually readily apparent on radiographs, but the radial head dislocation often goes unrecognized, even when radiographs include the elbow (Figs. 4–48 to 4–50). Whenever an ulnar fracture is seen, careful attention should be directed toward the radial head for evidence of dislocation. In the normal situation a line drawn through the proximal radial shaft and the radial head intersects the capitellum on both the anteroposterior and the lateral views (see Fig. 4–9);[48] any

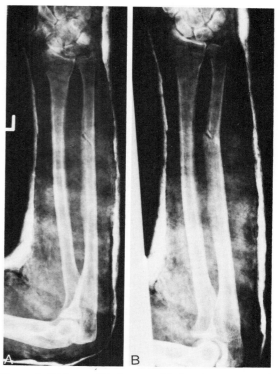

Figure 4–47. Loss of Reduction of Isolated Ulnar (Nightstick) Fracture. *A,* Original postcasting view shows essentially no angular deformity at the fracture site. *B,* Four days later angular deformity has developed.

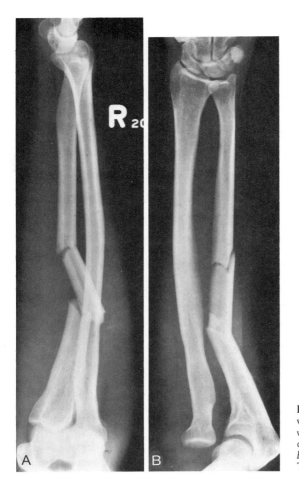

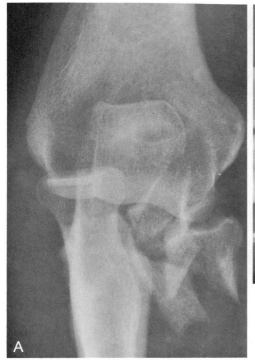

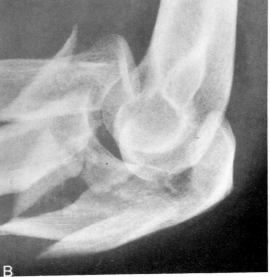

Figure 4–48. Monteggia Fracture (Lesion) Type I. *A*, The AP view (of the elbow) shows a segmental fracture of the ulna, with angular deformity. The radial head overlaps the capitellum despite the ulnar–humeral cartilage space being seen in profile. *B*, The lateral view shows angular deformity (apex anterior). The radial head dislocation is now evident.

Figure 4–49. Monteggia Fracture (Lesion) Type I. *A*, The AP view shows a comminuted olecranon fracture. The overlap of the radial head and the capitellum suggests radial head dislocation. *B*, The lateral view shows the anterior dislocation of the radial head.

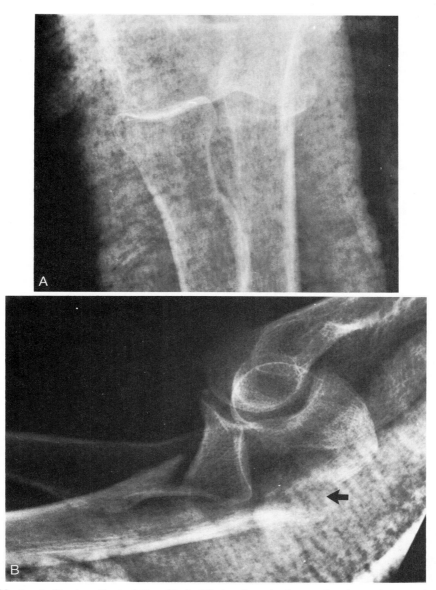

Figure 4–50. Monteggia Fracture (Lesion) Type II. *A,* AP view through plaster splint shows slight overlap of the radial head and the capitellum and lateral displacement of the radius. *B,* On lateral view, the posterior dislocation of the radius is seen. The ulna is fractured (arrow) but not dislocated.

deviation in this alignment suggests dislocation. In the type IV Monteggia lesion a radial fracture is present in addition to the radial dislocation. Thus finding a radial fracture should not dampen enthusiasm for seeking concomitant radial head dislocation. In fourteen patients with such type IV Monteggia lesions an accurate diagnosis on initial examination was made in only 58 percent of cases.

Treatment is controversial. Anderson notes the following factors to be important in achieving a good result in adults: (1) early accurate diag-nosis, (2) rigid internal fixation of the ulnar fracture, (3) complete reduction of the radial head dislocation, (4) cast immobilization in the appropriate position, and (5) early open reduction and internal fixation of the radial shaft fracture in type IV Monteggia lesions.[38]

Complications are similar to those of other forearm fractures and include infection, mal-union, and nonunion. The relationship of the radial head to the capitellum should be scrutinized on follow-up radiographs to exclude redislocation or subluxation.

Dislocations

Elbow dislocations are described by the direction in which the radius and ulna are displaced in relation to the distal humerus. The classification of adult elbow dislocations used by Eppright and Wilkins is as follows:[45]

Dislocation of both radius and ulna	Posterior (lateral or medial)
	Medial
	Lateral
	Anterior
	Divergent (anteroposterior or mediolateral)
Dislocation of radius only	Anterior
	Posterior
	Lateral
Dislocation of ulna only	Anterior
	Posterior

Dislocations of Both Radius and Ulna

Posterior Dislocation. Posterior and posterolateral dislocations account for 80 to 90 percent of all elbow dislocations.[45] These result from a fall on the outstretched hand with the arm in extension and abduction. There is damage to the collateral ligaments, the joint capsule, and the triceps insertion and disruption of the anterior capsule and the brachialis muscle by the displaced humerus. The diagnosis is usually evident clinically, but radiographic examination confirms the dislocation and any accompanying fractures (Figs. 4–51 to 4–53). Treatment usu-ally consists of closed reduction and short-term immobilization.

Medial and Lateral Dislocations. These injuries are most easily identified on AP radiographs, which show loss of normal alignment between the radius and the capitellum and between the ulna and the trochlea. The lateral view may not be strikingly abnormal. Closed reduction is the usual treatment.

Anterior Dislocations. These dislocations are very unusual injuries. The olecranon process impinges on the anterior aspect of the distal humerus on the lateral radiograph. Damage to the brachial artery or ulnar nerve may occur.[45]

Dislocations of Radius and Ulna in Different Directions. There are two types of dislocations, anteroposterior and mediolateral. The anteroposterior is the more common and consists of posterior dislocation of the ulna, with the coronoid process located in the olecranon fossa, and anterior dislocation of the radial head into the coronoid fossa.

Isolated Radial Head Dislocation

Radial head dislocation most often accompanies ulnar fracture (the Monteggia fracture dislocation); isolated radial head dislocation in an adult is very rare.

Isolated Ulnar Dislocation

The ulna alone may be dislocated anteriorly or posteriorly, the latter being the more frequent direction.

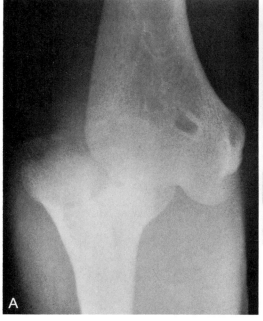
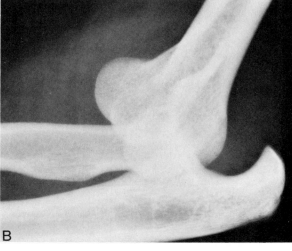

Figure 4–51. Posterolateral Dislocation. *A,* AP view shows lateral displacement of the radius and the ulna. *B,* Lateral view confirms posterior dislocation of both the radius and the ulna.

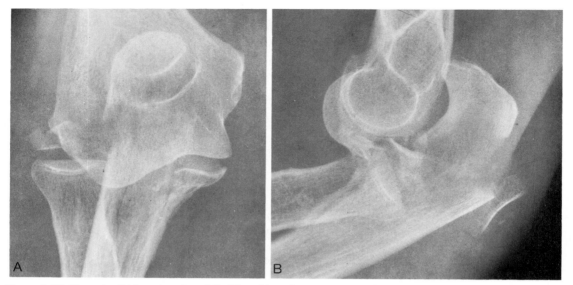

Figure 4–52. Posterior Dislocation. *A* and *B,* AP and lateral views, respectively, show posterior dislocation of the radius and the ulna and a comminuted fracture of the olecranon process. The lateral bony fragments most likely originate from the posterior capitellum.

Recurrent Dislocation

Recurrent dislocation of the elbow is a rare complication of acute dislocation and is usually of the posterior type. If a predisposing bony abnormality cannot be identified on standard radiographic examination, an arthrogram may be of help in identifying any associated or predisposing defects in the soft tissues or cartilage.[61]

Fractures accompanying elbow dislocation are frequent and include fractures of the medial epicondyle, coronoid process, lateral condyle, radial head, and capitellum.

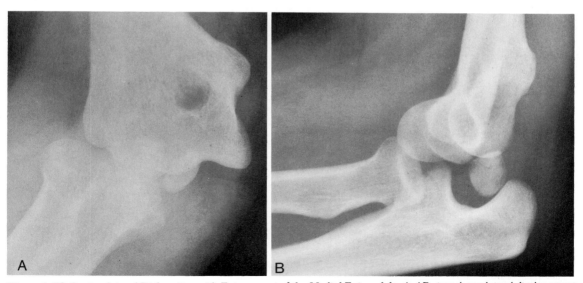

Figure 4–53. Posterolateral Dislocation with Entrapment of the Medial Epicondyle. *A,* AP view shows lateral displacement of the radius and the ulna. An oval density, most likely an ununited medial ossification center, has been pulled distally. *B,* Posterior displacement of the radius and the ulna is apparent. The ossicle overlies the olecranon fossa.

205

Complications of elbow dislocation include loss of motion, heterotopic bone formation in the joint capsule and ligaments (apparent on radiographs within 3 to 4 weeks after injury),[71] neural or vascular injury, and irreducibility.[45]

Tennis Elbow

Tennis elbow is a clinical syndrome consisting of pain over the lateral aspect of the elbow aggravated by active wrist extension.[74] A variety of names have been applied to this condition, including epicondylitis, radiohumeral bursitis, radiohumeral synovitis, tendinitis, and golfer's elbow. The multiplicity of titles results from the lack of agreement as to the pathogenesis of this condition. Among the etiologies suggested are small tears in the origin of the conjoined tendon of the extensors at the lateral epicondyle, periostitis due to partial tears of the origin of the extensor carpi radialis brevis, inflammation of a bursa under the conjoined tendon (although it is controversial whether such a bursa exists), calcific tendinitis of the conjoined tendon similar

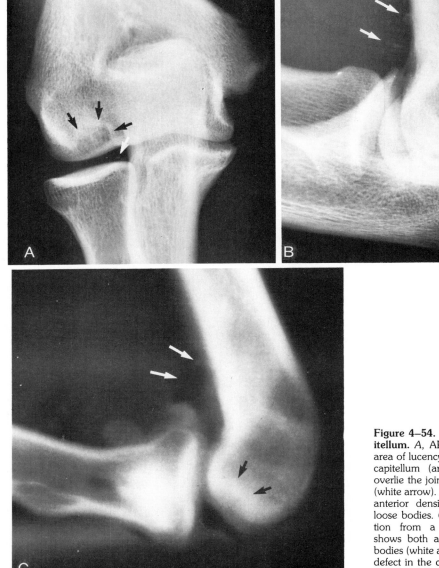

Figure 4–54. Avascular Necrosis of Capitellum. *A,* AP view shows a questionable area of lucency and adjacent sclerosis in the capitellum (arrows). Two small densities overlie the joint space just above the radius (white arrow). *B,* The lateral view shows two anterior densities (arrows) that could be loose bodies. *C,* A lateral tomographic section from a double-contrast arthrogram shows both anterior densities to be loose bodies (white arrows) and confirms the bony defect in the capitellum (black arrows) with slight irregularity of the overlying cartilage.

to that occurring in the shoulder, abnormalities in the annular ligament around the radial head, chondromalacia of the capitellum or radial head, localized synovitis, and nerve entrapment.[74, 76, 78]

Normally, loose areolar connective tissue is present under the common extensor tendon. Pathological examination of patients with tennis elbow has failed to show a separate bursa, periostitis, or tendon tears, but increased vascularity, edema, and granulation tissue have been seen in this subtendinous location.[75]

Clinically, pain is most often unilateral and gradual in onset and can be elicited by passive stretching of the extensor origin by forced pronation of the forearm while the hand and wrist are flexed and the elbow is extended.[74, 76]

Radiographic Findings

The diagnosis of tennis elbow is a clinical one, and in most series no specific radiological findings are discussed. However, Gondos noted that seven of twenty patients (35 percent) with a clinical diagnosis of tennis elbow demonstrated radiologically identifiable calcification adjacent to the lateral epicondyle.[76] Clinical and radiological parallels were noted to the calcific tendinitis occurring in the rotator cuff of the shoulder. Of particular interest to those evaluating routine radiographs of patients with this condition was the radiological study of anatomical specimens in which small bony projections from the lateral and medial epicondyles were noted that were thought to represent normal variations.[76]

Treatment

The majority of patients improve with no treatment or with conservative treatment. Recurrent or persistent cases may be treated with various surgical procedures involving the soft tissues, depending on the postulated underlying disturbance (e.g., bursal excision, radial nerve decompression).[74, 78]

Panner's Disease (AVN of the Capitellum)

Panner (1927 and 1929) reported the radiographic and clinical findings of three boys who developed mild elbow symptoms after trauma.[81, 82] Radiographs showed abnormalities limited to the capitellum consisting of rarefaction, irregularity, and decreased size of the ossification center; there was later improvement in radiographic appearance. Panner suggested that the clinical and radiologic features placed this condition (designated in his honor as Morbus Pannerii) in the group of epiphyseal disorders that

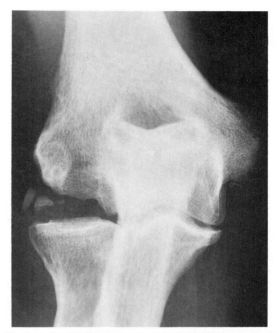

Figure 4–55. Avascular Necrosis of Capitellum (Panner's Disease). The capitellum is small and irregular. Multiple separate bony fragments (loose bodies) overlie the joint. There is hypertrophic lipping from the radial head and the ulnar-trochlear articular margins.

includes Legg–Calvé–Perthes disease, Köhler's disease, and the like.

This disorder seems to be uncommon, although it has been seen in patients with renal failure.[79] The radiographic findings are typical of avascular necrosis (AVN) (see Chapter 8) (Figs. 4–54 and 4–55). One patient with typical radiographic findings had increased radionuclide uptake on bone scan.[83] Arthrography may help to define defects in the overlying cartilage, the presence of intraarticular loose bodies, or both.

Total Elbow Prostheses

Total elbow prostheses are currently being developed for use in patients with severe sequelae (particularly pain) of rheumatoid arthritis or posttraumatic arthritis. The evolution of total elbow prostheses began with metal-to-metal hinge prostheses (e.g., Dee, Shiers, McKee), which were fixed to bone with methylmethacrylate cement.[85, 86] Later hinge prostheses include the Mayo prosthesis, in which the radiohumeral and the ulnar humeral joints are replaced. The Coonrad, Schlein, and GSB prostheses are similar metal hinges that replace only the ulnar-humeral joint. The Pritchard-Walker hinge pros-

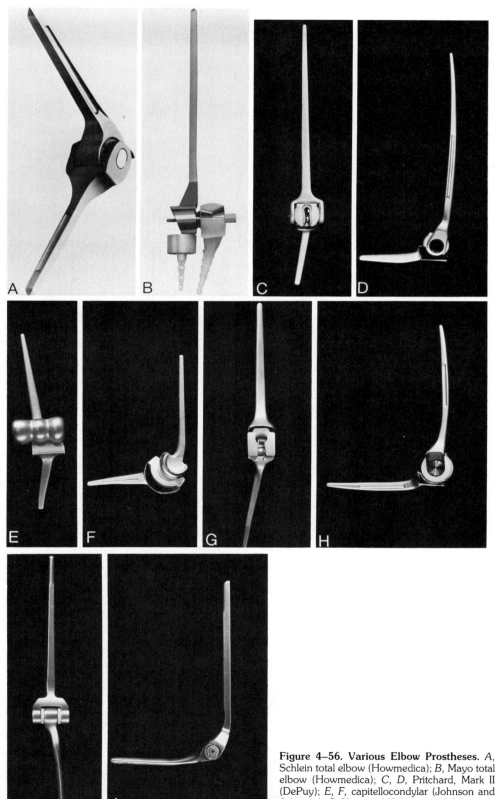

Figure 4–56. Various Elbow Prostheses. *A,* Schlein total elbow (Howmedica); *B,* Mayo total elbow (Howmedica); *C, D,* Pritchard, Mark II (DePuy); *E, F,* capitellocondylar (Johnson and Johnson); *G, H,* triaxial (Johnson and Johnson); *I, J,* Coonrad (Zimmer).

thesis allows a few degrees of varus-valgus motion in addition to flexion and extension. The triaxial prosthesis also allows rotational motion.[89] The capitellocondylar prosthesis is a semiconstrained nonhinged prosthesis that consists of a separate metal humeral component and a high-density polyethylene ulnar component that may have a metal backing (Fig. 4–56).[88]

The hinge prostheses with fixed axes of rotation are associated with loosening in about 19 percent of cases.[88] This complication is seen radiographically as widening of the cement-bone interface, particularly if it involves the entire extent of this interface (Fig. 4–57).

The recent trend toward less constrained prostheses (e.g., the triaxial and the capitellocondylar prostheses) should reduce the number of failures occurring because of loosening, and this has indeed been confirmed on follow-up studies.[88, 89] (Figures 4–58 and 4–59 show instances of failure.) With the nonconstrained capitellocondylar prosthesis, dislocation may, however, occur in either the anteroposterior or the medial lateral direction (Figs. 4–60 and 4–61).

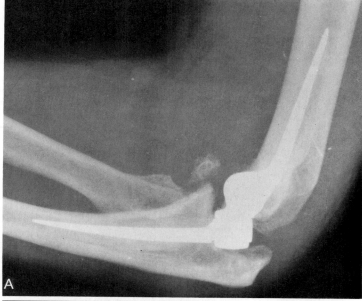

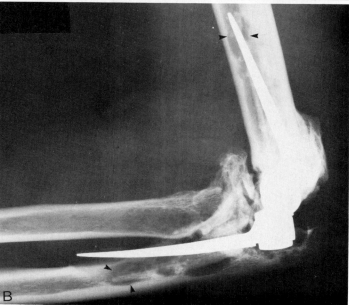

Figure 4–57. Loosening of Hinged Total-Elbow Prosthesis (GSB). *A,* A lateral view shortly after surgery shows the hinged total-elbow prosthesis with cement around each stem. There is no loosening. The radial head resection and the anterior ossification were stigmata of prior injury and surgery. *B,* Six years later the prosthesis is grossly loose, as evidenced by wide cement-bone lucencies (some shown by arrowheads), olecranon bone loss, and protrusion of the ulnar stem.

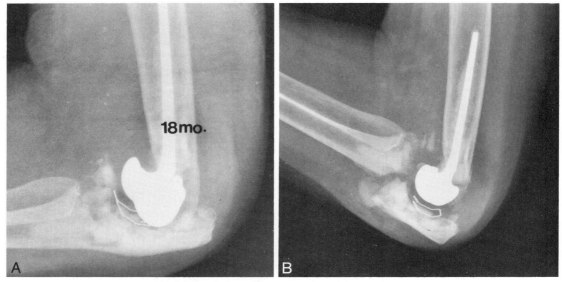

Figure 4–58. Loosening of the Total-Elbow Prosthesis (Capitellocondylar) with Olecranon Fracture. *A,* Eighteen months after total elbow replacement, there is evidence of loosening of the ulnar component with widening of the bone-cement interface, fragmentation of cement, and bone loss from the olecranon. *B,* Seven months later the olecranon has fractured and the ulnar component (indicated by the marker wire) has turned front-to-back as a result of loosening at the prosthesis-cement, as well as the cement-bone, interface.

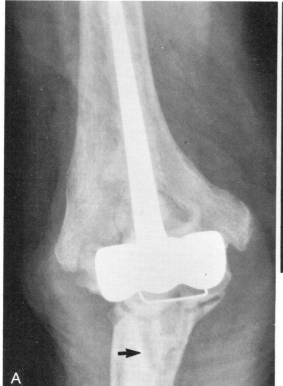

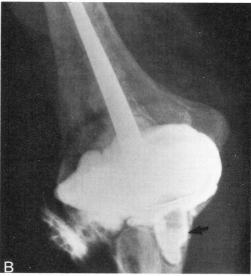

Figure 4–59. Loose Total-Elbow Prosthesis (Capitellocondylar) Confirmed on Arthrography. *A,* The preliminary AP view shows a wide cement-bone lucency around the ulnar prosthesis. *B,* The single-contrast arthrogram shows contrast medium filling the cement-bone interface (arrow). There has also been filling of the cement-bone interface in the supratrochlear region. (From the radiographic evaluation of total joint replacement. *In* Kelley EN et al., eds.: Textbook of Rheumatology. Philadelphia, WB Saunders, 1981.)

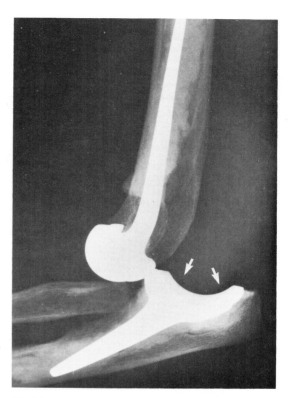

Figure 4–60. Posterior Dislocation of Total-Elbow Prosthesis. A lateral view shows the posterior position of the ulnar component (and the radius) in relation to the humeral component. The relatively lucent articular surface (arrows) of the ulnar component is well seen.

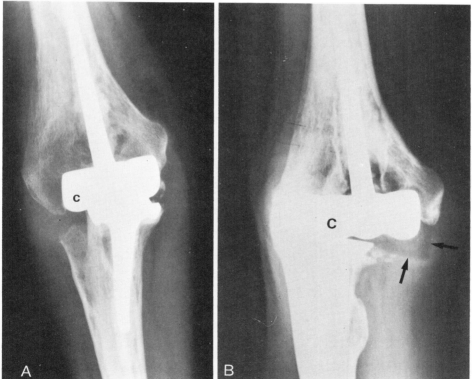

Figure 4–61. Lateral Dislocation of Total-Elbow Prosthesis. *A,* Usual AP view of a capitellocondylar prosthesis shows the "overhang" of the capitellar facet (C) in relation to the ulnar component. *B,* AP view in another patient shows the humeral component to be displaced medially (a lateral elbow dislocation) so that the trochlear facet is now uncovered. The plastic linear of the ulnar component (arrows) has dislocated into the joint. (C = capitellar facet.)

Additional complications that may be identified radiographically include infection, humeral and ulnar fractures, and fracture and malposition of the components.

References
Essential Anatomy
1. Barnard LB, McCoy SM: The supracondyloid process of the humerus. J Bone Joint Surg 28:845–850, 1946.
2. Feindel W, Stratford J: Cubital tunnel compression in tardy ulnar palsy. Can Med Assoc J 78:351–353, 1958.
3. Warwick R, Williams PL: Gray's Anatomy. 36th Br ed. Philadelphia, WB Saunders, 1982.
4. Kriss N: Clinical significance of the supracondyloid process of the humerus. Case report. AJR 76:1154–1156, 1956.
5. Morrey BF, Chao EYS: Passive motion of the elbow joint. J Bone Joint Surg (Am) 58:501–508, 1976.
6. Wadsworth TG: The Elbow. New York, Churchill Livingstone, 1982.
7. Wadsworth TG. The external compression syndrome of the ulnar nerve at the cubital tunnel. Clin Orthop 124:189–204, 1977.

Normal Radiographic Appearances
8. Beals RK: The normal carrying angle of the elbow. A radiographic study of 422 patients. Clin Orthop 119:194–196, 1976.
9. Keats TE, Teeslink R, Diamond AE, Williams JH: Normal axial relationships of the major joints. Radiology 87:904–907, 1966.
10. Rogers LF: Elbow. In Felson B, ed. Roentgenology of Fractures and Dislocations. New York, Grune & Stratton, 1978: 91–101.
11. Rogers LF, Malave S Jr, White H, Tachdjian MO: Plastic bowing, torus and greenstick supracondylar fractures of the humerus: Radiographic clues to obscure fractures of the elbow in children. Radiology 128:145–150, 1978.

Elbow Arthrography
12. Arvidsson H, Johansson O: Arthrography of the elbow-joint. Acta Radiol [Diagn] (Stockh) 43:445–452, 1955.
13. Ehrlich GE: Antecubital cysts in rheumatoid arthritis—a corollary to popliteal (Baker's) cysts. J Bone Joint Surg (Am) 54:165–169, 1972.
14. Eto RT, Anderson PW, Harley JD: Elbow arthrography with the application of tomography. Radiology 115:283–288, 1975.
15. Goode JD: Synovial rupture of the elbow joint. Ann Rheum Dis 27:604–609, 1968.
16. Hall FM: Elbow arthrography. Radiology 132:775, 1979.
17. Hudson T: The elbow. In Freiberger RH, Kaye JJ, eds. Arthrography. New York, Appleton-Century Crofts, 1979: 261–276.
18. Pavlov H, Ghelman B, Warren RF: Double-contrast arthrography of the elbow. Radiology 130:87–95, 1979.

Abnormal Soft Tissues (Periarticular Fat Pads)
19. Bledsoe RC, Izenstark JL: Displacement of fat pads in disease and injury of the elbow: A new radiographic sign. Radiology 73:717–724, 1959.
20. Bohrer SP: The fat pad sign following elbow trauma. Its usefulness and reliability in suspecting "invisible" fractures. Clin Radiol 21:90–94, 1970.

21. Jackman RJ, Pugh DG: The positive elbow fat pad sign in rheumatoid arthritis. AJR 108:812–818, 1970.
22. Kohn AM: Soft tissue alterations in elbow trauma. AJR 82:867–874, 1959.
23. Murphy WA, Siegel MJ: Elbow fat pads with new signs and extended differential diagnosis. Radiology 124:659–665, 1977.
24. Nelson SW: Some important diagnostic and technical fundamentals in the radiology of trauma, with particular emphasis on skeletal trauma. Radiol Clin North Am 42:241–259, 1966.
25. Norell HG: Roentgenologic visualization of the extracapsular fat. Its importance in the diagnosis of traumatic injuries to the elbow. Acta Radiol [Diagn] (Stockh) 42:205–210, 1954.
26. Rogers SL, MacEwan DW: Changes due to trauma in the fat plane overlying the supinator muscle: A radiologic sign. Radiology 92:954–958, 1969.
27. Saini M, Canoso JJ: Traumatic olecranon bursitis. Acta Radiol [Diagn] (Stockh) 23:255–258, 1982.
28. Smith DN, Lee JR: The radiological diagnosis of post-traumatic effusion of the elbow joint and its clinical significance. The 'displaced fat pad' sign. Injury 10:115–119, 1978.
29. Yousefzadeh DK, Jackson JH: Lipohemarthrosis of the elbow joint. Radiology 128:643–645, 1978.

Rheumatoid Arthritis, Bursitis, and Nodules
30. Berens DL, Lin RK: Roentgen Diagnosis of Rheumatoid Arthritis. Springfield, Ill. CC Thomas, 1969.
31. Ehrlich GE: Antecubital cysts in rheumatoid arthritis—a corollary to popliteal (Baker's) cysts. J Bone Joint Surg (Am) 54:165–169, 1972.
32. Goode JD: Synovial rupture of the elbow joint. Ann Rheum Dis 27:604–609, 1968.
33. Forrester DM, Nesson JW: The Radiology of Joint Disease. Philadelphia, WB Saunders, 1973.
34. Weston WJ, Palmer DG: Soft Tissues of the Extremities. A Radiologic Study of Rheumatic Disease. New York, Springer-Verlag, 1978.

Loose Bodies
35. Bassett LW, Mirra JM, Forrester DM, Gold RH, Bernstein ML, Rollins JS: Post-traumatic osteochondral "loose body" of the olecranon fossa. An entity which can be mistaken for a normal anatomical variant or osteoid osteoma. Radiology 141:635–638, 1981.
36. Milgram JW: The development of loose bodies in human joints. Clin Orthop 124:292–303, 1977.
37. Obermann WR, Loose HWC: The os supratrochleare dorsale: A normal variant that may cause symptoms. AJR 141:123–127, 1983.

Fractures and Dislocations
38. Anderson LD: Fracture of the Shafts of the Radius and Ulna. In Rockwood CA Jr, Green DP, eds. Fractures. Philadelphia, JB Lippincott, 1975: 441–485.
39. Bado JL: The Monteggia lesion. Clin Orthop 50:71–86, 1967.
40. Blecher KW, Saunders EA: Fractures of the radius and the ulna in adults. Am Surg 43:310–314, 1977.
41. Boyd HB, Boals JC: The Monteggia lesion. A review of 159 cases. Clin Orthop 66:94–100, 1969.
42. Brakenbury PH, Corea JR, Blakemore ME: Non-union of the isolated fracture of the ulnar shaft in adults. Injury 12:371–375, 1981.
43. Chessare JW, Rogers LF, White H, Tachdjian MO:

Injuries of the medial epicondylar ossification center of the humerus. AJR 129:49–55, 1977.

44. Colton CL: Fractures of the olecranon in adults: Classification and management. Injury 5:121–129, 1973.
45. Eppright RH, Wilkins KE: Fractures and dislocations of the elbow. *In* Rockwood CA Jr, Green DP, eds. Fractures. Philadelphia, JB Lippincott, 1975: 487–563.
46. Evans EM: Rotational deformity in the treatment of fractures of both bones of the forearm. J Bone Joint Surg 27:373–379, 1945.
47. Gartsman GM, Sculco TP, Otis JC: Operative treatment of olecranon fractures. Excision or open reduction with internal fixation. J Bone Joint Surg (Am) 63:718–721, 1981.
48. Giustra PE, Killoran PJ, Furman RS, Root JA: The missed Monteggia fracture. Radiology 110:45–47, 1974.
49. Gore RM, Rogers LF, Bowerman J, Suker J, Compere CL: Osseous manifestations of elbow stress associated with sports activities. AJR 134:971–977, 1980.
50. Grace TG, Eversmann WW: Forearm fractures. Treatment of rigid fixation with early motion. J Bone Joint Surg (Am) 62:433–438, 1980.
51. Greenspan A, Norman A: The radial head, capitellum view: Useful technique in elbow trauma. AJR 138:1186–1188, 1982.
52. Heppenstall RB: Fracture Treatment and Healing. Philadelphia, WB Saunders, 1980.
53. Horne JG, Tanzer TL: Olecranon fractures: A review of 100 cases. J Trauma 21:469–472, 1981.
54. Hughston JC: Fracture of the distal radial shaft. Mistakes in management. J Bone Joint Surg (Am) 39:249–264, 1957.
55. Knight RA: The management of fractures about the elbow in adults. AAOS Instructional Course Lectures 14:123–141, 1957.
56. Kulowski J: Fractures of the elbow joint: New classification and roentgenologic guide to major pitfalls of diagnosis and treatment. AJR 79:692–696, 1958.
57. Mason ML: Some observations on fractures of the head of the radius with a review of one hundred cases. Br J Surg 42:123–132, 1954.
58. Matthews WE, Saunders EA: Fractures of the radius and ulna: Part II. Am Surg 45:321–324, 1979.
59. Matthews LS, Kaufer H, Garver DF, Sonstegard DA: The effect on supination-pronation of angular malalignment of fractures of both bones of the forearm. An experimental study. J Bone Joint Surg (Am) 64:14–17, 1982.
60. Milch H: Fractures of the external humeral condyle. JAMA 160:641–647, 1956.
61. Mink JH, Eckardt JJ, Grant TT: Arthrography in recurrent dislocation of the elbow. AJR 136:1242–1244, 1981.
62. Muller ME, Allgower M, Schneider R, Willenegger H: Manual of Internal Fixation. Techniques Recommended by the AO Group. 2nd ed. New York, Springer-Verlag, 1979.
63. Patrick J: Fracture of the medial epicondyle with displacement into the elbow joint. J Bone Joint Surg 28:143–147, 1946.
64. Peltier LF: Eponymic fractures: Giovanni Battista Monteggia and Monteggia's fracture. Surgery 42:585–591, 1957.
65. Radin EL, Riseborough EJ: Fractures of the radial head (A review of eighty-eight cases and analysis of the indications for excision of the radial head and nonoperative treatment). J Bone Joint Surg (Am) 48:1055–1064, 1966.

66. Riseborough EJ, Radin EL: Intercondylar T fractures of the humerus in the adult. (A comparison of operative and nonoperative treatment in twenty-nine cases.) J Bone Joint Surg (Am) 51:130–141, 1969.
67. Rogers LF: Elbow. *In* Felson B, ed. Roentgenology of Fractures and Dislocations. New York, Grune & Stratton, 1978: 91–101.
68. Sarmiento A, Kinman P, Murphy RB, Phillips JG: Treatment of ulnar fractures by functional bracing. J Bone Joint Surg (Am) 58:1104–1107, 1976.
69. Swanson AB, Jaeger SH, La Rochelle D: Comminuted fractures of the radial head. The role of silicone-implant replacement arthroplasty. J Bone Joint Surg (Am) 63:1039–1049, 1981.
70. Teipner WA, Mast JW: Internal fixation of forearm diaphyseal fractures: Double plating versus single compression (tension band) plating—a comparative study. Orthop Clin North Am 11:381–391, 1980.
71. Thompson HC III, Garcia A: Myositis ossificans (aftermath of elbow injuries). Clin Orthop 50:129–134, 1967.
72. Wadsworth TG: Screw fixation of the olecranon after fracture or osteotomy. Clin Orthop 119:197–201, 1976.

Tennis Elbow

73. Boyd HB, McLeod AC: Tennis elbow. J Bone Joint Surg (Am) 1183–1187, 1973.
74. Friedlander HL, Reid RL, Cape RF: Tennis elbow. Clin Orthop 51:109–116, 1967.
75. Goldie I: Epicondylitis lateralis humeri (epicondylalgia or tennis elbow). A pathogenetical study. Acta Chir Scand [Suppl] 339:1–119, 1964.
76. Gondos B: Tennis elbow: A re-evaluation. AJR 79:684–691, 1958.
77. McCarty DJ: Tennis elbow (epicondylitis). *In* Hollander JL, McCarty DJ Jr, eds. Arthritis and Allied Conditions: A Textbook of Rheumatology. Philadelphia, Lea & Febiger, 1979: 995–996.
78. Roles NC, Maudsley RH: Radial tunnel syndrome: Resistant tennis elbow as a nerve entrapment. J Bone Joint Surg (Br) 54:499–508, 1972.

Panner's Disease

79. Kricun M, Resnick D: Elbow abnormalities in renal osteodystrophy. AJR 140:577–579, 1983.
80. Krebs C: Maladie de panner: une affection du condyle de l'humerus ressemblant à la maladie de Calvé-Perthes. Arch Franco-Belges de Chir 30:608–609, 1927.
81. Panner HJ: An affection of the capitulum humeri resembling Calvé-Perthes disease of the hip. Proceedings of the Northern Radiological Association, 1927. Acta Radiol [Diagn] (Stockh) 8:617–618, 1927.
82. Panner HJ: A peculiar affection of the capitulum humeri, resembling Calvé-Perthes disease of the hip. Acta Radiol [Diagn] (Stockh) 10:234–242, 1929.
83. Sty JR, Boedecker R: Panner's disease (osteonecrosis of the capitellum). Clin Nucl Med 3:117, 1978.

Total Elbow Replacement

84. Bryan RS, Dobyns JH, Linscheid RL, Peterson LFA: Preliminary Experiences with Total Elbow Arthroplasty. Symposium on Osteoarthritis. St. Louis, CV Mosby, 1974.
85. Dee R: Total replacement arthroplasty of the elbow for rheumatoid arthritis. J Bone Joint Surg (Br) 54:88–95, 1972.
86. Dee R: Total elbow replacement. J Bone Joint Surg (Br) 56:233, 1974.
87. Ewald FC, Scheinberg RD, Poss R, Thomas WH, Scott

RD, Sledge CB: Capitellocondylar total elbow arthroplasty. Two to five-year follow-up in rheumatoid arthritis. J Bone Joint Surg (Am) 62:1259–1263, 1980.

88. Ewald FC: Reconstructive surgery and rehabilitation of the elbow. *In* Kelley WN, Harris ED Jr, Ruddy S, Sledge CB, eds. Textbook of Rheumatology, Vol 2. Philadelphia, WB Saunders, 1981: 1921–1943.

89. Inglis AE, Pellicci PM: Total elbow replacement. J Bone Joint Surg (Am) 62:1252–1258, 1980.

90. London JT: Kinematics of the elbow. J Bone Joint Surg (Am) 63:529–535, 1981.

91. Morrey BF, Bryan RS: Total joint arthroplasty. The elbow. Mayo Clin Proc 54:507–512, 1979.

92. Souter WA: Arthroplasty of the elbow with particular reference to metallic hinge arthroplasty in rheumatoid patients. Orthop Clin North Am 4:395–413, 1973.

Chapter 5

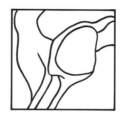

The
SHOULDER

Glenohumeral Joint

NORMAL STRUCTURE AND FUNCTION

Essential Anatomy
(Figs. 5–1 and 5–2)

The articular surface of the proximal humerus is directed medially, superiorly, and posteriorly (retroverted) about 20 degrees with relation to the transverse axis of the distal humerus.[1] The *anatomic neck* of the humerus is the area between the articular surface and the tuberosities and is the site of attachment of the joint capsule (Fig. 5–3). The *surgical neck* is the junction between the tuberosities and the humeral shaft and represents the level of anastomotic vessels

215

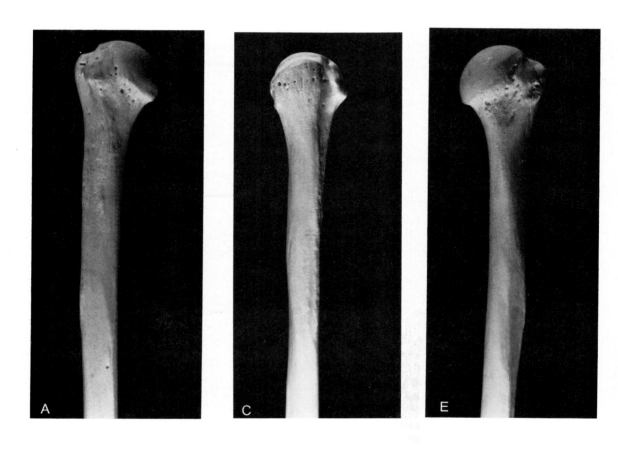

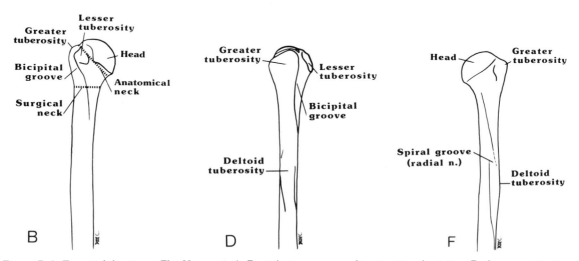

Figure 5–1. Essential Anatomy: The Humerus. *A,* Frontal view corresponding to external rotation; *B,* diagrammatic view of *A;* *C,* Frontal view corresponding to internal rotation; *D,* diagrammatic view of *C;* *E,* the posterior aspect; *F,* diagrammatic view of *E.*

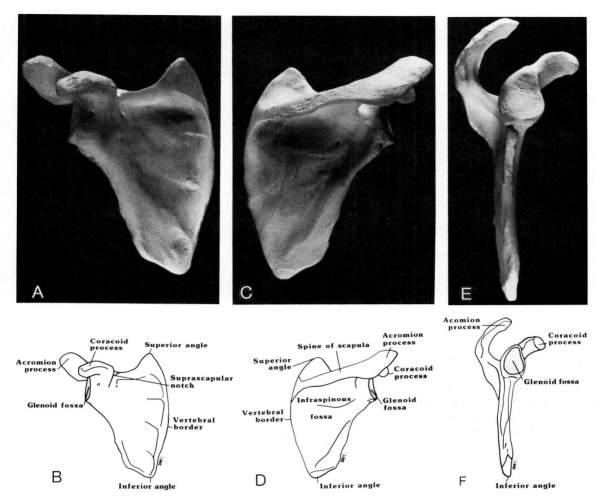

Figure 5–2. Essential Anatomy: the Scapula. *A,* Frontal view; *B,* diagrammatic representation of *A; C,* posterior aspect; *D,* diagrammatic representation of *C; E,* lateral view of scapula to show the glenoid surface; *F,* diagrammatic representation of *E.*

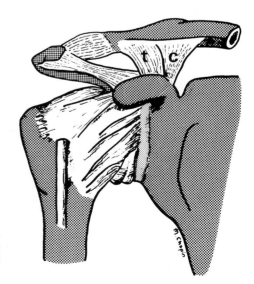

Figure 5–3. Joint Capsule. The joint capsule inserts along the anatomical neck of the humerus and along the neck of the glenoid. The coracoacromial and coracoclavicular ligaments (conoid [c] and trapezoid [t] portions) are shown.

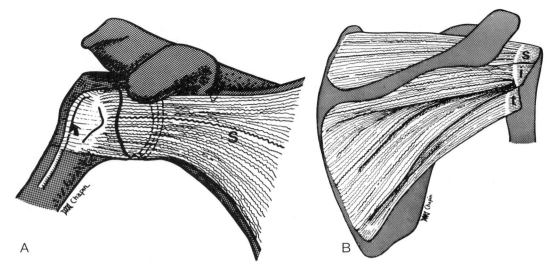

A   B

Figure 5–4. The Rotator Cuff. *A,* Frontal view of the shoulder shows the subscapularis muscle (S) inserting on the lesser tuberosity. The tendon of the long head of the biceps (in the bicipital groove) is seen (arrow). *B,* The posterior view shows the insertions of the supraspinatus (s), infraspinatus (i), and teres minor (t) muscles on the greater tuberosity.

(the posterior circumflex artery). Between these areas are the greater and lesser tuberosities, separated from each other by the bicipital groove, in which runs the tendon of the long head of the biceps.

The tuberosities provide insertion for the muscles of the rotator cuff: the subscapularis, supraspinatus, infraspinatus, and teres minor (Fig. 5–4). The supraspinatus tendon covers the superior aspect of the humeral head and inserts on the superior facet of the greater tuberosity. The infraspinatus tendon covers the superior and posterior aspects of the humeral head and inserts on the middle facet, which is distal to and more posterior than the superior facet. The teres minor is lower in position and inserts on the posterior, inferior facet of the greater tuberosity.[1] These muscles are external rotators. The supraspinatus initiates abduction by fixing the humeral head against the glenoid, thus providing a fulcrum for abduction. The subscapularis tendon is anterior to the humeral head and inserts on the lesser tuberosity; it functions to rotate the humerus internally. Knowledge of the positions of insertion of these tendons is helpful in localizing periarticular calcifications (see calcific tendinitis).

The glenoid cavity faces anteriorly; its long axis paralleling the vertebral border of the scapula. The shallow glenoid fossa is deepened by a fibrocartilaginous labrum, which attaches to the rim of the glenoid and is continuous with the joint capsule at the neck of the scapula. The tendon of the long head of the biceps blends with the labrum superiorly (Fig. 5–5).

Shoulder motion is a composite of motion at the sternoclavicular, acromioclavicular, scapulothoracic, and glenohumeral joints.[2, 3] Sternoclavicular motion is maximal early in the course of elevation of the arm and acromioclavicular motion is maximal later. With abduction of the arm

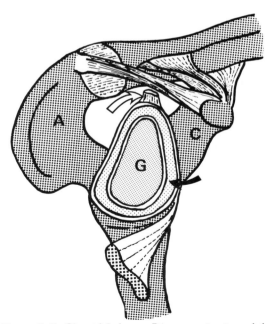

Figure 5–5. Glenoid Labrum. Diagrammatic view of the glenoid fossa en face shows the glenoid labrum (black arrow) arising from and encircling the margins of the fossa. The continuity of the tendon of the long head of the biceps (open arrow) with the labrum is evident. G = glenoid, C = coracoid process, A = acromion process.

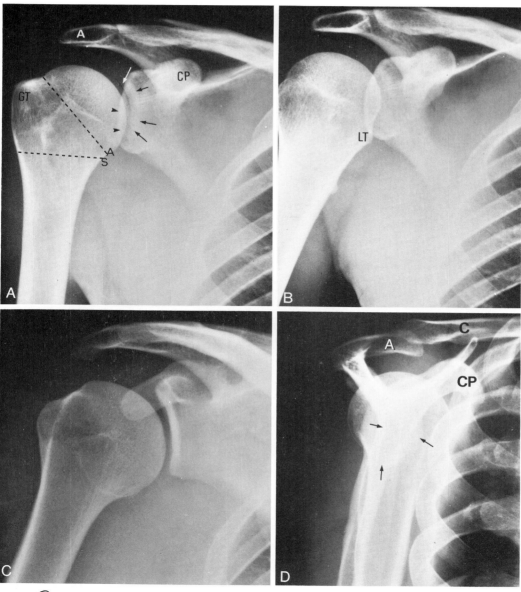

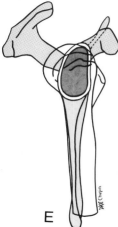

Figure 5–6. Normal Radiographic Examination. *A,* External rotation. The greater tuberosity (GT) is seen in profile. The humeral head normally overlaps the glenoid on this view. The anterior (small arrows) and posterior (arrowheads) glenoid margins are well seen and do not overlap owing to the anterior tilt of the glenoid. The anatomical (A, black) and surgical (S) necks of the humerus are indicated. CP = coracoid process, A (white) = acromion process. A vacuum phenomenon (white arrow) is present. *B,* Internal rotation. The overlap of the greater tuberosity and the humeral head produces a rounded appearance of the proximal humerus. LT = lesser tuberosity. A small exostosis is noted projecting from the humeral metaphysis. *C,* Posterior oblique. The glenohumeral cartilage space is seen in profile with no overlap of the humerus and glenoid. *D,* Normal scapular Y view. This true lateral view of the scapula (anterior oblique of the shoulder) shows the humeral head centered over the glenoid (arrows). A = acromion, C = clavicle, CP = coracoid process. *E,* Diagram of normal scapular Y.

Illustration continued on following page

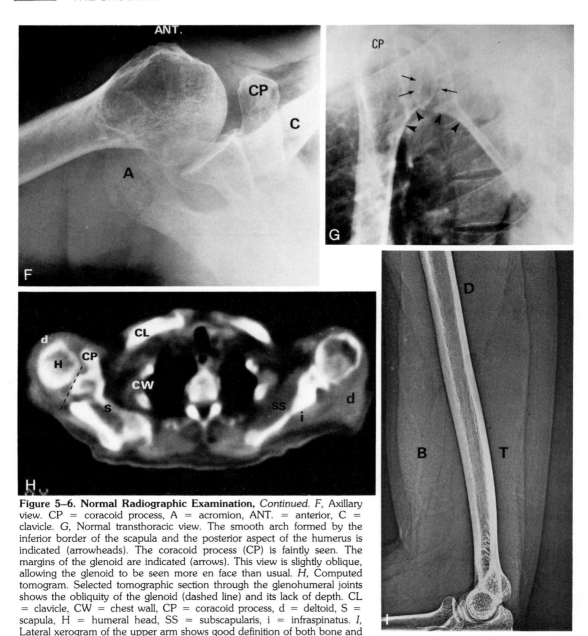

Figure 5–6. Normal Radiographic Examination, *Continued. F,* Axillary view. CP = coracoid process, A = acromion, ANT. = anterior, C = clavicle. *G,* Normal transthoracic view. The smooth arch formed by the inferior border of the scapula and the posterior aspect of the humerus is indicated (arrowheads). The coracoid process (CP) is faintly seen. The margins of the glenoid are indicated (arrows). This view is slightly oblique, allowing the glenoid to be seen more en face than usual. *H,* Computed tomogram. Selected tomographic section through the glenohumeral joints shows the obliquity of the glenoid (dashed line) and its lack of depth. CL = clavicle, CW = chest wall, CP = coracoid process, d = deltoid, S = scapula, H = humeral head, SS = subscapularis, i = infraspinatus. *I,* Lateral xerogram of the upper arm shows good definition of both bone and soft tissue structures. The biceps brachii (B), deltoid (D), and triceps (T) muscles are well delineated.

of less than 30 degrees the scapula moves only slightly, whereas with greater degrees of abduction scapulothoracic motion increases to a ratio of 1.25:1 between glenohumeral and scapulothoracic components.[3]

Normal Radiographic Appearances (Fig. 5–6)

Since the surface of the glenoid is obliquely oriented (tilted about 20 degrees anteriorly),

standard AP and lateral views are not tangential to the articular surface and do not adequately demonstrate the cartilage space or glenohumeral alignment. A posterior oblique view actually represents the true anteroposterior view of the glenohumeral joint. A 45- to 60-degree anterior oblique view (i.e., a true lateral view of the scapula) shows the glenoid en face.[4, 9, 10] A combination of these oblique views has been shown to be all that is necessary for diagnosis of most shoulder abnormalities.[10]

The posterior oblique view should show the glenohumeral joint space in profile with a 4- to 6-mm–thick cartilage space and no overlap of the humeral head and scapula. The inferior edge of the articular surface of the humerus may be a few millimeters higher than the inferior edge of the glenoid.

As seen on the anterior oblique projection, the scapula has a Y-configuration with the acromion process extending posteriorly, the coracoid process anteriorly, and the body of the scapula vertically and inferiorly. The glenoid fossa is at the junction of the three limbs of the Y, and the humeral head should be centered over it.[9]

Additional views with the humerus in internal or external rotation or an axillary view may supplement the oblique views when necessary.

Normal Soft Tissues

In the normal shoulder a thin lucent line may be seen paralleling the undersurface of the acromion process and then curving inferiorly along the lateral aspect of the proximal humerus (Fig. 5–7). According to Weston this represents extrasynovial fat around the collapsed subacromial subdeltoid bursa.[11] Since this bursa normally represents only a potential space, the two layers of fat are essentially in apposition.

Shoulder Arthrography

Technique. For single- or double-contrast arthrography needle placement under fluoroscopic control from an anterior approach has been quite satisfactory. The patient is placed supine

on the fluoroscopic table, with the humerus in slight external rotation. Although we routinely rotate the patient toward the involved side to obtain a tangential view of the glenohumeral joint, this is probably not necessary, and it is not recommended by Kaye and Schneider, since in this projection the needle tip may perforate the glenoid labrum.[7] They therefore recommend a straight supine position. Under fluoroscopic control a mark is then made directly over the glenohumeral joint space at the junction of its middle and lower thirds. Following skin preparation and anesthetic infiltration a 22-gauge needle is directed downward toward the glenohumeral joint space. The needle position is monitored intermittently by fluoroscopy, and the needle is repositioned if necessary so that the hub and tip are superimposed and overlie the joint space. A decrease in resistance is noted when the joint is reached, and on fluoroscopy the tip of the needle may be seen to bend slightly. If the needle meets resistance and if the position is directly vertical, overlying the joint space, and fairly deep, the needle tip should be withdrawn a few millimeters. An attempt is made to aspirate any effusion present. A trial injection of lidocaine (Xylocaine) may be done, and if the needle is in the joint, there is no resistance to injection. If the needle is not yet within the joint cavity or is imbedded in the articular cartilage, resistance to injection will be noted, and the needle should then be repositioned. As in arthrography of any joint, the injection of a few drops of contrast material under fluoroscopic

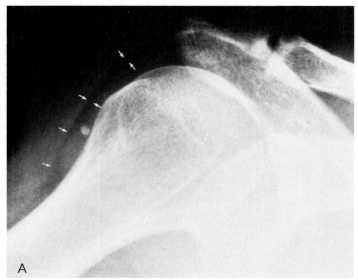

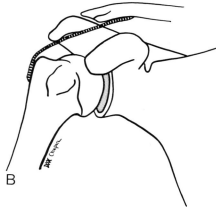

Figure 5–7. Normal Fat Lines. *A,* This internal rotation view of the humerus shows the apposed layers of fat (arrows) on either side of the subacromial-subdeltoid bursa. There is calcification in the subjacent rotator cuff. *B,* Diagram showing fat line. (Redrawn from Weston WJ. Br J Radiol 42:481, 1969, by permission.)

monitoring will confirm intraarticular needle position. The needle tip is intraarticular in location when contrast material flows away from the needle tip, either along the glenohumeral cartilage or into the axillary recess. If the position is extraarticular, the contrast material collects around the tip of the needle. When the needle is properly positioned, a mixture of Reno–M–60 and Xylocaine (16 ml of Reno–M–60 mixed with 4 ml of 1 percent Xylocaine) is injected until the patient has pain or until 10 to 12 ml of contrast is introduced.[8]

Injection technique for single- or double-contrast arthrography is identical. For double-contrast arthrography Goldman recommends that 3 to 4 ml of positive contrast medium be injected followed by 10 ml of room air.[5]

Following the injection of contrast material the needle is removed, and the joint is briefly examined fluoroscopically. Fluoroscopic spot films or overhead films with the humerus in internal and external rotation, and axillary and bicipital groove views are then obtained. A second set of internal and external rotation films is obtained after a few minutes of shoulder exercise, and if these are negative or if a partial rotator cuff tear is demonstrated, another series of films is done following additional exercise. For double-contrast examination upright views are obtained, with the tube angled 15 degrees toward the feet and with the patient holding a 5-lb sandbag.

Perhaps because of the injected Xylocaine, the patient usually experiences no discomfort at the time of the procedure. Increased pain is frequent, however, several hours after the study and may last for several days. Significant pain is less frequent after double-contrast than after single-contrast arthrography.[6]

Normal Arthrographic Anatomy (Figs. 5–8 and 5–9). The shoulder capsule attaches just medial to the glenoid labrum and along the anatomical neck of the humerus. The capsule is

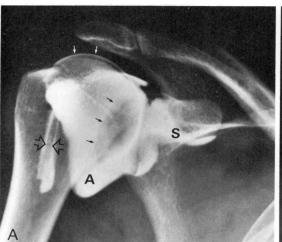

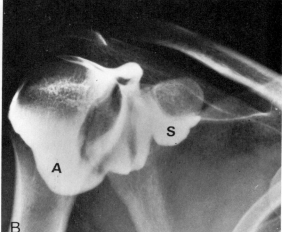

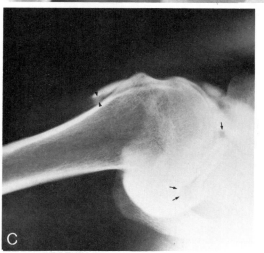

Figure 5–8. Normal Single-Contrast Arthrogram. External rotation *(A)* and internal rotation *(B)*. A = axillary recess, S = subscapularis recess, open arrows = tendon of long head of biceps within biceps sheath. The humeral articular cartilage is coated with contrast medium (white arrows). There is no contrast agent in the subacromial-subdeltoid bursa. The defect created by the glenoid labrum (arrows) is seen. Filling of the subscapularis recess is often poor on external rotation views because of bursal compression by the subscapularis muscle. In the axillary view (C) the anterior (single arrow) and posterior (double arrow) glenoid labral margins are seen. The biceps tendon (arrowheads) can be seen surrounded by contrast medium in the biceps tendon sheath. No contrast agent overlies the surgical neck of the humerus.

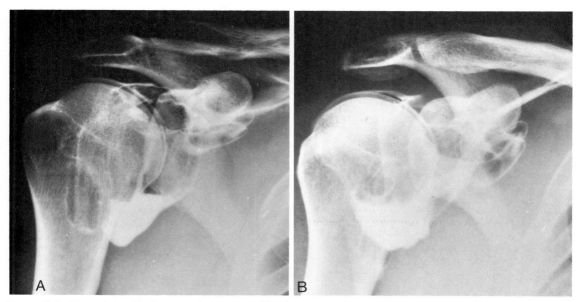

Figure 5–9. Normal Double-Contrast Arthrogram. Upright views with a sandbag suspended from the wrist and the humerus in external rotation *(A)* and internal rotation *(B)* show the structures noted on single-contrast examination and also allow better appreciation of the articular cartilages.

capacious inferiorly and medially (the axillary recess) to allow abduction of the arm. This recess is obliterated, therefore, when the arm is raised. Normally, the joint capsule communicates with the subscapularis recess anteriorly and medially (the recess lying between the scapula and subscapularis muscle). The entire capsule and the subscapularis recess are lined by a synovial membrane that also surrounds the proximal portion of the tendon of the long head of the biceps. As pointed out by Kaye and Schneider, the subscapularis recess and the synovial sheath around the long head of the biceps tendon represent the weakest areas of the joint, since they are covered only by the thin synovial membrane.[7] These areas are therefore the first to rupture when the joint is overdistended. The subcoracoid bursa lies anterior to the subscapularis muscle and under the coracoid process and is not opacified by contrast medium injected into the glenohumeral joint. Similarly, the subacromial bursa and its extension, the subdeltoid bursa, are normally separated from the joint capsule by the rotator cuff and should not be opacified after contrast agent injection into the joint.

External rotation views after arthrography show a thin layer of contrast medium along the articular surface of the humeral head. Contrast material surrounds the proximal portion of the tendon of the long head of the biceps, which will be seen in the bicipital groove laterally. The

origin of this tendon joins the superior margin of the glenoid labrum and produces a filling defect in the contrast medium just above the superior margin of the glenoid.[7] On external rotation views the subscapularis bursa may be only partially opacified because it is compressed by the subscapularis muscle.

Views in internal rotation should show the subscapularis bursa to be well filled, and there should be a clear indentation between it and the axillary recess. The tendon of the long head of the biceps is rotated to a more medial location. The posterior portion of the glenoid labrum produces a semicircular radiolucent filling defect. Contrast agent should not fill the area under the acromion (the subacromial-subdeltoid bursa).

The axillary view shows a thin layer of contrast along the articular cartilage. The subscapularis recess is seen anteriorly, and the posterior aspect of the joint capsule, the posterior recess, is seen to be lax. The biceps tendon sleeve can be followed anteriorly in the groove between the greater and lesser tuberosities. The glenoid labrum is seen as a radiolucent, triangular filling defects at the anterior and posterior glenoid margins. The posterior portion of the labrum may be rounded at its free margin, but the anterior portion has a sharply pointed contour. Tangential views of the bicipital groove should show contrast around the biceps tendon within the bicipital groove.

223

Table 5–1. Radiographic Findings Suggesting Distension of the Subdeltoid Bursa

Teardrop-shaped soft tissue density deep to the deltoid
Bulging of the deltoid contour

ABNORMAL CONDITIONS

Soft Tissue Swelling

Joint Effusion

Small amounts of fluid within the shoulder cannot be identified radiographically. Acute hemarthrosis can result in depression of the humeral head in relation to the glenoid, an appearance termed *pseudodislocation*.[12] Ultrasound examination has undergone preliminary investigation and appears to be of use in demonstrating fluid collections within and near the joint.[13]

Enlargement of the Subdeltoid Bursa
(Table 5–1)

Distension of the subdeltoid bursa, such as may be seen in patients with rheumatoid arthritis, produces separation of the previously described fat lines (Figs. 5–10 to 5–12). A teardrop-shaped soft tissue density outlined inferiorly by fat is produced between the greater tuberosity and the displaced deltoid muscle. The margin of the deltoid muscle, which usually appears flat at the level of the greater tuberosity, is displaced laterally and its contour bulges. Deltoid displacement, associated with a general increased density in this area, may suggest a distended subdeltoid bursa even when the fat lines are not well seen. Subsynovial masses of fat have been

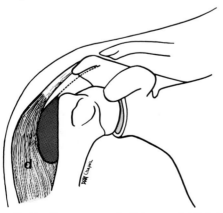

Figure 5–10. Distension of Subacromial-Subdeltoid Bursa. The distended bursa produces a teardrop-shaped tissue density (stippled area) that displaces adjacent fat and the deltoid muscle (d).

identified within the distended subdeltoid bursa in some patients with rheumatoid arthritis.[14]

Lipohemarthrosis (Fig. 5–13)

A fat-fluid level in the shoulder joint on upright (horizontal beam) radiographs is most commonly associated with acute fracture-dislocations. The fat in these cases is thought to originate from the bone marrow. Fat-fluid levels have also been reported accompanying simple fractures (even extraarticular ones) and dislocations of the humeral head without apparent fracture.[15, 17] In these cases it is postulated that there is disruption of the synovial membrane, allowing juxtaarticular fat to enter the joint.[16] The collected fat may have a configuration resembling two hills owing to the indentation produced by the tendon of the long head of the biceps.[14]

Calcific Tendinitis

Calcification in the tendons of the rotator cuff is the most common abnormality of the shoulder.[22] Although the sequence of events is controversial, degeneration of the tendons or muscles of the rotator cuff is probably the underlying abnormality, after which calcification in the form of calcium phosphate or calcium carbonate or both occurs.[24, 25]

Fluoroscopic study of 12,122 presumably normal shoulders yielded a 2.7 percent incidence of rotator cuff calcification.[18] The supraspinatus tendon is most frequently involved, followed by the infraspinatus, teres minor, and subscapularis in descending order.[24] Almost 50 percent of patients with calcification of one shoulder have bilateral deposits upon careful radiographic examination.[18, 19]

The areas of calcification may remain in the tendons for many years without any apparent symptoms.[23, 24] Rupture of the calcium salts into the adjacent bursa (usually the subacromial bursa) results in an acute, painful inflammatory reaction.

Radiographic Signs

Soft Tissue Swelling. Before calcification within the tendons is demonstrable, radiographic examination of the periarticular soft tissues may show blurring or absence of the normal fat planes around the subdeltoid bursa.[20] This finding correlates with clinical evidence of peritendinitis, whereas the presence or size of the calcification does not.[20, 22] Rarely, this fat zone may be displaced laterally.

Calcification

Appearance. Lippman reviewed the pathological sequence of events in calcific tendinitis

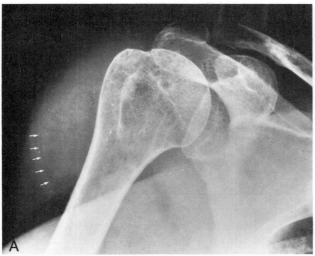

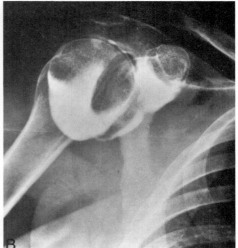

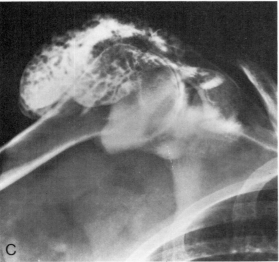

Figure 5–11. Distended Subacromial-Subdeltoid Bursa Caused by Rheumatoid Arthritis. *A*, AP radiograph shows a teardrop-shaped soft tissue density outlined by fat (arrows). The cartilage space is normal. *B*, Arthrogram shows no abnormality. *C*, Contrast agent injection into the subacromial-subdeltoid bursa shows abnormal bursal distension with multiple filling defects typical of rheumatoid arthritis. *D*, AP radiograph of another patient shows soft tissue swelling in the area of the deltoid. *E*, A subdeltoid bursogram shows multiple filling defects (arrows) and lymphatic and nodal filling (open arrows) typical of rheumatoid arthritis.

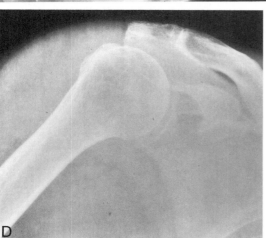

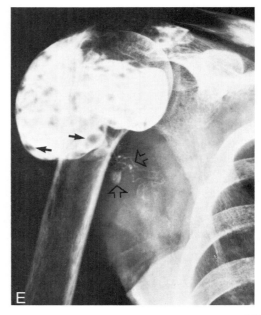

225

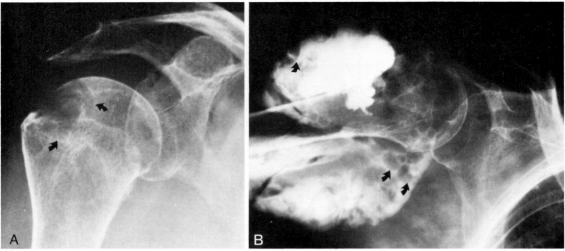

Figure 5–12. Tuberculous Bursitis and Arthritis. In an elderly woman who had experienced months of shoulder pain, frontal view *(A)* shows a large area of erosion (arrows) in the "bare area" of the humeral head, with undercutting of the cortex. The cartilage space is minimally narrow. Contrast medium injection into a massively enlarged subdeltoid bursa *(B)* shows nodular filling defects (arrows). Biopsy confirmed the diagnosis.

and correlated it with clinical and radiographic findings.[22] Early calcium deposits are chalk-like in consistency, firmly bound to the tendon fibrils, and unassociated with an inflammatory reaction. This calcification appears very dense and angular on radiographs.[19] Inflammatory changes re-

Figure 5–13. Lipohemarthrosis. There is a three-part humeral fracture. The humeral head is displaced inferiorly by the blood and fat within the joint, evidenced by fat-fluid levels (arrows). The upper fat-fluid level is within the subacromial bursa and suggests the presence of a rotator cuff tear.

sult in softening of the deposit to a more fluid (toothpaste-like) consistency, and its less firm adherence to the tendon. More frequent and more severe episodes of pain follow. Lippman notes that "impending disruption" of the deposit is associated with loss of the angular contour of the calcification, rounding of its borders due to distension, and development of peripheral radiolucent areas. The margins, however, remain sharp. Eventually, the deposit may rupture into adjacent areas of the tendon or into the overlying bursa, producing severe pain. Rupture into the adjacent tendon is suggested by increased, irregular areas of radiolucency or by a mottled pattern in the calcification and loss of definition of some of its borders (Fig. 5–14). Beginning discharge of the calcification into the bursa is seen as a "pseudopod" or "spray-like" extension into the area of the bursa and an outlining

Table 5–2. Radiographic Findings in Calcific Tendinitis

Chronic	Dense angular calcification
Acute	Blurring of adjacent fat lines
	Loss of angular contour of the calcification
	Decreased density with peripheral areas of lucency
	Eventual blurring of borders of the calcification
	Extension of calcification into the bursa

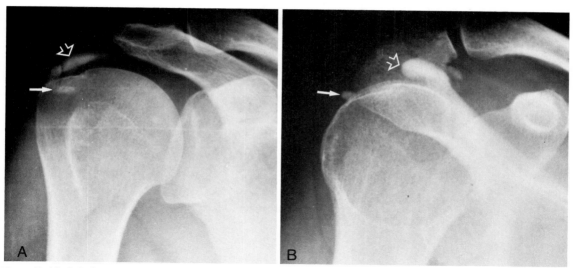

Figure 5–14. Calcific Tendinitis—Supraspinatus and Infraspinatus. *A,* External rotation view shows calcification projected over the base of the greater tuberosity (arrow) and above the greater tuberosity (open arrow). *B,* Internal rotation view projects the infraspinatus calcification (arrow) in profile and documents its posterior location. The supraspinatus calcification (open arrow) is rotated medially and maintains its superior location.

of the bursal floor (Table 5–2; Fig. 5–15). The calcifications in the bursa are then absorbed.

Localization. Knowledge of the paths and sites of insertion of the tendons about the shoulder make it possible to localize calcification to a particular tendon (Table 5–3).[26] Films in two projections are necessary, and views with the humerus in internal and external rotation are often available. The supraspinatus tendon inserts onto the promontory of the greater tuberosity.

Supraspinatus calcification will be seen in profile capping the greater tuberosity in external rotation (or in external oblique) views. When the arm is rotated internally the calcification will move medially (Figs. 5–15 and 5–16).

The tendons of the infraspinatus and teres minor muscles insert farther posteriorly on the greater tuberosity. Therefore, internal rotation of the arm projects them laterally and allows them to be more clearly seen (Fig. 5–17). Cal-

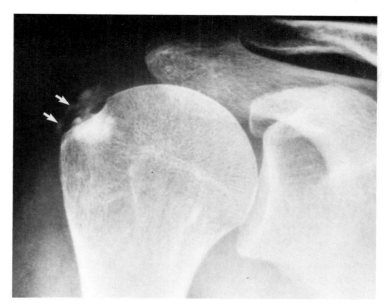

Figure 5–15. Calcific Tendinitis with Rupture into Bursa. Calcification is seen in the supraspinatus tendon with tracking into the subacromial bursa (arrows).

Table 5–3. **Calcific Tendinitis**

Tendon	Location of Calcification	Movement of Calcification With Arm Rotation	
		Internal	*External*
Supraspinatus	Greater tuberosity, upper third	Medial	Lateral
Infraspinatus	Greater tuberosity, middle third (posterior)	Lateral	Medial
Teres minor	Greater tuberosity, lower third (posterior)	Lateral	Medial
Subscapularis	Lesser tuberosity (anterior)	Medial	Lateral
Biceps:			
Long head	Superior glenoid rim	No change	No change
Short head	Inferior glenoid rim, tip of coracoid process	No change	No change

Source; Vigario GD, Keats TE: AJR 108:806, 1970.

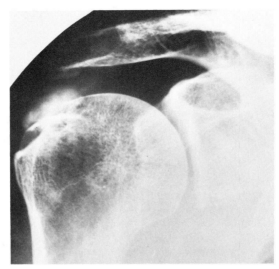

Figure 5–16. Acute Calcific Tendinitis of Supraspinatus. External rotation view shows calcification projected above the greater tuberosity. The poor definition of the calcification and the peripheral areas of radiolucency are typical changes associated with acute inflammation.

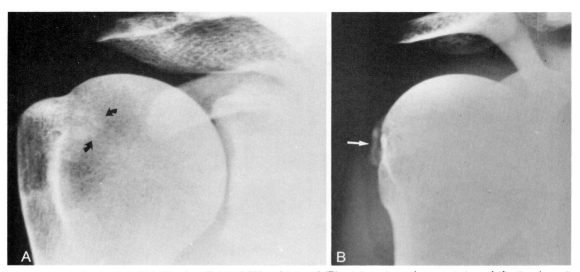

Figure 5–17. Infraspinatus Calcification. External *(A)* and internal *(B)* rotation views show posterior calcification (seen in profile on internal rotation [arrows]).

cification in the subscapularis tendon is anterior to the lesser tuberosity (Fig. 5–18). This calcification is seen to advantage on axillary views.

Calcification of the tendon of the long head of the biceps occurs near the superior edge of the glenoid fossa. Calcification of the short head of the biceps is usually seen near the inferior rim of the glenoid or near the tip of the coracoid process.

The identification of calcification within the expected area of a tendon is of some value in that it signifies tendon degeneration. However, calcification may be present without any clinical evidence of shoulder disability, and Olsson found no statistical correlation between the presence of calcific deposits and shoulder pain.[20] Golding found radiographically detectable calcification in only 62 of 198 patients clinically diagnosed as having tendinitis or bursitis and

noted that the clinical history (including the duration of symptoms) did not help in predicting which patients would have radiographically discernible calcifications and which would not.[21]

The clinical significance of precise localization of the calcific deposits is also debatable.[1, 21] The site selected for corticosteroid injections (if this treatment is utilized) depends on clinical localization of the tender area rather than on radiographic localization.[1]

Treatment

Conservative treatment, consisting of analgesics, immobilization in a sling, and cold packs, is used for mild cases. Moderate cases may also benefit from phenylbutazone for 4 to 5 days. In more severe cases injection of corticosteroids into the symptomatic site may be required. Surgical excision of the masses of calcific material with or

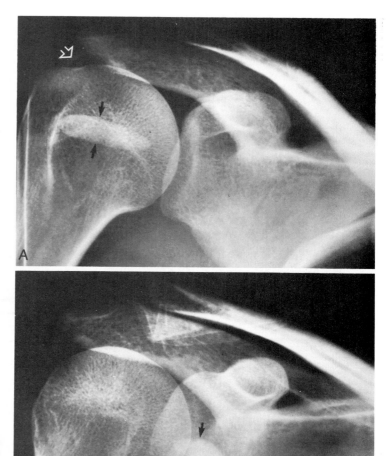

Figure 5–18. Calcific Tendinitis—Subscapularis. *A,* External rotation view shows calcification (arrows) overlying the humerus, along the course of the subscapularis. A small calcification is also noted in the supraspinatus tendon (open arrow). *B,* Internal rotation view confirms the anterior location of the calcification (arrows).

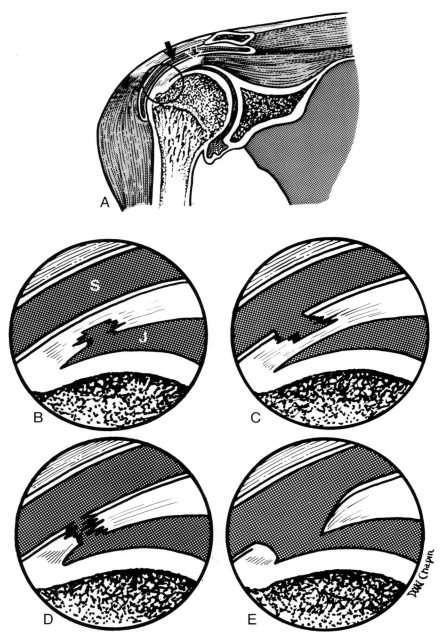

Figure 5–19. Rotator Cuff Tears. *A,* Diagram showing the intact tendons of the rotator cuff (open arrow) separating the shoulder joint from the subacromial-subdeltoid bursa (arrow). The circle indicates the critical area of the cuff, through which most tears occur. This is the area shown in parts *B* to *E. B,* A partial tear of the inferior aspect of the rotator cuff is shown. This tear would be demonstrated by shoulder arthrography. J = joint, S = subacromial-subdeltoid bursa. *C,* A partial tear of the superior aspect of the rotator cuff is shown. This tear would be demonstrable on bursography but not on arthrography. *D,* A complete tear of the cuff, with the irregular margins typical of an acute tear, is shown. A shoulder arthrogram would show filling of the subacromial-subdeltoid bursa. *E,* Chronic complete rotator cuff tear. The smoothly tapered margins are characteristic.

without partial anterior acromionectomy is occasionally necessary.

Rotator Cuff Tears

The tendons of the rotator cuff blend together and fuse with the underlying fibrous capsule of the shoulder. Below the rotator cuff is the synovial lining and joint space. Above it is the subacromial bursa and its extension, the subdeltoid bursa.

Classification

Rotator cuff tears have been classified anatomically as complete or incomplete (Fig. 5–19). Incomplete tears do not involve the entire thickness of the rotator cuff. They may be located on the superior or inferior surfaces or within the substance of the cuff. Complete tears involve the entire thickness of the rotator cuff, allowing communication between the subacromial bursa and the joint space; thus they are demonstrable on arthrography. Complete tears may be subdivided at the time of surgery into pure transverse ruptures, pure vertical or longitudinal tears, tears with retraction of the tendon edges, and massive avulsion of the cuff.[33]

Etiology

As summarized by Post, both acute trauma and chronic degeneration of the rotator cuff play a role in the genesis of a rotator cuff tear. The current feeling seems to be that rupture occurs when trauma is superimposed on an already weakened, degenerated rotator cuff.[1]

Clinical Symptoms

Patients with symptomatic rotator cuff tears are usually elderly. The history is one of chronic or recurrent attacks of shoulder pain, which may be worse at night. Weakness on abduction is present, and when the full thickness of the cuff is involved, there may be a popping or grating sensation.[1]

Radiologic diagnosis, particularly arthrography, is frequently used to confirm the clinical impression of a rotator cuff tear.

Radiographic Findings

Plain Film Findings. Plain film findings associated with tears of the rotator cuff include the following (Table 5–4; Fig. 5–20):[28–30]

1. *Sclerosis, atrophy, or irregularity of the greater tuberosity.* According to Skinner, the most marked bony changes associated with rotator cuff tears occur in the portion of the greater tuberosity that is exposed when the ruptured supraspinatus tendon retracts. Pathological examination in such cases reveals a rough, irregular, and pitted bony surface.[37] Cotton and Rideout noted that in the absence of other radiographic abnormalities sclerosis of the greater tuberosity is an unreliable sign of a rotator cuff tear.

2. *Cystic changes in the upper two thirds of the anatomical neck.* Cotton and Rideout found that all necropsy specimens with radiologically demonstrable cysts in the anatomical neck had tears of the rotator cuff, and, conversely, no cysts were seen in specimens without such tears.[28] The cysts occur under the cortical bone, just at the site of insertion of the inner fibers of the rotator cuff. They may be either single or multiple, and in most cases a communication exists between the cyst and the joint space, although the orifice may be pinpoint in size. Most of these "cysts" contain loose connective tissue.

3. *Notching between the humeral articular surface and the greater tuberosity.* This deformity is at the site of insertion of the rotator cuff tendons and results from tendon avulsion or bone resorption. The degree of excavation seems to correspond to the severity of the tear.[28] Sclerosis may also occur at this site.

Table 5–4. **Radiographic Features of Rotator Cuff Tears**

Plain Film Findings	Sclerosis, atrophy, or irregularity of greater tuberosity
	Cystic changes along upper two thirds of humeral neck
	Notching between greater tuberosity and articular surface
	Acromiohumeral distance < 6 mm
	Lateral new bone formation, erosion, and sclerosis of the undersurface of the acromion
	Absence of rotator cuff calcification
	Collapse of humeral head and abnormal glenohumeral joint (cuff tear arthropathy)
Arthrographic Findings	
Complete Tear	Filling of subacromial-subdeltoid bursa
	Filling of acromioclavicular joint
Partial Tear	Collection of contrast in area of rotator cuff

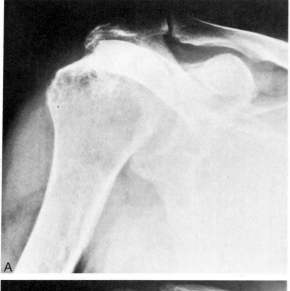

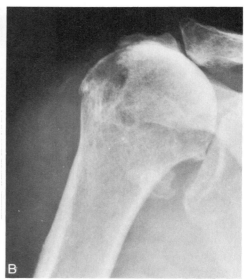

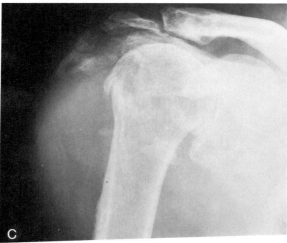

Figure 5–20. Rotator Cuff Tear. *A,* There is marked elevation of the humeral head in relation to the glenoid, and the acromiohumeral distance is reduced to less than 5 mm. There is erosion of the undersurface of the acromion process. All these findings suggest the presence of a rotator cuff tear. The flattening of the lateral aspect of the humerus is the result of prior anterior dislocation. *B* and *C.* Cuff tear arthropathy. There is marked elevation of the humeral head with loss of substance of the inferior aspect of the acromion process (*B*). Bony fragments are noted in the periarticular soft tissues. Three years later (*C*) fragmentation is more severe and a distended subacromial-subdeltoid bursa is present. The picture mimics that of a neuropathic shoulder.

4. *Narrowing of the distance between the acromion and the humeral head.* The space between the acromion process and the humerus is occupied by the tendons of the rotator cuff and the subacromial bursa. Normally, this interval measures between 6 and 14 mm.[28, 29, 38] Weiner and Macnab studied AP views of the shoulder in neutral rotation in 58 patients with rotator cuff tears and found 44 percent with intervals of 5 mm or less.[38] They postulated that the reduced interval is a late finding due to atrophy of the cuff, which decreases the thickness of soft tissues, and that this allows the unopposed pull of the deltoid muscle to move the humeral head proximally. The narrowing should also be present on both internal and external rotation views.[32] When the humeral head is so elevated that it articulates with the undersurface of the acromion, a complete rotator cuff tear is present.[28] This finding may be seen in patients with rheumatoid arthritis when destruction of the rotator cuff has occurred.

5. *New bone formation on the lateral margin of the acromion, sclerosis of the acromion, and erosion of the undersurface of the acromion.* Cotton and Rideout found irregularity of the lateral margin of the acromion in three necropsy cases, and in each case a complete tear of the rotator cuff was present.[28] Upward subluxation of the humeral head may produce chronic changes on the undersurface of the acromion process, including sclerosis, subchondral cyst formation, and eventual loss of bone, with a reversal of the normal acromial convexity.[32]

6. *Absence of rotator cuff calcification.* The combination of rotator cuff tears and rotator cuff

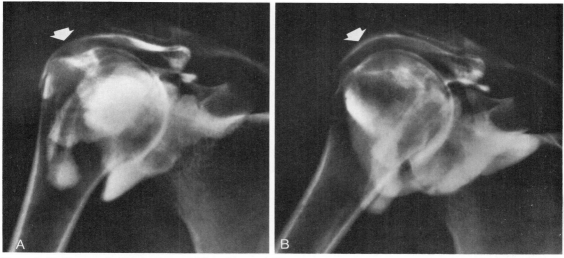

Figure 5–21. Rotator Cuff Tear. External (*A*) and internal (*B*) rotation views during a single-contrast arthrogram show filling of the subacromial-subdeltoid bursa (arrow), indicating a full-thickness rotator cuff tear.

calcification is very uncommon. The presence of such calcification is "reasonably strong evidence" against a rotator cuff tear.[34]

7. *Cuff tear arthropathy.* Massive tears of the rotator cuff can eventually lead to collapse and disorganization of the glenohumeral joint (Fig. 5–20). These severe changes have been termed "cuff tear arthropathy" by Neer and co-workers.[35]

Using the findings of narrowing of the acromiohumeral interval and reversal of the convexity of the undersurface of the acromion as indicators of a rotator cuff tear, Kotzen found only 23 percent of 48 surgically proven tears to have positive plain film examinations.[32] The interval from the onset of symptoms to the positive radiograph was 2 months to 4 years and was generally faster the larger the tear.

Thus the absence of abnormal findings does not exclude a rotator cuff tear, but the presence of the listed abnormalities (particularly an acromiohumeral interval of 6 mm or less or sub-

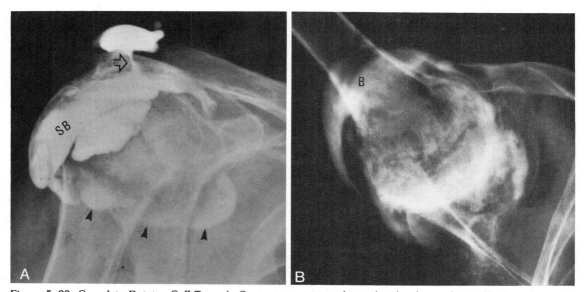

Figure 5–22. Complete Rotator Cuff Tear. *A,* Contrast agent injected into the glenohumeral joint fills the subacromial-subdeltoid bursa (SB) and the acromioclavicular joint (open arrow), indicating a complete rotator cuff tear. The joint capsule is faintly outlined (arrowheads). *B,* The axillary view (of another patient) shows the subacromial-subdeltoid bursa (B) to extend over the surgical neck of the humerus, an area not normally covered by the joint capsule.

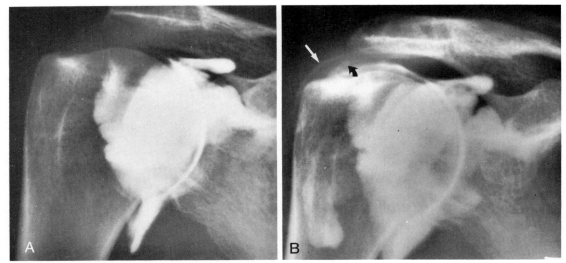

Figure 5–23. Rotator Cuff Tear Demonstrated after Exercise. *A,* External rotation view immediately after injection of 12 ml of positive contrast medium shows no filling of the biceps tendon sleeve or delineation of the superolateral articular cartilage. *B,* After exercise there is good filling of the biceps tendon sleeve. An irregular collection of contrast (curved arrow) demonstrates the site of rotator cuff tear, through which contrast medium leaks into the subacromial-subdeltoid bursa (straight arrow).

chondral cysts along the anatomical neck) should suggest the diagnosis.

Arthrographic Findings

Complete Rotator Cuff Tears *(Figs. 5–21 to 5–23).* Complete tears of the rotator cuff involve the entire thickness of the cuff and therefore

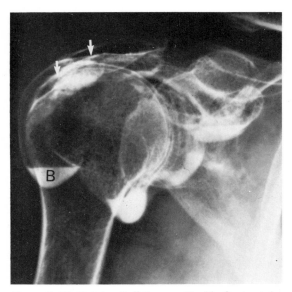

Figure 5–24. Rotator Cuff Tear on Double-Contrast Arthrogram. An upright, neutral rotation view shows filling of the subacromial-subdeltoid bursa (B) and outlines the triangular margins of the edges of the torn rotator cuff (arrows).

allow communication between the joint and the subacromial-subdeltoid bursa. This bursa is located under the acromion process and extends laterally and distally to a point below the greater tuberosity. Since the normal joint extends only to the anatomical neck, contrast medium that extends to the surgical neck (except for that around the biceps tendon) probably represents contrast medium within the subdeltoid bursa. Filling of the acromioclavicular joint following contrast agent injection into the shoulder also indicates the presence of a rotator cuff tear.

Double-contrast arthrography has an advantage over the single-contrast examination in that the double-contrast technique allows the size of the rotator cuff tear and the quality of the remaining tissues of the rotator cuff to be evaluated (Fig. 5–24). As summarized by Goldman, a traumatic tear has smooth margins, and the tendon is of normal thickness, occupying almost the entire space between the humeral head and the acromion process. Degenerative changes in the cuff are indicated on the arthrogram by irregularity at the margins of the tear; air, contrast agent, or both within the tendon fragments; and thinning of the torn tendons.[30] Some assessment of the size of the tear can also be obtained from the single-contrast study, since if only a small amount of contrast medium passes into the subacromial bursa or if contrast passes into the bursa only after exercise, the rotator cuff tear is probably small.

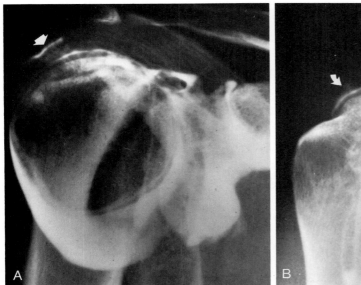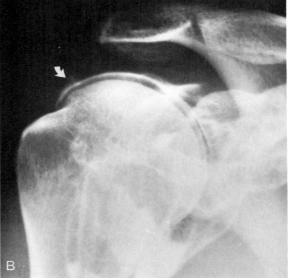

Figure 5–25. Partial Rotator Cuff Tear. *A*, An internal rotation view after injection of positive contrast agent and after exercise shows a linear collection of contrast medium in the area of the rotator cuff (arrow) but no filling of the subacromial-subdeltoid bursa. *B*, The external rotation view of another patient, after exercise, shows a small collection of contrast above the humeral head (arrow), in the region of the rotator cuff. No contrast extends into the subacromial-subdeltoid bursa; this is therefore an incomplete tear.

Partial Rotator Cuff Tears (Fig. 5–25). Partial rotator cuff tears do not extend through the full thickness of the rotator cuff. They are identifiable on arthrography only if they involve the inferior surface of the cuff adjacent to the injected shoulder joint. In these cases the arthrogram shows a small collection of contrast material in the area of the cuff; this material is usually seen to advantage on external rotation views. The postexercise films are of particular importance because many partial rotator cuff tears are seen only on the postexercise films, and, in some cases, what appears to be a partial rotator cuff tear before exercise is seen to be a full-thickness tear on the postexercise films.[36] When the arthrogram is normal, contrast injection into the subacromial bursa allows identification of partial tears of the superior surface of the rotator cuff.

Impingement Syndrome

Impingement of the rotator cuff between the coracoacromial arch and the tuberosity during abduction or elevation of the arm may cause chronic shoulder pain.[38b, 40] The anatomical lesions associated with this syndrome include chronic tendinitis, partial or complete tears of the supraspinatus tendon, and tears of the adjacent rotator cuff.[39]

Review of 100 dissected scapular specimens showed alterations thought to be due to me-chanical impingement in 11 instances.[39] The characteristic finding was a ridge of proliferative spurs from the undersurface of the anterior portion of the acromion process, thought to be the result of repeated impingement of the rotator cuff and humeral head, with traction on the coracoacromial ligament. Eburnation and erosion of the acromion was less common. Neer emphasizes that it is the undersurface of the anterior acromion that is involved.

Radiographic examination may show new bone proliferation along the anterior edge of the acromion and cysts or sclerosis of the greater tuberosity (Table 5–5). Arthrography may delineate a rotator cuff tear (see arthrography of rotator cuff tears). Injection of contrast medium into the subacromial bursa has been suggested as a means of evaluating patients with clinically suspected impingement syndrome.[41] The normal subacromial bursa can accommodate 5 to 10 ml of contrast material. An abnormally small bursa (or, in experienced hands, inability to locate and inject the bursa) suggests that symp-

Table 5–5. **Radiographic Findings Associated With Impingement Syndrome**

Hypertrophic spurs from acromion process
Cysts or sclerosis of the greater tuberosity
With or without rotator cuff tear on arthrography
Small subacromial bursa on bursography

toms may be due to impingement, whereas patients with normal bursograms probably do not have this syndrome. A combination of arthrography and bursography allows both the superior and the inferior aspects as well as the thickness of the rotator cuff to be evaluated. The arthrogram is done first, and if this is normal, a bursogram is then done. The treatment advocated by Neer consists of removal of the anterior edge and the undersurface of the anterior part of the acromion, and the attached coracoacromial ligament.

Adhesive Capsulitis (Frozen Shoulder)

The term *adhesive capsulitis* refers to a frequent and disabling malady in which, without demonstrable intrinsic cause, the shoulder gradually becomes stiff and painful. Inflammatory synovitis is present in only a minority of cases.[48] In most cases the joint capsule is reduced in size, and there is absence of its normal outpouchings—the axillary and the subscapularis recesses. Adhesions may be present between the synovial surfaces, but, according to McLaughlin, these alone do not account for the observed restriction in joint motion.

Adhesive capsulitis of the shoulder can result in confusing clinical symptoms mimicking disorders originating in the neck, chest wall, or heart. McLaughlin postulated that prolonged dependency and immobility due to a variety of painful conditions result in changes in the collagenous tissues around the shoulder with consequent

Table 5–6. **Radiographic Features of Adhesive Capsulitis**

Plain Films	Osteopenia
	Limited motion
Arthrography	Small joint capacity
	Constricted capsule
	Absent filling of subscapularis and axillary recesses
	Small or absent biceps tendon sleeve
	Contrast extravasation
	Irregular capsular margin
	Reflux of contrast through puncture site

joint stiffening.[48] Bicipital tenosynovitis often accompanies a frozen shoulder.[1]

Radiographic Findings (Fig. 5–26)

Plain film examination is usually unrewarding, showing only osteopenia and any decrease in motion that can be identified on the standard views.

Arthrography. The findings on arthrography are characteristic (Table 5–6).[49] Intraarticular needle placement may be more difficult in these patients because of the tight joint capsule. Only a small amount of contrast material (5 or 6 ml) can be injected before the patient complains of pain and a feeling of tightness. The joint capsule typically appears small and constricted with absence of filling of the subscapularis and axillary recesses. There is often a decrease in size or a lack of filling of the biceps tendon sleeve. Leakage of contrast medium from the subscapularis

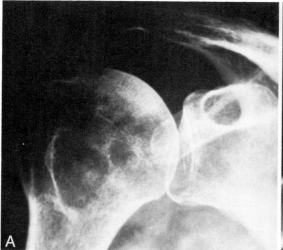
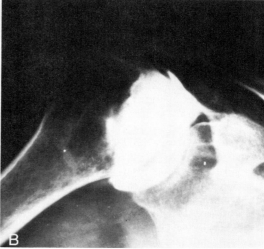

Figure 5–26. Adhesive Capsulitis. *A,* External rotation view shows osteopenia. The cartilage space is normal. *B,* A single-contrast arthrogram shows filling of a very small joint capsule. There is no filling of the biceps tendon sleeve or subscapularis recess. The axillary pouch is small.

recess or the biceps tendon is more frequent in patients with adhesive capsulitis but is not, in itself, an abnormal finding. According to Kaye and Schneider, leakage of contrast agent back through the needle puncture site is indicative of increased pressure within the joint and is not seen in patients with a normal joint capacity.[47] In addition, the insertion of the capsule onto the humerus may be irregular.

Treatment

This condition is usually self-limited, and after 3 to 12 months or more of pain and disability spontaneous recovery ensues.[46] Treatment in the early phases consists of analgesics and exercises. In long-standing cases refractory to conservative measures, manipulation under anesthesia is sometimes done. Reeves has noted that at the time of open manipulation increased abduction is associated with rupture of the inferior capsule close to the glenoid margin. Improvement in external rotation is produced by rupture of the subscapularis tendon and the underlying capsule. Arthrographic examination confirms capsular disruption.[49] Andrén and Lundberg and others have used arthrography, not only as a diagnostic technique, but as a therapeutic one.[42, 43] Particularly in mild or moderate cases gradual distension of the joint with a mixture of Xylocaine or bupivicaine (Marcaine), contrast agent, and saline may result in increased mobility.

Arthritis

Osteoarthritis

Primary degenerative arthritis leading to joint incongruity is less frequent in the glenohumeral joint than in weight-bearing joints. It is not rare, however, to have some abnormality of this joint in older patients. Correlation of radiographic abnormalities and clinical symptoms is imperfect, and cartilage narrowing and hypertrophic lipping may be noted in asymptomatic patients. In addition, hypertrophic changes of the humeral head and bicipital groove may be associated with adjacent soft tissue abnormalities in the rotator cuff or biceps tendon rather than with isolated degenerative arthritis of the glenohumeral joint.[57]

Secondary Osteoarthritis. Younger patients with evidence of glenohumeral osteoarthritis should be evaluated for possible underlying diseases that damage the articular cartilage or the underlying cancellous bone of the humeral head. Rheumatoid arthritis, gout, ochronosis,[58]

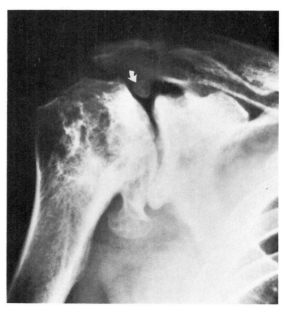

Figure 5–27. Osteoarthritis (Acromegaly). There is severe cartilage loss with sclerosis and flattening of articular surfaces. A very large osteophyte projects from the humerus inferiorly and a loose body (arrow) is noted superiorly. (Courtesy of Dr. Manorama Saini, Boston, Mass.)

acromegaly, avascular necrosis, radiation changes, and prior humeral neck fractures or dislocations are possible underlying conditions (Fig. 5–27).

Rheumatoid Arthritis (Fig. 5–28)

Early soft tissue swelling is difficult to identify, but eventually distension of the subdeltoid bursa may be detectable (see soft tissue swelling).[59] Bony alterations can often be best seen on the external rotation or the posterior oblique view, since early erosion often involves the lateral aspect of the humeral head, just medial to the greater tuberosity. Erosion progresses in the area of the anatomical neck, especially superolaterally under the rotator cuff but also medially and circumferentially. Irregularity of the articular surface of the humerus and glenoid occurs, and bone loss may be striking, but, in contrast to osteoarthritis, no new bone formation occurs. Cartilage-space narrowing ensues. Elevation of the humeral head due to attrition and rupture of the rotator cuff may occur and may precede erosive changes.[58]

Typical findings on shoulder arthrography include diffuse nodular filling defects involving the joint and the subdeltoid bursa (visible if a rotator cuff tear is present), irregularity of the capsular attachment, and opacification of draining lymphatics. Rotator cuff tears and arthrographic

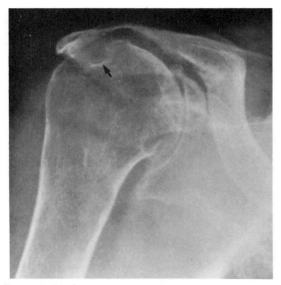

Figure 5–28. Rheumatoid Arthritis. There is severe glenohumeral cartilage space narrowing with little osteophytic lipping. There is erosion of the humeral head (arrow). The marked elevation of the humeral head and bone loss from the undersurface of the acromion is due to the associated rotator cuff damage.

Table 5–7. Radiographic Features of Neuropathic Arthropathy

Soft tissue swelling
Destruction
Debris and fragmentation
Subluxation
Sclerosis
Absence of osteopenia

findings of adhesive capsulitis are seen in a minority of patients. A unique localized dilatation of the biceps tendon sheath may be demonstrated.[51]

Neuropathic Arthropathy
(Fig. 5–29)

The primary factors leading to the development of a neuropathic joint are absent or decreased pain sensation and continued activity.[50, 52] According to Post, syphilis and diabetic neuropathy are uncommon causes of upper extremity changes, but 25 percent of patients with cervical syringomyelia develop upper extremity joint destruction, particularly involving the shoulder.[1]

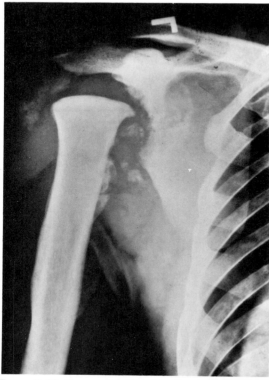

Figure 5–29. Neuropathic Shoulder Due to Syringomyelia. AP view shows many of the hallmarks of a neuropathic joint, including severe joint destruction, soft tissue debris, and sclerosis rather than osteopenia.

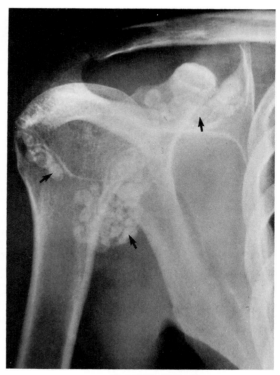

Figure 5–30. Synovial Osteochondromatosis. A 34-year-old man with a 6-month history of shoulder pain and swelling. A radiograph (without contrast) shows multiple calcified densities (arrows) that conform to the shape of the joint capsule, a virtually diagnostic appearance of synovial osteochondromatosis.

Table 5–8. **Radiographic Findings in "Milwaukee Shoulder"**

Plain Films	Cystic changes in tuberosities
	Roughening or erosion at rotator cuff insertion
	Osteoarthritic changes of glenohumeral joint
	Osteoarthritic changes of AC joint
	Calcific tendinitis and periarticular calcification
	Upward subluxation of humerus
Arthrography	Rotator cuff tears
	Filling defects

Radiographic findings of persistent soft tissue swelling, bone destruction, fragmentation and disruption of articular surfaces, subluxation, and sclerosis are noted. In the shoulder (and the hip) rapid bone loss without the other characteristic features of a neuropathic joint may occur (Table 5–7).

Synovial Osteochondromatosis
(Fig. 5–30)
See the discussion of synovial osteochondromatosis of the knee in Chapter 9.

"Milwaukee Shoulder"
"Milwaukee shoulder" refers to a conglomerate of findings including (1) complete tear of the rotator cuff and (2) noninflammatory joint fluid containing hydroxyapatite crystals within microspheroids; activated collagenase; and neutral protease.[53-55]

On radiographic examination periarticular calcifications, elevation of the humerus, degenerative changes of the glenohumeral or the acromioclavicular joint or both, and the nonspecific findings that accompany rotator cuff tears are seen. Arthrography may show intraarticular filling defects in addition to the rotator cuff tear (Table 5–8).

Fractures

Proximal Humeral Fractures
(Figs. 5–31 to 5–37)
Neer developed the classification of proximal humeral fractures that is in general use today.[60] It is based on the number of fracture fragments that are displaced or angulated and the location of the fracture lines. The four major fragments to be analyzed are the humeral head, the lesser tuberosity, the greater tuberosity, and the humeral shaft. Displaced fractures are designated as two-part, three-part, or four-part based on the number of fracture fragments that are displaced more than 1 cm or angulated more than 45 degrees. Thus a humeral fracture with the greater tuberosity displaced and the humeral shaft angulated more than 45 degrees is a three-part fracture. The same fracture lines without angulation or displacement of one of the fragments would be a two-part fracture. The appropriate Neer classification is determined from the prereduction radiographs and is summarized in Table 5–9.

Nondisplaced fractures are by far the most common, representing about 85 percent of all proximal humeral fractures. Of the displaced fractures most are two-part fractures.[60, 61] The position of fracture fragments after injury is determined by the integrity of the adjacent soft tissue structures (i.e., periosteum and joint capsule) and the pull of attached muscles. For example, in displaced surgical neck fractures with intact or nondisplaced tuberosities, the humeral head remains in neutral rotation. This is a clue that one is dealing with a two-part frac-

Text continued on page 248

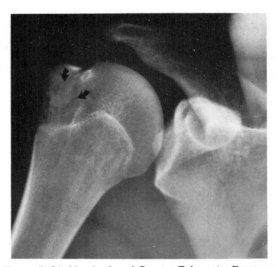

Figure 5–31. Nondisplaced Greater Tuberosity Fracture. Fracture lines are seen through the greater tuberosity (arrows), but there is no displacement or angular deformity. This could be called a one-part fracture, although that terminology is not preferred, since it is hard to conceive of a fracture with only one part. The absence of the clavicle in this patient is due to cleidocranial dysostosis.

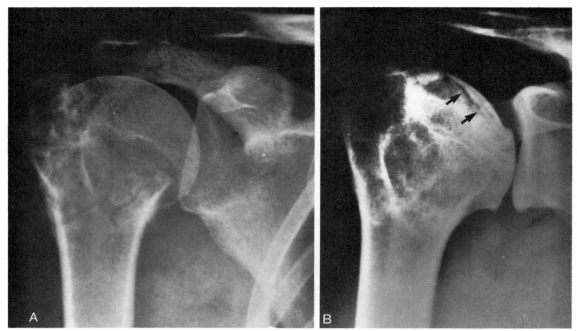

Figure 5–32. Avascular Necrosis Following Anatomical Neck Fracture. *A,* Initial radiograph shows fractures through the anatomical neck (minimally displaced) and greater tuberosity (displaced), a two-part fracture. *B,* Radiograph 2 years later shows flattening of the articular surface and a lucent crescent sign (arrows), indicating the presence of osteonecrosis. The fractures have healed. (Courtesy of Dr. Alan Naimark, University Hospital, Boston, Mass.)

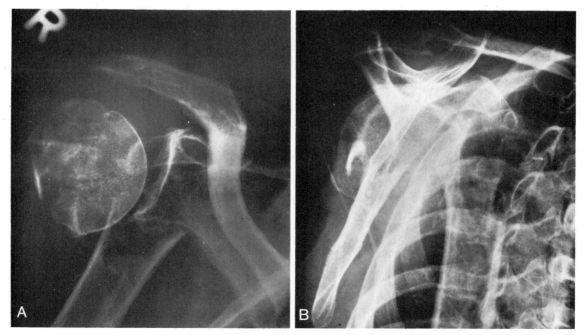

Figure 5–33. Two-Part Surgical Neck Fracture (Group 3). Posterior oblique *(A)* and anterior oblique *(B)* views show a fracture through the surgical neck of the humerus with the shaft displaced anteriorly and medially. The Y view *(B)* shows the humeral head centered over the glenoid; therefore dislocation is excluded.

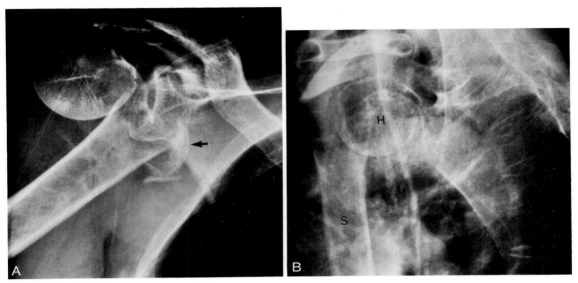

Figure 5–34. Three-Part Fracture (Group 5). Anteroposterior *(A)* and transthoracic *(B)* lateral radiograph. H = humeral head, S = humeral shaft. The humeral head is rotated so that the articular surface faces inferiorly. The lesser tuberosity (arrow) is separated and medially displaced.

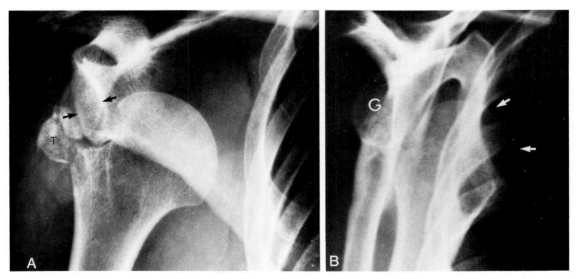

Figure 5–35. Two-Part Fracture Dislocation. *A*, AP view shows the inferior and medial position of the humeral head and a displaced fracture of the greater tuberosity (T). Arrows indicate the glenoid margins. The coracoid process is superimposed on the glenoid. *B*, The scapular Y view confirms anterior dislocation of the humeral head (arrows on anterior humerus) from the glenoid (G).

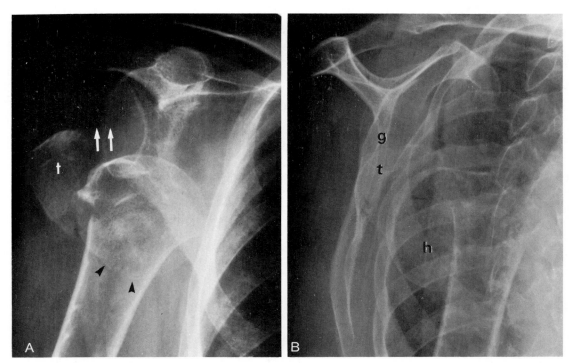

Figure 5–36. Three-Part Anterior Fracture Dislocation. *A*, AP view shows inferior displacement of the humeral head and a separated greater tuberosity (t). The surgical neck fracture is shown by overlap of the head and shaft (arrowheads). A fat-fluid level is faintly seen (white arrows). *B*, The scapular Y view confirms the anterior and inferior displacement of the humeral head (g = glenoid, h = humeral head, t = greater tuberosity).

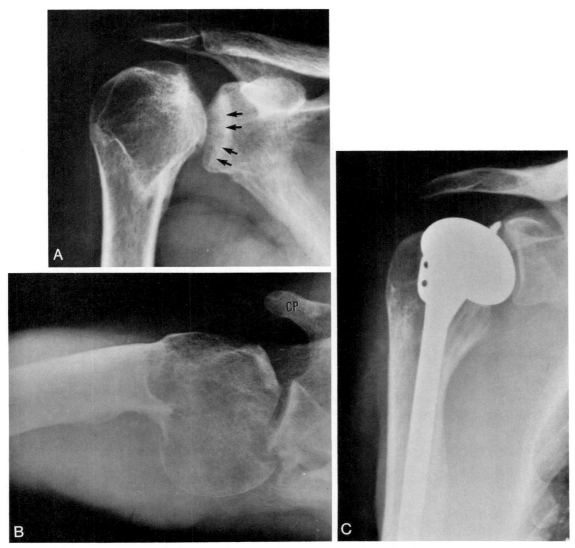

Figure 5–37. Posterior Fracture-Dislocation. *A,* Anteroposterior view several months after injury shows the humeral head to be in internal rotation. There is a wide (more than 6 mm) separation between the humeral head and the anterior glenoid margin (arrows). *B,* The axillary view shows deformity from the prior "head-splitting" fracture. The posterior aspect of the glenoid impinges on the fracture site. The glenoid cartilage, outlined by a vacuum phenomenon within the joint, appears normal. CP = coracoid process. *C,* A noncemented proximal humeral component (Neer II) was inserted. The tip of a screw in the coracoid is seen.

Table 5–9. Neer Classification of Proximal Humeral Fractures

Group	Description	Significance
Minimal or no displacement		
I	Includes all fractures regardless of level or number of fracture lines with no segment displaced >1 cm and no angulation >45°	Represents >85% of proximal humeral fractures
		Requires brief immobilization, then early functional exercises
Displaced fractures		
II Anatomical neck fracture with articular segment displaced	Fractures with displacement at anatomical neck	Need external rotation view of humerus
	No other displaced fractures (all are therefore 2-part fractures)	May develop malunion or avascular necrosis
III Surgical neck fracture with shaft displacement	Surgical neck fracture with >1 cm displacement or >45° angulation (all are two-part)	Rotator cuff intact
	Three subdivisions	
	Angulation >45°	Residual angulation results in limited abduction and elevation
	Separated shaft displaced medially and anteriorly by pectoralis	Often unstable after closed reduction

Comminuted distally

± Neurovascular damage. May get nonunion

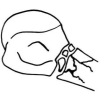

IV Greater tuberosity fracture with displacement

Greater tuberosity displaced >1 cm from lesser tuberosity

Always have longitudinal tear of rotator cuff

Two-part fracture when only greater tuberosity displaced or when *minimally* displaced surgical neck fracture

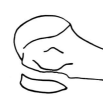

Three-part when displaced greater tuberosity fracture and *displaced* surgical neck fracture

Good blood supply

Need open reduction

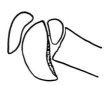

Four-part when lesser tuberosity also displaced

Blood supply to humeral head severed

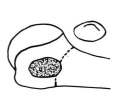

V Lesser tuberosity fracture with displacement

Two-part when displaced lesser tuberosity ± *nondisplaced* fracture of surgical neck

Table continued on following page

Table 5–9. **Neer Classification of Proximal Humeral Fractures** *Continued*

Group		Description	Significance
		Three-part when displaced lesser tuberosity and displaced surgical neck fracture; head rotated externally and abducted; articular surface faces *anteriorly*	
		Four-part when displaced lesser tuberosity, greater tuberosity, and surgical neck fractures (same as Group IV, four-part)	Blood supply to humeral head severed
VI Fracture-dislocations		Anterior, posterior, or superior dislocation of humeral head	Suggests injury to periarticular structures
		Two-part: dislocation and displaced tuberosity fracture. (anterior, posterior)	Blood supply intact

Three-part: dislocation, displaced tuberosity, and displaced surgical neck fracture (greater tuberosity fractured in anterior dislocations and lesser tuberosity fractured in posterior dislocations)

Four-part: dislocation, displaced greater and lesser tuberosity fractures, and displaced surgical neck fracture. (anterior, posterior)

Neurovascular symptoms may occur

Includes impacted fractures associated with dislocations (e.g., Hill-Sachs)

Redislocation when >20° of articular surface involved

Unstable joint when >50% articular surface involved

Articular surface fractures

Head-splitting fractures

Adapted from Neer CS II: J Bone Joint Surg (Am) 52:1077, 1970.

ture. When the greater tuberosity is also displaced, the pull of the subscapularis (remaining on the attached lesser tuberosity) rotates the humeral head internally, causing the articular surface to face posteriorly (a three-part fracture). When the displaced or angulated surgical neck fracture is associated with a displaced fracture of the lesser tuberosity, the unopposed pull of the supraspinatus and external rotators on the attached greater tuberosity will produce external rotation and abduction of the humeral head and will position the articular surface anteriorly (another three-part fracture).

Fractures are also classified by their location as anatomical neck, surgical neck, and the like. Although the anatomical definitions of the anatomical and surgical neck areas is clear, localization of the fracture site to one or both of these areas from preoperative radiographs may be difficult. The fracture may seem to involve both these areas. The presence of a fracture through the anatomical neck is important, however, since the possibility of subsequent avascular necrosis is then raised (Fig. 5–32).

True dislocation is usually established by noting an anterior or posterior position of the humeral head in relation to the glenoid. In anterior three-part fracture-dislocations the greater tuberosity is detached, and the lesser tuberosity remains intact. Conversely, in posterior three-part fracture-dislocations the greater tuberosity remains attached to the humeral head (Figs. 5–36 and 5–37).[60]

Compression fractures of the articular surface may accompany anterior dislocations (the Hill-Sachs deformity) or posterior dislocations. Any compression fracture involving more than 20 percent of the articular surface tends to result in redislocation, and when more than 50 percent

of the articular surface is involved, the joint will be unstable.[60]

Humeral Shaft Fractures

Shaft fractures are usually the result of direct trauma, although they may also result from indirect trauma, such as a fall on the outstretched hand[1, 62] or violent muscular contraction. Fractures caused by direct trauma tend to be transverse or comminuted;[1] indirect injuries typically result in oblique or spiral fractures. Pathological fractures most often involve the proximal portion of the humerus, and traumatic fractures most commonly involve the junction of the mid- and distal thirds.

Fracture Deformity (Fig. 5–38). The direction of angular displacement will depend on the level of fracture and the muscular forces acting on the fracture fragments. Thus when the fracture occurs above the insertion of the deltoid muscle, the distal fragment will be pulled laterally by the attached deltoid. The proximal fragment will be pulled inward by the pectoralis major, the latissimus dorsi, and the teres major. When the fracture is below the deltoid insertion, the proximal fragment will be displaced laterally by the deltoid and the coracobrachialis, and the distal fragment will be pulled proximally by the biceps and triceps muscles.[1]

Treatment. Most humeral fractures are treated with closed methods, and healing ensues in more than 90 percent of patients. Contact of one fourth to one third of the fracture surfaces is required. Considerable angular deformity (20 degrees of anterior bowing or 30 degrees of varus) is apparently acceptable and unassociated with cosmetic or functional deficit. Some of the closed methods of treatment used include the following.

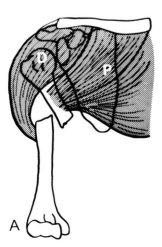

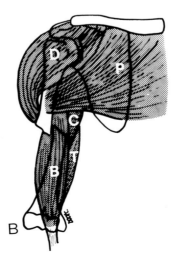

Figure 5–38. Displacement of Humeral Shaft Fractures. *A*, Fractures proximal to the deltoid are associated with lateral displacement of the distal fragment because of the pull of the attached deltoid muscle. The proximal fragment is pulled medially. *B*, When the fracture occurs distal to the deltoid insertion, the proximal fragment is displaced laterally by the deltoid muscle and coracobrachialis, and the distal fragment will be pulled proximally by the biceps and the triceps muscles. D = deltoid, P = pectoralis major, C = coracobrachialis, B = biceps, T = triceps.

Hanging Cast. According to Heppenstall, this method is more suitable for injuries with long fracture surfaces than for simple transverse fractures.[62] The method consists of applying a cast that immobilizes the elbow and extends from the metacarpophalangeal joints to just below the axilla. The weight of the cast is important; one that is too heavy may cause distraction of fracture fragments, whereas one that is relatively light helps to correct angular deformity without producing undue distraction. The proximal edge of the cast should not overlie the fracture line; otherwise the cast may act as a fulcrum at the fracture site and interfere with healing.[62]

Functional Bracing.[65] Functional bracing allows contraction of muscles near the fracture site, and this is thought to have a beneficial effect on healing. Large bulky callus is formed that is apparently stronger than the smaller callus produced when rigid immobilization techniques are used.

Elephant Tongs. This term refers to a U-shaped plaster splint that extends from under the axilla, around the elbow, and up the lateral aspect of the humerus to the shoulder. Flexion at the elbow and motion at the shoulder are possible. Angular deformity is controlled, and distraction does not occur.

Healing. Healing with closed methods occurs in more than 90 percent of patients. The average time to fracture healing is 10 weeks.[62]

Open reduction and internal fixation are considered when soft tissues are interposed between fracture fragments, when vascular injury is present, when delayed union or nonunion has occurred, when there is a spiral fracture of the distal third of the humerus with radial nerve paresis, when a pathologic fracture due to malignancy is present, when the patient has Parkinson's disease, or when satisfactory position cannot be obtained or maintained.[62] Compression plates and rods have been used for fixation.

Complications. Injury to the radial nerve occurs in between 5 and 10 percent of humeral shaft fractures.[1] Medial and ulnar nerve damage may also occur. Damage may be reversible, and

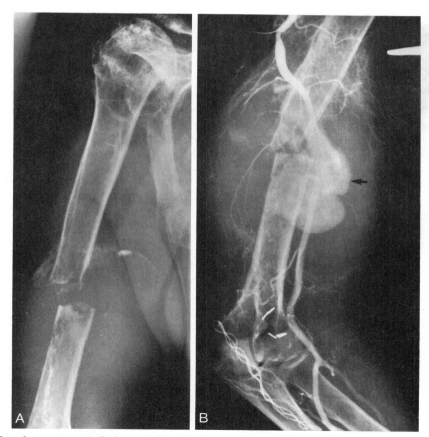

Figure 5–39. Pseudoaneurysm. *A,* Radiograph 2 weeks after a midhumeral fracture shows periosteal reaction and a large soft tissue mass around the fracture site. *B,* Selective intraoperative brachial arteriogram shows arterial disruption, with filling of a large pseudoaneurysm (arrow). The large hematoma is reflected by the displacement and stretching of adjacent vessels.

therefore conservative treatment is usually appropriate, with exploration and repair at a later date if healing does not occur. Vascular injuries usually require primary operative repair (Fig. 5–39).

Delayed union and nonunion occur most often in transverse fractures of the mid-diaphysis. When healing has not occurred after 4 to 5 months of conservative treatment, delayed union is present. Surgical intervention may then be necessary to establish contact between the fracture surfaces, obtain rigid internal fixation, and apply bone graft (Fig. 5–40).[1]

Glenohumeral Dislocations

Pseudodislocation (Inferior Subluxation of the Humeral Head, or "Drooping Shoulder") (Fig. 5–41)

Inferior displacement of the humeral head without anterior or posterior subluxation or dislocation has been termed pseudodislocation. This

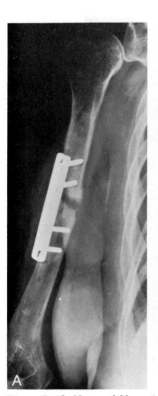
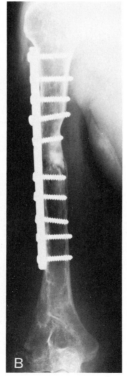

Figure 5–40. Humeral Nonunion. *A,* A frontal view after attempted repair of a humeral nonunion shows a wide separation of fracture fragments, with sclerosis across the medullary canals indicative of nonunion. There is resorption about the hardware, confirming loosening. *B,* Follow-up film after bone grafting and internal fixation shows healing.

condition has been noted to accompany injury of the brachial plexus or axillary nerve, proximal humeral head fracture, and hemarthrosis due to hemophilia. Months after humeral neck fractures such downward displacement of the shoulder has been attributed to gradual stretching of supporting musculature. Subluxation following acute fracture may be due to partial detachment of the capsule anteriorly and inferiorly or to associated hemarthrosis.[67]

When this relatively benign pseudodislocation is associated with the acute fractures, its differentiation from the more serious true fracture-dislocation is of considerable importance. Pseudodislocation is confirmed if oblique views show the absence of anterior or posterior displacement or if repeat radiographs with the arm supported in a sling show improvement in position. If doubt remains, aspiration of the hemarthrosis with return of the humeral head to a more normal position will establish the diagnosis.

True glenohumeral dislocations may be divided into four groups: anterior, posterior, inferior, or superior, depending upon the final position of the humeral head.

Anterior Dislocation

Anterior dislocations represent about 95 percent of all shoulder dislocations and occur most frequently in males. The vast majority of cases are post-traumatic. Rowe noted that patients with atraumatic dislocations (only 6 percent of his series) differed from those with post-traumatic dislocations by their greater likelihood of having an associated anatomical variation of the articular or soft tissue structures, instability in more than one direction, voluntary dislocation and reduction in some, and an unpredictable response to surgery.[90] In contrast patients in whom the first dislocation is due to trauma usually have instability in only one direction and do well after surgery.

Mechanism of Injury. Most anterior dislocations are the result of a force that produces abduction and external rotation of the arm. The surgical neck of the humerus impinges on the acromion process and levers the head out of the glenoid fossa anteriorly and inferiorly.[80] The greater the degree of abduction, the more the head is forced inferiorly.[1] Dislocation may also occur from a fall backward on the point of the elbow with the shoulder in extension or from a direct blow on the shoulder posteriorly that forces the humerus out of the glenoid.[80, 87]

Anatomical Changes Related to Dislocation. Following anterior dislocation, damage can occur to the soft tissues anterior or posterior to

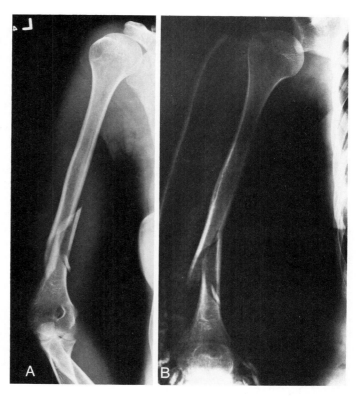

Figure 5–41. Pseudodislocation. *A,* AP film immediately after injury shows a spiral fracture of the humerus. The glenohumeral relationships appear normal. *B,* Follow-up examination 1 week later (in a U-shaped plaster splint) shows inferior displacement of the humeral head in relation to the glenoid.

the joint as well as to the bony structures. The soft tissues anterior to the joint, collectively termed the anterior soft tissue mechanism, consist of the glenoid labrum, the anterior capsule, the synovial lining and its recesses, and the subscapularis muscle and tendon.[80, 82] The "posterior soft tissue mechanism" consists of the posterior capsule and the labrum; the synovial membrane; and the supraspinatus, the infraspi-

natus, and the teres minor muscles and tendons (Fig. 5–42).

With dislocation, various anatomically demonstrated abnormalities occur, including the following:[68, 70, 71, 76, 80, 82, 90]

1. Tearing and stretching of both anterior and posterior soft tissues

2. Detachment of the anterior glenoid labrum (present in about 85 percent of patients with

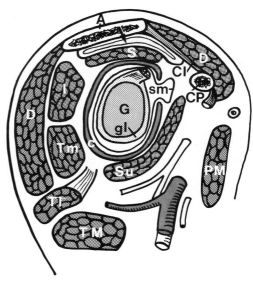

Figure 5–42. Periarticular Soft Tissues. A cross section through the glenoid fossa shows the adjacent soft tissues. A = acromion; arrow = subacromial-subdeltoid bursa; c = capsule; CP = coracoid process; Cl = coracoacromial ligament; D = deltoid; G = glenoid fossa; gl = glenoid labrum; I = infraspinatus; PM = pectoralis major S = supraspinatus; sm = synovial membrane; Su = subscapularis; Tl = triceps, long head; Tm = teres minor; TM = teres major. (Redrawn from Snell RS: Clinical Anatomy for Medical Students. Boston, Little, Brown, 1981.)

Table 5–10. **Factors of Importance in Recurrent Dislocation**

Anatomical		
	Soft tissue abnormalities	Bankart lesion
		Weakness of posterior muscles
		Weakness of subscapularis
		Elongation of the posterior capsule
		Large joint capacity
		Formation of ant. pouch of joint capsule
	Bony abnormalities	Relatively large diameter humeral head
		Increased retroversion of humerus
		Hill-Sachs deformity
Clinical		Age under 20 years
		Epilepsy
		Electric shock

Sources: Post M: The Shoulder. Philadelphia, Lea & Febiger, 1978; Bankart ASB: Br Med J [Clin Res] 2:1132, 1923; Bankart ASB: Br J Surg 26:23, 1938; Moseley HF: Surg Clin North Am 43:1631, 1963; Rowe CR: J Bone J Surg. (Am) 38:957, 1956; Rowe CR: Surg Clin North Am 43:1609, 1963; Rowe CR, Pierce D: J Bone Joint Surg (Am) 47:1670, 1965; Rowe RC, Sakellarides HT: Clin Orthop 20:40, 1961; Saha AK: Acta Orthop Scand 38:479, 1967.

recurrent dislocation), detachment of the anterior capsule from the neck of the scapula, or avulsion of the glenoid rim

3. Formation of an anterior pouch from stretching of the glenohumeral ligament and capsule

4. Laxity and stretching of the subscapularis tendon with detachment from the anterior aspect of the scapula and, often, elevation of the periosteum

5. Compression fracture of the humeral head.

Recurrent Anterior Dislocation. Several anatomical features seem to be important in allowing recurrent dislocation after an initial injury (Table 5–10). At the time of injury there usually is stripping of the capsule from the anterior neck of the scapula and detachment of the glenoid labrum. In 1923 Bankart noted that the essential feature of recurrent dislocation was a detachment of the capsule from the glenoid labrum.[70] This was modified in 1938, when he reported that the typical lesion of recurrent dislocation was in fact detachment of the labrum from the anterior rim of the glenoid.[71] This latter defect is usually termed the Bankart lesion,[1] and it is present in the majority of patients with recurrent dislocation.[71, 75, 76] In addition, the posterolateral aspect of the humeral head may be compressed against the glenoid (the Hill-Sachs deformity), and the subscapularis tendon may be stretched and continue to be lax after reduction.[79, 92] The torn capsule and the laxity of the subscapularis contribute to a decrease in the normal restraining mechanisms that keep the humeral head within the glenoid fossa.[1] Developmental bony abnormalities, including a relatively large humeral head[93] and an abnormal tilt of the glenoid or

the proximal humerus, have been postulated as predisposing factors. In addition to anatomical factors, several clinical factors seem to predispose to recurrent dislocation. Rowe and Sakellarides noted, for example, that the age of the patient at the time of the first dislocation was particularly important in determining the incidence of recurrence. Ninety-four percent of patients who had their first dislocation under the age of 20 had subsequent recurrences, whereas the patients with dislocation occurring after the age of 40 had only a 14 percent recurrence rate.[92] Also, patients with epilepsy had a very high recurrence rate as well as a high incidence of humeral-head compression fractures.

Radiographic Features of Anterior Dislocation

Abnormal Position of the Humeral Head. Depending on the final position of the humeral head, dislocations can be subdivided into four varieties: subcoracoid, subglenoid, subclavicular, and intrathoracic. The subcoracoid anterior dislocations in which the humeral head is displaced anteriorly, under the coracoid process, is the most frequent.[1] Frontal radiographs will show the humeral head to be medially positioned (Fig. 5–43). An anterior oblique or an axillary view confirms the abnormal anterior location of the humeral head. Transthoracic lateral views will show disruption of the smooth curve that is usually present between the inferior margin of the scapula and the posterior margin of the humerus.

Following reduction of an anterior dislocation, the position of the humeral head should be confirmed on oblique or on AP views. A post-reduction axillary view is to be avoided, since

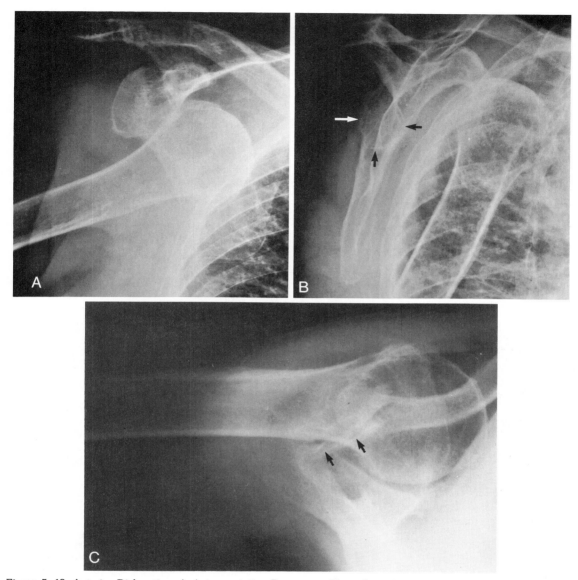

Figure 5–43. Anterior Dislocation. *A*, Anteroposterior, *B*, anterior oblique (scapular Y), and *C*, axillary, views show the humeral head displaced anteriorly and medially. Arrows indicate glenoid margins.

abduction of the arm may result in redislocation.[77]

Associated Fractures

Greater Tuberosity Fractures. According to Moseley, there is a higher incidence of fracture of the greater tuberosity and avulsion of the rotator cuff with subglenoid as compared with other dislocations.[82] Greater tuberosity fractures were noted in 37 percent of 119 patients with anterior dislocation reviewed by Hill and Sachs.[79] Rowe and Sakellarides noted a definite decrease in the tendency to develop recurrent

subluxation in patients with greater tuberosity fractures; they suggested that the increased trauma and resulting increase in scar tissue and, often, the advanced age of those patients may play roles in lowering the recurrence rate.[92]

Hill-Sachs Deformity. In 1940 Harold Hill and Maurice Sachs reviewed 119 cases of shoulder dislocation and noted bony injury to the humerus or scapula on radiographic examination in more than two thirds.[79] In particular the wedge-shaped defect of the posterolateral aspect of the humeral head was evaluated in detail.

253

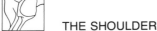
This defect (now called the Hill-Sachs lesion) is a compression fracture that occurs when the posterolateral aspect of the dislocated humeral head impacts on the glenoid rim.

Radiographic examination with the humerus in external rotation frequently obscures the lesion and may show only slight lucency in the area medial to the greater tuberosity. With the humerus internally rotated (a variable amount but usually optimal at between 60 and 70 degrees), the affected posterolateral surface is brought into profile, and the defect is seen to advantage.[69] Several additional radiographic views have been suggested specifically to identify the Hill-Sachs lesion, including the Didiee view, the Hermoddson view, and the notch view.[80]

The Hill-Sachs lesion consists of (1) a flattened or indented area at the level of the greater tuberosity, (2) a sharp, dense vertical line of condensation that extends from the top of the humeral head distally and represents the compressed bone along the medial aspect of the defect, and (3) a dense inferior border (Fig. 5–44).

These lesions occurred in 21 percent of all dislocations and in 74 percent of patients with recurrent dislocation studied by Hill and Sachs.[79] Other authors have found this fracture to be even more frequent. For example, Adams found such a defect in 82 percent of patients thought to have had adequate radiographic examination.[69, 80]

As pointed out by Hill and Sachs and others, the defect may occur after a single dislocation.[69, 92] Following multiple dislocations, it may remain stable or may enlarge.[79]

Abnormalities of the Glenoid Rim. Bankart emphasized that recurrent dislocations result from detachment of the labrum from the glenoid

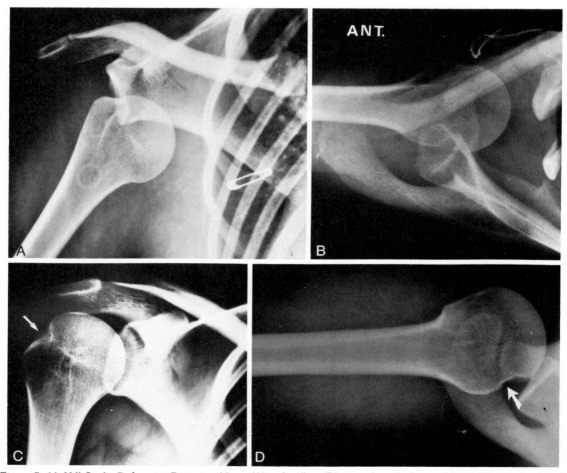

Figure 5–44. Hill-Sachs Deformity. Posterior oblique *(A)* and axillary *(B)* views show the humeral head dislocated anteriorly and inferiorly, perched on the anterior glenoid rim. Postreduction internal rotation *(C)* and axillary *(D)* views show the compression fracture of the humeral head (arrow), the Hill-Sachs lesion.

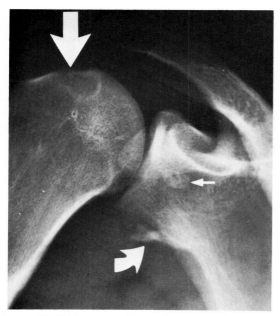

Figure 5–45. Stigmata of Prior Anterior Dislocation. A lucency in the humeral head (large arrow) was shown on additional views to be a Hill-Sachs defect. There is irregularity along the inferior aspect of the scapular neck (curved arrow) at the site of capsular insertion. A presumed loose body (small arrow) is noted in the area of the subscapularis recess.

rim.[71] A fracture along the anterior-inferior rim of the glenoid (the Bankart fracture) may occur in association with this soft tissue injury. Rounding or eburnation of the glenoid margin may result.[68] Periosteal new bone may be deposited in the area of detachment of the glenoid labrum, capsule, and periosteum from the anterior surface of the scapula (Figs. 5–45 and 5–46).[76] The axillary view shows the anterior margin of the glenoid to advantage.[80] A modified axillary view (the West Point view) shows the anterior inferior glenoid rim in profile and may show anteriorly located bone or calcification that cannot be demonstrated on other views. The presence of this calcification establishes a diagnosis of prior subluxation or dislocation.[86, 88]

False Joint Formation on the Anterior Aspect of the Scapula. With recurrent dislocation a sclerotic pseudojoint may develop.[1]

Loose Bodies. Loose bodies occur in about 8 percent of dislocations.[1, 72]

Arthrography. Deformity of the anterior capsule resulting from recurrent anterior dislocation can be documented on arthrography. On the internal rotation view the notch normally seen between the subscapularis and the axillary recesses will be absent in such cases.[100]

Double-contrast arthrography provides addi-

tional information concerning the integrity of the articular cartilage and the glenoid labrum. Goldman suggests that the anterior glenoid labrum may be evaluated on the supine axillary view following double-contrast arthrography. In patients in whom posterior abnormality is suspected the prone axillary view should be done.[97] Mink and associates, however, suggest that the supine view is of help for evaluation of the posterior glenoid labrum and the prone view for evaluation of the anterior glenoid labrum. This latter technique would surround the labrum with contrast medium in a manner similar to a single-contrast study.[99] El-Khoury and colleagues used hypocycloidal tomography in the axial projection, after injection of 4 ml of Renografin-60 and 10 ml of air into the joint, to study the labrum.[96, 98] Braunstein uses hypocycloidal tomography in a posterior oblique projection (Fig. 5–47).[95]

When available, computed tomography following double-contrast arthrography is an excellent method of evaluating the integrity of the glenoid labrum (Fig. 5–47). The procedure is highly accurate, adds no discomfort to the arthrographic study, and is lower in radiation exposure than is complex-motion tomography.

The glenoid labrum is a circular rim of tissue that inserts on the circumference of the glenoid cavity. It is triangular in cross section. As seen on the arthrogram, the normal anterior labrum appears as a lucent triangular area, sharply pointed. The free margin of the posterior labrum is more rounded in contour.[96] The base of the labrum is continuous with the articular cartilage of the glenoid (see Figs. 5–8 and 5–47). Several abnormalities in the labrum have been demonstrated, and these appear to correlate well with surgical findings.[98] The abnormalities include (1) change in the shape, blunting, or irregularity of the free margin of the labrum indicating a tear of its substance (see Fig. 5–47), and (2) leakage of contrast material outside the joint. It is uncertain whether this leakage represents capsular detachment or merely overdistension of the joint. Small Hill-Sachs deformities, loose bodies, enlargement of the anterior capsule, and rotator cuff tears can be demonstrated during the examination.[100]

Double-contrast arthrography with special attention to the glenoid labrum has been used to (1) confirm clinically and radiographically undocumented, repeated dislocation or subluxation; (2) evaluate patients with unexplained shoulder pain that may be due to capsular abnormalities; and (3) document the direction of instability.[96, 99]

Text continued on page 260

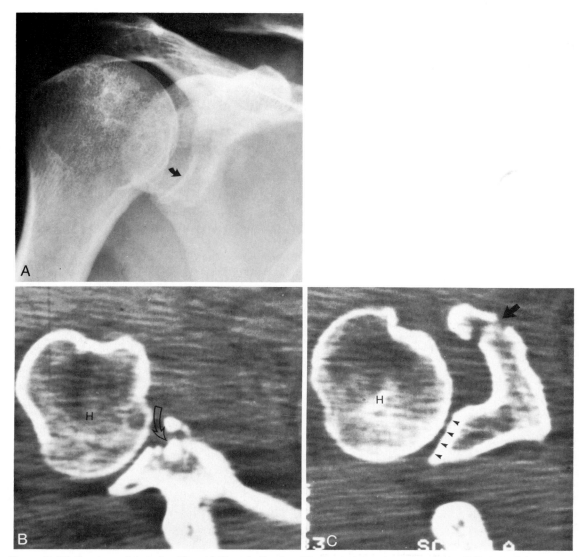

Figure 5–46. Fracture of Anterior Glenoid Rim. *A*, Routine AP view in internal rotation shows deformity of the anterior glenoid rim (arrow). *B*, A CT scan better shows the extent of damage to the anterior glenoid (arrow). No dislocation is present now. H = humeral head. *C*, A CT scan above that in *B* shows a previously unrecognized coracoid process fracture (arrow). Arrowheads indicate glenoid fossa. H = humeral head.

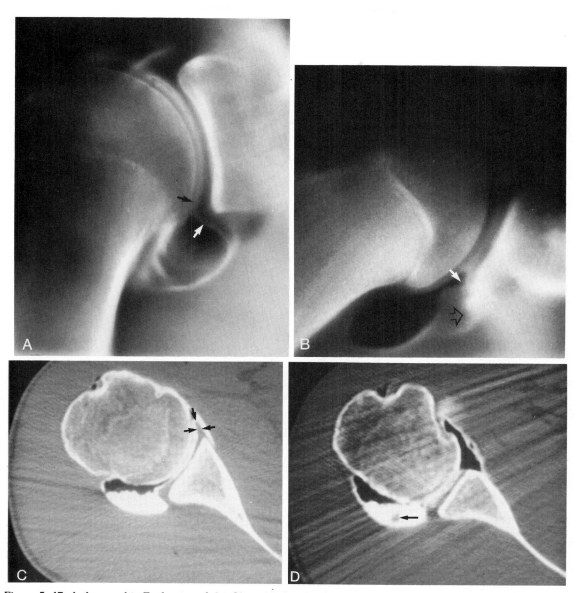

Figure 5–47. Arthrographic Evaluation of the Glenoid Labrum. *A,* Normal glenoid labrum on posterior oblique double contrast arthrotomography. Tomographic section through the anterior margin of the glenoid in the posterior oblique position shows smooth articular cartilage on the humeral head and glenoid and a smooth contour to the glenoid labrum (arrows). *B,* Abnormal glenoid labrum. Tomographic section shows a triangular defect in the labrum (arrow). The bony margin of the glenoid is also noted to be irregular (open arrow). The patient had suffered a single anterior dislocation. (Courtesy of Dr. Ethan Braunstein, Brigham and Women's Hospital, Boston, Mass.) *C,* Normal glenoid labrum on computed tomography following double contrast arthrography. The sharply pointed anterior (arrows) and the slightly rounder posterior margins of the labrum are well seen. *D,* Computed arthrotomogram shows absence of the anterior labrum and a loose body (arrow) posteriorly. (*C* and *D* courtesy of Arthur Newberg, M.D., Boston, Mass.)

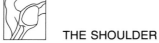

Table 5–11. **Surgical Procedures for Recurrent Anterior Dislocation**

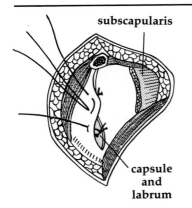

subscapularis

capsule
and
labrum

Method: Bankart, repair of anterior capsule mechanism.

Operation: reattachment of anterior capsule to anterior glenoid.

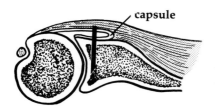

capsule

Method: DuToit and Roux.

Operation: detached labrum or torn capsule fixed to glenoid rim with 1 to 3 staples.

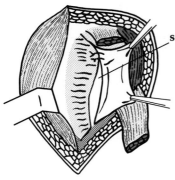

subscapularis tendon and
underlying capsule

Method: Putti-Platt, shortening of subscapularis.

Operation: transection of lateral part of subscapularis and attachment of lateral inch of tendon to anterior glenoid rim.

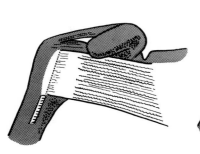
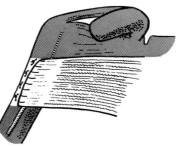

Method: Magnuson-Stack, transfer of subscapularis.

Operation: distal and lateral transfer of subscapularis tendon across bicipital groove.

Table continued on opposite page

Table 5–11. **Surgical Procedures for Recurrent Anterior Dislocation** *Continued*

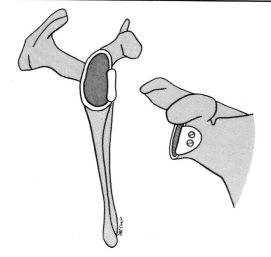

Method: Eden-Hybinette, anterior glenoid bone block.

Operation: iliac grafts to buttress the anterior glenoid.

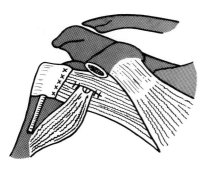

Method: Bristow-Helfet, coracoid transfer.

Operation: transfer of coracoid and conjoined tendon to anterior glenoid.

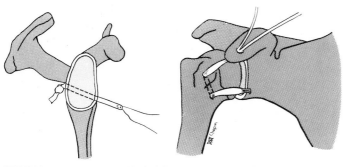

Method: Gallie-LeMesurier, fascial repair.

Operation: use of autogenous fascia lata to reconstruct new ligaments between the anterior-inferior capsule and the neck of humerus.

Source: Modified from Post M: The Shoulder. Philadelphia, Lea & Febiger, 1978.

Complications of Anterior Dislocation. Radiographically identifiable complications include rotator cuff tears, adhesive capsulitis, and myositis ossificans.[1]

Surgical Procedures for Recurrent Dislocation. According to Post, operative treatment is indicated when three or more dislocations have occurred in a reasonably short period of time.[1] Documentation of dislocation and the direction of dislocation is important, and when this is absent clinically, fluoroscopic examination during attempted voluntary subluxation may be helpful. Demonstration of the Hill-Sachs defect or the anterior compression fracture that accompanies posterior dislocation provides presumptive evidence of prior dislocation.

Multiple surgical procedures are in use, and the choice is guided by the anatomical lesions present (Table 5–11). Whatever procedure is used, however, defects in the anterior capsule are closed or buttressed by scar tissue. Glenoid-bone blocks[1] or metal may be used to reconstruct the glenoid margin.[82] The coracoid process may be divided to facilitate exposure; it is screwed or sutured in place at the end of the procedure (Fig. 5–48).

Posterior Dislocation

Posterior dislocation is decidedly less common than anterior, accounting for less than 5 percent of all dislocations.[89] However, the actual incidence may be underestimated, since the diagnosis may be missed on clinical and radiographic examination. Clinically, posterior dislocations are subdivided into acute, chronic, and recurrent categories. The chronic group is of considerable interest, since these patients may have mild pain and some limitation of motion for days, months, or years before the diagnosis is made. As with anterior dislocations, recurrence is more frequent in patients whose initial dislocation occurs before age 20.[105]

Posterior dislocations may also be subdivided according to the final position of the humeral head into (1) subacromial—humeral head behind the glenoid and below the acromion, (2) posterior subglenoid—humeral head behind and inferior to the glenoid, and (3) subspinous—humeral head under the spine of the scapula.[114] The vast majority of posterior dislocations are of the subacromial variety. Trauma, in which there is a fall on the outstretched hand resulting in sudden internal rotation, adduction, and flexion of the arm, is the most frequent mechanism of injury.[1] Rarely, direct trauma to the front of the shoulder may dislocate the humerus posteriorly. Posterior dislocation also occurs in association with epilepsy and electro-shock therapy, with congenital abnormalities such as the Ehlers-Danlos and Marfan syndromes, and with cerebral palsy.[1, 103, 105, 108] Bilateral posterior dislocations are usually the result of violent muscular

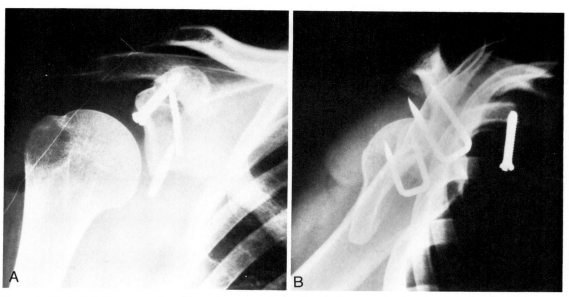

Figure 5–48. DuToit Reconstruction. The anterior capsule was bunched up and fixed to the glenoid with two staples. A screw holds the surgically created coracoid process fracture fragments. Mild inferior subluxation is present. *A,* External rotation; *B,* Y view.

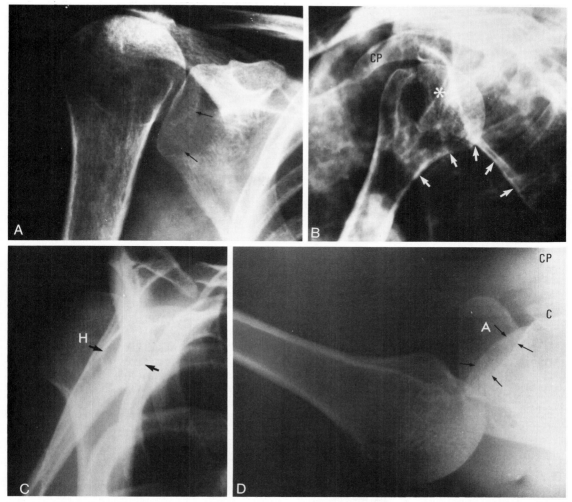

Figure 5–49. Posterior Dislocation. *A*, Anteroposterior view in a woman with systemic lupus erythematosus and shoulder pain shows the humeral head to be internally rotated and elevated. The wide separation between the anterior glenoid rim (arrows) and the humeral head suggests the diagnosis of posterior dislocation. *B*, The transthoracic lateral view confirms the posterior displacement of the humeral head. This view, however, may be difficult to interpret, and the anterior oblique or axillary views are more likely to be confirmatory. The arch formed by the humerus and scapula is pointed (arrows) superiorly rather than smoothly arched. CP = coracoid process; asterisk = location of glenoid. *C*, The anterior oblique (scapular Y) view of another patient shows the humeral head (H) to be centered behind the glenoid (arrows). *D*, An axillary view confirms the posterior location of the humeral head. CP = coracoid process; C = clavicle; A = acromion process; arrows = glenoid fossa.

contraction such as occurs with seizures or electric shock.[115] In some cases voluntary dislocation is possible.

Pathological Abnormalities. Bony and soft tissue abnormalities associated with posterior dislocation include

1. Detachment and laxity of the posterior part of the joint capsule
2. Detachment or tear of the posterior glenoid labrum
3. Anteromedial compression fracture of the humeral head

4. Fracture of the posterior aspect of the glenoid fossa
5. Congenital abnormalities of the joint, among them excessive retrotilt of the glenoid fossa and excessive retroversion of the humeral head.[1, 89]

Radiographic Findings (Fig. 5–49)

Abnormal Position of the Humeral Head. Frontal radiographs reflect the fact that the humerus is held in the neutral or internally rotated position and the arm is adducted. In fact, if the patient is able to externally rotate the arm, a

THE SHOULDER

traumatic posterior dislocation is virtually excluded.[1, 104] The position of the humeral head may be abnormally high or low. Bloom and Obata suggest two views that can be used to demonstrate the abnormal location of the humeral head, even in the patient whose shoulder is immobilized by a bandage.[102] Anterior oblique views or an axillary view will confirm the posterior location of the humeral head. Axillary views can be obtained even if abduction of the arm is not possible.[118] It is important to remember that usually the head is only partially displaced posteriorly and is actually impacted against the posterior glenoid rim.

Widening of the Joint Space on the AP View (Positive Rim Sign). In patients with posterior dislocation the distance between the anterior rim of the glenoid fossa and the medial aspect of the humeral head may be widened, an appearance termed a positive rim sign by Arndt and Sears.[101] Separation of these structures by more than 6 mm is considered abnormal. Review of radiographs in 48 published cases of posterior dislocation yielded 31 cases in which the rim sign was positive. False negative cases were attributed to medial displacement of the humeral head due to associated fractures or to notching of the humeral head. Rotation toward the posterior oblique view will also produce a falsely negative rim sign.

Brown suggests that a single anteroposterior view of the upper chest and shoulders, using a short tube–film distance and centering near the top of the sternum, should be taken. In this way both shoulders are included on the same film, allowing comparison between them.[103]

Absence of a "Half-moon" Overlap on the Anteroposterior View. As stated by Nobel, the medial aspect of the humeral head normally overlaps the glenoid fossa on AP views, producing a shadow resembling a half-moon, which reaches down to the lower border of the glenoid fossa.[114] In patients with posterior dislocation this overlap shadow may be absent. Sixteen of 48 cases of posterior dislocation reviewed by Arndt and Sears displayed this finding.[101]

Abnormal Arch on the Transthoracic Lateral View. The normal arch made by the axillary margin of the scapula and the medial posterior aspect of the humerus may be disrupted, with the top of the curve more narrowed than usual. In practice, the transthoracic view is often difficult to interpret.[103]

Overlap of the Humeral Head and Glenoid on the Posterior Oblique View. The posterior oblique projection usually shows the cartilage space in tangent, and therefore no overlap of the humeral head and the glenoid is expected. In the presence of posterior dislocation of the humerus with an impaction fracture, the humeral head is displaced medially and may overlap the glenoid on this view.

Compression Fracture of the Humeral Head (the Trough Line) *(Fig. 5–50).* As a consequence of posterior dislocation, the humeral head may be impacted on the posterior

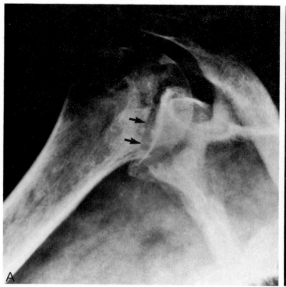
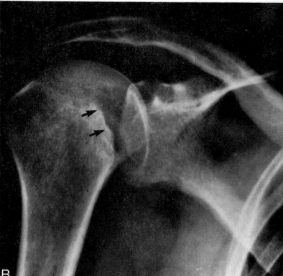

Figure 5–50. Posterior Dislocation—Trough Sign. *A,* The posterior oblique view shows abnormal overlap between the humeral head and glenoid as well as elevation of the humeral head. A line (arrows) with increased density lateral to it (trough sign) indicates an impacted fracture of the humeral head. *B,* Anteroposterior view shows the area of impaction (arrows), as well as the abnormal position of the humeral head.

262

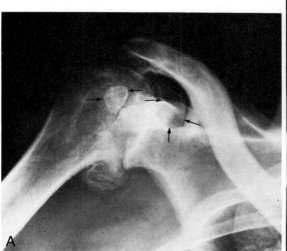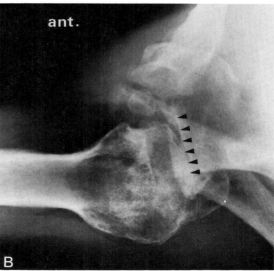

Figure 5–51. Chronic Posterior Dislocation. An elderly man with chronic shoulder pain after injury. The posterior dislocation was not recognized. *A,* Posterior oblique view shows apparent marked narrowing of the glenohumeral cartilage space and a large osteophyte or loose body at the inferior humeral margin. Two smooth ossicles (arrows) are thought to represent old fractures of the lesser (smaller fragment) and greater tuberosities. *B,* Axillary view confirms the posterior subluxation of the humeral head in relation to the glenoid (arrowheads). There is severe cartilage loss as a result of secondary osteoarthritis; ant. = anterior.

aspect of the glenoid, producing a compression fracture of the humeral head analogous to the Hill-Sachs lesion that follows anterior dislocation. Three of 10 patients with posterior dislocation studied by Rowe had such defects,[89] and Arndt and Sears observed it in 22 of 48 cases of posterior dislocation.[101] Cisternino and colleagues noted that a dense line (the trough line), roughly paralleling the articular surface of the humerus, can be seen on frontal radiographs; this corresponds to the impacted fracture noted pathologically. This sign was seen in 75 percent of 20 posteriorly dislocated shoulders.[104]

Notch Defect. With marked internal rotation the compression fracture of the anterior aspect of the humeral head may be brought into profile and will appear as a notch on the medial surface of the humerus.[104]

Fractures. Fractures of the humeral head, the lesser tuberosity, the humeral neck or shaft, the scapula, and the glenoid margin may accompany posterior dislocation.[104] Fractures of the humeral head were seen in 10 of 48 patients with posterior dislocation, and in 7 patients the dislocation was overlooked (Fig. 5–51).[101]

Surgical Procedures. *Acute traumatic* posterior dislocations are usually treated by closed reduction and immobilization.[1, 105] Wilson noted that redislocation may occur if external immobilization alone is used and suggested crossed wires to fix the humeral head to the acromion

process during healing.[119] According to McLaughlin, the prognosis becomes less favorable and therapeutic difficulties increase in direct proportion to the length of time the posterior dislocation remains unrecognized.[111] Within 2 weeks closed reduction may be attempted, but after 2 to 4 weeks open reduction is necessary.

Recurrent posterior dislocation is treated surgically when recurrences are frequent or when the joint produces painful or disabling symptoms (Fig. 5–52). Available surgical procedures include

1. Reverse Bankart procedure to repair the posterior capsule

2. Reverse Putti-Platt procedure, in which the infraspinatus muscle is shortened or plicated

3. Posterior capsulorrhaphy and transfer of the long head of the biceps to the posterior glenoid rim

4. Opening posterior wedge osteotomy

5. Combined soft tissue and bone procedure

6. McLaughlin procedure, in which a large compression defect in the humeral head is filled either by the transplanted end of the subscapularis tendon or by the tendon and lesser tuberosity—the Neer modification.[1, 87, 108, 111, 117]

The presence of anterior medial humeral head fractures and deformity of the posterior glenoid must be demonstrated on preoperative radiographs so that the appropriate surgical technique can be chosen.

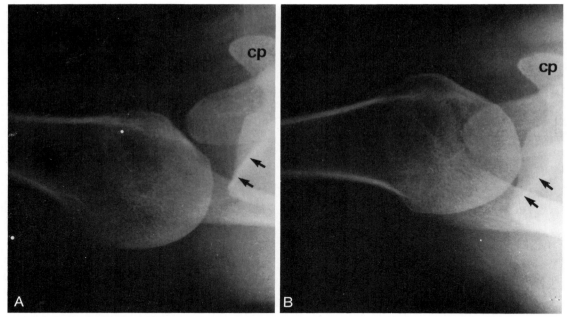

Figure 5–52. Recurrent Posterior Subluxation. This young nurse noted increasing pain and instability after an episode of heavy lifting. Axillary views show the humeral head in the posteriorly subluxed *(A)* and reduced *(B)* positions; CP = coracoid process, arrows = glenoid margin.

Surgical treatment is not usually applied to cases of *voluntary* dislocation.

Complications of Posterior Dislocation. Damage to neurovascular structures is an unlikely consequence of posterior dislocation. Soft tissue calcification may be seen. Following surgical correction of a posterior dislocation, anterior dislocation may occasionally occur.[119]

Inferior and Superior Dislocations[107]

Inferior dislocation (luxatio erecta) is an uncommon dislocation resulting from hyperabduction of the arm (Fig. 5–53). The humeral head is positioned below the glenoid fossa with the humeral articular surface facing inferiorly and the humeral shaft directed upward. There may be a fracture of the greater tuberosity. Closed reduction is usually effective.

Superior dislocation is rare. The humeral head is above the glenoid, and fractures of the acromion or clavicle or disruption of the AC joint may occur.

Anterior Capsular Derangement[120, 121]

The anterior capsular mechanism consists of the soft tissues extending from the neck of the glenoid to the lesser tuberosity, including the insertions of the glenohumeral ligaments, the sub-

scapularis tendon, and the glenoid labrum. Kummel noted a particular constellation of findings in patients in whom capsular tears and avulsions, abnormalities of the glenoid labrum,

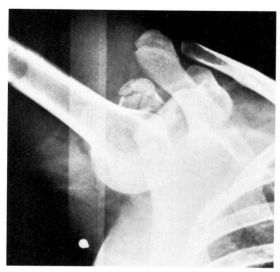

Figure 5–53. Luxatio Erecta. The humerus is fixed in an abducted position with the humeral head beneath the glenoid fossa. Fracture fragments, most likely from the greater tuberosity, are seen.

and irregularities in the subscapularis tendon were found at surgery. The clinical syndrome included a history of pain and instability with normal range of motion on physical examination and pain on abduction and external rotation. A palpable click could be produced on the anterior aspect of the shoulder at a level below the coracoid process. Single-contrast arthrography was performed in these patients, and it was suggested that bilateral examinations should be done to evaluate subtle abnormalities. According to Kummel, three types of defects were seen on arthrography: (1) filling of an anterior-inferior pouch representing a defect in the capsule, (2) extravasation of contrast beyond the capsule, and (3) an enlarged and irregular axillary pouch.

Total Shoulder Replacement

Total shoulder replacement is a relatively recent technique used primarily in patients with incapacitating pain and secondarily for improvement in function. Normally, the stability of the glenohumeral joint is provided largely by the joint capsule and rotator cuff. Since in some of the diseases treated with these prostheses (e.g.,

rheumatoid arthritis) there is associated damage to these structures, either the structures must be repaired or their functions must be replaced or augmented by the prostheses.

Cofield has categorized the currently available prostheses into three groups:[124] (1) prostheses that replace the articular surfaces of the joint (e.g., Neer; Fig. 5–54);[122, 125] (2) prostheses that replace the articular surfaces and provide some additional stability (e.g., Gristina; Fig. 5–55); and (3) prostheses that replace the articular surface and replace the constraining functions of the soft tissues (e.g., Stanmore and Michael Reese; Fig. 5–56).[126, 127]

The Neer prosthesis is the one most frequently used at the Brigham and Women's Hospital. It consists of a chromium-cobalt humeral component (the same component used in hemiarthroplasty) and a dish-shaped, high-density polyethylene glenoid component which may have a metal backing. The glenoid component is fixed to the glenoid with methyl methacrylate.[125]

Postoperative radiographic examination should include a posterior oblique view (approximately 45 degrees) to evaluate the components in profile as well as internal rotation and axillary views. Usually, the inferior aspect of the humeral

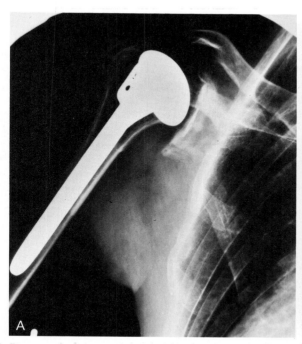
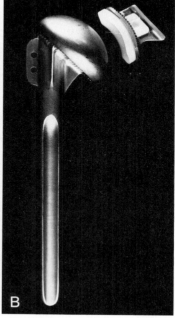

Figure 5–54. Total Shoulder Prosthesis (Neer). A, This posterior oblique view shows the nonopaque polyethylene glenoid component and the metallic humeral component in profile. Opaque cement is present under the glenoid component. Erosion of the clavicle and acromion due to severe rheumatoid arthritis and rotator cuff damage can be seen. There is slight superior subluxation of the humeral component. (Same patient as in Figure 5–28.) B, Photograph of the prosthesis, which has a metal-backed glenoid component.

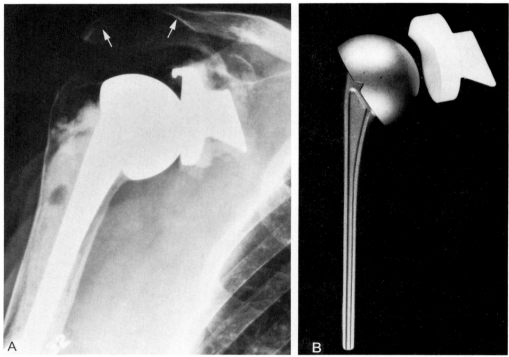

Figure 5–55. Total-Shoulder Prosthesis (Gristina). *A*, Posterior oblique radiograph shows the components in profile with opaque cement around them. The glenoid component is metal-backed. Severe erosion of the undersurface of the clavicle and acromion (arrows) is present as a consequence of rheumatoid arthritis and severe rotator cuff damage. *B*, Photograph of the prosthesis shows the glenoid component with its superior lip, used to limit upward subluxation of the humerus in patients with rheumatoid arthritis. The metal backing is not shown.

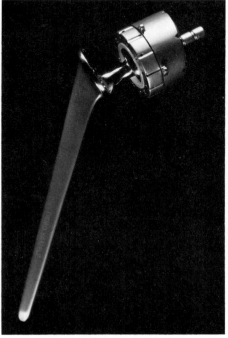

Figure 5–56. Total-Shoulder Prosthesis (Michael-Reese).

component is aligned with the inferior edge of the glenoid component. The glenoid component is placed parallel to the vertebral border of the scapula. Medial tilting of its superior aspect may occur in patients with rheumatoid arthritis, as a consequence of bone loss from the upper glenoid, and predisposes to upward subluxation of the humeral component. A modified glenoid component includes a superior lip to limit such upward subluxation. The humeral component is placed as in a hemiarthroplasty so that the edge of the head of the prosthesis is parallel to the cut surface of the neck, the holes of the lateral stabilizing fin are well seated in cancellous bone, and the component is in 30 to 40 degrees of retroversion. Retroversion can be documented with a fluoroscopic method analogous to the method for determining femoral anteversion. The patient lies supine on the fluoroscopic table with the humerus parallel to the table top and the elbow flexed to 90 degrees. The forearm is rotated until the neck of the prosthesis is seen in profile. The measured angle from the vertical to the forearm is the angle of retroversion (Fig. 5–57).

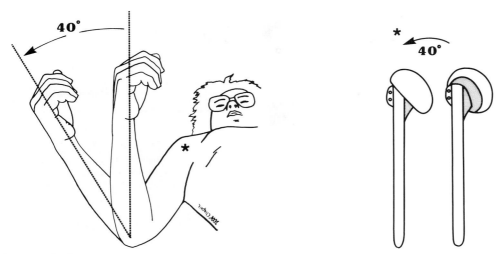

Figure 5–57. Measuring Retroversion of the Humeral Component. The patient lies supine on the fluoroscopic table, with the humerus parallel to the table top and the elbow flexed to 90 degrees. The forearm is then rotated until the humeral component is seen in profile. The measured angle from the vertical to the forearm is the angle of retroversion or anteversion. If the humeral component (inset) is brought into profile by external rotation of the arm, the component is retroverted.

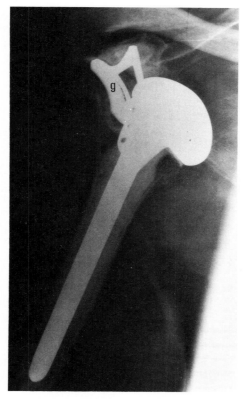

Figure 5–58. Anterior Dislocation of Total-Shoulder Prosthesis. The prosthetic humeral head lies inferior and medial to the glenoid component (g). The nonopaque glenoid articular surface cannot be seen. Axillary and anterior oblique views confirmed the anterior displacement of the humerus.

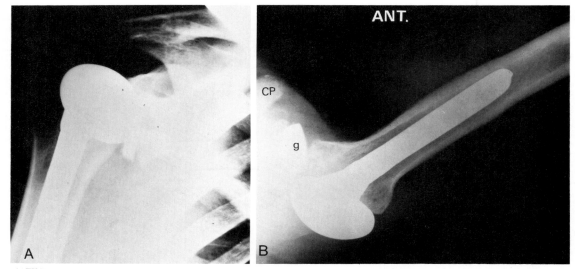

Figure 5–59. Posterior Dislocation of Total-Shoulder Prosthesis. *A,* A posterior oblique view shows the humeral component to be high in position and to overlie the glenoid. In the posterior oblique projection this overlap strongly suggests dislocation. *B,* The axillary view confirms posterior dislocation of the humeral component. CP = coracoid process, g = glenoid, ANT. = anterior.

Complications that may be detected radiographically include dislocation, upward subluxation of the humeral component, heterotopic bone formation, and widening of the cement-bone lucency around the glenoid component indicative of loosening or infection (Figs. 5–58 and 5–59). Averill and co-workers noted radio-lucent zones of 1 mm or less at the cement-bone interface in 74 percent of their patients. Six percent had lucent zones of 2 mm or more; in these patients the prostheses are presumed to be loose, although the patients are thus far pain-free (Fig. 5–60).[123]

Clavicle and Acromioclavicular Joint

NORMAL STRUCTURE AND FUNCTION

Essential Anatomy

The acromioclavicular (AC) joint is a true synovial joint surrounded by a capsule that is strengthened above and below by superior and inferior acromioclavicular ligaments. An articular disc is present in most joints but is usually incomplete (Fig. 5–61).[159] The inferior aspect of the joint is in direct contact with the subacromial bursa. The coracoclavicular ligament, consisting of trapezoid and conoid portions, connects the clavicle to the coracoid process of the scapula and keeps the clavicle and acromion in contact.[141] The coracoacromial ligament extends from the acromion process to the superolateral border of the coracoid process and provides additional support for the humeral head.

Motion at the AC joint includes forward and backward gliding, hinge-like abduction and adduction, and rotation about the long axis of the clavicle.[159] Motion at the AC and sternoclavicular joints is necessary for scapulothoracic motion to occur; therefore, surgical fusion of the AC joint or disorders that interfere with acromioclavicular motion may limit arm motion as well.

Normal Radiographic Anatomy

The subcutaneous fat adjacent to the aponeurosis linking the trapezius and deltoid muscles can be seen above the AC joint on normal frontal radiographs. Fibers of this aponeurosis are intimately related to the underlying acromioclavicular ligaments.[11, 157] The inferior aspect of the AC joint is adjacent to the extrasynovial fat around the subacromial-subdeltoid bursa.

The AC joint space is normally between 2 and 5 mm in width. The bony margins should be smooth and may be straight, notched, con-

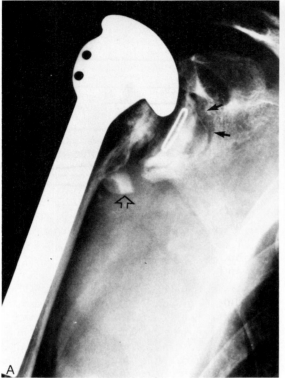

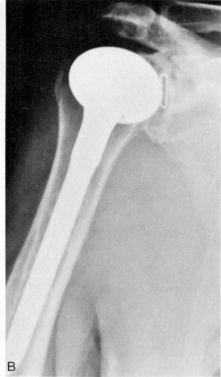

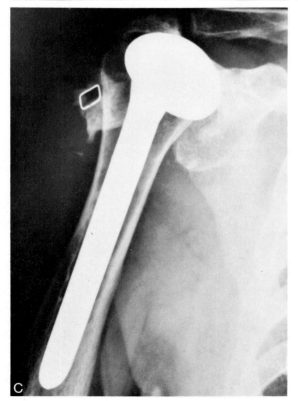

Figure 5–60. Subluxation and Loosening of Total-Shoulder Prosthesis. *A,* Examination 6 months after total shoulder replacement for rheumatoid arthritis shows upward position of the humerus due to glenoid malposition and rotator cuff damage. There is loosening of the glenoid component, indicated by the wide cement-bone lucent zone (arrows). A dislodged fragment of cement is seen (open arrow). *B,* An AP view of the shoulder of another patient shows no apparent complication following total shoulder arthroplasty. The wire marker of the glenoid component is in its expected location. *C,* A routine follow-up examination shows that the glenoid component and attached cement have been dislodged and are now within a distended subdeltoid bursa.

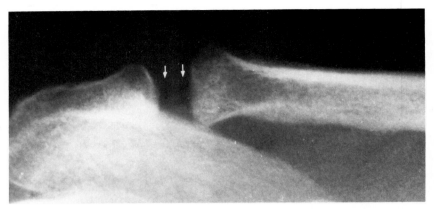

Figure 5–61. Acromioclavicular Joint. Gas (arrows) in the joint, as a result of the vacuum phenomenon, outlines the central meniscus and peripheral articular cartilage.

cave, or convex and asymmetrical in appearance.[149]

ABNORMAL CONDITIONS

Arthritis Affecting the AC Joint

Rheumatoid Arthritis (RA)
(see Fig. 5–28)
The earliest radiographic finding of RA in the AC joint consists of soft tissue swelling superior to the bony margins of the joint. Early bone erosion involves the distal clavicle first but may progress to involve both bones, producing apparent joint-space widening. Clavicular erosion usually predominates and may be extensive, with loss of 1 to 2 cm of bone from the lateral clavicle. Erosion also involves the inferior aspect of the clavicle at the insertions of the coracoclavicular ligaments. In contrast to the usual irregular erosion associated with rheumatoid arthritis elsewhere, the erosion of the distal or inferior clavicle has a smooth appearance.

Osteoarthritis
According to Zanca, degenerative changes of the AC joint may be seen on radiographs of asymptomatic patients as a consequence of aging, and in his series of 100 unselected patients 12.7 percent had an acromioclavicular joint abnormality.[161] Worcester and Green noted that radiographic examination is not a particularly good indicator of symptomatic disease in this area.[159] Oppenheimer, however, found no abnormalities in the AC joints of 50 individuals who had no shoulder pain or disability.[149]

Clinical symptoms may be diffuse and not well localized to the AC joint. Findings of tenderness over the joint, pain on forced shoulder abduction, and pain relief after injection of local anesthetic are important in diagnosis.[159]

Radiographic findings of advanced osteoarthritis include sclerosis and roughening of the bony surfaces, osteophytic lipping, and joint-space narrowing.[149] Osteophytic lipping from the inferior margin of the joint may produce impingement on the subjacent supraspinatus tendon, leading to attritional changes, rupture, and pain. These osteophytes may be demonstrated on AP radiographs taken with the tube angled 15 degrees cephalad.

Trauma

Acromioclavicular Sprains
Classification. Acromioclavicular sprains have been classified by Allman according to the extent of injury to the AC joint and adjacent ligaments.[129]

Grade I—These injuries involve only a few fibers of the acromioclavicular ligament and capsule. There is no laxity of the acromioclavicular joint.

Grade II—These sprains are the result of a force that produces rupture of the capsule and the acromioclavicular ligament. This injury is referred to as subluxation.

Grade III—These sprains are dislocations of the joint. They result from severe injury that produces a rupture of the acromioclavicular and coracoclavicular ligaments.

Allman also notes that posterior displacement of the distal end of the clavicle may follow a direct blow or a fall on the posterosuperior aspect of the shoulder. This possibility is sug-

Table 5–12. **Plain Film Findings in Acromioclavicular Sprains**

Classification	Signs
Grade I	Soft tissue swelling Periosteal reaction on delayed films
Grade II	As in I Elevation of clavicle by less than width of clavicle
Grade III	As in I Elevation of distal clavicle above superior aspect of acromion Increased (>1.7 cm) clavicle-coracoid distance

gested when there is an increase in the width of the acromioclavicular joint space but a normal alignment of the acromion process and clavicle on AP views.[129, 156] The deformity may be palpable clinically.

Mechanism of Injury. Most injuries of the acromioclavicular joint result from a fall onto the point of the involved shoulder. Less commonly,

injury is the result of force transmitted from a fall on the elbow or the outstretched hand.[1, 129]

Radiographic Examination (Table 5–12). If there is any question of abnormality localized to the acromioclavicular area, special views are recommended. An anteroposterior view with the beam angled 15 degrees toward the feet allows better visualization of the subacromial space,

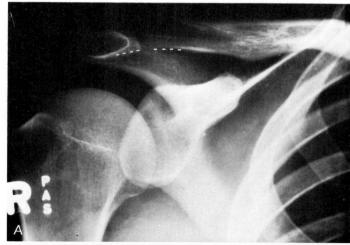

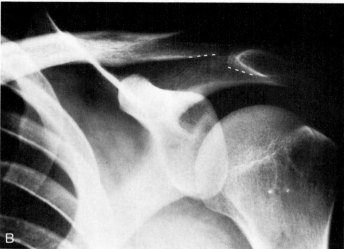

Figure 5–62. Grade II Acromioclavicular Separation. Views of each side with weights suspended from the patient's wrists show normal alignment of the inferior aspect (dashed lines) of the acromion and clavicle on the right (A). On the left (B) the mild elevation of the clavicle in relation to the acromion indicates a grade II AC sprain.

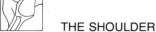

and AP views with cranial angulation (10 to 35 degrees) may also help.[145, 161] Anteroposterior views that include both shoulders with and without 5 to 15 pounds of weight suspended from each wrist are recommended in cases of trauma. Post suggests that it is more accurate to suspend the weights from the wrists, since weights placed in the hand elicit a tendency to lift the arm involuntarily, with possible decrease in the observed AC joint separation.[1]

The normal AC joint space ranges from 2 to 5 mm.[148] The normal coracoclavicular space measures 1.1 to 1.3 cm.[135] Usually, in a normal AC joint the inferior aspect of the clavicle will be aligned with the inferior aspect of the acromion process.

Grade I Sprains. Grade I injuries are suggested by the presence of soft tissue swelling around the joint but no widening of the joint or abnormality in alignment. Follow-up examination may show subperiosteal new bone formation around the distal end of the clavicle.

Grades II and III Sprains

Soft Tissue Changes. Weston has described three soft tissue changes that occur with subluxation or dislocation of the AC joint. The first is increase in soft tissue density under the AC joint with separation and loss of parallelism between the inferior surface of the joint and the extrasynovial fat around the subacromial-subdeltoid bursa. The second finding is a soft tissue mass over the superior aspect of the AC joint, resulting from edema and hemorrhage deep to the aponeurosis. Three or 4 weeks after trauma, the soft tissue swelling decreases and, according to Weston, only then may the alignment abnormality become apparent. The third soft tissue sign of subluxation or dislocation is change in the contour of the origin of the deltoid. The deltoid origin from the acromion process is delineated superiorly by subcutaneous fat and inferiorly by extrasynovial fat around the subdeltoid bursa. The soft tissue swelling that accompanies AC subluxation or dislocation extends beneath the aponeurosis to the origin of the deltoid muscle. This produces a squaring-off of the normally beak-shaped deltoid origin.[11, 157]

Bony Changes. Grade II sprains (subluxation) show the clavicle to be higher than the acromion, usually by less than the width of the clavicle, even on weight-bearing views. Bearden and co-workers note that with suspension of weights from the wrists an increase in the coracoclavicular space of up to 4 mm above the normal 1.1 to 1.3 cm indicates subluxation (Fig. 5–62).[135]

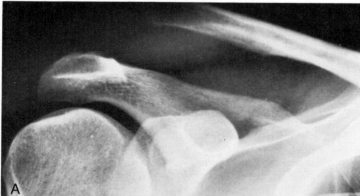

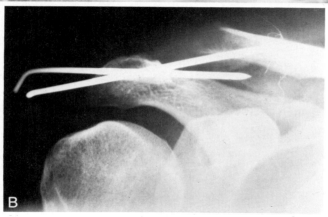

Figure 5–63. Grade III Acromioclavicular Sprain. *A*, Frontal radiograph confirms the marked superior displacement of the distal clavicle, indicating rupture of the acromioclavicular and coracoclavicular ligaments. *B*, Attempted fusion of the acromioclavicular joint was unsuccessful (demonstrated by loss of reduction at the AC joint and pulling-out of the pins from the clavicle). The loss of reduction is evidence that motion of the AC joint accompanies other motions of the shoulder girdle.

In grade III sprains (dislocation) the distal end of the clavicle is above the superior aspect of the acromion. The distance between the clavicle and the coracoid process is increased by more than 40 to 50 percent of the normal measurements (Fig. 5–63).[1] Associated fractures of the coracoid process should be sought.[153]

Arthrography Following AC Injury. Arthrography has been suggested as a method of evaluating the extent of ligamentous injury accompanying acromioclavicular dislocation (grade III sprains).[160] This examination is not often necessary, as diagnosis is usually possible from the clinical findings and the radiographic techniques previously described.

The normal joint cavity has an L shape and a 1 ml capacity, and may have a meniscus dividing it partially or completely.[11, 139] Zachrisson and Ejeskar injected 5 ml of contrast agent into the involved joint 1 to 8 days after injury. Antero-

posterior projections with 0, 15, and 30 degrees of cranial angulation proved to be the most useful views. Positive findings included (1) leakage of contrast medium around the lateral end of the clavicle, indicating detachment of the clavicle from the adjacent soft tissues; and (2) leakage of contrast material toward the coracoid process. If this contrast extended beyond the medial aspect of the coracoid, complete rupture of the coracoclavicular ligaments was identified at subsequent surgery. Incomplete ligamentous rupture was associated with contrast leakage that did not extend as far medially.[160]

Treatment. Grades I and II sprains are treated conservatively. Grade I sprains are protected from injury until they are asymptomatic and strength and function have returned. Grade II sprains are treated with reduction and immobilization for about 3 weeks, with periodic radiographic examinations to confirm that reduction

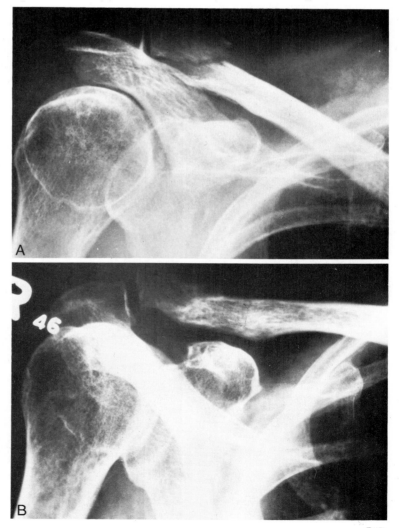

Figure 5–64. Distal Clavicular Fracture (Type I). *A,* Initial film after injury shows an oblique fracture of the distal clavicle without marked elevation of the clavicle or extension into the acromioclavicular joint. *B,* Three months later there is complete healing.

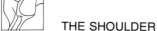

is maintained.[129] Grade III sprains may be treated conservatively with immobilization for 6 to 8 weeks. Surgical treatment is preferred by some and is used by others when conservative treatment fails, when deformity is unacceptable, or when the patient is not a candidate for closed treatment.[1] Several types of repair may be used:

1. Repair, fixation, or reconstruction of the coracoclavicular ligament. An example of this is the Bosworth method, in which a screw is placed through the superior clavicle into the coracoid process.[138]

2. Acromioclavicular repair, internal fixation, or reconstruction. Wires or pins may be placed across the joint.

3. Excision of the distal clavicle.

4. Dynamic muscle transfers.

Radiographically identifiable complications include residual subluxation, iatrogenic fracture, soft tissue calcification, infection, and complications associated with inserted hardware, including metal fracture, migration of pins, and loosening of screws.

Fractures of the Clavicle

Fractures of the clavicle may be grouped anatomically as those involving (1) the middle third (80 percent), (2) the distal clavicle (15 percent), and (3) the proximal end of the clavicle (5 percent). When displacement is present, the proximal fragment is usually elevated, and the distal fragment and shoulder are displaced downward and medially. Radiographic examination is important to confirm the diagnosis and document the degree of displacement.

Fractures of the distal clavicle have been subdivided by Neer into two types: Type I fractures have intact coracoclavicular ligaments (Fig. 5–64). Type II fractures are associated with disruption of the coracoclavicular ligaments and therefore exhibit greater displacement of the proximal fragment posteriorly and superiorly. Delayed radiographs in these cases may show calcification in the coracoclavicular ligaments, confirming damage to these structures.[146] If ligamentous damage is not obvious (i.e., there is no calcification, and the proximal fragment is

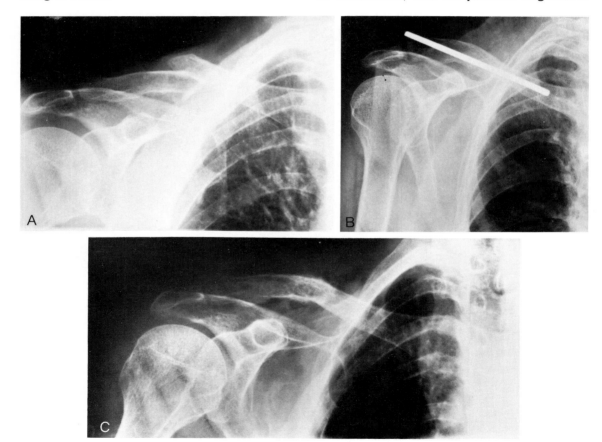

Figure 5–65. Nonunion of Midclavicular Fracture. Examination 2 years after injury. *A*, The midclavicular fracture margins are smooth and corticated. The proximal shaft is displaced upward. There was continued pain. *B*, The fracture margins were resected and an intramedullary rod was inserted. *C*, Examination 3 months after that shown in *B*. The rod had been removed because of pain associated with a change in its position. There is, however, healing across the fracture site.

not markedly elevated), views with the patient holding a 10-pound sandbag or with a 10-pound weight strapped to each wrist should be done. These will show any increased separation between the coracoid and clavicle in comparison with preliminary films and with simultaneously taken films of the opposite side and thereby confirm any ligamentous disruption.[107] Type II fractures are associated with a higher incidence of nonunion, and it is suggested that they are best treated by internal fixation, in contrast to the closed methods of treatment that are used in fractures with intact ligaments. Damage to the distal articular surface may occur and should be defined by tomographic study, if necessary.

Fractures of the proximal end of the clavicle are uncommon, and there is little or no displacement if the costoclavicular ligament remains intact and attached to the lateral fragment.[129] Damage to the articular surface may occur.

Radiographically identifiable complications of clavicular fractures include malunion, nonunion, refracture, and post-traumatic arthritis (Fig. 5–65).

References

General Reference

1. Post M: The Shoulder. Surgical and Nonsurgical Management. Philadelphia, Lea & Febiger, 1978.

Essential Anatomy

2. Inman VT, Saunders JB deC M, Abbott LC: Observations on the function of the shoulder joint. J Bone Joint Surg 26:1–30, 1944.
3. Poppen NK, Walker PS: Normal and abnormal motion of the shoulder. J Bone Joint Surg (Am) 58:195–201, 1976.

Normal Radiographic Appearances

4. DeSmett AA: Axillary projection in radiography of the nontraumatized shoulder. AJR 134:511–518, 1980.
5. Goldman AB: Double contrast shoulder arthrography. In Freiberger RH, Kaye JJ, eds. Arthrography. New York, Appleton-Century-Crofts, 1979: 165–188.
6. Hall FM, Rosenthal DI, Goldberg RP, Wyshak G: Morbidity from shoulder arthrography: Etiology, incidence, and prevention. AJR 136:59–62, 1981.
7. Kaye JJ, Schneider R: Positive contrast shoulder arthrography. In Freiberger RH, Kaye JJ, eds. Arthrography. New York, Appleton-Century-Crofts, 1979: 137–164.
8. Neviaser JS: Arthrography of the Shoulder. The Diagnosis and Management of the Lesions Visualized. Springfield, Ill, CC Thomas, 1975.
9. Rubin SA, Gray RL, Green WR: The scapular "y": A diagnostic aid in shoulder trauma. Radiology 110: 725–726, 1974.
10. Slivka J, Resnick D: An improved radiographic view of the glenohumeral joint. J Can Assoc Radiol 30: 83–85, 1979.
11. Weston WJ, Palmer DG: Soft Tissues of the Extremities: A Radiographic Study of Rheumatic Disease. New York, Springer-Verlag, 1978.

Soft Tissue Swelling
Joint Effusion

12. Laskin RS, Schreiber S: Inferior subluxation of the humeral head: The drooping shoulder. Radiology 98:585–596, 1971.
13. Seltzer SE, Finberg HF, Weissman BN: Arthrosonography: Technique, sonographic anatomy and pathology. Invest Radiol 15:19–28, 1980.
14. Weston WJ, Palmer DG: Soft Tissues of the Extremities. A Radiologic Study of Rheumatic Disease. New York, Springer-Verlag, 1978.

Lipohemarthrosis

15. Arger PH, Oberkircher PE, Miller WT: Lipohemarthrosis. AJR 121:97–100, 1974.
16. Saxton HM: Lipohaemarthrosis. Br J Radiol 35:122–127, 1962.
17. Weston WJ: Recurrent dislocation of the shoulder with an intracapsular lipohaemarthrosis. Australas Radiol 15:52–54, 1971.

Calcific Tendinitis

18. Bosworth BM: Calcium deposits in the shoulder and subacromial bursitis: A survey of 12,122 shoulders. JAMA 116:2477–2482, 1941.
19. Bosworth BM: Examination of the shoulder for calcium deposits: Technique of fluoroscopy and spot film roentgenography. J Bone Joint Surg 23:567–577, 1941.
20. Deichgräber E, Olsson B: Soft tissue radiography in painful shoulder. Acta Radiol [Diagn] (Stockh) 16:393–400, 1975.
21. Golding FC: The shoulder—the forgotten joint. Br J Radiol 35:149–158, 1962.
22. Lippman RK: Observations concerning the calcific cuff deposit. Clin Orthop 20:49–59, 1961.
23. Moseley HF: The natural history and clinical syndromes produced by calcified deposits in the rotator cuff. Surg Clin North Am 43:1489–1493, 1963.
24. Pederson HE, Key JA: Pathology of calcareous tendinitis and subdeltoid bursitis. Arch Surg 62:50–63, 1951.
25. Pinals RS, Short CL: Calcific periarthritis involving multiple sites. Arthritis Rheum 9:566–574, 1966.
26. Vigario GD, Keats TE: Localization of calcific deposits in the shoulder. AJR 108:806–811, 1970.

Rotator Cuff Tears

27. Bosworth DM: An analysis of twenty-eight consecutive cases of incapacitating shoulder lesions radically explored and repaired. J Bone Joint Surg 22:369–392, 1940.
28. Cotton RE, Rideout DF: Tears of the humeral rotator cuff: A radiological and pathological necropsy survey. J Bone Joint Surg (Br) 46:314–328, 1964.
29. Golding FC: The shoulder—the forgotten joint. Br J Radiol 35:149–158, 1962.
30. Goldman AB: Double Contrast Shoulder Arthrography. In Freiberger RH, Kaye JJ, eds. Arthrography. New York, Appleton-Century-Crofts, 1979.
31. Goldman AB, Ghelman B: The double-contrast shoulder arthrogram. Radiology 127:655–663, 1978.
32. Kotzen LM: Roentgen diagnosis of rotator cuff tear: Report of 48 surgically proven cases. AJR 112:507–511, 1971.
33. McLaughlin HL: Lesions of the musculotendinous cuff of the shoulder. I. The exposure and treatment of tears with retraction. J Bone Joint Surg 26:31–49, 1944.
34. McLaughlin HL: Rupture of the rotator cuff. An AAOS

instructional course lecture. J Bone Joint Surg (Am) 44:979–983, 1962.

35. Neer CS II, Craig EV, Fukuda H, Mendoza FX: Cuff Tear Arthropathy. Paper presented at the annual meeting, American Academy of Orthopedic Surgeons, New Orleans, 1982.

36. Schneider R, Kaye JJ: Positive Contrast Shoulder Arthrography. In Freiberger RH, Kaye JJ, Arthrography. New York, Appleton-Century-Crofts, 1979.

37. Skinner HA: Anatomical considerations relative to rupture of the supraspinatus tendon. J Bone Joint Surg 19:137–151, 1937.

38. Weiner DS, Macnab I: Superior migration of the humeral head. A radiological aid in the diagnosis of tears of the rotator cuff. J Bone Joint Surg (Br) 52:524–527, 1970.

Luxatio Erecta

38a. Downey EF Jr, Curtis DJ, Brower AC: Unusual dislocations of the shoulder. AJR 140:1207–1210, 1983.

Impingement Syndrome

38b. Cone RO III, Resnick D, Danzig L: Shoulder impingement syndrome: radiographic evaluation. Radiology 150:29–33, 1984.

39. Neer CS II: Anterior acromioplasty for the chronic impingement syndrome in the shoulder. A preliminary report. J Bone Joint Surg (Am) 54:41–50, 1972.

40. Penny JN, Welsh RP: Shoulder impingement syndromes in athletes and their surgical management. Am J Sports Med 9:11–15, 1981.

41. Strizak AM, Danzig L, Jackson DW, Greenway G, Resnick D, Staple T: Subacromial bursography. J Bone Joint Surg (Am) 64:196–201, 1982.

Adhesive Capsulitis

42. Andrén L, Lundberg BJ: Treatment of rigid shoulders by joint distension during arthrography. Acta Orthop Scand 36:45–53, 1965.

43. Gilula LA, Schoenecker PL, Murphy WA: Shoulder arthrography as a treatment modality. AJR 131:1047–1048, 1978.

44. Goldman AB, Ghelman B: The double-contrast shoulder arthrogram. Radiology 127:655–663, 1978.

45. Goldman AB: Double Contrast Shoulder Arthrography. In Freiberger RH, Kaye JJ, eds. Arthrography. New York, Appleton-Century-Crofts, 1979.

46. Jayson MIV: Frozen shoulder: Adhesive capsulitis. Br Med J 283:1005–1006, 1981.

47. Kaye JJ, Schneider R: Positive Contrast Shoulder Arthrography. In Freiberger RH, Kaye JJ, eds. Arthrography. New York, Appleton-Century-Crofts, 1979.

48. McLaughlin HL: The "frozen shoulder." Clin Orthop 20:126–131, 1961.

49. Reeves B: Arthrographic changes in frozen and posttraumatic stiff shoulders. Proc R Soc Med 59:827–830, 1966.

Arthritis

50. Brower AC, Allman RM: Pathogenesis of the neurotrophic joint: Neurotraumatic vs. neurovascular. Radiology 139:349–354, 1981.

51. DeSmett AA, Ting YM, Weiss JJ: Shoulder arthrography in rheumatoid arthritis. Radiology 116:601–605, 1975.

52. Freiberger RH, Edeiken J, Jacobson HG, Norman A: Bone Disease Syllabus, 2nd Series. American College of Radiology, Ill., 1976.

53. Garancis JC, Cheung HS, Halverson PB, McCarty DJ:

"Milwaukee shoulder"—Association of microspheroids containing hydroxyapatite crystals, active collagenase, and neutral protease with rotator cuff defects. III. Morphologic and biochemical studies of an excised synovium showing chondromatosis. Arthritis Rheum 24:484–491, 1981.

54. Halverson PB, Cheung HS, McCarty DH, Garancis J, Mandel N: "Milwaukee shoulder"—Association of microspheroids containing hydroxyapatite crystals, active collagenase, and neutral protease with rotator cuff defects. II. Synovial fluid studies. Arthritis Rheum 24:474–483, 1981.

55. McCarty DJ, Halverson PB, Carrera GF, Brewer BJ, Kozin F: "Milwaukee shoulder"—association of microspheroids containing hydroxyapatite crystals, active collagenase, and neutral protease with rotator cuff defects. I. Clinical aspects. Arthritis Rheum 24:464–473, 1981.

56. McNair MM, Boyle JA, Buchanan WW, Davidson JK: A clinical and radiological study of rheumatoid arthritis with a note on the findings in osteoarthrosis. I. The shoulder joint. Clin Radiol 20:269–277, 1969.

57. Neer CS II: Degenerative lesions of the proximal humeral articular surface. Clin Orthop 20:116–125, 1961.

58. Neer CS II: Reconstructive Surgery and Rehabilitation of the Shoulder. In Kelley WN, Harris ED Jr, Ruddy S, Sledge CB, eds. Textbook of Rheumatology. Philadelphia, WB Saunders, 1981: 1944–1959.

59. Weston WJ: The enlarged subdeltoid bursa in rheumatoid arthritis. Br J Radiol 42:481–486, 1969.

Fractures

Proximal Humeral Fractures

60. Neer CS II: Displaced proximal humeral fractures. I. Classification and evaluation. J Bone Joint Surg (Am) 52:1077–1089, 1970.

61. Pavlov H, Freiberger RH: Shoulder. In Felson B, ed. New York, Grune & Stratton, 1978: 79–90.

Humeral Shaft Fractures

62. Heppenstall RB: Fracture Treatment and Healing. Philadelphia, WB Saunders, 1980: 424–438.

63. Research Committee, Pennsylvania Orthopedic Society. Fresh midshaft fractures of the humerus in adults. Evaluation of treatment in Pennsylvania during 1952–1956. Penn Med 62:848–850, 1959.

64. Holm CL: Management of humeral shaft fractures: Fundamental nonoperative technics. Clin Orthop 71:132–139, 1970.

65. Sarmiento A, Kinman PB, Glavin EG, et al: Functional bracing of fracture of the shaft of the humerus. J Bone Joint Surg (Am) 59:596–601, 1977.

66. Stewart MJ, Hundley JM: Fractures of the humerus: A comparative study in methods of treatment. J Bone Joint Surg (Am) 37:681–692, 1955.

Dislocation

Pseudodislocation

67. Laskin RS, Schreiber S: Inferior subluxation of the humeral head: The drooping shoulder. Radiology 98:585–586, 1971.

67a. Lev-Toaff, AS, Karasick, D, Madan Rao, V: "Drooping shoulder"—Nontraumatic Causes of Glenohumeral Subluxation Skeletal Radiol 12:34–36, 1984.

Anterior Dislocation

68. Adams JC: Recurrent dislocation of the shoulder. J Bone Joint Surg (Br) 30:26–38, 1948.

69. Adams JC: The humeral head defect in recurrent anterior dislocation of the shoulder. Br J Radiol 23:151–156, 1950.

70. Bankart ASB: Recurrent or habitual dislocation of the shoulder-joint. Br Med [Clin Res] J 2:1132–1133, 1923.

71. Bankart ASB: The pathology and treatment of recurrent dislocation of the shoulder-joint. Br J Surg 26:23–29, 1938.

72. Brav EA: Recurrent dislocation of the shoulder: Ten years' experience with the Putti-Platt reconstruction procedure. Am Surg 100:423–430, 1960.

73. Carter C: Recurrent dislocation of the patella and of the shoulder: Their association with familial joint laxity. J Bone Joint Surg (Br) 42:721–727, 1960.

74. Cotton FJ, Morrison GM: Recurrent dislocation of the shoulder. N Engl J Med 210:1070–1072, 1934.

75. DuToit GT, Roux D: Recurrent dislocation of the shoulder. J Bone Joint Surg (Am) 38:1–12, 1956.

76. Eyre-Brook AL: Recurrent dislocation of the shoulder: Lesions discovered in seventeen cases, surgery employed, and intermediate report on results. J Bone Joint Surg (Br) 30:39–46, 1948.

77. Freiberger RH, Edeiken J, Jacobson HG, Norman A: Bone Disease Syllabus, 2nd Series. American College of Radiology, Chicago, Ill., 1976.

78. Golding C: Radiology and orthopaedic surgery. J Bone Joint Surg (Br) 48:320–332, 1966.

79. Hill HA, Sachs MD: The grooved defect of the humeral head: A frequently unrecognized complication of dislocations of the shoulder joint. Radiology 35:690–700, 1940.

80. MacDonald FR: Intra-articular fractures in recurrent dislocation of the shoulder. Surg Clin North Am 43:1635–1645, 1963.

81. Morrey BF, Janes JM: Recurrent anterior dislocation of the shoulder: Long-term follow-up of the Putti-Platt and Bankart procedures. J Bone Joint Surg (Am) 58:252–256, 1976.

82. Moseley HF: The basic lesions of recurrent anterior dislocation. Surg Clin North Am 43:1631–1634, 1963.

83. Nicola T: Anterior dislocation of the shoulder: The role of the articular capsule. J Bone Joint Surg 24:614–616, 1942.

84. Nidecker A, Cooke GM: Hill-Sachs deformity with an unusually large defect. J Can Assoc Radiol 30:116–117, 1979.

85. Osmond-Clarke H: Habitual dislocation of the shoulder: The Putti-Platt operation. J Bone Joint Surg (Br) 30:19–25, 1948.

86. Protzman RR: Anterior instability of the shoulder. J Bone Joint Surg (Am) 62:909–918, 1980.

87. Rockwood CA Jr, Green DP, eds.: Fractures. Vol. I. Philadelphia, JB Lippincott, 1978.

88. Rokous JR, Feagin JA, Abbott HG: Modified axillary roentgenogram: A useful adjunct in the diagnosis of recurrent instability of the shoulder. Clin Orthop 82:84–86, 1972.

89. Rowe CR: Prognosis in dislocations of the shoulder. J Bone Joint Surg (Am) 38:957–976, 1956.

90. Rowe CR: Anterior dislocations of the shoulder: Prognosis and treatment. Surg Clin North Am 43:1609–1614, 1963.

91. Rowe CR, Pierce D: The enigma of voluntary recurrent dislocation of the shoulder. J Bone Joint Surg (Am) 47:1670, 1965.

92. Rowe CR, Sakellarides HT: Factors related to recurrences of anterior dislocation of the shoulder. Clin Orthop 20:40–47, 1961.

93. Saha AK: Anterior recurrent dislocation of the shoulder. Acta Orthop Scand 38:479–493, 1967.

94. Turkel SJ, Panio MW, Marshall JL, Girgis FG: Stabilizing mechanisms preventing anterior dislocation of the glenohumeral joint. J Bone Joint Surg 63:1208–1217, 1981.

Shoulder Arthrography in Dislocation

95. Braunstein EM, O'Connor G: Double-contrast arthrotomography of the shoulder. J Bone Joint Surg (Am) 64:192–195, 1982.

96. El-Khoury GY, Albright JP, Yousef MMA, Montgomery WJ, Tuck SL: Arthrotomography of the glenoid labrum. Radiology 131:333–337, 1979.

97. Goldman AB: Double contrast shoulder arthrography. In Freiberger RH, Kaye JJ, eds. Arthrography. New York, Appleton-Century-Crofts, 1979.

97a. Haynor DR, Shuman WP: CT arthrography of the shoulder. Radiographics 4:411–421, 1984.

97b. Kleinman PK, Kanzaria PK, Goss TP, et al.: Axillary arthrotomography of the glenoid labrum. AJR 141:993–999, 1984.

98. McGlynn FJ, El-Khoury G, Albright JP: Arthrotomography of the glenoid labrum in shoulder instability. J Bone Joint Surg (Am) 64:506–518, 1982.

99. Mink JH, Richardson A, Grant TT: Evaluation of glenoid labrum by double-contrast shoulder arthrography. AJR 133:883–887, 1979.

100. Reeves B: Arthrography of the shoulder. J Bone Joint Surg (Br) 48:424–434, 1966.

100a. Shuman WP, Kilcoyne RF, Matsen FA, et al.: Double-contrast computed tomography of the glenoid labrum. AJR 141:581–584, 1983.

Posterior Dislocation

101. Arndt JG, Sears AD: Posterior dislocation of the shoulder. AJR 94:639–645, 1965.

102. Bloom MH, Obata WG: Diagnosis of posterior dislocation of the shoulder with use of Velpeau axillary and angle-up roentgenographic views. J Bone Joint Surg (Am) 49:943–949, 1967.

103. Brown WH, Dennis JM, Davidson CN, Rubin PS, Fulton H: Posterior dislocation of the shoulder. Radiology 69:815–822, 1957.

104. Cisternino SJ, Rogers LF, Stufflebam BC, Kruglik GD: The trough line: A radiographic sign of posterior shoulder dislocation. AJR 130:951–954, 1978.

105. Detenbeck LC: Posterior dislocations of the shoulder. J Trauma 12:183–192, 1972.

106. Fagerlund M, Ahlgren O: Axial projection of the humeroscapular joint. Acta Radiol [Diagn] (Stockh) 22:203–205, 1981.

107. Heppenstall RB: Fracture Treatment and Healing. Philadelphia, WB Saunders, 1980.

108. Kretzler HH Jr, Blue AR: Recurrent posterior dislocation of the shoulder in cerebral palsy. J Bone Joint Surg (Am) 48:1221, 1966.

109. Lindholm TS: Recurrent posterior dislocation of the shoulder. Acta Chir Scand 140:101–106, 1974.

110. May H: Nicola operation for posterior subacromial dislocation of the humerus. J Bone Joint Surg 25:78–84, 1943.

111. McLaughlin HL: Posterior dislocation of the shoulder. J Bone Joint Surg (Am) 34:584–590, 1952.

112. McLaughlin HL: Follow-up notes on articles previously published in the journal: Posterior dislocation of the shoulder. J Bone Joint Surg (Am) 44:1477, 1962.

113. Neviaser JS: Posterior dislocations of the shoulder: Diagnosis and treatment. Surg Clin North Am 43:1623–1630, 1963.

114. Nobel W: Posterior traumatic dislocation of the shoulder. J Bone Joint Surg (Am) 44:523–537, 1962.

115. Pear BL: Bilateral posterior fracture dislocation of the

shoulder—an uncommon complication of a convulsive seizure. N Engl Med 283:135–136, 1970.

116. Pear BL: Dislocation of the shoulder: X-ray signs. N Engl J Med 283:1113, 1970.

117. Scott DJ Jr: Treatment of recurrent posterior dislocations of the shoulder by glenoplasty: Report of three cases. J Bone Joint Surg (Am) 49:471–476, 1967.

118. Warrick CK: Posterior dislocation of the shoulder joint. Br J Radiol 38:758–761, 1965.

119. Wilson JC, McKeever FM: Traumatic posterior (retroglenoid) dislocation of the humerus. J Bone Joint Surg (Am) 31:160–172, 1949.

Anterior Capsular Derangement

120. Kummel BM: The syndrome of anterior-capsular derangement of the shoulder. Orthop Rev 1:7–12, 1972.

121. Kummel BM: Arthrography in anterior capsular derangements of the shoulder. Clin Orthop 83:170–176, 1972.

Total Shoulder Replacement

122. Amstutz HC, Sew Hoy AL, Clarke IC: UCLA Anatomic total shoulder arthroplasty. Clin Orthop 155:7–20, 1981.

123. Averill RM, Sledge CB, Thomas WH: Neer total shoulder arthroplasty. Paper presented at the 44th annual meeting of the American Rheumatism Association, May 23–31, 1980, Atlanta.

124. Cofield RH: Status of total shoulder arthroplasty. Arch Surg 112:1088–1091, 1977.

124a. Cofield RH: Total shoulder arthroplasty with the Neer prosthesis. J Bone Joint Surg (Am) 66:899–906, 1984.

125. Neer CS II: Replacement arthroplasty for glenohumeral osteoarthritis. J Bone Joint Surg (Am) 56:1–13, 1974.

126. Post M, Haskell SS, Jablon M: Total shoulder replacement with a constrained prosthesis. J Bone Joint Surg (Am) 62:327–335, 1980.

127. Post M, Jablon M, Miller H, Singh M: Constrained total shoulder joint replacement: A critical review. Clin Orthop 114:135–150, 1979.

Acromioclavicular Joint

128. Alldredge RH: Surgical treatment of acromioclavicular dislocations. J Bone Joint Surg (Am) 47:1278, 1965.

129. Allman FL Jr: Fractures and ligamentous injuries of the clavicle and its articulation. J Bone Joint Surg (Am) 49:774–784, 1967.

130. Arner O, Sandahl U, Öhrling H: Dislocation of the acromioclavicular joint: Review of the literature and a report on 56 cases. Acta Chir Scand 113:140–152, 1957.

131. Aufranc OE, Jones WN, Harris WH: Complete acromioclavicular dislocation. JAMA 180:681–683, 1962.

132. Badgley CE: Sports injuries of the shoulder girdle. JAMA 172:444–448, 1960.

133. Barnhart JM: Acromioclavicular joint injuries. Clin Orthop 81:199, 1970.

134. Bateman JE: Athletic injuries about the shoulder in throwing and body-contact sports. Clin Orthop 23:75–83, 1962.

135. Bearden JM, Hughston JC, Whatly GS: Acromioclavicular dislocation. Method of treatment. J Sports Med Phys Fitness 1:5–17, 1973.

136. Behling F: Treatment of acromioclavicular separations. Orthop Clin North Am 4:747–757, 1973.

137. Bloom FA: Wire fixation in acromioclavicular dislocation. J Bone Joint Surg 27:273–276, 1945.

138. Bosworth BM: Acromioclavicular separation: New method of repair. Surg Gynecol Obstet 73:866–871, 1941.

139. Brosgol MP: Traumatic acromioclavicular sprains and subluxations. Clin Orthop 20:98–107, 1961.

140. Bundens WD Jr, Cook JT; Repair of acromioclavicular separation by deltoid-trapezius imbrication: Clin Orthop 20:109–114, 1961.

141. Goss CM, ed. Gray's Anatomy of the Human Body. 29th Am. ed. Philadelphia, Lea & Febiger, 1973.

142. Imatani RJ, Hanlon JJ, Cady GW: Acute complete acromioclavicular separation. J Bone Joint Surg (Am) 57:328–332, 1975.

143. Jacobs B, Wade PA: Acromioclavicular-joint injury: An end-result study. J Bone Joint Surg (Am) 48:475–486, 1966.

144. Laing PG: Transplantation of the long head of the biceps in complete acromioclavicular separations. J Bone Joint Surg (Am) 41:1677–1678, 1969.

145. Meuli HC, Hafner E: Radiologic Examination in Orthopaedics. Baltimore, University Park Press, 1976.

146. Neer CS II: Nonunion of the clavicle. JAMA 172:1006–1011, 1960.

147. Neer CS II: Anterior acromioplasty for the chronic impingement syndrome in the shoulder. J Bone Joint Surg (Am) 54:41–50, 1972.

148. Oppenheimer A: Arthritis of the acromioclavicular joint. J Bone Joint Surg 25:867–870, 1943.

149. Oppenheimer A: Lesions of the acromioclavicular joint causing pain and disability of the shoulder. AJR 51:699–706, 1944.

150. Patterson WP: Inferior dislocation of the distal end of the clavicle: A case report. J Bone Joint Surg (Am) 49:1184–1186, 1967.

151. Pillay VK: Significance of the coraco-clavicular joint. J Bone Joint Surg (Br) 49:390, 1967.

152. Powers JA, Bach PJ: Acromioclavicular separations: Closed or open treatment? Clin Orthop 104:213–223, 1974.

153. Protass JJ, Stampfli FV, Osmer JC: Coracoid process fracture diagnosis in acromioclavicular separation. Radiology 116:61–64, 1975.

154. Quigley TB: Injuries to the acromioclavicular and sternoclavicular joints sustained in athletics. Surg Clin North Am 43:1551–1554, 1963.

155. Tossy JD, Mead NC, Sigmond HM: Acromioclavicular separations: Useful and practical classification for treatment. Clin Orthop 28:111–119, 1963.

156. Urist MR: Complete dislocations of the acromioclavicular joint: The nature of the traumatic lesion and effective methods of treatment with an analysis of forty-one cases. J Bone Joint Surg 28:813–837, 1946.

157. Weston WJ: Soft tissue signs in recent sub-luxation and dislocation of the acromio-clavicular joint. Br J Radiol 45:832–834, 1972.

158. Wilson FC Jr, Prothero SR: Results of operative treatment of acute dislocations of the acromioclavicular joint. J Trauma 7:202–209, 1967.

159. Worcester JN Jr, Green DP: Osteoarthritis of the acromioclavicular joint. Clin Orthop 58:69–73, 1968.

160. Zachrisson BE, Ejeskär A: Arthrography in dislocation of the acromioclavicular joint. Acta Radiol [Diagn] (Stockh) 20:81–87, 1979.

161. Zanca P: Shoulder pain: Involvement of the acromioclavicular joint (analysis of 1,000 cases). AJR 112:493–505, 1971.

Chapter 6

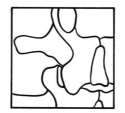

The
LUMBAR SPINE

NORMAL STRUCTURE AND FUNCTION

The lumbar spine transmits load through the sacroiliac (SI) joints to the lower extremities via a series of biomechanical units termed vertebral motion segments, made up of two adjacent vertebrae, the intervening disc, and the associated ligaments.[3]

Essential Anatomy

Vertebrae (Fig. 6–1)

The kidney-shaped vertebral bodies consist largely of cancellous bone and are bordered superiorly and inferiorly by cortical end plates that are important in load bearing.[1] Each cortical end plate has a concave surface that is covered by a hyaline cartilage end plate. The posterior elements of each vertebra consist of the pedicles, the superior and inferior articular processes, the laminae, and the spinous process. The spinal canal is bounded by these bony structures and is oval in shape at the upper levels and somewhat triangular, or deltoid, at the lower levels.[6] The vertebrae articulate with each other via the intervertebral disc and the superior and inferior articular processes (forming the facet, or zygapophyseal, joints). The facet joints are true synovial joints.

279

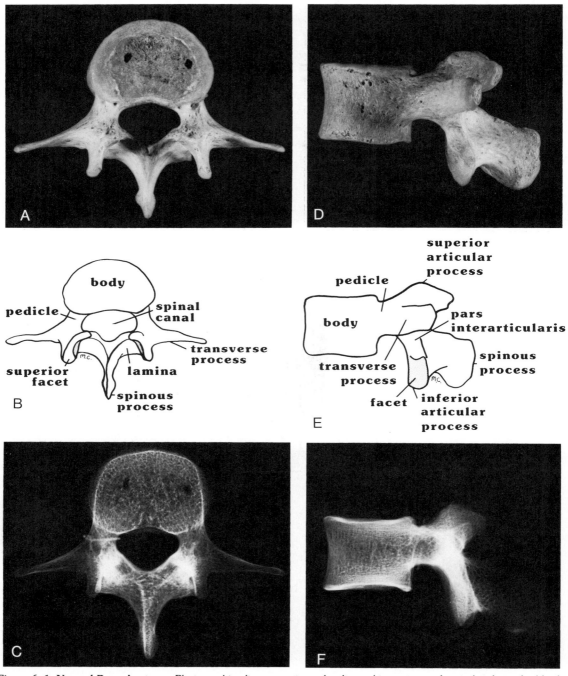

Figure 6–1. Normal Bony Anatomy. Photographic, diagrammatic, and radiographic anatomy of an isolated vertebral body (L3). *A, B, C,* from above; The holes in the body are artefacts. *D, E. F,* lateral.

Illustration continued on opposite page

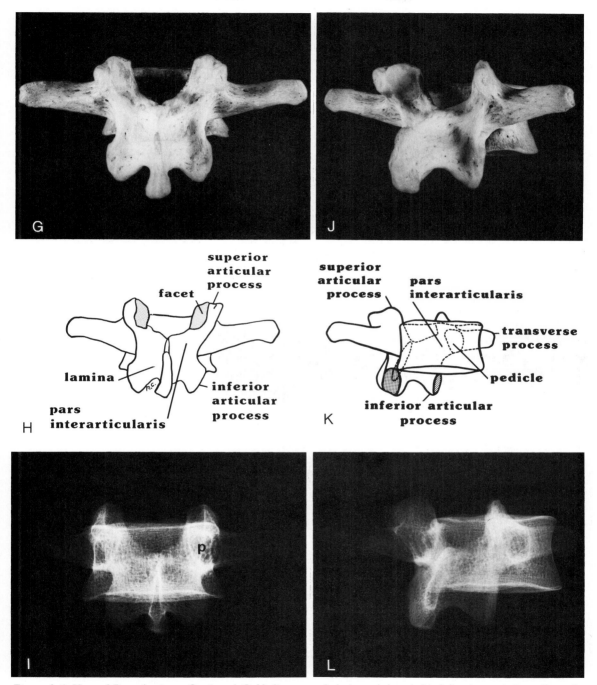

Figure 6–1. Normal Bony Anatomy *Continued. G, H,* diagram and photograph from behind; *I,* anteroposterior radiograph; *J, K, L,* left posterior oblique (LPO). A thin wire loop has been placed around the left pedicle of the radiographed specimen.

281

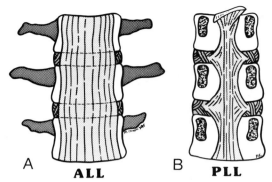

Figure 6–2. Anterior and Posterior Longitudinal Ligaments. *A,* The anterior longitudinal ligament (ALL) covers almost the entire anterior disc surface. *B,* The posterior longitudinal ligament (PLL) is narrower than the anterior.

Soft Tissues

Ligaments. The anterior longitudinal ligament runs the entire length of the spine (Fig. 6–2). Fibers of the anterior and posterior longitudinal ligaments blend with the anulus fibrosus of the disc and extend, via Sharpey's fibers, to the vertebral bodies (Fig. 6–3). Of the two ligaments, anterior and posterior, the anterior is the stronger and the wider.

Intervertebral Discs.[1, 2] The disc in the adult is an avascular structure that is nourished by diffusion from adjacent bones and soft tissues.[3, 7] It consists of an inner nucleus pulposus, derived from the notochord, and an outer anulus fibrosus, derived from the fibroblastic extension of the vertebral bodies. Some authors include the hyaline cartilage vertebral end plates as part of the disc structure.

Cartilage End Plates. Each vertebral body is covered centrally along its superior and inferior surfaces by a hyaline cartilage end plate. The end plate does not cover the entire surface but ends peripherally at the attachment of the ring epiphysis (Fig. 6–3).[1] In childhood the end plates are perforated by blood vessels that pass from the vertebral body to the disc. These are obliterated in later life but leave a potential site of weakness through which the nucleus pulposus may later herniate to form Schmorl's nodes.[4, 8] Three functions are attributed to the cartilage end plate: (1) growth of the vertebral body, (2) anchorage for the disc, and (3) barrier between the disc and the vertebral body.[4]

Anulus Fibrosus. The anulus fibrosus consists of fibrous and fibrocartilaginous lamellae. The fibers are directed obliquely but with changing

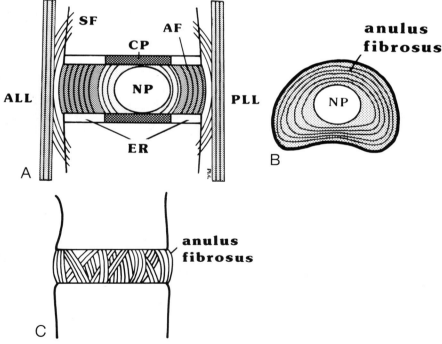

Figure 6–3. Diagram of Discovertebral Anatomy. *A,* Fibers from anterior and posterior longitudinal ligaments and outer anulus fibrosus (Sharpey's fibers) penetrate adjacent vertebral bodies. Each vertebral end plate consists of a central hyaline cartilage plate and a peripheral epiphyseal ring. The central nucleus pulposus and outer anulus fibrosus are shown. *B,* Cross section through the disc shows the central nucleus pulposus and the peripheral anulus fibrosus. *C,* The crisscrossing pattern of anular fibers is shown. AF = anulus fibrosus, ALL = anterior longitudinal ligament, CP = cartilage end plate, ER = epiphyseal ring, NP = nucleus pulposus, PLL = posterior longitudinal ligament, SF = Sharpey's fibers. (Adapted from MacNab, I: Backache. Baltimore, Williams & Wilkins, 1977.)

orientation and are attached to the hyaline cartilage end plates, the anterior and posterior longitudinal ligaments, and the adjacent vertebral bodies about 3 mm from the vertebral margin.[1, 4] The anulus functions to contain the nucleus pulposus and to limit displacement of the nucleus during flexion, extension, and load bearing.

Nucleus Pulposus. The nucleus pulposus is a gelatinous structure with loose fibrous strands coursing through it. The ground substance is made primarily of proteoglycan and water.[1] The nucleus is not distinctly marginated but blends with the fibers of the anulus fibrosus.[2] In youth the nucleus is relatively smooth and homogenous. Vertical sections through the spine show bulging of the nucleus pulposus, termed turgor. This state is an inherent property of the nucleus itself by virtue of the physicochemical properties of the proteoglycan molecule. As in articular cartilage, the proteoglycan molecule of the nucleus is constrained from occupying its full vol-

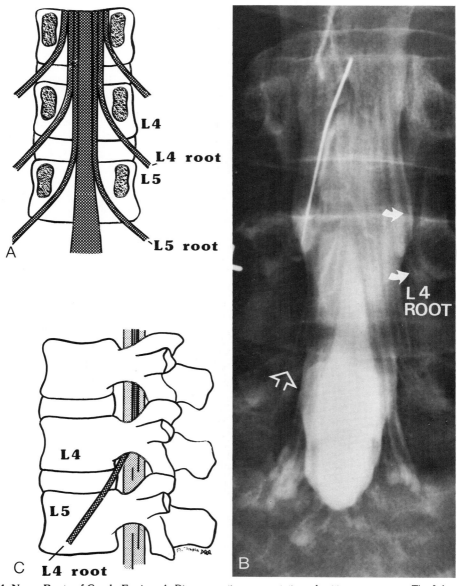

Figure 6–4. Nerve Roots of Cauda Equina. *A,* Diagrammatic representation of exiting nerve roots. The L4 root exits under the L4 pedicle, the L5 root under the L5 pedicle, and so on. *B,* Metrizamide myelogram demonstrates the relationship of exiting nerve roots to the pedicles. The slight decrease in filling of the left L5 root (open arrow) was later confirmed to be the result of compression by a herniated disc. *C,* Lateral diagram shows the exiting L4 nerve root. The proximity of the posterior aspect of the vertebral body, the disc, and the facets to the nerve root explains possible root compression in patients with osteophytic lipping or disc herniation. *(A and C adapted from MacNab I: Backache. Baltimore, Williams & Wilkins, 1977.)*

ume in fluid. When constraint is lost by damage to the hyaline cartilage end plate or anulus, swelling results.

Lumbar and Sacral Nerve Roots (Figs. 6–4 and 6–5).[5] The spinal cord usually ends at the level of the L1–L2 disc. The spinal canal distal to this contains the sensory (dorsal) and motor (ventral) roots of the spinal nerves. These roots fuse to form the spinal nerves, which exit through the intervertebral foramina.

Each lumbar nerve leaves the dural sac at about the level of the intervertebral disc of the segment above, then descends obliquely to exit through the foramen, the L4 roots exiting under the L4 pedicles, the L5 roots under the L5 pedicles, and so on. The foramina of L1 to L4 are directed laterally and are well seen on the lateral view. The L5–S1 foramen is directed anterolaterally and may therefore appear smaller on the lateral radiographs than it actually is.

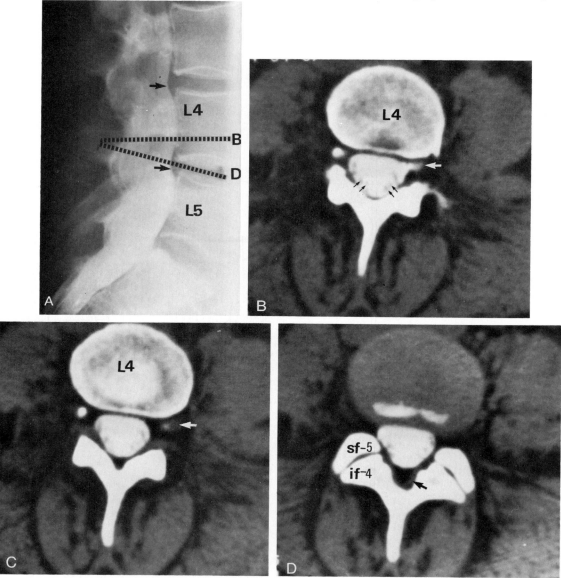

Figure 6–5. Computed Tomographic Anatomy of L4 Nerve Roots. *A*, Lateral view during metrizamide myelogram shows indentations on the anterior aspect of the contrast column (arrows) at L3–L4 and L4–L5 resulting from bulging intervertebral discs. The levels for subsequent computed tomograms *B* and *D* are marked. *B*, CT section through the L4 vertebra and L4–L5 foramina 1 hour after a metrizamide myelogram shows contrast agent filling the left axillary pouch (white arrow) and the right nerve-root sleeve. Small arrows indicate the filling defects produced by the remaining nerve roots. *C*, CT section slightly more distal than *B* shows the L4 nerve root ganglia (left ganglion indicated by arrow). *D*, Section through the L4–L5 disc and the posterior inferior body of L4 shows an abnormally bulging disc without compression of the subarachnoid space. The ligamentum flavum on the left (arrow), the superior facet of L5 (sf-5), and the inferior facet of L4 (if-4) are indicated.

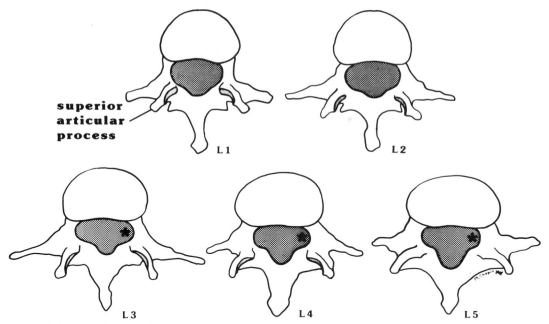

Figure 6–6. Lateral Recesses. Diagrammatic representation of the lumbar vertebrae from above shows the increased prominence of the lateral recesses (asterisk) at the lower levels.

Each nerve passes through the foramen along the medial and inferior surface of the pedicle, within a sulcus termed the lateral recess (Fig. 6–6). This sulcus is more prominent at the L4 and L5 levels. The nerve roots occupy only the upper half of each foramen.

Normal Radiographic Examination

Role of Radiography

Considerable literature is available regarding the role of the radiologic examination in patients with low back pain. It is generally agreed that a number of findings are not significantly more frequent in patients with low back pain as compared with control subjects. These incidental findings include transitional vertebrae, spina bifida occulta, asymmetrical facet joint orientation, facet joint osteophytes, Schmorl's nodes, increased lordosis, acute lumbosacral angle, and osteophytic lipping from vertebral bodies (Fig. 6–7). Which findings are of significance is more controversial. Bone destruction from tumor or infection, spondylolisthesis,[22, 33] and disc narrowing at multiple levels[14, 33] are considered significant. In addition, congenital or traumatic kyphosis, severe scoliosis, osteoporosis, ankylosing spondylitis, and Scheuermann's disease are very

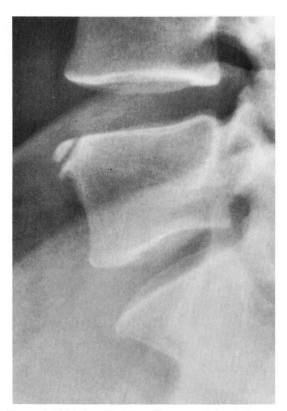

Figure 6–7. Limbus Vertebra. The separated anterior corner of the vertebral body (limbus vertebra), analogous to a Schmorl's node, is probably the result of anterior disc herniation into the vertebral body.

285

Table 6–1. **The Significance of Radiographic Findings in the Lumbar Spine**

Probably significant findings	Spondylolisthesis Disc narrowing at multiple levels Congenital or traumatic kyphosis Scheuermann's disease Ankylosing spondylitis Osteoporosis
Findings of questionable significance	Spondylolysis Mild spondylolisthesis Severe kyphosis Retrolisthesis $< 80°$ lumbar scoliosis in adults Severe lordosis Decreased lordosis
Inconsequential findings	Transitional vertebrae Spina bifida occulta Increased lordosis Acute lumbosacral angle Facet joint orientation Schmorl's nodes Osteophytic lipping Accessory ossicles Facet joint osteophytes Disc calcification Pseudospondylolisthesis Single disc narrowing

likely to be associated with back pain (Table 6–1).[25, 33] None of these findings, however, can be considered certain to be the source of a particular patient's pain, and the major role of the radiographic examination is the exclusion of potentially serious disease such as fracture, infection, or metastasis.

Radiographic examination of the low back is the largest single source of gonadal irradiation in the United States; therefore its use should be carefully considered.[28] The question as to which radiographic views are necessary has received moderate attention in the literature. A study of compensation-related low back examinations in Veterans Administration hospitals concluded that 99.3 percent of the sought-for abnormalities were demonstrated by a combination of AP and lateral views centered just above the iliac crest.[12] Rhea and co-workers also concluded that the oblique views were unnecessary for the initial evaluation of an adult patient.[11] Of 200 patients reviewed, there were only 4 instances in which the radiographic diagnosis was changed by the availability of the oblique projection; in three

patients spondylolysis was detected, and in the fourth a pseudarthrosis following spinal fusion was noted. Similar results are found in the pediatric age group.[27] Other studies do, however, attach greater importance to the oblique views.[14a, 20a] These studies are of particular importance, since oblique views contribute more to the gonadal dose than does either the AP or the lateral projection.[27] The total gonadal dose from a five-view (AP, lateral, coned lateral, and both oblique views) lumbar spine examination is calculated to be 75 mrad in men and 382 mrad in women.[26] In comparative terms even a three-view lumbosacral spine examination provides the same female gonadal irradiation as would many years of daily chest radiographs.[18]

Indications for radiographic examination are controversial, but the following guidelines, proposed by Macnab, seem rational.[20, 22]

1. Severe back pain following significant trauma

2. Incapacitating back pain

3. History suggesting vertebral compression due to osteoporosis or malignancy

Figure 6–8. Normal Radiographic Examination. *A,* Anteroposterior view. *B,* Lateral view. Note the usual mild lordosis, the normal increase in disc-space height from L1 to L5 with a slightly more narrow L5–S1 disc space, and the slight concavity of the inferior aspect of L5. *C,* Right posterior oblique view shows the right posterior elements. b = vertebral body of L4, f = foramen, if = inferior articular process, l = lamina, p = pedicle(s), pi = pars interarticularis, s = spinous process, sf = superior articular process, t = transverse process,)(= interpediculate distance. *D,* Left posterior oblique (LPO) view shows the left facet joint, pedicle, and pars interarticularis to advantage.

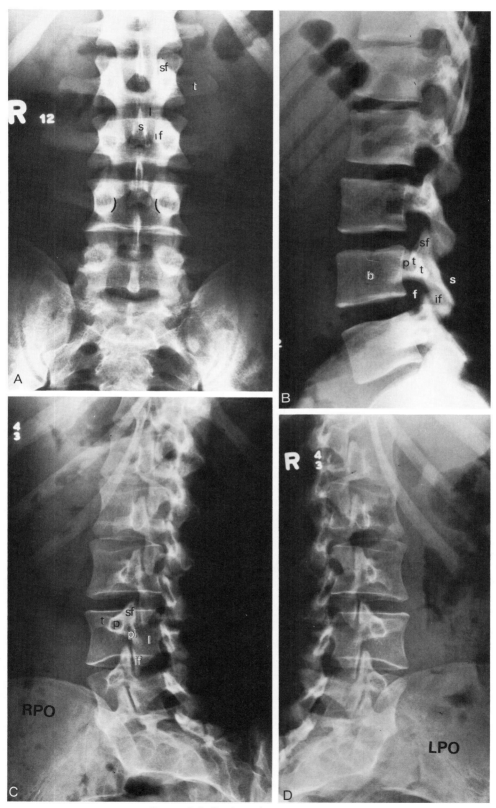

Figure 6–8. *See legend on opposite page.*

4. An excessively anxious patient

5. Suspected ankylosing spondylitis

6. Clinically apparent spinal deformity

7. Significant root tension or impaired root conduction

8. Persistent pain for more than 2 weeks, despite treatment.

Computed tomography is being used more frequently for the diagnosis of back disorders, including spinal stenosis, herniated nucleus pulposus, and facet joint abnormalities. Such examinations can result in a dose of 6 rads per study.[10]

Normal Radiographic Anatomy

Standard lumbar spine radiographs usually consist of an anteroposterior (AP) and two lateral views, one of the entire lumbar spine and one centered at the L5–S1 disc space (Fig. 6–8). Additional oblique views, supine and/or standing lateral views, lateral views in flexion and extension and angled views[9] may be done as needed. The bony structures seen on standard radiographic examination are shown in Figure 6–1. The anatomy on oblique views has been clarified by Etter and Carabello.[13] In the left posterior oblique (LPO) view or in the right anterior oblique (RAO) view, the left pedicle, lamina, pars interarticularis, and facets are seen to advantage. Thus as the patient turns toward the left side, the left posterior elements are optimally seen. The appearance of these structures on the oblique view (see Fig. 6–1) has been likened to that of a "Scottie" dog with an eye (the pedicle), nose (the transverse process), ear (the superior articular process), neck (the pars interarticularis), leg (the inferior articular process), and back (the lamina).

Normally, on the lateral view the disc spaces widen from the upper to the lower levels, with the widest disc space at L4–L5. The L5–S1 disc space may normally be slightly narrower. The

Table 6–2. **Minimal Normal Values in True Millimeters of the Sagittal Diameter of the Spinal Canal Obtained by Anatomic and Tomographic Measurements**

	L1	L2	L3	L4	L5
Huizinga	14	13	12	11	12
Davatchi	12.3	12.3	12.3	10.7	11.5
Guillaume	14	13	12	13	14
De Berail	16	14	15	14	12

Source: Roulleau J, Guillaume J: Plain x-ray diagnosis of developmental narrow lumbar canal. *In* Wackenheim A, Babin E, eds. The Narrow Lumbar Canal. Radiologic Signs & Surgery. New York, Springer-Verlag, 1980. Used with permission.

Table 6–3. **Interpediculate Distance in True Millimeters (Corrected Values)**

	L1	L2	L3	L4	L5
Delmas and Pineau	19	20	19	18	20
Huizinga	19	20	20	19	20
Roulleau	19	18	17	20	22
De Berail	17	19	19	20	23
Elsberg and Dyke	17	18	18	18	20

Source: Roulleau J, Guillaume J: Plain x-ray diagnosis of developmental narrow lumbar canal. *In* Wackenheim A, Babbin E, eds. The Narrow Lumbar Canal. Radiologic Signs & Surgery. New York, Springer-Verlag 1980. Used with permission.

disc spaces are often wider anteriorly than posteriorly.[15] A lordotic curve of about 40 degrees is normally present.[21] This can be measured as the angle of intersection of perpendiculars to the end plates of L3 and the upper surface of S1. The lordosis increases on standing.

The sagittal diameter of the spinal canal may be difficult to evaluate on a routine lateral projection. It is measured as the shortest midline perpendicular distance from the vertebral body to the inner surface of the back of the neural arch (spinolaminar line). Minimal normal values have been compiled by Roulleau and Guillaume (Table 6–2)[29] and by Hinck, Hopkins, and Clark.[17]

The interpediculate distance generally increases toward L5. Normal measurements, corrected for magnification, are shown in Table 6–3.

ABNORMAL CONDITIONS

Scoliosis

Definitions

Scoliosis is defined as "an appreciable lateral deviation in the normally straight vertical line of the spine."[36] *Kyphosis* is derived from the Greek word for *humpback* and refers to an increase in the posterior angulation of the spine. Its opposite, *lordosis,* refers to an increase in anterior angulation of the spine.[36] Lumbar lordosis of more than 40 degrees is considered abnormal.[43]

Lateral bending films demonstrate the flexibility of a curve. A structural scoliosis is not fully correctable on lateral bending films and is accompanied by fixed vertebral rotation. Compensatory curves may occur above or below the structural curve. The terms *primary, major,* and *minor,* tend no longer to be used.[44]

The term *balance* refers to the observation

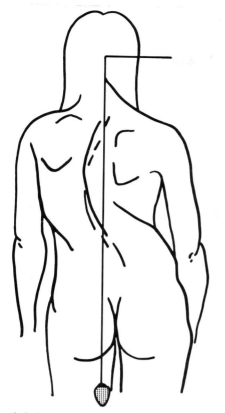

Figure 6–9. Balance. In the normal situation a plumb line placed at the occiput falls over the gluteal crease. The spine pictured is therefore unbalanced. (Adapted from an original painting by Frank H. Netter, M.D., from CLINICAL SYMPOSIA, copyright by CIBA Pharmaceutical Company, Division of CIBA-GEIGY Corporation.)

that a plumb line dropped from the midocciput or C7 spinous process normally falls over the midline gluteal crease (Fig. 6–9). Balance is evaluated radiographically by drawing a straight line upward from the midsacrum parallel to the side of the x-ray film. Deviation of this line from the midpoint of the T1 vertebral body is measured and can be graded as grade 1—<1.5 cm, grade 2—1.6–3 cm, grade 3—2.1–5 cm, and grade 4—>5 cm.

Etiology and Classification

Scoliosis is not only a problem in childhood; in fact, some forms of scoliosis appear to have an increased incidence in the elderly. In one study this increased incidence was attributed to the presence of osteoporosis or osteomalacia,[50] a finding that was not, however, confirmed by Robin and colleagues.[48] Nor could the possibility that degenerative disc disease was the underlying factor in the development of late-onset scoliosis be documented; therefore the cause of scoliosis in this population remains unknown. The increased frequency of dorsal scoliosis in comparison with lumbar curves and the predominant right dorsal, left lumbar pattern is seen both in the elderly and in children with idiopathic scoliosis. One classification of scoliosis based on etiology has been presented by McAlister and Shackelford (Table 6–4).[44]

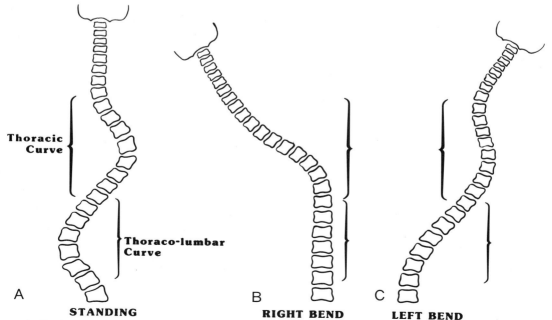

Figure 6–10. Diagram of Side Bending. *A,* The standing view shows a thoracolumbar scoliosis convex to the right and a thoracic scoliosis convex to the left. *B,* Right-bending view shows complete correction of the lower curve; therefore it is flexible. *C,* On a left-bending view the thoracic curve does not completely correct; therefore it is a structural curve. (After Keim HA: CIBA Clinical Symposia 24:1, 1972.)

Table 6–4. **Classification of Spinal Curves**

Curve	Type or Cause	Examples
Scoliosis		

Idiopathic	Infantile
	    Resolving
	    Progressive
	Juvenile
	Adolescent	

Congenital anomaly	Deformity due to abnormal
	    bone development
	    Failure of formation
	        Complete unilateral
	            (hemivertebrae)
	        Partial unilateral (wedge)
	    Failure of segmentation
	        Partial or unilateral (bar)
	        Complete or bilateral (bloc)
	    Mixed, miscellaneous, and
	        congenital syndromes
		Spondylocostal dysostosis,
		    oculovertebral syndrome,
		    Klippel-Feil syndrome,
		    Sprengel's deformity, caudal
		    regression syndrome

	Abnormal bony or neural
	    development
	    Myelodysplasia
	    Miscellaneous
		Diastematomyelia, tethered cord,
		    lateral or anterior meningocele,
		    neurenteric cyst

	Extravertebral	Congenital posterior rib fusions,
		    hypoplastic lungs, myositis
		    ossificans progressiva

Neuromuscular		Poliomyelitis, syringomyelia,
		    cerebral palsy, Duchenne's
		    muscular dystrophy

Skeletal dysplasias
Developmental ectodermal or
    mesodermal defects
		Neurofibromatosis, Marfan's
		    syndrome, Ehlers-Danlos
		    syndrome, arthrogryposis,
		    homocystinuria

Radiographic Examination

In adults preoperative examination usually includes standing AP and lateral views on 14 × 36-inch (36 × 91-cm) film. The occiput and sacrum should be included. The use of a gradient intensifying screen can help to show the entire spine well on a single film.[47] In addition, the use of appropriate screens may decrease radiation exposure.

Lateral bending films are done to evaluate the flexibility of a curve. When the patient bends toward the convex side of the curve, a structural curve will be incompletely corrected, whereas a flexible curve will disappear (Figs. 6–10 and 6–11). Additional studies, multidirectional tomography, for example, are indicated for evaluation of congenital lesions, such as bony bars or segmentation failures, or for evaluation of acquired bone lesions, such as osteoid osteoma.

Measurement

The two most frequently used methods of measuring spinal curvature are those of Cobb and of Ferguson (Figs. 6–12 and 6–13).

The Cobb Method. This method is the standard measurement technique of the Scoliosis Research Society.[35, 42] It is preferred because it is more reproducible and gives larger angles in severe cases.[41] It is most accurate for measuring curves of greater than 50 degrees. The standard deviation of the Cobb method is 2 to 3 degrees,[41] and therefore differences of up to 6 degrees may be accepted as resulting from the measurement technique itself.

The technique of measurement involves the following steps:

1. *Drawing lines along the superior end plate of the uppermost vertebra and the inferior end plate of the lowermost vertebra.* The uppermost

Table 6–4. **Classification of Spinal Curves** *Continued*

Curve	Type or Cause	Examples
Post-traumatic	Vertebral	Fracture; irradiation; surgery, including intrathecal shunts
	Extravertebral	Thoracoplasty, burns
Inflammatory and neoplastic disease involving the spine		Tuberculosis, osteoid osteoma, osteoblastoma, rheumatoid arthritis, histiocytosis
Spinal cord lesion and/or canal lesions, excluding myelodysplasia		Astrocytoma, arachnoid cyst, lipoma, neurofibroma
Bone-softening disease		Osteoporosis, osteomalacia, rickets, hyperparathyroidism, Cushing's disease, disease from use of steroids
Miscellaneous		Larsen's syndrome, familial dysautonomia
Kyphosis		
Adolescent or Scheuermann's disease		
Congenital	Failure of vertebral body formation	
	Failure of vertebral body segmentation	
	Mixed	
Neuromuscular		
Bone-softening diseases		
Skeletal dysplasia		
Trauma		
Inflammatory diseases		
Arthritides		
Tumors		
Miscellaneous		Stickler's syndrome
Lordosis		
Congenital		
Acquired		Spondylolisthesis, neuromuscular, skeletal dysplasia

Source: McAlister WH, Shackelford GD: Radiol Clin North Am 13:93, 1975.

vertebra of the curve is the highest in which the superior surface tilts toward the concave aspect of the curve. The lowermost vertebra is that in which the inferior surface tilts toward the concavity of the curve. All of the levels within the curve will show widening of the intervertebral disc spaces on the convex side of the curve. Similarly, the distance between the pedicles on the convex side of the curve is widened. These observations help to determine which vertebrae are included in the curve.

2. *Drawing lines perpendicular to those indicating the upper- and lowermost aspects of the curve.* The angle between the perpendiculars is the measured angle of scoliosis.

The Ferguson Method[42]

1. *The vertebrae at each end of the curve are located.* These are noted to be the least rotated vertebral bodies.

2. *The apical vertebra is located.* This is the vertebral body at the apex of the curve that is the most rotated.

3. *The centers of the chosen vertebrae are marked.* In cases with minimal deformity diagonal lines through the corners of the vertebral bodies will indicate the center. Where greater vertebral deformity is present, this method is inaccurate, and finding the centers of the vertebral bodies is a matter of judgment.

4. *The angle of the curve* is that formed by the intersection of lines drawn from the uppermost vertebra to the apical vertebra and from the apical vertebra to the lowermost vertebra.

Because of the difficulty in determining the midportion of the vertebrae, the Ferguson method is least accurate for measuring curves of greater than 50 degrees.[42] In addition, the calculated angle is smaller than that formed by

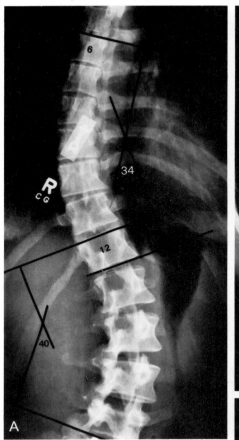

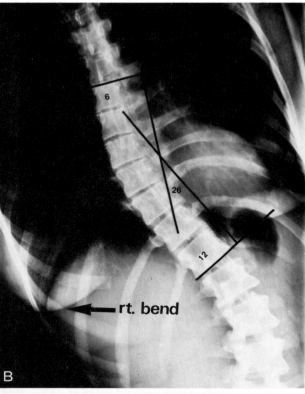

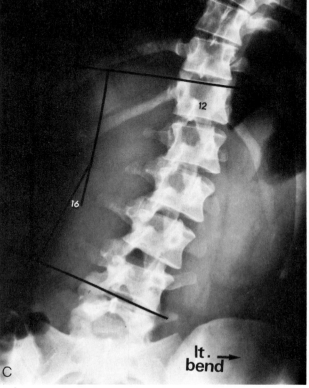

Figure 6–11. Scoliosis, Standing, and Bending Films. *A,* Standing view shows a 34° thoracic scoliosis, convex right, and a 40° thoracolumbar scoliosis, convex left. *B,* Right-bending view shows incomplete correction of the dorsal curve, which therefore is a structural curve. Note that the levels used for measurement are the same as those used in *A. C,* Left-bending view shows improvement, but not complete correction, of the lumbar curve, which therefore is also a structural curve.

Figure 6–12. Measuring Scoliosis. *Ferguson Method*: (1) The vertebrae at each end of the curve are located. (These are noted to be the least rotated vertebral bodies.) (2) The apical vertebra, the vertebral body at the apex of the curve that is the most rotated, is located. (3) The centers of the chosen vertebra are marked. In patients with minimal deformity diagonal lines through the corners of vertebral bodies will indicate the center. When greater vertebral deformity is present, this method is inaccurate, and finding the center of a vertebral body is a matter of judgement. (4) Angles of the curves are those formed by the intersection of lines drawn from the uppermost vertebra to the apical vertebra and from the apical vertebra to the lowermost vertebra. *Cobb Method*: (1) Lines are drawn along the superior end plate of the uppermost vertebra and the inferior end plate of the lowermost vertebra of the curve. The top vertebra is the highest one in which the superior surface tilts toward the concave aspect of the curve. The lowermost vertebra is the one in which the inferior surface tilts toward the concavity of the curve. All the vertebrae within the curve will show widening of the intervertebral disc spaces on the convex side of the curve. This finding may help in deciding which are the uppermost and the lowermost involved vertebrae. Similarly, the distance between the pedicles on the convex side of the curve is widened and this factor may also help to determine which vertebrae are included in the curve. (2) Lines are drawn perpendicular to the lines that indicate upper- and lowermost aspects of the curve. The angle between the perpendiculars is the measured angle of scoliosis. Differences of 6° or less may be accepted as the result of the measurement technique itself.

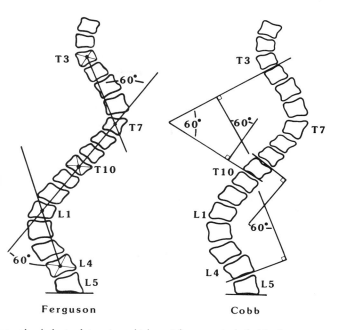

Ferguson   Cobb

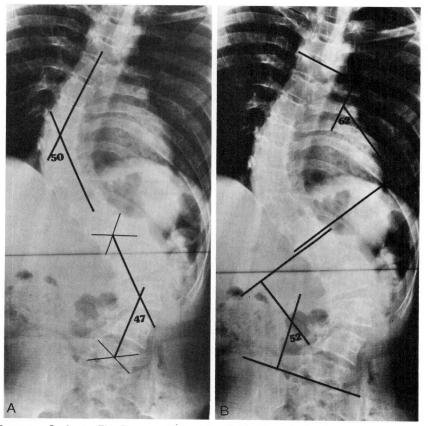

Figure 6–13. Measuring Scoliosis. The Ferguson *(A)* and the Cobb *(B)* methods of measurement are shown. Note the smaller angles obtained when the Ferguson method is used.

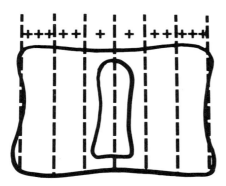

Figure 6–14. Vertebral Rotation, Spinous Process Measurements. The degree of rotation can be estimated as 1+, 2+, or 3+ by the position of the spinous process in relation to the superimposed vertebral body.

other methods because the measured angle lies on the concavity of the curve rather than on its convexity.[41]

Computerized Method. Using a computer program, Jeffries and co-workers have developed a method of measuring scoliosis that is easier and apparently more reproducible than the hand-drawn methods described earlier.[41] When the computer method is used, a change in the angle of scoliosis of more than 2 degrees is significant.

Kyphosis. The degree of kyphosis can be measured by using a modified Cobb technique. Lines are drawn along the upper edge of the proximal vertebra and the lower edge of the

distal vertebra. Perpendiculars are drawn to these lines, and the angle they form is the degree of kyphosis. The end vertebrae are those most tilted from the horizontal. Twenty to 40 degrees is considered a normal amount of dorsal kyphosis (or lumbar lordosis).

Vertebral Rotation.[46] The degree of vertebral rotation can theoretically be determined by the following:

1. *The location of the spinous process.* The spinous process on a straight AP view should be midline in relation to the vertebral body. As rotation occurs, the spinous process shifts toward the concavity of the curve, and the amount of shift relates to the amount of rotation (Fig. 6–14).

2. Evaluation of the *position and symmetry of the pedicles.* In the anteroposterior view the pedicles are normally projected as symmetrical oval structures at equal distances from the lateral margins of the vertebral bodies. As rotation occurs, the pedicles on the convex side shift toward the midline and change their configuration (Fig. 6–15). These observations, however, provide an inaccurate measure of the degree of rotation, since the appearance of the pedicle varies in different individuals and with the tilt of the vertebra in the sagittal and frontal planes.[34] It has been suggested, therefore, that pedicle offset should not be used for precise evaluation of rotation either on a single radiograph or on comparison radiographs.

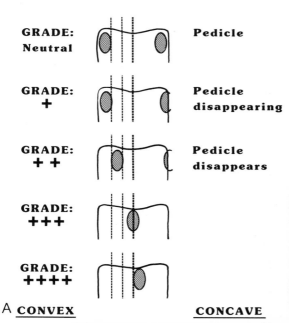
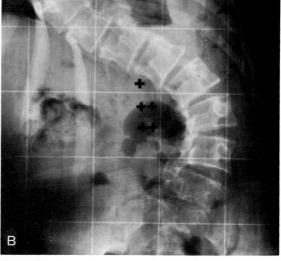

Figure 6–15. Pedicle Method of Determining Vertebral Body Rotation. *A,* The degree of rotation can be graded by noting the pedicle position and appearance. *B,* Example of grading vertebral rotation in a patient with scoliosis. (From Nash CL Jr, Moe JH: J Bone Joint Surg (Am) 51:228, 1969.)

Surgical Correction

Indications for surgery in the adult include unremitting back pain, progression of curvature, severe curves, cardiopulmonary symptoms, and sometimes patient appearance.[45, 49] The source of the pain is unclear. Lateral vertebral subluxation and degenerative changes in the facet joints on the concave side of the curve have been found in patients with painful lumbar scoliosis. However, no clear relationship between the occurrence of pain and the presence of these radiographic findings can be confirmed.[49]

The goal of surgery is a fused, balanced, and painless spine, rather than maximum correction of the spinal curvature.[49] Spinal fusion is now commonly accompanied by internal fixation of the spine, with the advantages of better correction of the scoliosis, earlier postoperative ambulation, and a decreased incidence of pseudarthrosis.[45] In all of these instrumentation procedures, the internal fixation provides stability while the bone graft is solidifying. Ultimate stability will depend on the bone graft, rather than on the fixation device. There are three major types of instrumentation in use.

Harrington Rods (Distraction and Compression).[40, 51] This procedure involves removal of the spinous processes, decortication of the laminae, removal of cartilage from the facet joints, and placement of autogenous bone graft along these areas for fusion. The hooks of the distraction rod are inserted under the laminae of the upper and lower ends of the curve concavity. Distraction is accomplished at the upper end of the rod, where the hook is advanced on a ratchet, in an action similar to that of an automobile jack. When the hook can no longer be advanced, a collar of wire is placed around the rod, beneath the upper hook. Multiple distraction rods may be used, and if necessary, they may be bent to conform to the shape of the spine. In addition, compression rods may be used along the convexity of the curve, with the hooks usually placed around the transverse processes, rather than around the laminae.[38, 51]

Dwyer Fusion.[37] This technique of anterior spine fusion is especially useful in treating patients who have severe paralytic curves, absent posterior elements, or cerebral palsy.[39] Depending on the site to be corrected, the procedure is performed through an anterior, a retroperitoneal, or a thoracic approach, or a combination of these. The intervertebral discs and vertebral end plates are removed, and bone graft from an excised rib is inserted between the vertebrae. A staple and a screw are placed in each vertebral body along the convex side of the curve. The screw should be long enough to go through both cortices of the vertebra and should parallel the end plates. A cable runs along the convex side, through each screw. Tension is applied at each level and maintained by crimping the screw heads on the cable. Both Dwyer instrumentation and Harrington rod application may be used in the same patient.

Segmental Spinal Instrumentation (Luque Rod Fixation; Fig. 6–16). This is a relatively new technique that is currently used in adults with flexible idiopathic curves, supple paralytic curves, or kyphosis and in patients who would tolerate immobilization poorly. The procedure consists of posterior spinal fusion and insertion posteriorly of a prebent rod that is held to the vertebrae by a series of wires placed around the laminae. The stability that this system provides markedly decreases the necessary postoperative immobilization.

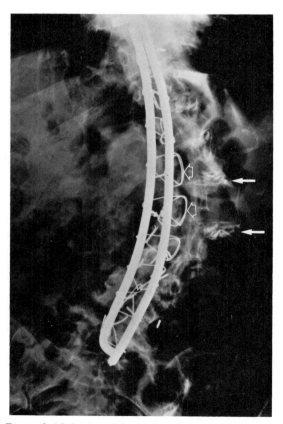

Figure 6–16. Luque Rods. Anterior fusion was attempted, and the bone graft replacing the discs is well seen (arrows). Attempted placement of Dwyer instrumentation was unsuccessful because of severe osteoporosis, and Luque rods were wired to the laminae at a second operation. Open arrows indicate some of the wires that encircle the laminae and the rods.

295

Radiographically Identifiable Complications. The overall complication rate of scoliosis surgery is high, particularly in the adult. Radiographically identifiable complications include the general problems of pulmonary embolic disease, gastric distension, ileus, and superior mesenteric artery syndrome. Retroperitoneal fibrosis and ruptured aortic aneurysm have been reported following Dwyer instrumentation.[39] In addition, local complications include the following:

1. *Loss of correction.* Swank and colleagues noted postoperatively a loss of correction of

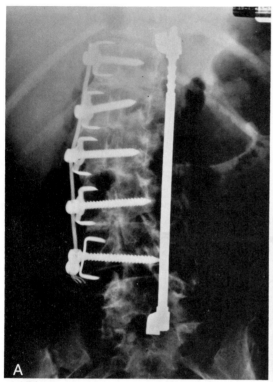

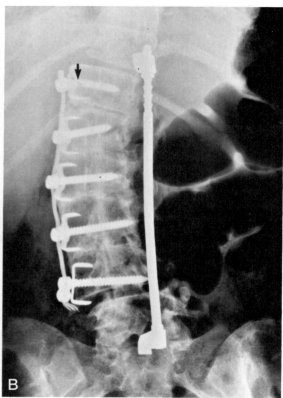

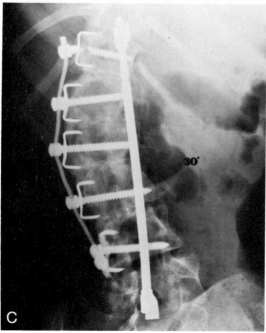

Figure 6–17. **Dwyer Instrumentation and Anterior Fusion with Break in Upper Screw.** *A,* Frontal view after Dwyer instrumentation and anterior fusion and posterior Harrington distraction rod insertion and fusion. *B,* Seven months later there is a break in the uppermost screw (T12), and there is nonunion across the T12–L1 disc space. *C,* The oblique view better demonstrates the break in the upper screw.

approximately 6 degrees in patients with idiopathic scoliosis. After the bone graft solidifies (6 to 9 months), increase in the curvature by more than 10 degrees suggests the possibility of pseudarthrosis.[39, 49]

2. *Pseudarthrosis.* In 6 to 9 months the graft material, which is present largely on the concave side of the curve, should appear solid, and areas of sparse graft or defects in the graft should be noted.[49, 51] Swank and associates define *pseudarthrosis* as a defect in the fusion mass present more than 1 year after surgery.[49] Pseudarthrosis should be suspected when there is a loss of correction of more than 10 degrees or fracture or disruption of the internal fixation apparatus, especially if the broken ends of the rod overlap.[40] An increased rate of pseudarthrosis has been noted in adults; the rate apparently increases with age. In one series a 2 percent incidence of pseudarthrosis was noted in patients in their 20s, 18 percent in those in their 30s, and 22 percent in patients older than 40.[49]

3. *Fracture of hardware.* Fracture of the internal fixation device often, but not always, indicates pseudarthrosis (Fig. 6–17). In one series 6 of 15 patients with fractured Harrington rods had no apparent pseudarthrosis.[49] Harrington rods usually break at the junction of the solid and notched parts.

4. *Displacement of hardware.* Early in the postoperative course, this complication may result from injudicious patient handling or inadequate immobilization (Fig. 6–18).

Disc Degeneration

Pathological Anatomy

Degenerative changes occur normally with aging and involve the cartilage end plates, the anulus, and the nucleus pulposus. With increasing age there is fibrillation and then thinning of the

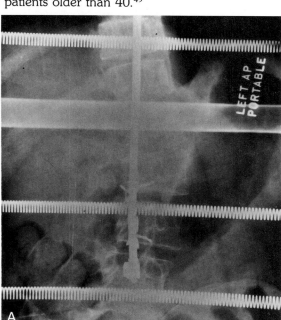
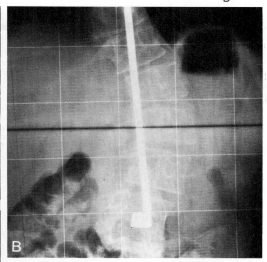
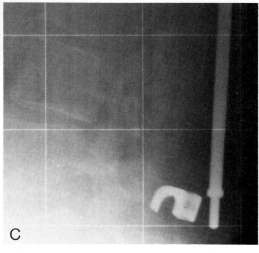

Figure 6–18. Displacement of Lower Hook of a Harrington Rod. *A,* Immediate postoperative film shows the Harrington rod with the lower hook on the L4 lamina. *B,* Repeat AP view prior to discharge shows the hook apparently lateral to the end of the rod. *C,* Lateral view confirms the separation of the hook from the rod and the lamina, necessitating reoperation.

Table 6–5. Findings in Disc Degeneration

Disc-space narrowing
Vacuum discs
Vertebral sclerosis
Osteophytes
Osteoarthritis of facet joints
Subluxation of facet joints

cartilage end plates, and granulation tissue grows into them from the adjacent vertebral body, sometimes extending into the nucleus pulposus. Herniation of nuclear material into the vertebral bodies (Schmorl's nodes) may accompany the thinning of the end plates.[64, 71]

When a person is approximately age 30, the water content of the nucleus pulposus is maximal. Specimens at this age, however, already show some fragmentation of the posterior fibers of the anulus fibrosus. The anulus fibrosus loses its lamellar character, and posterior protrusion of the anulus and disc narrowing occur.[54] The water content of the nucleus pulposus becomes markedly reduced, and cleft formation, degeneration, and calcium salt deposition occur. The loss of fluid results in loss of turgor in the nucleus. Findings of disc degeneration are usually greatest in the more distal lumbar levels.[64]

A review of the postulated causes of disc degeneration is presented by Lipson.[64]

Radiological Findings
(Table 6–5; Fig. 6–19)

Disc-Space Narrowing. From L1 to L5 the heights of the intervertebral disc spaces normally increase.[55] The L5–S1 disc space may normally be narrower than that of L4–L5. Disc narrowing is a common accompaniment of degenerative disc disease but is uncommon in herniation of the nucleus pulposus (herniated disc).

Vacuum Discs. Gas within the disc space (the vacuum phenomenon) is seen in about 2 percent of lumbar spine radiographs obtained in flexion.[56, 66] The incidence of detection can be increased, however, if films are taken with the spine in extension.[62]

Analysis has shown that over 90 percent of the gas present is nitrogen, which presumably enters the spaces created by disc degeneration, a process apparently analogous to the gas seen in more peripheral joints with distraction or relaxation.[56] Pathological studies by Resnick and co-workers have shown that the most common site for this gas to accumulate is in the nucleus pulposus, where the dehydration that normally occurs with aging results in small clefts in the nuclear substance.[72] These clefts progress pe-

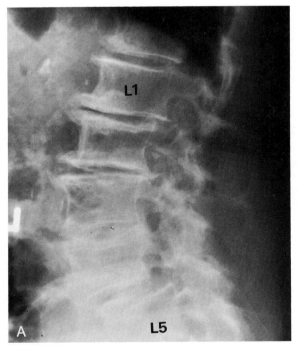

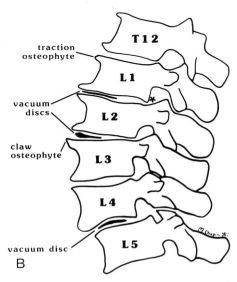

Figure 6–19. Degenerative Disc Disease. *A*, Lateral radiograph of an elderly woman's spine demonstrates many of the findings of disc degeneration, including vacuum phenomena at L1–L2, L2–L3, and L3–L4; retrolisthesis of L1 on L2; degenerative (pseudo-) spondylolisthesis L4–L5, and claw spondylophytes, especially at L1–L2. *B*, Diagram of the same patient's spine. Asterisk indicates retrolisthesis.

ripherally to involve the anulus fibrosus. Both these sites correspond to the round or linear gas collections demonstrable on radiographs. The degenerative etiology of this phenomenon is substantiated by the strikingly increased incidence of the vacuum phenomenon in the elderly[58] and by the coincident findings of disc narrowing, vertebral sclerosis, and osteophytic lipping typical of degenerative disc disease.[55, 59] Tears of the peripheral fibers of the anulus fibrosus (degenerative or traumatic) may be associated with localized peripheral collections of gas.[72]

Conditions associated with secondary disc degeneration, including calcium pyrophosphate dihydrate deposition and ochronosis, can produce vacuum phenomena. In patients with ochronosis the abnormality involves most intervertebral discs and may precede radiographically identifiable disc calcification (Fig. 6–20). Tumors that involve adjacent vertebral bodies may interfere with disc nutrition and result in secondary disc degeneration, sometimes with a vacuum phenomenon.

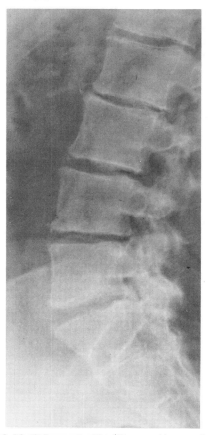

Figure 6–20. Ochronosis. This 40-year-old patient's father and brother have ochronosis. There are multiple narrowed discs with vacuum phenomena.

Since the presence of fluid in a joint or in the disc will prevent the creation of any potential space, disc infection should not be accompanied by a vacuum phenomenon. In fact, the presence of a vacuum phenomenon essentially excludes acute infection at that level.

Discogenic Vertebral Sclerosis (Fig. 6–21). Sclerosis of adjacent vertebral bodies may follow disc degeneration. Such degeneration probably underlies a number of previously reported conditions in which sclerosis and lysis of vertebral bodies are the major radiographic findings. These conditions are, therefore, probably best termed discogenic vertebral sclerosis.

Williams and colleagues referred to this condition in 1968, when they noted pre- and postoperative patients who developed lytic lesions of the vertebral bodies adjacent to the disc, followed by progressive vertebral sclerosis and disc narrowing.[72] It was suggested that these lesions represented low-grade infections, although there was no evidence of fever, or elevation of the white blood cell count or erythrocyte sedimentation rate. Cultures were negative in cases in which biopsy was done.

Eight years later Martel and associates described similar lesions of the discovertebral junction and postulated that they were post-traumatic in origin.[67] Three categories of radiological abnormality were noted—lytic, sclerotic, and mixed. The lytic lesions represented intravertebral disc herniations (Schmorl's nodes). The superior aspect of the vertebral body is usually involved in these cases, and there is associated disc-space narrowing. The absence of a paraspinal mass and the preservation of the adjacent vertebral body end plate helped to distinguish this lytic lesion from an infection.

Mixed lytic and sclerotic and purely sclerotic lesions were postulated to be the sequelae of fractures of the vertebral end plates, with subsequent disc degeneration and secondary vertebral sclerosis. The sclerosis was noted to involve a wide area in the anterior portion of the vertebral body at the location of the attachment of Sharpey's fibers into the vertebra. The anterior-inferior aspect of the vertebra (usually L4) was most often involved, and disc-space narrowing and anterior periosteal reaction were frequently present (Table 6–6).[73]

Thus, it would seem that degenerative changes in the disc may produce abnormal stress on the attachment of the adjacent soft tissue to bone and the subsequent sclerotic reaction. The associated lytic areas represent intravertebral disc herniation.[73] Mixed lesions may radiologically suggest the possibility of infection, but they

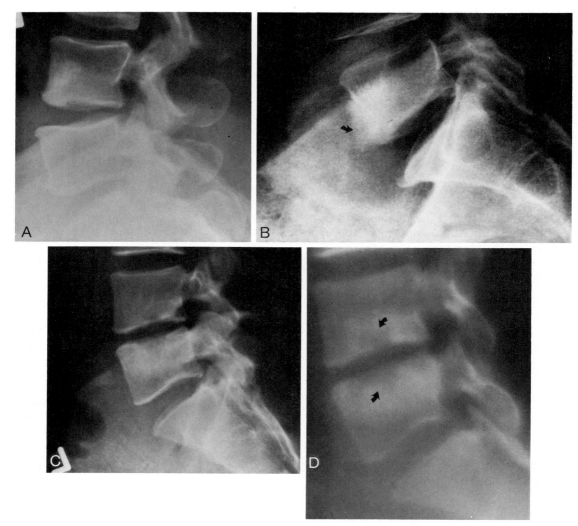

Figure 6–21. Various Examples of Discovertebral Sclerosis. *A,* A 39-year-old obese woman with a 14-year history of low back pain. Sclerosis is noted along the inferoanterior aspect of L4, and there is a little hypertrophic lipping anteriorly from L4 and L5. The L4–L5 disc space is mildly narrowed. There is mild retrolisthesis of L4 on L5. Bone and gallium scans were not consistent with active infection, and there has been no change in the appearance of the area in 1 year. A biopsy was nondiagnostic. *B,* A middle-aged male piano mover with low back pain. There is marked sclerosis of the anterior aspect of L5, with bone extending anteriorly (arrow). Small osteophytes are present. There was no clinical evidence of infection and a biopsy specimen grew no organisms. *C,* Young man with back pain. Lateral radiograph demonstrates disc narrowing and well-defined lucency centrally involving the adjacent end plates of L4 and L5. Notice that there is no destruction anteriorly. The radiographic features are however, worrisome since they suggest infection. *D,* Tomography confirms sclerosis and Schmorl's nodes (arrows). Biopsy showed no evidence of infection.

Table 6–6. **Typical Radiographic Features in Discogenic Vertebral Sclerosis**

Location of Sclerosis	Usually anterior third of vertebral body (79%)
	L4–5 (58%) or L5–S1 (26%)
	Adjacent aspects of both vertebrae involved (86%)
Associated Lucency	Central lucency (Schmorl's node) (75%)
Disc Abnormalities	Narrowed disc (100%)
	Vacuum disc (44%)
Hypertrophic Lipping Vertebral Body Height	Normal (100%)
Paraspinal Mass	Absent (100%)

Source: Sauser DD, Goldman AB, Kaye, JJ: J Can Assoc Radiol 29:44, 1978.

may be distinguished by absence of a paraspinal soft tissue mass, of clinical evidence of infection, and of progression of radiological findings. Resolution of sclerosis may be noted on follow-up radiographs. Although Williams and co-workers noted no elevation of the erythrocyte sedimentation rate, this finding was present in almost one fourth of patients with discogenic vertebral sclerosis studied by Sauser and colleagues.[73]

Osteophytes. Two types of osteophytes are recognized radiographically (Fig. 6–22). The first, called claw spondylophyte by Macnab, extends horizontally from the vertebral body several millimeters from its corner.[65] It then courses vertically across the disc space, sometimes joining a similar osteophyte arising from the adjacent vertebral body. This type of osteophyte is associated with prolapse of the anulus fibrosus, elevation of the anterior longitudinal ligament, and traction at the site of ligamentous attachment to the vertebral body.[52, 70] These osteophytes predominate on the anterior and lateral aspects of the spine. They are not related to degenerative disc disease nor are they associated with disc-space narrowing or vertebral sclerosis.

The second type of osteophyte (called a traction spur by Macnab) develops about 1 mm away from the corner of the vertebral body and projects horizontally.[65] These are usually small.

It is thought that they are caused by degenerative changes in the disc that allow abnormal motion to occur between vertebrae, producing a traction strain on the outermost fibers of the anulus fibrosus. Other findings of disc degeneration, including disc-space narrowing, reactive sclerosis, Schmorl's nodes, and vacuum phenomena, are the usual accompanying findings.

Differentiation of Osteophytes and Syndesmophytes. Osteophytes can be distinguished from the bony bridges, termed syndesmophytes by Forestier, that are seen in ankylosing spondylitis.[57] Syndesmophytes result from ossification of the anulus fibrosus and adjacent connective tissue. Therefore, the classic syndesmophyte extends from the "margin" (corner) of one vertebral body to the margin of the next vertebral body (Fig. 6–23).[68] Occasionally, ossification also occurs in the deep portions of the overlying anterior longitudinal ligament.[53] In contrast to syndesmophytes, osteophytes characteristically originate at right angles to the vertebral body, usually do not completely bridge the disc space, and consist of cortical and cancellous bone—the latter being continuous with the cancellous bone of the vertebral body.

Bony bridging in spondylitis. Several types of bony bridging have been described in patients with ankylosing spondylitis and the spondylitis accompanying inflammatory bowel disease, pso-

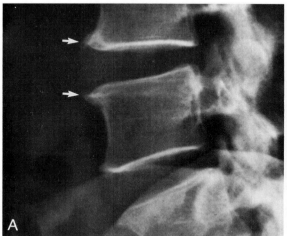

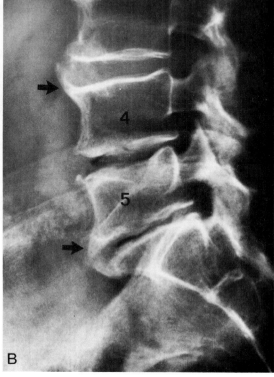

Figure 6–22. Osteophytes. *A,* Traction osteophytes. These small bony projections (arrows) arise just below the corners of the vertebrae and suggest abnormal motion at that level. *B,* Claw osteophytes. These large bony projections extend from the corners of vertebrae (arrows) and are associated with stretching of the anterior longitudinal ligament by a bulging anulus. Vacuum phenomena are noted at L4–L5 and L5–S1.

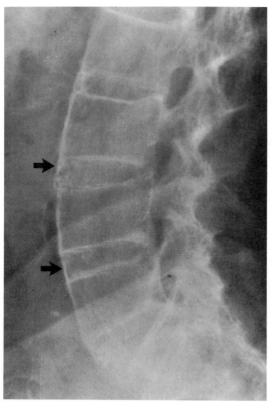

Figure 6–23. Ankylosing Spondylitis. This lateral view of a patient with late-stage ankylosing spondylitis demonstrates typical syndesmophytes (arrows) that extend between edges of the vertebral bodies. The facet joints are also fused.

riasis, and Reiter's syndrome. McEwen and associates analyzed the bony bridging in patients with these disorders and found that marginal bridging (syndesmophytes) occurs most frequently in ankylosing spondylitis and ulcerative colitis. Although similar marginal bridging predominated in patients with spondylitis accompanying psoriasis or Reiter's syndrome, nonmarginal bony bridging, comma-shaped excrescences, and bridging extending between the midportions of vertebral bodies and separated from the vertebrae by a clear space (Bywaters-Dickson syndesmophytes) were commonly seen in these disorders (Fig. 6–24). Approximately 25 percent of patients with spondylitis accompanying psoriasis or Reiter's syndrome had only the classic marginal syndesmophytes described for ankylosing spondylitis.[68]

Apophyseal Joint Changes. Degenerative changes in the apophyseal joints are accelerated by degenerative changes in the intervertebral disc. According to Harris and Macnab, the nucleus pulposus functions as a ball bearing, with the vertebral bodies rolling over the nucleus

during flexion. The posterior joints guide and steady the motion.[60] Disc degeneration leads to irregular, abnormal motion and sometimes to a shift of the axis of motion to the facet joints. These then develop the changes of osteoarthritis, with joint-space narrowing, sclerosis, and osteophytic lipping.

Subluxation of the posterior joints tends to occur as a consequence of the loss of height of the disc space (Fig. 6–25). This subluxation leads to further damage to the facet joints. The subluxation may be a relatively early finding in disc degeneration and can be identified on radiographs as follows.[60]

Lateral View. The tip of the superior facet will be seen to extend more than a few millimeters above the posterior inferior border of the vertebral body proximal to it. Thus a line drawn along the inferior aspect of the proximal vertebral body will intersect the middle of the superior facet rather than its tip.[65]

Anteroposterior View. As subluxation proceeds, the distance from the superior facet to the pedicle above diminishes, so that the tip of the facet may impinge on the pedicle above.

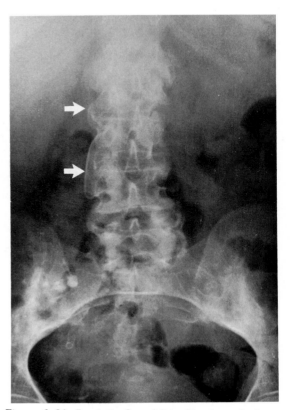

Figure 6–24. Psoriatic Spondylitis. The bony bridging (arrows) is asymmetrical and nonmarginal (i.e., it does not begin at the corners of the vertebrae). Bilateral sacroiliac involvement is present.

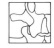

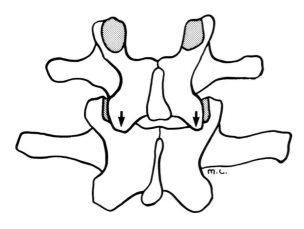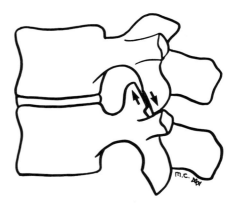

Figure 6–25. Facet Joint Subluxation Due to Disc Degeneration. Loss of height of the disc leads to facet joint damage and subluxation. (Redrawn from MacNab I: Backache. Baltimore, Williams & Wilkins, 1977.)

Oblique View. The subluxed facets will be seen to articulate with the adjacent laminae rather than with the facet, and a ridge of hypertrophic bone may form from the laminar surfaces.

Retrolisthesis. At the level of disc degeneration, the upper vertebral body may be subluxed downward and backward. This malposition tends to displace the nerve roots cranially, so that they may be compressed between the capsule of the facet joint and the superior articular facet of the lower vertebra.[60] This compression may be further increased by coincidental bulging of the disc owing to degenerative changes in the anulus.

Increased Flexion-Extension Motion. Disc degeneration allows abnormal amounts of flexion-extension motion to occur. This, along with anterior-posterior subluxation of the involved vertebrae, may be noted before disc narrowing is apparent.[60]

Relation of Radiological Findings of Disc Degeneration to Symptoms. Radiological evidence of disc degeneration is common. In a large population study, changes such as those noted previously were found in 65 percent of men and 52 percent of women over age 35.[63] Symptoms may occur with disc degeneration because of the damaged disc itself or, more commonly, from secondary effects on the paraspinal soft tissues, facet joints, and nerve roots.[60] However, Hussar and Guller studied 500 male hospital employees and were unable to demonstrate a positive correlation between the presence of back pain and the presence or severity of x-ray changes indicative of disc degeneration.[61] Most patients with these radiographic findings will be asymptomatic. In both the cervical and the lumbar areas, the presence of these x-ray findings becomes more frequent with increasing age. The L5–S1 disc space is involved earliest, but according to Macnab, seldom gives rise to prolonged symptoms.[65] The L4–L5 level is much more commonly responsible for pain.[65] Discography has been suggested for localization of symptoms to a specific degenerated disc and is thought to be particularly helpful if the patient's symptoms are recreated by disc distension with saline or contrast material.[65]

Disc Herniation

Definition

Disc herniation may be defined as the rupture of nuclear material through a tear in the anulus fibrosus.[77] The nuclear material may remain confined by the outermost fibers of the anulus (prolapse), or it may be extruded through the anulus, often posteriorly, with the fragment lying under the posterior longitudinal ligament or displaced through the posterior longitudinal ligament to lie within the spinal canal (a sequestered fragment) (Fig. 6–26).[87] Diffuse or localized bulging of a disc is differentiated from true disc herniation by the presence of intact anular fibers around the bulging disc.

Relevant Anatomy

Each lumbar nerve root leaves the dural sac at about the level of the intervertebral disc of the segment above.[85] An extension of the dura covers the roots and blends with them distally. The nerve exits through the foramen of the vertebra below. Thus the L4 nerve root passes under the pedicle of L4 and out of the foramen

ANTERIOR

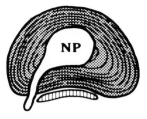

PROLAPSED   **EXTRUDED**   **SEQUESTRATED**

Figure 6–26. Disc Herniation. In all these circumstances the nucleus pulposus (NP) herniates through a tear in the anulus fibrosus. In prolapse the outermost fibers of the anulus remain intact, whereas in an extruded disc the outer anular fibers are disrupted. In sequestration a fragment of the disc is displaced into the spinal canal. (Modified from MacNab I: Backache. Baltimore, Williams & Wilkins, 1977.)

between L4 and L5. The nerve actually occupies only the upper half of the neural foramen (see Fig. 6–4).[85]

In 1934 Mixter and Barr published their historic article in which nerve root compression was documented to be caused by herniation of nuclear material through the anulus fibrosus.[89] There are, however, other causes of nerve root compression, including kinking of the nerve root as it exits under the pedicle, compression by osteophytes from the posterior aspects of the vertebral bodies or facet joints, subluxation of the facet joints, and congenital or acquired spinal stenosis. Of interest is the observation that pressure on a peripheral nerve produces paresthesias, rather than pain. It has been suggested that the pain seen with disc herniation is the result of a secondary inflammatory reaction that occurs around the nerve root.[87] Most disc herniations occur at the L4–L5 or L5–S1 levels.[82] Disc herniation at the L5–S1 level usually compresses the S1 nerve root, whereas herniation at L4–L5

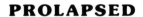

Figure 6–27. Disc Herniation. Often an L4–L5 disc herniation will compress the L5 root; an L5–S1 herniation will compress the S1 root. (Modified from MacNab I: Backache. Baltimore, Williams & Wilkins, 1977.)

usually compresses the L5 root (Figs. 6–27 and 6–28).[87]

Plain Film Examination

This examination is more important for eliminating other causes of low back pain than for identifying disc herniation.[82] Identification of disc narrowing does not necessarily indicate that this is the site of disc herniation, and, conversely, disc herniation often occurs with a normal disc space. Review of the plain films of 300 instances of disc herniation showed no abnormality in 65 percent of patients.[82] The L5–S1 interspace was narrowed in 16 percent of patients with disc herniation at that level and in 45 percent of L4–L5 disc herniations. In 15 percent of patients with L5–S1 disc herniation, the L4 interspace appeared narrow.

Computed Tomography

Normal Examination. Technological improvements in computed tomography have made possible the identification of the dural sac and adjacent structures. The availability of a scout lateral view allows the scan to be angled along the disc space or spaces of interest. Computed tomograms that are not parallel to the disc may give an erroneous impression of disc herniation.[84]

Normally, computed tomograms through the level of the disc show the dural sac and the ligamentum flavum. At the L4–L5 level the posterior margin of the disc is slightly concave. There is almost no epidural fat between the disc and the dural sac in the midline, but epidural fat is seen laterally. The nerve roots are not usually identified at the level of the L4–L5 disc.[93] At L5–S1 there is considerable epidural fat around the dural sac, with fat filling the space between the disc and the dural sac. The S1 nerve roots are easily seen (Fig. 6–29).

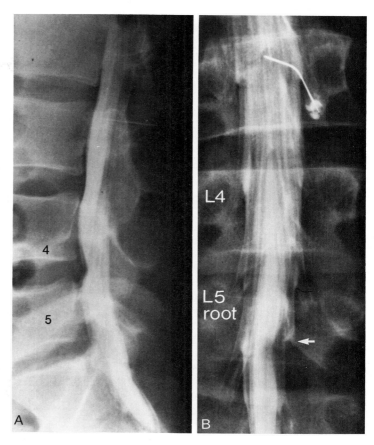

Figure 6–28. Herniated L5–S1 Disc: Metrizamide Myelogram. A 35-year-old man having a 5-year history of low back pain with intermittent exacerbations. *A,* Lateral view shows a ventral impression on the contrast at the L4–L5 level caused by a bulging disc. *B,* Frontal view shows no abnormality at L4–L5. At L5–L1 on the left there is an extradural defect with compression of the left S1 nerve root (arrow). An L5–S1 herniated disc was proved at surgery.

Computed Tomographic Findings in Cases of Disc Herniation. As summarized by Williams, Carrera, and their colleagues, the following findings may be seen with disc herniation.[77, 93]

1. Abnormal posterior disc margin with displacement of epidural fat
2. Indentation on the dural sac
3. Calcification within the posterior disc protrusion
4. Compression or displacement of nerve-root sleeves
5. A free disc (soft tissue) fragment
6. Displacement of the dural sac by soft tissues.

Displacement of epidural fat by the posterior disc margin and indentation on the dural sac are the most frequently seen findings (Fig. 6–30).[93] Bulging discs usually exhibit circumferential, symmetrical displacement of the disc margin, whereas a herniated disc is characterized by a focal, usually asymmetrical, bulge in the disc contour.[83] Comparison studies of myelography and CT have been done.[83, 90] Haughton and associates found that CT demonstrates lumbar-disc herniation as well as does myelography.

Laminectomy for Removal of Prolapsed Intervertebral Disc

Surgical Procedure (Fig. 6–31). In order to see the posterior aspect of the disc, an opening is made in the ligamentum flavum. The opening is then usually enlarged by removal of the inferior part of the lamina above. In some cases the entire lamina or both laminae and the spinous process may be removed. The dural sac is then gently displaced medially in order that the nerve root and any prolapsed or extruded disc material can be seen. If the disc material has not extruded through the posterior longitudinal ligament, this ligament is incised, and the degenerated disc material is then removed. If the disc herniation is central, rather than posterolateral, incision of the dural sac may be necessary. Central herniations occur in 5 to 12 percent of patients.[93]

Complications.[87] Failure to relieve sciatic pain may be the result of (1) incorrect preoperative diagnosis in which, for example, nerve root entrapment has been overlooked; or (2) technical failures, such as the failure to remove a sequestered fragment or the incomplete removal

305

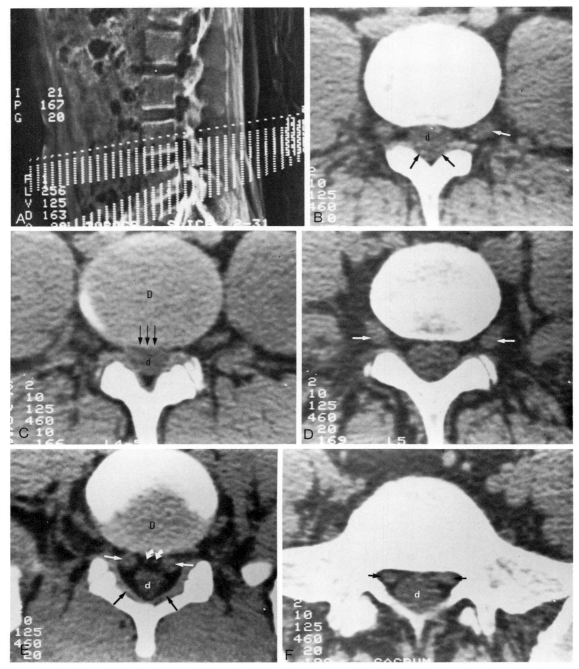

Figure 6–29. Normal Disc Anatomy on CT. *A,* Scout view. The chosen sections (dashed lines) can be planned and angled along the plane of the discs. *B,* CT scan through the L4 vertebral body shows the neural foramina and the L4 nerve root ganglia (white arrow on left ganglion). The dural sac (d) and ligamenta flava (black arrows) are shown. *C,* CT scan through the L4–L5 disc (D) shows very little fat between the posterior margin of the disc (arrows) and the dural sac (d). The nerve roots are not clearly seen. *D,* CT scan through the L5 vertebral body and foramina shows the L5 nerve root ganglia (arrows). *E,* CT scan through the L5–S1 disc (D) space shows the L5 nerve roots (arrows), the dural sac (d), and the ligamenta flava (black arrows). Small epidural veins are noted (curved arrows). *F,* At the S1 level the S1 nerve roots (arrows) and dural sac (d) are well seen.

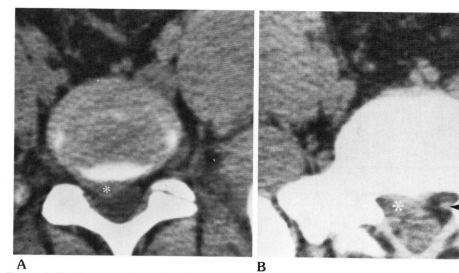

A　　　　　　　　　　　　**B**

Figure 6–30. Herniated Disc with Nerve Root Compression. *A,* Computed tomogram through L5–S1 disc shows a localized bulge of disc material (asterisk) posteriorly compressing the thecal sac. *B,* At the S1 level the normal left S1 nerve root is seen (arrow), but the right nerve root is compressed by soft tissue (herniated disc; asterisk).

of degenerated disc material, so that extrusion of more disc material occurs postoperatively.

Sciatic pain may recur postoperatively because of (1) recurrent disc herniation, usually at another level; (2) marked disc narrowing following surgery, causing bony compression of the nerve root; or (3) development of fibrosis around the dural sac, the nerve roots, or both.

Radiographic Findings
Plain Film Findings. Plain film findings after laminectomy are often minimal. The surgical defect in the lamina is frequently difficult to see because of the small amount of cortical bone removed.

Computed Tomography. Computed tomography allows the preoperative diagnosis to be more complete and accurate, thus helping to avoid an incorrect or incomplete preoperative diagnosis. Computed tomography may also define postoperative complications, including the presence of soft tissue (fibrous tissue or disc material) compressing a nerve root or the bony compression of a nerve root.

Spinal Fusion
Surgical Procedures. There are three basic types of fusion: intertransverse, posterior, and anterior intervertebral.

Intertransverse Fusion (Fig. 6–32). There are several modifications of this procedure. In one method grafts are fashioned to fit between the transverse processes of the segments to be fused.[75] An alternative procedure involves placing bone graft along the prepared surfaces of the posterior lateral aspects of the facet joints and laminae as well as along the transverse processes.[88]

Posterior Fusion. The *Hibbs fusion* consists of removal of the spinous processes, excision of

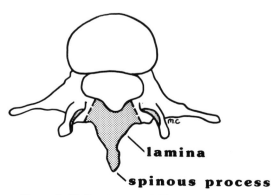
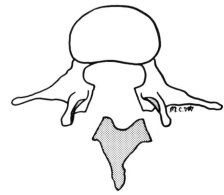

Figure 6–31. Laminectomy. The spinous process and laminae are removed. The facet joints remain intact.

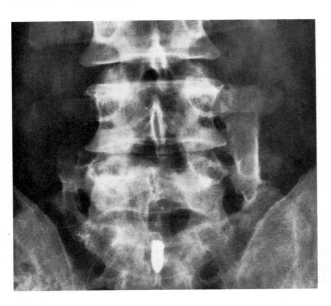

Figure 6–32. Intertransverse Fusion. Bone graft unites the left L4–L5 and the right L5 transverse processes to the sacrum. Laminectomy and posterior fusion have also been done (best seen on lateral and oblique views).

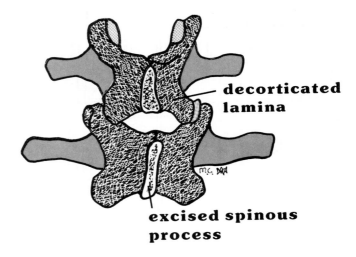

decorticated lamina

excised spinous process

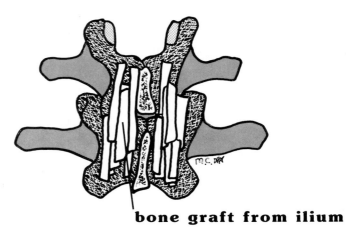

Figure 6–33. Posterior Fusion. The spinous processes are removed, the facet joints excised, and the laminae denuded of cortical bone. Bone graft is placed over the prepared surfaces.

bone graft from ilium

the facet joints, and scraping of the laminae, followed by interdigitation of a number of small bone slivers that are raised from the laminae, spinous processes, and articular facets.[80] Additional bone graft may be added (Fig. 6–33).

The *Albee fusion* involves uniting the spinous processes, using graft obtained from the tibia.[10]

Anterior Intervertebral Fusion. With this technique an attempt is made to fuse the vertebral bodies by placing blocks of cancellous bone between the vertebrae after the discs have been removed and the vertebral end plates have been resected and shaped to receive the graft.[75]

Complications of Fusion

Pseudarthrosis. The incidence of pseudarthrosis varies, depending on the operator and the technique used. Fusion of two vertebrae (single-segment fusion) is more likely to be successful than is more extensive fusion.[88] Pseudarthrosis is less common in fusion for disc degeneration than in that for spondylolisthesis.[88] Comparison of techniques for two-segment fusion (L4–S1) in patients with degenerative disc

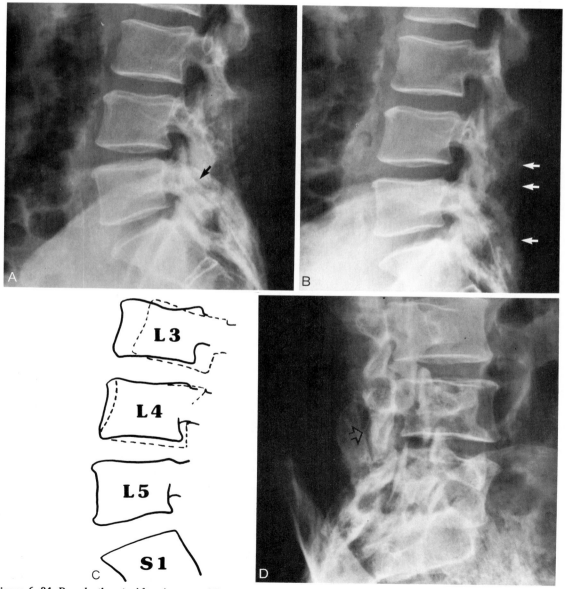

Figure 6–34. Pseudarthrosis After Attempted Posterior Fusion of L3 to Sacrum. *A,* Lateral view in extension shows the posterior fusion mass without definite defect but with apparently open facets at L4–L5 (arrow). *B,* Flexion view. The graft (arrows) looks solid. *C,* Superimposition of flexion and extension views demonstrates motion occurring at the L4–L5 level, thus documenting a pseudarthrosis. *D,* Oblique view shows a defect in the fusion mass (arrow).

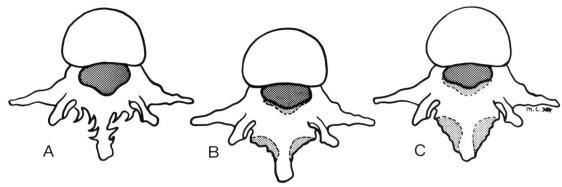

Figure 6–35. Narrowing of Spinal Canal After Posterior Fusion. *A,* For posterior fusion the posterior aspects of the laminae and spinous processes are feathered (and bone graft is applied). *B,* With healing there is overgrowth of the inner as well as the outer surfaces of the laminae (lightly stippled areas). *C,* Narrowing of the spinal canal may become significant. (Redrawn from MacNab I: Backache. Baltimore, Williams & Wilkins, 1977.)

disease showed that pseudarthrosis developed in 30 percent of anterior interbody fusions, 17 percent of posterior fusions, and 7 percent of intertransverse fusions.[88]

Pseudarthrosis may be difficult to demonstrate radiographically, and when demonstrated, it may or may not be the cause of pain.[87] Lateral views in flexion and extension may help to detect motion at the site of attempted fusion (Fig. 6–34). Tomography can demonstrate areas at which the bone graft is discontinuous, and, if necessary, tomography in the lateral projection in both flexion and extension will show movement at the level of the pseudarthrosis. Documentation of progressive deformity indicates pseudarthrosis. Computed tomography with direct coronal images may be helpful. Technetium bone scanning may show increased uptake at the site of a pseudarthrosis.

According to Macnab, discography at the level of a pseudarthrosis will be painful, whereas when pseudarthrosis is not present, the injection of contrast is painless. The reported accuracy of this procedure is about 80 percent.[87]

Root Compression (Iatrogenic Spinal Stenosis). Decortication and grafting of the laminae at the time of posterior fusion may lead to overgrowth of the internal as well as the external aspects of the laminae, sometimes compromising the spinal canal (Figs. 6–35 and 6–36).[81, 86, 87] This can be detected on computed tomography.[91]

Ruptured Disc. Disc rupture is uncommon under a solid spine fusion, but a ruptured disc may accompany pseudarthrosis.

Spondylolysis. Several cases have been reported in which spondylolysis has developed above or below the site of an otherwise successful spinal fusion.[76, 78, 80] These defects presumably represent fractures through areas in

which stress is increased as a consequence of the fusion. Spondylolysis was seen in about 1 percent of cases of two- and three-segment spinal fusions performed for degenerative disc

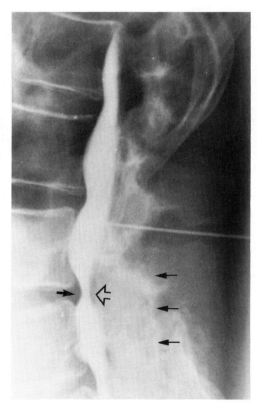

Figure 6–36. Spinal Stenosis Due to Bulging Discs and (Possibly Hypertophied) Posterior Bone Graft. A 53-year-old woman with prior laminectomy, excision of a herniated disc, and L4–sacrum fusion. After many years without symptoms, left leg and back pain occurred. Lateral view during myelography shows the narrowing of the spinal canal at L3–L4 as a result of graft material posteriorly (open arrow) and bulging discs anteriorly (closed arrow). Small arrows indicate bone graft.

disease or spondylolisthesis.[2, 87] It is, however, not seen after intertransverse fusions since the graft in that type of fusion includes and supports the area of the pars interarticularis.[87]

Spondylolisthesis

Spondylolisthesis refers to an abnormal sliding of one vertebral body over the next. The word is derived from the Greek *spondylos,* meaning *vertebra,* and *olisthanein,* meaning *to slip.*[97] Spondylolysis refers to a defect in the pars interarticularis (isthmus), which may be unilateral or bilateral and may or may not be accompanied by spondylolisthesis.

Classification

Wiltse and associates noted five types of spondylolisthesis that are summarized as follows:[120]

Dysplastic—resulting from congenital dysplasia of the upper sacrum or the L5 neural arch.

Isthmic—caused by an abnormality of the pars interarticularis.

Degenerative—resulting from disc degeneration and secondary segmental instability.

Traumatic—caused by severe trauma with fracture of the posterior elements—usually the pedicles or the facets—or from facet dislocation. Acute traumatic fractures of the pars interarticularis are rare.[104]

Pathological—a result of localized or generalized bone disease involving the pars, the pedicles, or the articular facets (e.g., osteomalacia, Paget's disease).

In adults, the isthmic and the degenerative forms are most commonly encountered.

Isthmic Spondylolisthesis

The term *isthmic spondylolisthesis* is used by Wiltse and co-workers to indicate spondylolisthesis caused by abnormalities in the pars interarticularis (the isthmus), including (1) elongation and attenuation of the pars, (2) lytic defects in the pars, and (3) acute fractures of the pars.[120] Other authors use this term to refer only to the first subgroup and the term *spondylolytic spondylolisthesis* to refer to the second subgroup.[104] Elongation of the pars interarticularis may either precede[104] or result from[119] spondylolysis.

In spondylolytic spondylolisthesis the defect in the pars is thought to be the primary abnormality. Numerous theories have been advanced regarding the pathogenesis of this defect. Since both halves of the neural arch develop from one ossification center, failure of ossification centers to unite is an implausible theory. A familial tendency has been noted, and it is thought most likely that the etiology of the defect is twofold, resulting from a hereditary predisposition and from superimposed strain, producing a stress fracture.[98, 101, 109, 110, 114, 118, 119]

It is interesting to note that spondylolysis does not occur in the newborn but first appears in childhood, with spondylolisthesis usually occurring between the ages of 10 and 15[104] and usually stabilizing by the age of 20.[119] About 50 percent of children with spondylolysis will develop spondylolisthesis.[119]

Preemployment radiographic examination of 32,600 men between the ages of 18 and 35 has disclosed a 7.2 percent incidence of spondylolysis.[108] Seventy-four percent of the defects were bilateral, and the last lumbar vertebra was involved in 91.2 percent of cases. The incidence of this defect varies depending on race; consequently, one study reports an incidence of 6.4 percent in white males, compared with 2.8 percent in black males, and an incidence of 2.3 percent in white females, compared with 1.1 percent in black females.[113] A 26.3 percent incidence of these defects has been found in Alaskan skeletal remains.[116]

Pathological studies have shown fibrous tissue or fibrocartilage bridging the area of spondylolysis,[100, 119] and when the edges of the defect are close together, a hyaline cartilage pseudarthrosis may be noted.[119] There is no evidence of callus to support the currently popular theory of a stress fracture.[116, 119]

Radiographic Findings. Radiographic findings are of two types: one, the demonstration of the spondylolysis, and two, the demonstration of the spondylolisthesis.

Spondylolysis (Fig. 6–37). The defect in the pars interarticularis can often be seen on the lateral radiograph. Oblique views may show this defect to advantage and in some cases the oblique views are the only ones that demonstrate a spondylolysis.[96, 112] Lateral views in flexion may show widening of the pars defect (instability) as compared with similar films in extension. On the side opposite a unilateral pars defect, increased sclerosis, presumably in response to the increased stress placed on the intact side, has been observed (Fig. 6–38).[115, 117] Rotation of the posterior elements occurs, with the result that the spinous process of the involved vertebra appears to have shifted away from the side of a unilateral spondylolytic defect or, in the case of bilateral pars defects,[111, 105] to have shifted away from the more separated side. This deviation of the spinous process may suggest the appropriate diagnosis on the AP radiograph.

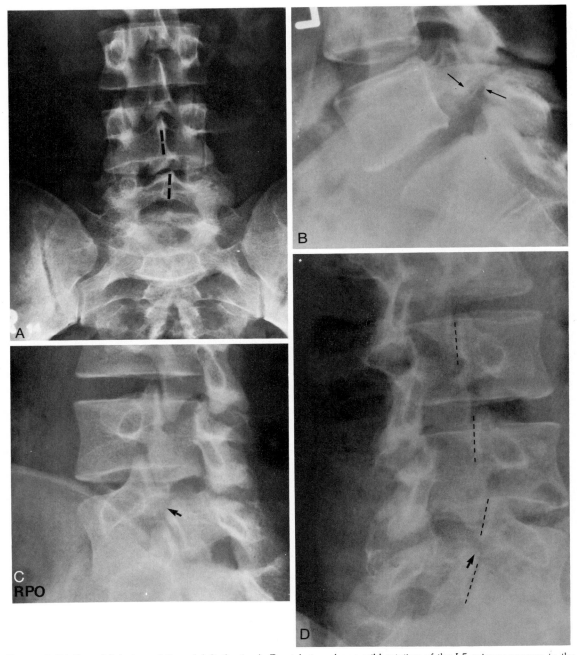

Figure 6–37. Spondylolysis and Spondylolisthesis. *A,* Frontal view shows mild rotation of the L5 spinous process to the left (dashed lines on L4 and L5 spinous processes). *B,* Lateral view confirms grade 1 spondylolisthesis of L5 on S1. The bilateral spondylolytic defects of L5 are well seen on this view (arrows). *C, D,* Oblique views clearly demonstrate the areas of spondylolysis (arrows) and the malalignment of the facet joints (dashed lines).

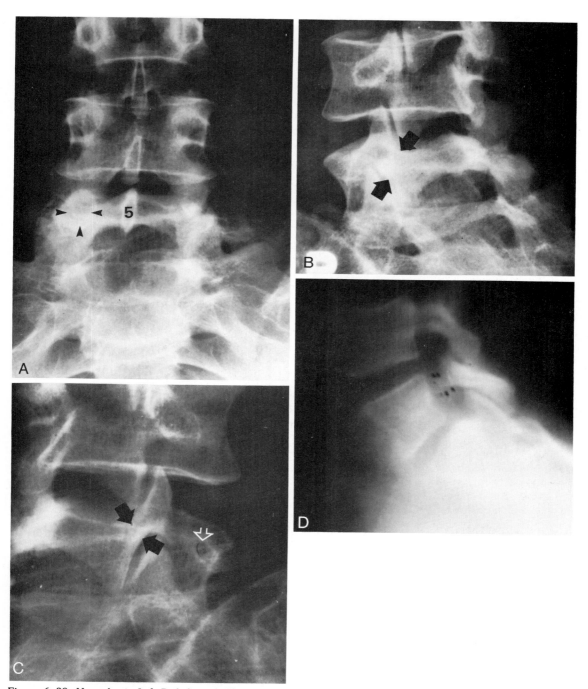

Figure 6–38. Hypoplastic Left Pedicle with Hypertrophy of the Contralateral Pedicle. *A*, AP view shows increased density of the right pedicle and of L5 (arrowheads) and no visible left pedicle; 5 = L5 spinous process. *B*, Right posterior oblique view shows sclerosis of the inferior portion of the right pedicle and of the pars interarticularis (arrows indicate the latter). *C*, Left posterior oblique view shows an intact pars interarticularis (arrows) and a small left pedicle (white arrow). *D*, Tomogram shows only a small ossicle in the expected location of the left pedicle (whiskers).

THE LUMBAR SPINE

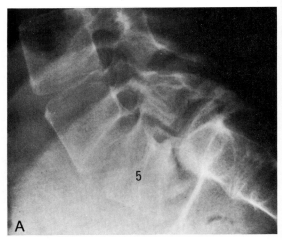

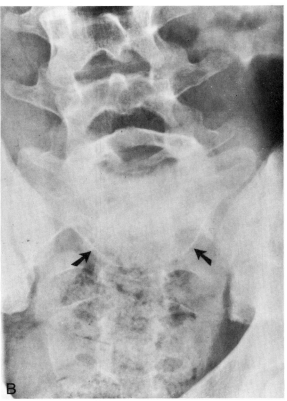

Figure 6–39. Grade 4 Spondylolisthesis with "Gendarme's Hat" Sign. *A,* A 21-year-old man. Lateral view demonstrates the grade 4 spondylolisthesis of L5 on S1, with chronic changes of sclerosis and rounding of the adjacent vertebral margins. *B,* Frontal view. The subluxed body of L5 produces an appearance similar to an inverted Napoleon's or gendarme's, hat. (From Sarokhan CT, Weisman BNW: Consultant, December 1981.)

One case has been reported in which arthrography of the L4–L5 facet joint demonstrated a previously unsuspected spondylytic defect in the pars of the lower vertebra.[99]

Spondylolisthesis. Spondylolisthesis is usually apparent on lateral views. The posterior margin of the vertebral body is noted to be displaced anteriorly in relation to the posterior margin of the subjacent vertebra. The vertebral body and the spine above the level of the pars defect are displaced forward, while the inferior facets, laminae, spinous process, and subjacent vertebrae are not displaced (Fig. 6–39). The amount of subluxation can be expressed as a percentage of the articular surface of the lower vertebra.[102] Meyerding divided the end plate of the lower vertebra into four equal parts. The degree of subluxation was termed grade 1 if the posterior portion of the anteriorly displaced vertebra was slipped forward by less than one fourth of the end-plate surface. In grade 2 the slip amounts to between one fourth and one half of the lower vertebral surface, and so on (Fig. 6–40).[107] In some cases spondylolisthesis is just apparent or noted to be increased on lateral films taken with the patient standing as compared with lateral films taken with the patient

supine.[102, 106] The oblique view will confirm malalignment of the facets.[94]

The significance of the radiographic demonstration of spondylolisthesis varies. The condi-

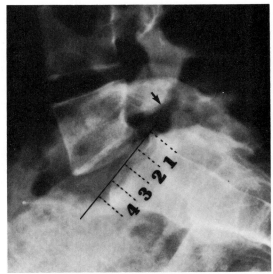

Figure 6–40. Meyerding Grading of Spondylolisthesis. The degree of spondylolisthesis can be graded by noting the position of the posterior aspect of the slipped vertebra in relation to the superior surface of the lower vertebra. This is a grade 1 spondylolisthesis. The spondylolytic defects are apparent (arrow).

tion may be entirely asymptomatic. When back pain is present at the level of a spondylolysis, spondylolisthesis, or both, the pain may be a result of instability at the spondylolysis; nerve root compression at, or distal to, the foramen; or disc degeneration.[104] Disc herniation above or below the slip, disc degeneration above the slip, or totally unrelated disorders may also produce pain. In patients with back pain spondylolisthesis has been noted in 18.9 percent of patients under age 25, 7.6 percent of patients 26 to 39, and 5.2 percent of patients over age 40.[104] Comparison of these findings with the approximately 6 percent incidence of spondylolysis in the North American Caucasian population led Macnab to conclude: "If the x-ray of a patient with back pain shows a spondylolisthesis, and if the patient is under 26 the defect is probably the cause of the symptoms; between 26 and 40 it is only possibly the cause; over 40

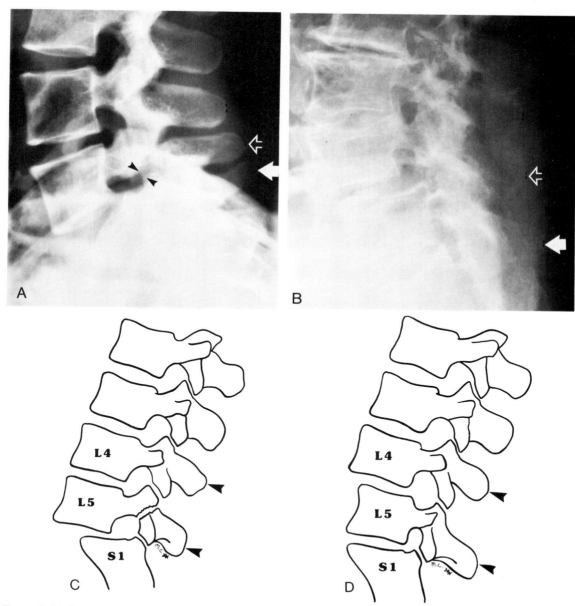

Figure 6–41. Spinous Process Sign. *A*, Spondylolytic spondylolisthesis. The spinous process of the involved vertebra (open arrow) remains in normal alignment in relation to the spinous process below (closed arrow). The spondylolysis is seen (arrowheads). *B*, Degenerative (pseudo-) spondylolisthesis. The spinous process of the involved vertebra (open arrow) is shifted anteriorly in relation to the one below (closed arrow). *C*, Spondylolytic spondylolisthesis. Note the lack of forward displacement of the L5 spinous process. *D*, Degenerative spondylolisthesis. Note the forward displacement of the L4 spinous process and those above in comparison with the L5 spinous process (arrowheads).

it is rarely, if ever, the sole cause of symptoms."[104]

Degenerative
(Pseudo-) Spondylolisthesis

The terms *degenerative* and *pseudo-* spondylolisthesis refer to anterior subluxation of one vertebral body on the vertebra below as a consequence of degenerative disease in the intervening disc and facets. Normally, the axis of flexion-extension motion passes through the nucleus pulposus.[103] When disc degeneration occurs, the axis of motion shifts posteriorly to the facet joints, allowing abnormal motion at these joints. It is postulated that such abnormal rocking motion eventually leads to degenerative changes in the facets, which in turn lead to vertebral subluxation. The anterior displacement finally becomes fixed because of increasing facet deformity with a more horizontal orientation to the facet joints than normal.

Degenerative spondylolisthesis is not uncommon. It is seen most frequently at the L4–L5 level, especially in women over the age of 50, and is not seen in patients under 40.[104] The degree of subluxation is usually minor, seldom greater than 30 percent.[120]

Back pain may occur as a result of the abnormal motion and facet joint damage. Nerve-root entrapment may be a consequence of the subluxation, of bulging of the anulus fibrosus at the involved level, of redundancy of the ligamentum flavum, or of osteophytic lipping from the facet joint margins.[104]

Radiographic Findings. As in spondylolytic spondylolisthesis, in degenerative spondylolisthesis a vertebra slips anteriorly over the one below. In contrast to the findings in spondylolytic spondylolisthesis, however, no defect in the pars interarticularis is demonstrable in patients with degenerative spondylolisthesis. Evaluation of the relative positions of the spinous processes may be helpful: in degenerative spondylolisthesis the spinous process is shifted anteriorly along with the vertebral body, whereas in "true" (spondylolytic) spondylolisthesis the spinous process remains normally positioned while the superior articular facets, pedicles, and vertebral body are displaced anteriorly (Fig. 6–41).[95] Narrowing, sclerosis, and osteophytic lipping are often present in the facet joints. The angle between the inferior articular process and the pedicle is said to be increased (normally it is 90 degrees) as a consequence of degenerative joint disease.[103] The findings of disc degeneration (disc-space narrowing, osteophytic lipping, and vertebral sclerosis) are also present.

Facet Arthropathy

Facet joint abnormalities may be responsible for back pain, sciatica,* or both.[126] Standard radiographic examination is inadequate for tracing the source of pain to these joints, since radiographs often show degenerative changes in asymptomatic individuals, and, conversely, normal radiographs may be found in symptomatic patients. Computed tomography aids greatly in the evaluation of these joints.[123]

Injection of local anesthetic and corticosteroids into the facet joints may be done for diagnostic and therapeutic purposes. Arthrography may be performed in conjunction with such injection, particularly to confirm needle placement and to define the location of injected anesthetic.[121, 122, 124, 125] Since the normal facet joint capsule accommodates only a few ml of fluid, injection of more than 3 to 5 ml invariably leads to capsular rupture, usually from the inferior recess. Most of the injected material actually enters the adjacent soft tissues, including the epidural space or the foramina.

Injection of the facet joints is accomplished fairly easily with fluoroscopic monitoring. In some cases the facet joints are curved, and the posterior portions may lie within the sagittal plane, making them visible on the frontal radiograph (Fig. 6–42). The anterior portion of the joint is best seen on the oblique views. Since

---

*Low back pain radiating to one leg along the course of the sciatic nerve.

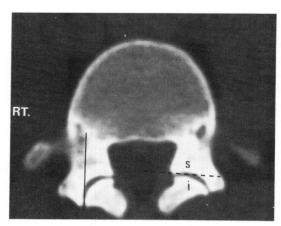

Figure 6–42. Facet Joint Orientation. Computed tomogram through the L5 vertebra and pedicles and the L4–L5 facet joints demonstrates the relatively horizontal orientation of the anterior aspect of these joints (dashed line) in comparison with the vertical alignment of the posterior portion of the joints (solid line). The posterior part of the right facet joint would optimally be seen on a straight posteroanterior (or anteroposterior) radiograph rather than on an oblique projection; i = inferior facet of L4, s = superior facet of L5.

the posterior portion is the portion to be injected, positioning in or near the prone position is optimal. Thus, if the facet joints are well seen on the straight frontal view, then this position should be used for injection. If the joints are best seen in the oblique projection, then the patient should be placed in the least rotated position possible for needle placement.[125]

Spinal Stenosis

Classification

The term *spinal stenosis* is a general one, referring to any soft tissue or bony abnormality that narrows the spinal canal, nerve root canals, or intervertebral foramina.[130] Spinal stenosis is classified according to cause as follows:[130]

Congenital Stenosis
    Idiopathic
    Achondroplastic
Acquired Stenosis
    Degenerative
        Central portion of the spinal canal
        Lateral portion of the spinal canal
        Degenerative spondylolisthesis
    Combined—any combination of congenital, degenerative, and disc herniations
    Spondylolytic, spondylolisthetic
    Iatrogenic
        Postlaminectomy
        Postfusion
        Postchemonucleolysis
    Post-traumatic
    Miscellaneous
        Paget's disease
        Fluorosis

Clinical Picture

Patients with spinal stenosis generally have a long history of back pain. Two major clinical presentations are noted: narrow lumbar canal syndrome with neurogenic claudication; and narrow radicular canal syndrome with root pain.[127] Neurogenic claudication refers to pain

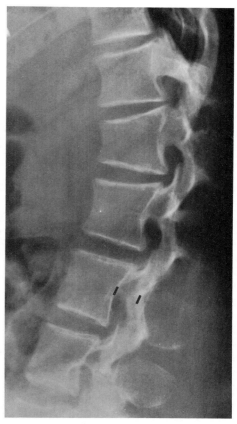

Figure 6–43. Achondroplasia. The typical short pedicles are evident on this lateral view. This, combined with a small interpediculate distance, thickened laminae, and bulging intervertebral discs, decreases the size of the spinal canal. A method of measuring the AP diameter of the spinal canal as the distance from the posterior aspect of the vertebra to the spinous process is shown.

and paresthesias that occur in the legs with walking. Whereas vascular claudication is relieved by stopping the activity, neurogenic claudication is relieved, not by standing still, but by flexing the spine, as in sitting. Patients with neurogenic claudication typically can walk uphill more easily than down and can bicycle, since these are activities in which the spine is flexed. Bowel and bladder symptoms may occur. In

Table 6–7. **Plain Film and Tomographic Findings Indicating a Narrow Lumbar Canal**

Projection	Finding
Lateral	Narrow sagittal diameter of spinal canal
	Narrow foramina
	Short pedicles
	Narrow lateral recess
AP	Small interpediculate distance
	Hypertrophy of pedicles
	Visibility of too many facet joints
	Inferior articular processes too near midline

Source: Epstein BS, Epstein JA, Jones MD: Radiol Clin North Am 15:227, 1977.

Table 6–8. **CT Findings in Spinal Stenosis**

Sagittal diameter of canal	Definite narrowing: < 10 mm Borderline narrowing: 10 to 15 mm
Lateral recess	No stenosis: > than 5 mm Possible stenosis: 3 to 5 mm Definite stenosis: ≤ 3 mm
Trefoil configuration of spinal canal	

contrast to lower lumbar disc herniations, straight leg raising is usually normal, and root involvement occurs at multiple levels.

Radicular pain due to degenerative spinal stenosis generally affects individuals over age 50. Disc herniation is the most common cause of radicular pain in patients under age 50.[130]

Macnab has classified nerve-root entrapment syndromes occurring with degenerative disease into several categories based on the location of root compression.[131] Central stenosis, subarticular stenosis (lateral recess syndrome), foraminal narrowing, and pedicular kinking are differentiated.

Radiological Findings

Radiological findings depend on the type and the location of the abnormality (Table 6–7).

Congenital Spinal Stenosis. Congenital spinal stenosis is typified by the changes of achondroplasia, in which premature fusion and abnormal endochondral bone formation result in thick neural arches, narrowed interpediculate distances, and a trefoil configuration of the spinal canal, demonstrable on computed tomography (Fig. 6–43). The anteroposterior diameter of the spinal canal is normally greater than 15 mm.[128] A diameter of 10 to 15 mm is suggestive of narrowing, and a diameter of less than 10 mm

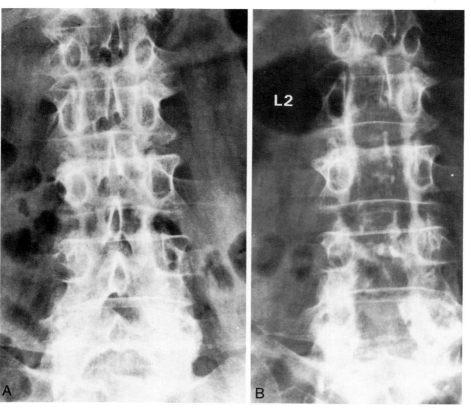

Figure 6–44. Laminectomy. A, Frontal radiograph of patient with degenerative spinal stenosis. B, A postoperative film shows the extensive decompression, with removal of laminae and spinous processes from L2 to L5.

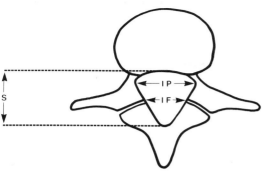

Figure 6–45. Canal Measurement with CT. The interpediculate (IP), interfacet (IF), and sagittal (S) diameters of the spinal canal can be measured with CT. (Redrawn from Lee BCP, Kazam E, Newman AD: Radiology 128:95, 1978.)

as the shortest midline perpendicular distance from the vertebral body to the inner surface of the neural arch.[128, 131] Surgical observation has led to the conclusion that a sagittal diameter of less than 10 mm indicates absolute spinal stenosis and that 10 to 12 mm indicates relative stenosis.[133] If these figures are to be applied to radiographic studies, correction for magnification must be made by dividing the measured number by the magnification factor (up to 1.15 to 1.20) (see Table 6–2).

The shape of the spinal canal can be better assessed by CT examination (Fig. 6–45).[132, 135] Normally, the spinal canal changes in configuration from from an oval to a triangular or trefoil shape, and the interfacet and interpediculate distances increase from more cranial to more caudal levels. The sagittal and transverse diameters of the spinal canal (Table 6–8),[135] and any hypertrophic lipping from the facets or the vertebral bodies that may produce focal narrowing can be evaluated on CT.

Lateral-Recess Narrowing. The lateral recess is the space bounded posteriorly by the superior articular facet and the lamina, laterally by the pedicle, and anteriorly by the vertebral body and the adjacent disc (see Fig. 6–6).[132, 135] The recess is normally more shallow at the L5 and S1 levels than at the upper levels. The most frequent site of abnormal narrowing is at L5, where the superior facet of L5 narrows the recess at the level of the upper border of the pedicle, compressing the L5 root and sometimes the S1 root as well.

It is often difficult to evaluate lateral-recess narrowing on a standard lateral radiograph. Polytomography in the lateral projection allows accurate measurement of the space between the

indicates definite narrowing (see Table 6–2).[131, 133] On the midsagittal lateral tomogram, the diameter of the canal is measured at the same level from the most anterior aspect of the neural arch to the back of the vertebral body along a line perpendicular to the long axis of the spinal canal.[127] The result is divided by the magnification factor.

Degenerative Spinal Stenosis. Advancing disc degeneration and its sequelae may result either in central compression of the cauda equina or in more lateral nerve-root compression.[130] These changes may be further compromise an already congenitally narrow spinal cord.

Routine radiographs show the changes of disc degeneration, including disc-space narrowing, facet joint damage, retrolisthesis, and spondylolisthesis (pseudospondylolisthesis) (Fig. 6–44). However, such findings are frequent and are commonly seen in asymptomatic individuals. The AP diameter of the spinal canal is measured

Figure 6–46. Lateral Recess. The depth of the lateral recess (dashed line) is measured from the posterior aspect of the vertebral body to the anteromedial aspect of the superior facet at the level of the superior border of the pedicle.

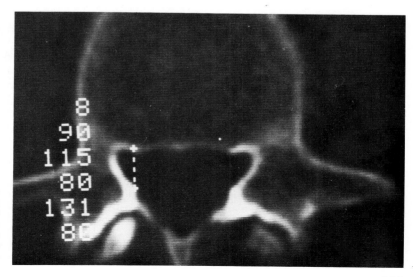

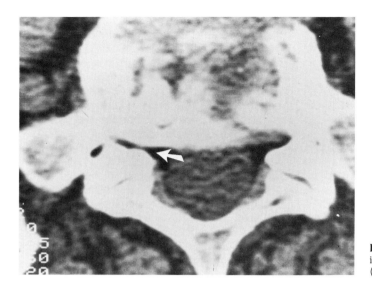

Figure 6–47. Lateral Recess Stenosis. There is marked narrowing of the right lateral recess (arrow).

most anterior portion of the superior facet and the posterior border of the spinal canal at the level of the superior margin of the pedicle. Measurement of the depth of the lateral recess can accurately be done on computed tomograms (Fig. 6–46). Definite stenosis is said to be present if the recess is less than, or equal to, 3 mm; possible stenosis is present if the recess

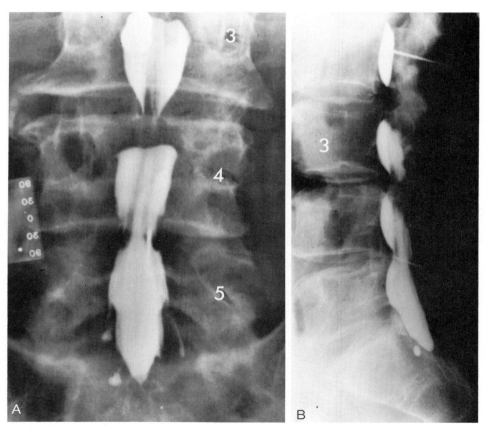

Figure 6–48. Degenerative Spinal Stenosis. Posteroanterior (A) and lateral (B) views taken during a metrizamide myelogram show marked narrowing of the dural sac at the level of the discs, producing an hourglass configuration. There is complete blockage of the flow of contrast at L2–L3. (From Sarokhan CT. Weissman BNW: Consultant, December 1981.)

measures 3 to 5 mm; no stenosis is present if the recess measures more than 5 mm (corrected for magnification) in either of these studies (Fig. 6–47).

Metrizamide (Amipaque) myelography can demonstrate flattening of the involved nerve root, an extradural defect resulting from compression by the hypertrophied facet joint or from partial or complete block (Fig. 6–48). [132] CT or polytomography, however, are the most accurate means of diagnosis.

Postfusion Stenosis. Following posterior fusion, overgrowth of the internal diameter of the laminae may occur. CT is of particular help in these cases, since, in addition to the central structures,[134] the nerve roots and the neural foramina can be seen well.

Laminectomy for Spinal Stenosis

Surgical Procedure. The surgical procedure consists of unroofing the spinal canal by removing the laminae and ligamenta flava at each level involved. The level to be decompressed is judged from preoperative radiographs and visual

assessment of the bony constriction of the dural sac at the time of surgery.[126a] Return of pulsations to the dural sac indicates that the space is adequate. The lateral dimensions of the canal may be enlarged at surgery, but the facet joints are usually left undisturbed (see Fig. 6–44).

Complications. (1) The decompression may be incomplete, with residual nerve root compression. This may be due, for example, to entrapment of the nerve root at more than one site or to involvement of more than one nerve root. (2) Instability may occur because of resection of the facet joints. (3) Postoperative fibrosis may occur around the dura and nerve roots.

Diffuse Idiopathic Skeletal Hyperostosis (DISH, Forestier's Disease)

Diffuse idiopathic skeletal hyperostosis is a condition characterized radiographically by the presence of "flowing" calcification and ossification along the anterolateral aspects of vertebrae (particularly in the cervical and thoracic areas), large osteophytes with relatively normal heights

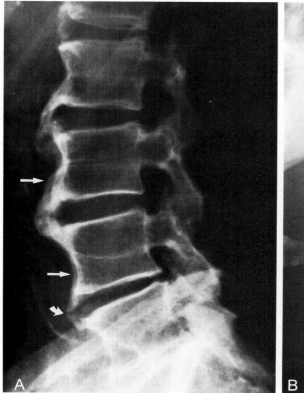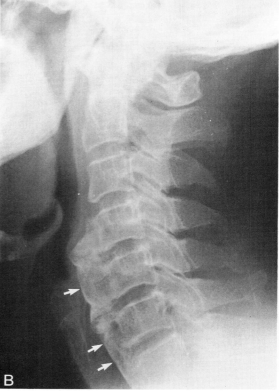

Figure 6–49. DISH (Diffuse Idiopathic Skeletal Hyperostosis; Forestier's Disease). *A*, Lumbar spine. The characteristic "flowing" calcification or ossification (straight arrows) is seen. The lucency at the level of the disc (curved arrow) is caused by intervening disc material. The disc spaces are characteristically normal, although in this case the L4–L5 and L5–S1 interspaces are narrow. *B*, Cervical spine. The ossification (arrows) is more prominent.

of disc spaces, and the absence of apophyseal joint abnormalities or sacroiliitis (Fig. 6–49). Extraspinal abnormalities in patients with DISH include bony proliferation at tendon insertions and ligamentous calcification.

According to Resnick, DISH is a common entity found in 12 percent of randomly selected autopsies.[137] The condition is usually detected in older males, the mean age being 66 years. A majority of patients have symptoms such as spinal stiffness, restricted motion, and tendinitis. Back pain is usually mild, nonradiating, and intermittent. Dysphagia may occur because of compression of the hypopharynx by large cervical osteophytes.

Calcification or ossification of the posterior longitudinal ligament may accompany the marked hyperostosis noted in DISH. Such calcification or ossification was found in the cervical spine in 50 percent of a group of patients with DISH.[138] In this same group 41 percent had hyperostosis of the posterior aspect of the cervical vertebrae, and 34 percent had posterior spinal osteophytes. Any of these deformities might narrow the spinal canal.[136a]

Vertebral Osteomyelitis

Vertebral osteomyelitis is usually the result of hematogenous spread of organisms to the vertebral bodies, most often from the genitourinary tract, skin, or respiratory system.[147] *Staphylococcus aureus* and Enterobacteriaceae are the most frequent organisms responsible. *Pseudomonas, Serratia,* and *Candida* are frequently found in the vertebral osteomyelitis occurring in heroin users.

Radiological Findings

Diagnosis is suggested clinically by the presence of back pain and fever. In other cases diagnosis is more obscure, and symptoms and signs may be nonspecific. Radiographic diagnosis is even more crucial in these clinically confusing cases but is hampered by the fact that radiographic findings are delayed, taking 2 to 8 weeks after clinical presentation to become apparent.[147] Radiographic findings include the following (Fig. 6–50).

1. Paravertebral soft tissue swelling
2. Disc-space narrowing
3. Bone destruction usually involving the anterior portions of the vertebral bodies adjacent to the disc
4. Progressive bone destruction accompanied by increasing new bone production
5. Bony bridging between involved vertebrae or fusion of adjacent vertebral bodies.

Several radiographic features have been suggested for distinguishing between tuberculous

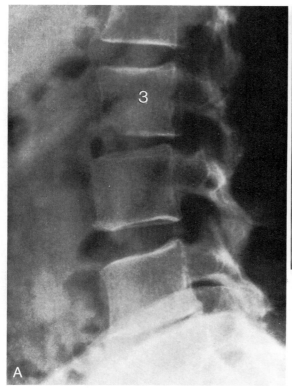

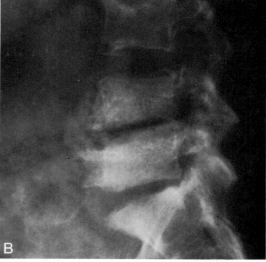

Figure 6–50. Osteomyelitis. *A,* Lateral view of lumbar spine in a middle-aged woman with severe back pain. Note destruction of the anterior inferior margin of L3 and mild L3–L4 disc narrowing, typical of infection. The disc narrowing and hypertrophic lipping at L5–S1 is incidental. *B,* Another patient with osteomyelitis *(Escherichia coli)* under treatment shows some new bone anteriorly. Severe bone loss from the adjacent vertebrae and the disc-space narrowing are apparent. The activity of infection cannot be assessed from the radiographic appearance alone. (From Sarokhan CT, Weissman BNW: Consultant, December 1981.)

and pyogenic infections. Thus in pyogenic infection (1) paravertebral masses are small or absent; (2) the course of bone destruction is more rapid; (3) total destruction is less severe; (4) marked osteoblastic response is more frequent, occurring within 4 to 6 weeks after onset of symptoms; and (5) the posterior elements may be involved, with or without vertebral body

involvement.[148] These findings were reviewed by Allen, Cosgrove, and Millard, and they concluded, "No radiological pattern was completely reliable in distinguishing tuberculosis from nontuberculous infection, but in white patients the formation of new bone certainly suggests a pyogenic lesion."[44]

Computed tomography may be a useful ad-

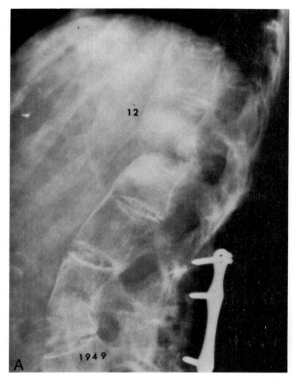

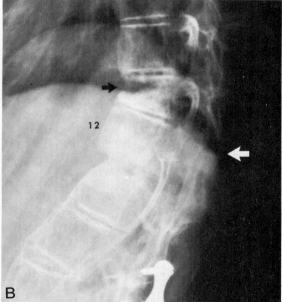

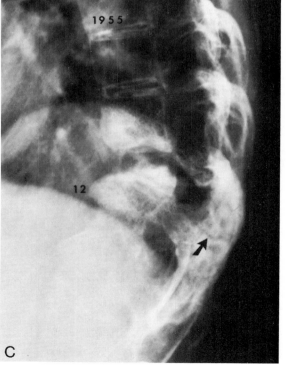

Figure 6–51. Pseudoinfection in Ankylosing Spondylitis. A, Lateral radiograph taken in 1949 shortly after osteotomy (L3) to correct deformity shows bone erosion and sclerosis around the T12–L1 disc space, suggesting infection or pseudarthrosis. The spine is otherwise completely fused—anteriorly by syndesmophytes and posteriorly by facet joint fusion. At this time there was no clinical evidence of infection. B, In a film taken several years later the T12–L1 site of pseudarthrosis has healed (presumably as a consequence of the change in stress resulting from the osteotomy). A fracture through the body and posterior elements of T11 (arrows) has occurred. C, In this view from 1955 there is increased destruction and displacement at the pseudarthrosis site. The posterior fracture is well seen (arrow).

junct in establishing the diagnosis of osteomyelitis.[146, 149] The presence of osteomyelitis increases the attenuation coefficient of the marrow space, possibly owing to increased vascularity or edema.[146] In addition, paravertebral abscesses and the extent of bone destruction can be evaluated.

Response to therapy should be measured on clinical grounds. Radiological examination may show progression of findings during treatment, but these findings can be safely ignored if there is clinical indication of improvement.[145] Com-

puted tomography can show the diminishing size of paravertebral abscesses in successfully treated cases.

Destructive Lesions in Ankylosing Spondylitis[150–157]

Destructive vertebral lesions occur occasionally in ankylosing spondylitis and may involve localized areas or most of a vertebral body end plate. The diffuse lesions are of particular importance, since their appearance may closely mimic that of infection. These lesions occur most frequently

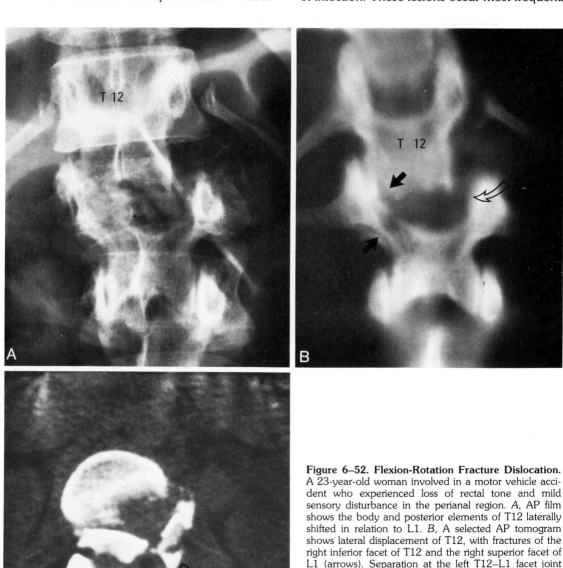

Figure 6–52. Flexion-Rotation Fracture Dislocation. A 23-year-old woman involved in a motor vehicle accident who experienced loss of rectal tone and mild sensory disturbance in the perianal region. *A,* AP film shows the body and posterior elements of T12 laterally shifted in relation to L1. *B,* A selected AP tomogram shows lateral displacement of T12, with fractures of the right inferior facet of T12 and the right superior facet of L1 (arrows). Separation at the left T12–L1 facet joint (open arrow) is apparent. *C,* Computed tomogram at the level of the upper portion of L1 shows a highly comminuted fracture of the vertebral body, with displacement of fragments into the spinal canal. The separation of the left articular facets (arrow) is contrasted to the normal apposition on the other side; s = superior facet of L1, i = inferior facets of T12.

in patients with long-standing disease and ankylosed spines. Irregular destruction and sclerosis of adjacent vertebral body end plates are noted (Fig. 6–51).

The hypothesis that these lesions represent fractures through areas of prior ankylosis, with formation of a pseudarthrosis, is supported by the prior history of trauma that is often elicited and by the presence of fractures of the posterior elements that may accompany the anterior defects.

Acute fractures through previously fused areas can occur after relatively minor trauma. The cervical region is most often affected, and neurological sequelae can be mild or severe. Treatment is controversial.[153a]

Fractures and Dislocations

Most spine fractures involve the distal thoracic and the lumbar areas, with more than 50 percent of vertebral body fractures occurring between T12 and L2.[169]

Classification

As summarized by Kaufer, the pattern of injury can be explained by the initiating force.[169]

Hyperflexion. Most lumbar and thoracic spine fractures result from hyperflexion, which results in crushing of the anterior portion of the vertebral body. Usually, the posterior cortex of the vertebra is spared, although it may be involved in severe injuries, when displacement of these posterior fragments may produce neurological deficit. Because the axis of flexion is near the center of the disc, the anterior portion of the vertebral body is subjected to a compressive load four times greater than the tensile load on the spinous processes and adjacent ligaments. Therefore, posterior-element avulsion fracture or ligamentous rupture does not occur. Usually these injuries do not result in neurological deficit and are not acutely unstable.

Hyperextension. Hyperextension injuries are uncommon in the lumbar spine. They can be detected on radiographs by the presence of an avulsion fracture of the anterior portion of a vertebral body or a fracture through the pars interarticularis. The injury is usually stable and neurological deficit is uncommon.

Excessive Lateral Bending. These injuries, too, are uncommon. They result in lateral wedge fractures and are usually stable, without associated neurological deficit.

Rotation. Most injuries that occur as the result of rotation are actually caused by a combination of rotation and flexion; this is the most frequent cause for dislocations and fracture-dislocations

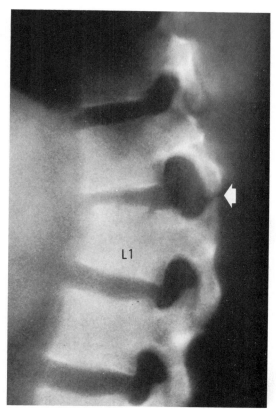

Figure 6–53. Dorsolumbar Fracture Dislocation. A selected lateral tomogram shows a wedge fracture of L1 and the left T12 inferior facet perched on the superior L1 facet (arrow).

of the thoracolumbar spine (Figs. 6–52 and 6–53).[169] The flexion component is shown by a crush fracture of the vertebral body. The rotation component is indicated by an oblique vertebral body fracture with lateral displacement. Flexion stress alone does not result in disruption of the neural arch; however, the combination of flexion and rotation may.

These lesions are often unstable and are associated with neurological abnormality. Spontaneous reduction may occur when the patient is placed in the supine position for radiography, and radiographs therefore may show little or no displacement. Damage to the vertebral body and the posterior elements should be sought, since damage to both of these structures indicates instability.

Shear Fractures. Shear fractures are identified by the presence of translational displacement without evidence of rotation, of a wedge fracture, or of angular displacement to suggest flexion. These fractures are unstable, and neurological deficit is common.

Compression Fractures. Compression fractures are caused by excessive vertical loading,

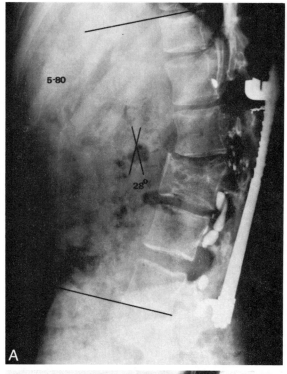

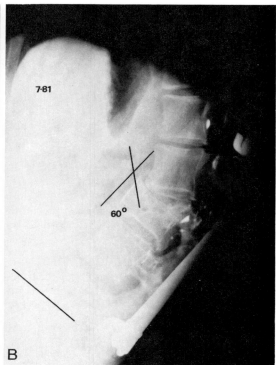

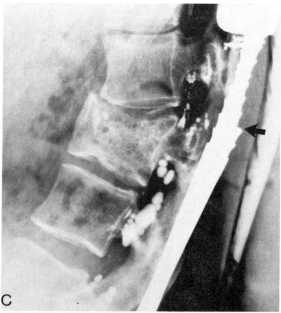

Figure 6–54. Compression Fracture with Loss of Reduction. *A,* Lateral view taken in May 1980, after attempted posterior fusion and Harrington distraction rod instrumentation, shows a compression fracture of L3 and a 28 degree kyphosis. *B,* Lateral view taken in July 1981 shows an increase in kyphosis, suggesting development of a pseudarthrosis. *C,* Coned lateral view taken in July 1981 shows the break that occurred in one of the rods (arrow). Pseudarthrosis was confirmed at surgery.

which produces central fracture of a vertebral end plate as a result of the impact on the vertebra from the nucleus pulposus of the disc. The superior end plate is most often affected (Fig. 6–54). These fractures are stable, since the posterior portions of the spine are intact; neurological deficit is rare. However, with severe compression the vertebral body may be split in

two, and neurological deficit may result from displacement of the posterior fragment.

Fractures Caused by Distraction. When a person wearing a lap-seatbelt experiences sudden deceleration, a distraction fracture may result. Flexion occurs, but since the spinal column is posterior to the axis of flexion (at the junction of the seatbelt and the abdominal wall), the

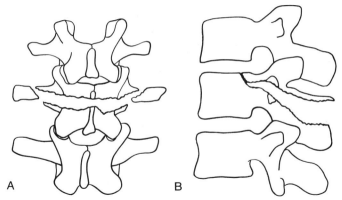

Figure 6–55. Chance Fracture. G. Q. Chance described this fracture as consisting of "horizontal splitting of the spine and neural arch, ending in an upper surface of the body just in front of the neural foramen." *A,* Diagram of AP radiograph. *B,* Diagram of lateral radiograph. (Redrawn from Chance GQ: Br J Radiol 21:452, 1948.)

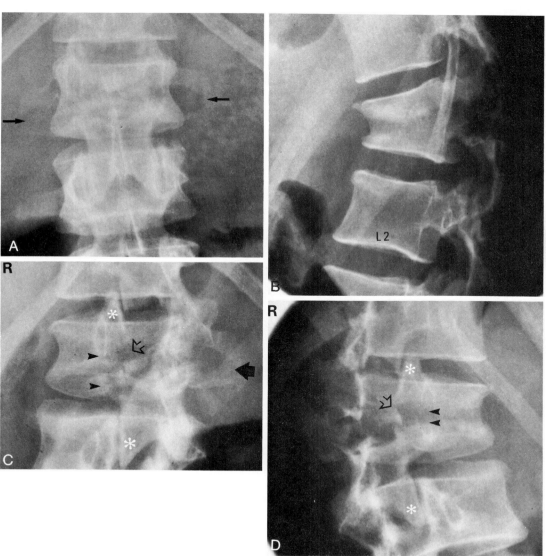

Figure 6–56. Chance Fracture of L1. *A,* AP view shows fractures across each pedicle, making the pedicles appear elongated. The partes interarticulares, transverse processes (arrows) and the L1 spinous process are split. *B,* Lateral view. The L1 body and the upper aspect of the L2 body are wedged. Right posterior oblique view *(C)* and left posterior oblique view *(D)* better demonstrate the pars (open arrow), pedicle (arrowheads), and transverse process (arrow) fractures. (Asterisks indicate superior and inferior facets of L1; R = right side.)

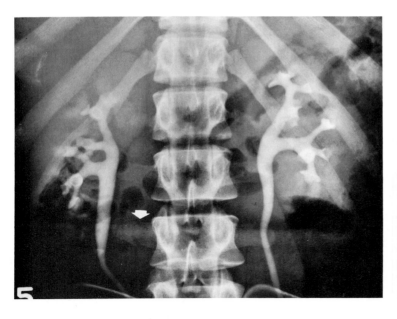

Figure 6–57. Transverse Process Fractures and Retroperitoneal Hematoma. This 24-year-old man fell from a ladder, striking his right flank on a bedframe. Film taken during an intravenous pyelogram confirms fractures of the L3 transverse process (arrow). The L4 transverse process fracture is not well seen. There is lateral deviation of the proximal right ureter, caused by a retroperitoneal hematoma.

vertebral column is subjected to tensile stress. This is the type of injury described by Chance,[160] and it is not usually associated with neurological sequelae (Figs. 6–55 and 6–56). Chance fractures are transverse, noncomminuted fractures of the vertebral body and posterior elements and are usually stable because of the relative integrity of the ligamentous structures and the interdigitation of fracture surfaces. The presence of dislocation associated with distraction is, however, an unstable situation.

Avulsion Fractures. These are usually avulsion fractures of the transverse processes (Fig. 6–57).[165]

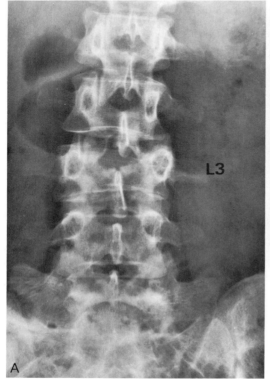

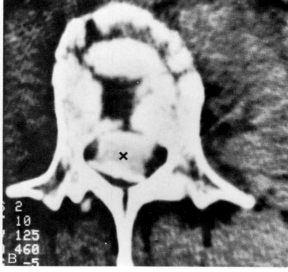

Figure 6–58. Comminuted Fracture of L3. A, AP view shows widening of the interpediculate distance of L3, loss of height of the body of L3, and a vertical lucency at the superior aspect of the spinous process. (Lateral view showed decreased height of L3. No bone fragments could be identified in the spinal canal.) B, CT through the pedicles and the body of L3 shows a highly comminuted fracture, with a large fragment (x) displaced into the spinal canal. The split at the origin of the spinous process is seen.

Radiological Evaluation

Stability.[169] A spinal fracture or dislocation is considered to be unstable if, during healing, its fragments are capable of displacement that might result in neural injury. Acute instability refers to the possibility of displacement at the level of injury that may produce neurological deficit during the early period after injury. Acute instability is possible if there is damage to both anterior structures (vertebral bodies and discs) and posterior structures (the neural arch, articular processes, and ligaments). The presence of vertebral displacement, a widened interspinous space, widened apophyseal joint(s), or a widened spinal canal indicates instability.[164]

Chronic instability refers to the possibility of progressive deformity in the months or years after injury. It is diagnosed by the gradual increase in angular deformity that occurs.

Tomography. Complex motion tomography can be extremely helpful in the evaluation of vertebral injuries. Anteroposterior and lateral tomography is suggested, since false-negative studies can result if only the anteroposterior study is done. Three-mm tomographic intervals are suggested for evaluation of the posterior elements on anteroposterior tomographs, but larger intervals will suffice for study of the vertebral bodies.

Computed Tomography. Advantages of computed tomography in patients with spine trauma include the following:[158, 161, 162, 168, 172, 174]

1. Detection of fractures not apparent on plain films, such as posterior arch fractures

2. Identification of displaced bone fragments that may not be apparent on either plain films or conventional tomography (Fig. 6–58).

3. Localization of bone and bullet fragments within the spinal canal, the lateral recesses, or both

4. Detection of paraspinal abnormalities

5. Demonstration of intraspinal soft tissue abnormalities, including intramedullary hematomas, herniated discs, and post-traumatic syrinxes

6. Differentiation of spinal cord swelling from extrinsic cord compression if intrathecal metrizamide is used.

Because of these advantages and because of the disadvantages of obtaining multiple studies, computed tomography, when it is available, is suggested as the next step after routine radiography in patients with spinal trauma.[166]

Postoperative Evaluation

Spinal fusion may be used for the treatment of unstable injuries. Surgical planning usually requires preoperative multidirectional tomography, CT of the area, or both. In addition, standard radiographs of the entire spine to help exclude other areas of injury are recommended.

Foley and colleagues reviewed the radiographic findings of 206 patients who underwent thoracic or lumbar spine fusion after severe trauma.[163] Posterior fusions were performed in cases in which there were gross disruptions of posterior elements with anterior displacement of the vertebral bodies above the level of injury and intact anterior longitudinal ligaments. Harrington distraction rods were used most often and were hooked to the laminae of the second intact vertebra below the level of injury and the facet joints of the second vertebra above the level of instability. Harrington compression rods were primarily used for stabilization of multiple, severe anterior compression deformities or for distraction injuries with kyphosis. Other forms of posterior stabilization, combined methods, and additional anterior fusion or (rarely) isolated anterior fusion were done as necessary. Postoperative complications included unhooking of Harrington distraction rods, overdistraction when the Harrington distraction rod was used, fracture of the rod, incorrect placement of the hooks, and loss of reduction with progressive deformity (kyphosis).

Despite the presence of metal, computed tomography can be used to evaluate persistent postoperative spinal cord or nerve root compression due to residual bone fragments in the spinal canal.[166] Later in the postoperative period, exuberant callus and pseudarthrosis may be detected with this technique.

References
Essential Anatomy

1. Coventry MB: Anatomy of the intervertebral disk. Clin Orthop 67:9–15, 1969.
2. Epstein BS: The Spine. A Radiological Text and Atlas. Philadelphia, Lea & Febiger, 1976.
3. Grabias SL, Mankin HJ: Pain in the lower back. Arthritis Fdtn, Bull Rheum Dis 30:1040–1045, 1979–80.
4. Harris RI, Macnab I: Structural changes in the lumbar intervertebral discs: Their relationship to low back pain and sciatica. J Bone Joint Surg (Br) 36:304–322, 1954.
5. Inman VT, Saunders JB: The clinico-anatomical aspects of the lumbosacral region. Radiology 38:669–678, 1942.
6. Lee BCP, Kazam E, Newman AD: Computed tomography of the spine and spinal cord. Radiology 128:95–102, 1978.
7. Nachemson AL: The lumbar spine, an orthopaedic challenge. Spine 1:59–71, 1976.
8. Resnick D, Niwayama G: Intravertebral disc herniations: Cartilaginous (Schmorl's) nodes. Radiology 126:57–65, 1978.

Normal Radiographic Examination

9. Abel MS, Smith GR: Visualization of the posterolateral elements of the lumbar vertebrae in the anteroposterior projection. Radiology 122:824–825, 1977.

10. Carrera GF, Williams AL, Haughton VM: Computed tomography in sciatica. Radiology 137:433–437, 1980.

11. Eisenberg RL, Hedgcock MW, Gooding GAW, DeMartini WJ, Akin JR, Ovenfors CO: Compensation examination of the cervical and lumbar spines: Critical disagreement in radiographic interpretation. AJR 134:519–522, 1980.

12. Eisenberg RL, Hedgcock MW, Williams EA, Lyden BJ, Akin JR, Gooding GAW, Ovenfors CO: Optimum radiographic examination for consideration of compensation awards: II. Cervical and lumbar spines. AJR 135:1071–1074, 1980.

13. Etter LE, Carabello NC: Roentgen anatomy of oblique views of the lumbar spine. AJR 61:699–705, 1949.

14. Fullenlove TM, Williams AJ: Comparative roentgen findings in symptomatic and asymptomatic backs. Radiology 68:572–574, 1957.

14a. Gehweiler Jr JA, Daffner, RH: Low back pain: the controversy of radiologic evaluation. AJR 140:109–112, 1983.

15. Grabias SL, Mankin HJ: Pain in the lower back. Arthritis Fdtn, Bull Rheum Dis. 30:1040–1045, 1979–80.

16. Hall FM: Back pain and the radiologist. Radiology 137:861–863, 1980.

17. Hinck VC, Hopkins CE, Clark WM: Sagittal diameter of the lumbar spinal canal in children and adults. Radiology 85:929–937, 1965.

18. Hall FM: Overutilization of radiological examinations. Radiology 120:443–448, 1976.

19. La Rocca H, Macnab I: Value of pre-employment radiographic assessment of the lumbar spine. Can Med Assoc J 101:49–54, 1969.

20. Liang M and Komaroff AL: Roentgenograms in primary care patients with acute low back pain. A cost-effectiveness analysis. Arch Intern Med 142:1108–1112, 1982.

20a. Libson E, Bloom RA, Dinari G, et al.: Oblique lumbar spine radiographs: Importance in young patients. Radiology 151:89–90, 1984.

21. McAlister WH, Shackelford GD: Classification of spinal curvatures. Radiol Clin North Am 13:93–112, 1975.

22. Macnab I: Backache. Baltimore, Williams & Wilkins, 1977.

23. Magora A, Schwartz A: Relation between the low back pain syndrome and x-ray findings: 2. Transitional vertebra (mainly sacralization). Scand J Rehabil Med 10:135–145, 1978.

24. Magora A, Schwartz A: Relation between the low back pain syndrome and x-ray findings. I. Degenerative osteoarthritis. Scand J Rehabil Med 8:115–125, 1976.

25. Nachemson AL: The lumbar spine, an orthopaedic challenge. Spine 1:59–71, 1976.

26. Rhea JT, DeLuca SA, Llewellyn HJ, Boyd RJ: The oblique view: An unnecessary component of the initial adult lumbar spine examination. Radiology 134:45–47, 1980.

27. Roberts FF, Kishore PRS, Cunningham ME: Routine oblique radiography of the pediatric lumbar spine: Is it necessary? AJR 131:297–298, 1978.

28. Rockey PH, Tompkins RK, Wood RW, Wolcott BW: The usefulness of x-ray examinations in the evaluation of patients with back pain. J Fam Pract 7:455–465, 1978.

29. Roulleau J, Guillaume J: Plain x-ray diagnosis of developmental narrow lumbar canal. In Wackenheim A, Babin E, eds. The Narrow Lumbar Canal, Radiologic Signs and Surgery. New York, Springer-Verlag, 1980.

30. Scavone JG, Latshaw RF, Rohrer GV: Use of lumbar spine films: Statistical evaluation at a university teaching hospital. JAMA 246:1105–1108, 1981.

31. Splithoff CA: Lumbosacral junction: Roentgenographic comparison of patients with and without backaches. JAMA 152:1610–1613, 1953.

32. Stapleton JG: Letter to the editor: Pre-employment radiographs of the lumbar spine. J Can Assoc Radiol 29:4–5, 1978.

33. Torgerson WR, Dotter WE: Comparative roentgenographic study of the asymptomatic and symptomatic lumbar spine. J Bone Joint Surg (Br) 58:850–853, 1976.

Scoliosis

34. Benson DR, Schultz AB, Dewald RL: Roentgenographic evaluation of vertebral rotation. J Bone Joint Surg (Am) 58:1125–1129, 1976.

35. Cobb JR: Outline for the study of scoliosis. AAOS Instructional Course Lectures, 5:261–275, 1948.

36. Dorland's Illustrated Medical Dictionary, 26th ed. Philadelphia, WB Saunders, 1981.

37. Dwyer AF: Experience of anterior correction of scoliosis. Clin Orthop 93:191–206, 1973.

38. Goldstein LA: The surgical treatment of idiopathic scoliosis. Clin Orthop 93:131–157, 1973.

39. Hall JE: Current concepts review: Dwyer instrumentation in anterior fusion of the spine. J Bone Joint Surg (Am) 63:1188–1190, 1981.

40. Harrington PR, Dickson JG: An eleven-year investigation of Harrington instrumentation: A preliminary report on 578 cases. Clin Orthop 93:113–130, 1973.

41. Jeffries BF, Tarlton M, DeSmet AA, Dwyer SJ III, Brower AC: Computerized measurement and analysis of scoliosis: A more accurate representation of the shape of the curve. Radiology 134:381–385, 1980.

42. Kittleson AC, Lim LW: Measurement of scoliosis. AJR 108:775–777, 1970.

43. McAlister WH, Shackelford GD: Measurement of spinal curvatures. Radiol Clin North Am 13:113–121, 1975.

44. McAlister WH, Shackelford GD: Classification of spinal curvatures. Radiol Clin North Am 13:93–112, 1975.

45. Micheli LJ, Riseborough EJ, Hall JE: Scoliosis in the adult. Orthop Rev 6:27–39, 1977.

46. Nash CL, Moe JH: A study of vertebral rotation. J Bone Joint Surg (Am) 51:223–229, 1969.

47. Ritter EM, Wright CE, Fritz SL, Kirchmer NA, DeSmet AA: Use of a gradient intensifying screen for scoliosis radiography. Radiology 135:230–232, 1980.

48. Robin G, Span Y, Makin M, Steinberg R: Scoliosis in the elderly: Idiopathic or osteoporotic? Zorao, PA, ed. Proceedings of 5th Symposium, Brompton Hospital, London, 1976.

49. Swank S, Lonstein JE, Moe JH, Winter RB, Bradford DS: Surgical treatment of adult scoliosis: A review of two hundred and twenty-two cases. J Bone Joint Surg (Am) 63:268–287, 1981.

50. Vanderpool DW, James JIP, Wynne-Davies R: Scoliosis in the elderly. J Bone Joint Surg (Am) 51:446–455, 1969.

51. Wilkinson RH, Willi UV, Gilsanz V, Mulvihill D: Radiographic evaluation of the spine after surgical correction of scoliosis. AJR 133:703–709, 1979.

Disc Degeneration

52. Bick EM: Vertebral osteophytosis: Pathologic basis of its roentgenology. AJR 73:979–983, 1955.
53. Berens DL: Roentgen features of ankylosing spondylitis. Clin Orthop 74:20, 1971.
54. Coventry MB: Anatomy of the intervertebral disc. Clin Orthop 67:9–15, 1969.
55. Edeiken J, Pitt MJ: The radiologic diagnosis of disc disease. Orthop Clin North Am 2:405–417, 1971.
56. Ford LT, Gilula LA, Murphy WA, Gado M: Analysis of gas in vacuum lumbar disc. AJR 128:1056–1057, 1977.
57. Forestier J: The importance of sacroiliac changes in the early diagnosis of ankylosing spondyloarthritis. Radiology 33:389, 1939.
58. Gershon-Cohen J, Schraer H, Sklaroft DM, Blumberg N: Dissolution of the intervertebral disk in the aged normal. Radiology 62:383–387, 1954.
59. Gershon-Cohen J: The phantom nucleus pulposus. AJR 56:43–48, 1946.
60. Harris RI, Macnab I: Structural changes in the lumbar intervertebral discs: Their relationship to low back pain and sciatica. J Bone Joint Surg (Br) 36:304–322, 1954.
61. Hussar AE, Guller EJ: Correlation of pain and the roentgenographic findings of spondylosis of the cervical and lumbar spine. Am J Med Sci 232:518–527, 1956.
62. Knutsson F: The vacuum phenomenon in the intervertebral discs. Acta Radiol 23:173–179, 1942.
63. Lawrence JS: Disc degeneration: Its frequency and relationship to symptoms. Ann Rheum Dis 28:121–137, 1969.
64. Lipson SJ: Low back pain. In Kelley WN, Harris ED Jr, Ruddy S, Sledge CB, eds. Textbook of Rheumatology. Philadelphia, WB Saunders 1981:451–471.
65. Macnab I: Backache. Baltimore, Williams & Wilkins, 1977.
66. Marr JT: Gas in intervertebral discs. AJR 70:804–809, 1953.
67. Martel W, Seeger JF, Wicks JD, Washburn RL: Traumatic lesions of the discovertebral junction in the lumbar spine. AJR 127:457–464, 1976.
68. McEwen C, DiTata D, Lingg C, et al: Ankylosing spondylitis and spondylitis accompanying ulcerative colitis, regional enteritis, psoriasis and Reiter's disease. Arthritis Rheum 14:291–317, 1971.
69. Raines JR: Intervertebral disc fissures (vacuum intervertebral disc). AJR 70:964–966, 1953.
70. Resnick D: Osteophytes, syndesmophytes and other "phyghtes." Postgrad Radiol 1:217–232, 1981.
71. Resnick D, Niwayama G: Intervertebral disc herniations: Cartilaginous (Schmorl's) nodes. Radiology 126:57–65, 1978.
72. Resnick D, Niwayama G, Guerra J Jr, Vint V, Usselman J: Spinal vacuum phenomena: Anatomical study and review. Radiology 139:341–348, 1981.
73. Sauser DD, Goldman AB, Kaye JJ: Discogenic vertebral sclerosis. J Can Assoc Radiol 29:44–50, 1978.
74. Williams JL, Moller GA, O'Rourke TL: Pseudoinfections of the intervertebral disk and adjacent vertebrae? AJR 103:611–615, 1968.

Disc Hereniation

75. Adams JC: Standard Orthopaedic Operations. New York, Churchill Livingstone, 1980.
75a. Braun IF, Lin JP, Benjamin MV, et al.: Computed tomography of the asymptomatic postsurgical lumbar spine: analysis of the physiologic scar. AJR 142:149–152, 1984.

76. Calabrese AS, Freiberger RH: Acquired spondylolysis after spinal fusion. Radiology 81:492–494, 1963.
77. Carrera GF, Williams AL, Haughton VM: Computed tomography in sciatica. Radiology 137:433–437, 1980.
78. Chandler FA: Lesions of the "isthmus" (pars interarticularis) of the laminae of the lower lumbar vertebrae and their relation to spondylolisthesis. Surg Gynecol Obstet 53:273–306, 1931.
79. DePalma AF, Marone PJ: Spondylolysis following spinal fusion. Clin Orthop 15:208–211, 1959.
80. Edmonson AS, Crenshaw AH: Campbell's Operative Orthopaedics. St. Louis, CV Mosby, 1980.
81. Eismont FJ, Simeone FA: Bone overgrowth (hypertrophy) as a cause of late paraparesis after scoliosis fusion. J Bone Joint Surg (Am) 63:1016–1019, 1981.
82. Epstein BS: Herniation of the intervertebral discs. In Epstein BS, ed. The Spine: A Radiological Text and Atlas, 4th ed. Philadelphia, Lea & Febiger, 1976:632–677.
83. Haughton VM, Eldevik OP, Magnaes B, Amundsen P: A prospective comparison of computed tomography and myelography in the diagnosis of herniated lumbar discs. Radiology 142:103–110, 1982.
84. Hirschy JC, Leue WM, Berninger WH, Hamilton RH, Abbott GF: CT of the lumbosacral spine: Importance of tomographic planes parallel to vertebral end plate. AJR 126:47–52, 1981.
85. Inman VT, Saunders JB: The clinico-anatomical aspects of the lumbosacral region. Radiology 38:669–678, 1942.
86. Kestler OC: Overgrowth (hypertrophy) of lumbosacral grafts, causing a complete block. Bull Hosp Jt Dis Orthop Inst 27:51–57, 1966.
87. Macnab I: Backache. Baltimore, Williams & Wilkins, 1977.
88. Macnab I, Dall D: The blood supply of the lumbar spine and its application to the technique of intertransverse lumbar fusion. J Bone Joint Surg (Br) 53:628–638, 1971.
89. Mixter WJ, Barr JS: Rupture of the intervertebral disc with involvement of the spinal canal. N Engl J Med 211:210–215, 1934.
90. Raskin SP, Keating JW: Recognition of lumbar disc disease: Comparison of myelography and computed tomography. AJR 139:349–355, 1982.
91. Sheldon JJ, Sersland T, Leborgne J: Computed tomography of the lower lumbar vertebral column. Radiology 124:113–118, 1977.
91a. Teplick JG, Haskin, ME: Computed tomography of the postoperative lumbar spine. AJR 141:865–884, 1983.
92. Williams AL, Haughton VM, Daniels DL, Thornton RS: CT recognition of lateral lumbar disc herniation. AJR 139:345–347, 1982.
93. Williams AL, Haughton VM, Syvertsen A: Computed tomography in the diagnosis of herniated nucleus pulposus. Radiology 135:95–99, 1980.

Spondylolisthesis

94. Appleby A, Stabler J: A new sign of spondylolisthesis. Clin Radiol 20:315–319, 1969.
95. Bryk D, Rosenkranz W: True spondylolisthesis and pseudospondylolisthesis: The spinous process sign. J Can Assoc Radiol 20:53–56, 1969.
96. DeLuca SA, Rhea JT: Are routine oblique roentgenograms of the lumbar spine of value? J Bone Joint Surg 63:846, 1981.
97. Dorland's Illustrated Medical Dictionary, 26th Edition. Philadelphia, WB Saunders, 1981.

98. Fullenlove TM, Wilson JG: Traumatic defects of the pars interarticularis of the lumbar vertebrae. AJR 122:634–638, 1974.

99. Ghelman B, Doherty JH: Demonstration of spondylolysis by arthrography of the apophyseal joint. AJR 130:986–987, 1978.

100. Gill GG, Manning JG, White HL: Surgical treatment of spondylolisthesis without spine fusion. Excision of the loose lamina with decompression of the nerve roots. J Bone Joint Surg (Am) 37:493–520, 1955.

101. Harris RI, Wiley JJ: Acquired spondylolysis as a sequel to spine fusion. J Bone Joint Surg (Am) 45:1159–1170, 1963.

102. Lowe RW, Hayes TD, Kaye J, Bagg RJ, Luekens CA Jr: Standing roentgenograms in spondylolisthesis. Clin Orthop 117:80–84, 1976.

103. Macnab I: Spondylolisthesis with an intact neural arch—the so-called pseudo-spondylolisthesis. J Bone Joint Surg (Br) 32:325–333, 1950.

104. Macnab I: Backache. Baltimore, Williams & Wilkins, 1977.

105. Maldague BE, Malghem JJ: Unilateral arch hypertrophy with spinous process tilt: A sign of arch deficiency. Radiology 121:567–574, 1976.

106. Meschan I: A radiographic study of spondylolisthesis with special reference to stability and determination. Radiology 47:249–262, 1946.

107. Meyerding HW: Spondylolisthesis. Surg Gynecol Obstet 34:371–377, 1932.

108. Moreton RD: Spondylolysis. JAMA 195:671–674, 1966.

109. Munster JK, Troup JDG: The structure of the pars interarticularis of the lower lumbar vertebrae and its relation to the etiology of spondylolysis—With a report of a healing fracture in the neural arch of a fourth lumbar vertebra. J Bone Joint Surg (Br) 55:735–741, 1973.

110. Nathan H: Spondylolysis: Its anatomy and mechanism of development. J Bone Joint Surg (Am) 41:303–320, 1959.

111. Ravichandran G: A radiologic sign in spondylolisthesis. AJR 134:113–117, 1980.

112. Rhea JT, DeLuca SA, Llewellyn HJ, Boyd RJ: The oblique view: An unnecessary component of the initial adult lumbar spine examination. Radiology 134:45–47, 1980.

113. Roche MB, Rowe GG: The incidence of separate neural arch and coincident bone variations. A survey of 4,200 skeletons. Anat Rec 109:233–255, 1951.

114. Schneider CC, Melamed A: Spondylolysis and spondylolisthesis. Case report clarifying the etiology of spondylolysis. Radiology 69:863–866, 1957.

115. Sherman FC, Wilkinson RH, Hall JE: Reactive sclerosis of a pedicle and spondylosis in the lumbar spine. J Bone Joint Surg (Am) 59:49–54, 1977.

116. Stewart TD: The age incidence of neural-arch defects in Alaskan natives, considered from the standpoint of etiology. J Bone Joint Surg (Am) 35:937–950, 1953.

117. Wilkinson RH, Hall JE: The sclerotic pedicle: Tumor or pseudotumor? Radiology 111:683–688, 1974.

118. Wiltse LL: The etiology of spondylolisthesis. J Bone Joint Surg (Am) 44:539–560, 1962.

119. Wiltse LL, Widell EH, Jackson DW: Fatigue fracture: The basic lesion in isthmic spondylolisthesis. J Bone Joint Surg (Am) 57:17–22, 1975.

120. Wiltse LL, Newman PH, Macnab I: Classification of spondylolysis and spondylolisthesis. Clin Orthop 117:23–28, 1976.

Facet Arthropathy

121. Carrera GF: Lumbar facet joint injection in low back pain and sciatica: Description of technique. Radiology 137:661–664, 1980.

122. Carrera GF: Lumbar facet joint injection in low back pain and sciatica: Preliminary results. Radiology 137:665–667, 1980.

123. Carrera GF, Haughton VM, Syvertsen A, Williams AL: Computed tomography of the lumbar facet joints. Radiology 134:145–148, 1980.

124. Dory MA: Arthrography of the lumbar facet joints. Radiology 140:23–27, 1981.

125. Maldague B, Mathurin P, Malghem J: Facet joint arthrography in lumbar spondylolysis. Radiology 140:29–36, 1981.

126. Mooney V, Robertson J: The facet syndrome. Clin Orthop 115:149–156, 1976.

Spinal Stenosis

126a. Dorwart RH, Vogler III JB, Helms CA: Spinal stenosis. Radiol Clin North Am 21:301–325, 1983.

127. Epstein BS, Epstein JA, Jones MD: Lumbar spinal stenosis. Radiol Clin North Am 15:227–239, 1977.

128. Hinck VC, Hopkins CE, Clark WM: Sagittal diameter of the lumbar spinal canal in children and adults. Radiology 85:929–937, 1965.

129. Lee BCP, Kazam E, Newman AD: Computed tomography of the spine and spinal cord. Radiology 128:95–102, 1978.

130. Lipson SJ: Low back pain. In Kelley WN, Harris ED Jr, Ruddy S, Sledge CB, eds. Textbook of Rheumatology. WB Saunders, 1981:451–471.

131. Macnab I: Backache. Baltimore, Williams & Wilkins, 1977.

132. Mikhael MA, Ciric I, Tarkington JA, Vick NA: Neuroradiological evaluation of lateral recess syndrome. Radiology 140:97–107, 1981.

133. Roulleau J, Guillaume J: Plain x-ray diagnosis of developmental narrow lumbar canal. In Wackenheim A, Babin E, eds. The Narrow Lumbar Canal. Radiologic Signs and Surgery. New York, Springer-Verlag, 1980.

134. Sheldon JJ, Sersland T, Leborgne J: Computed tomography of the lower lumbar vertebral column. Radiology 124:113–118, 1977.

135. Ullrich CG, Binet EF, Sanecki MG, Kieffer SA: Quantitative assessment of the lumbar spinal canal by computed tomography. Radiology 134:137–143, 1980.

136. Verbiest H: Chap. 16. Neurogenic intermittent claudication in cases with absolute and relative stenosis of the lumbar vertebral canal (ASLC and RSLC), in cases with narrow lumbar intervertebral foramina, and in cases with both entities. Clin Neurosurg 20:204–214, 1973.

Diffuse Idiopathic Skeletal Hyperostosis (DISH)

136a. Alenghat JP, Hallett M, Kido DK: Spinal cord compression in diffuse idiopathic skeletal hyperostosis. Radiology 142:119–120, 1982.

137. Resnick D: Diffuse idiopathic skeletal hyperostosis (DISH). Semin Arthritis Rheum 3:153–186, 1978.

138. Resnick D, Guerra J Jr, Robinson CA, Vint VC: Association of diffuse idiopathic skeletal hyperostosis (DISH) and calcification and ossification of the posterior longitudinal ligament. AJR 131:1049–1053, 1978.

139. Resnick D, Niwayama G: Radiographic and pathologic features of spinal involvement in diffuse idiopathic skeletal hyperostosis (DISH). Radiology 119:559–568, 1976.
140. Resnick D, Shaul SR, Robins JM: Diffuse idiopathic skeletal hyperostosis (DISH): Forestier's disease with extraspinal manifestations. Radiology 115:513–524, 1975.
141. Rosenthal M, Bahous I, Muller W: Increased frequency of HLA B8 in hyperostotic spondylosis. J Rheumatol [4 Suppl] 3:94–96, 1977.
142. Sebes JI, Nasrallah NS, Rabinowitz JG, Masi AT: The relationship between HLA-B27 positive peripheral arthritis and sacroiliitis. Radiology 126:299–302, 1978.
143. Tsukamoto Y, Onitsuka H, Lee K: Radiologic aspects of diffuse idiopathic skeletal hyperostosis in the spine. AJR 129:913–918, 1977.

Vertebral Osteomyelitis

144. Allen EH, Cosgrove D, Millard FJC: The radiological changes in infections of the spine and their diagnostic value. Clin Radiol 29:31–40, 1978.
145. Butt WP: The radiology of infection. Clin Orthop 96:20–30, 1973.
146. Kuhn JP, Berger PE: Computed tomographic diagnosis of osteomyelitis. Radiology 130:503–506, 1979.
147. Waldvogel FA, Vasey H: Osteomyelitis: The past decade. N Engl J Med 303:360–363, 1980.
148. Wear JE, Baylin GJ, Martin TL: Pyogenic osteomyelitis of the spine. AJR 67:90–94, 1952.
149. Wilson JS, Korobkin M, Genant HK, Bovill EG Jr: Computed tomography of musculoskeletal disorders. AJR 131:55–61, 1978.

Ankylosing Spondylitis

150. Cawley MID, Chalmers TM, Kellgren JH, Ball J: Destructive lesions of vertebral bodies in ankylosing spondylitis. Ann Rheum Dis 31:345–358, 1972.
151. Gelman MI, Umber JS: Fractures of the thoracolumbar spine in ankylosing spondylitis. AJR 130:485–491, 1978.
152. Good AE: Nontraumatic fracture of the thoracic spine in ankylosing spondylitis. Arthritis Rheum 10:467–469, 1967.
153. Hansen ST Jr, Taylor TKF, Honet JC, Lewis FR: Fracture-dislocations of the ankylosed thoracic spine in rheumatoid spondylitis. J Trauma 7:827–837, 1967.
153a. Hunter T, Dubo HIC: Spinal fractures complicating ankylosing spondylitis. A long-term follow-up study. Arthritis Rheum 26:751–758, 1983.
154. Kanefield DG, Mullins BP, Freehafer AA, Furley JG, Horenstein S, Chamberlin WB: Destructive lesions of the spine in rheumatoid ankylosing spondylitis. J Bone Joint Surg (Am) 51:1369–1375, 1969.
155. Lorber A, Pearson CM, Rene RM: Osteolytic vertebral lesions as a manifestation of rheumatoid arthritis and related disorders. Arthritis Rheum 4:514–532, 1961.
156. Rivelis M, Freiberger RH: Vertebral destruction at unfused segments in late ankylosing spondylitis. Radiology 93:251–256, 1969.
157. Wholey MH, Pugh DG, Bickel WH: Localized destructive lesions in rheumatoid spondylitis. Radiology 74:54–56, 1960.

Fractures and Dislocations

158. Brant-Zawadzki M, Miller EM, Federle MP: CT in the evaluation of spine trauma. AJR 136:369–375, 1981.
159. Brant-Zawadzki M, Jeffrey Jr RB, Minagi H, et al.: High resolution CT of thoracolumbar fractures. AJR 138:699–704, 1982.
160. Chance GQ: Note on a type of flexion fracture of the spine. Br J Radiol 21:452–453, 1948.
161. Colley DP, Dunsker SB: Traumatic narrowing of the dorsolumbar spinal canal demonstrated by computed tomography. Radiology 129:95–98, 1978.
162. Faerber EN, Wolpert SM, Scott RM, Belkin SC, Carter BL: Computed tomography of spinal fractures. J Comput Assist Tomogr 3:657–661, 1979.
163. Foley, MJ, Calenoff L, Hendrix RW, Schafer MF: Thoracic and lumbar spine fusion: Postoperative radiologic evaluation. Postoperative radiologic evaluation. AJR 141:373–380, 1983.
164. Gehweiler Jr JA, Daffner RN, Osborne Jr RH: Relevant signs of stable and unstable thoracolumbar vertical column. Trauma. Skeletal Radiol 7:179–183, 1981.
165. Gilsanz V, Miranda J, Cleveland J, Willi U: Scoliosis secondary to fractures of the transverse processes of lumbar vertebrae. Radiology 134:627–629, 1980.
166. Golimbu C, Firooznia H, Kafii M, et al.: CT of thoracic and lumbar spine fractures that have been treated with Harrington instrumentation. Radiology 151:731–733, 1984.
167. Gverra Jr J, Garfin SR, Resnick D: Vertebral burst fractures: CT analysis of the retropulsed fragment. Radiology 153:769–772, 1984.
168. Handel SF, Twiford TW Jr, Reigel DH, Kaufman HH: Posterior lumbar apophyseal fractures. Radiology 130:629–633, 1979.
169. Kaufer H: 2: The Thoracolumbar Spine. In Rockwood CA Jr, Green DP, eds. Fractures. Philadelphia, JB Lippincott, 1975: 861–884.
170. Kilcoyne RF, Mack LA, King HA, et al.: Thoracolumbar spine injuries associated with vertical plunges: reappraisal with computed tomography. Radiology 146:137–140, 1983.
171. O'Callaghan JP, Ullrich CG, Yuan HA, et al.: CT of facet distraction in flexion injuries of the thoracolumbar spine: the "naked" facet. AJR 134:563–568, 1980.
172. Roub LW, Drayer BP: Spinal computed tomography: limitations and applications. AJR 133:267–273, 1979.
173. Smith GR, Northrop CH, Loop JW: Jumpers' fractures: patterns of thoracolumbar spine injuries associated with vertical plunges. Radiology 122:657–663, 1977.
174. Tadmor R, Davies KR, Roberson GH, et al.: Computed tomographic evaluation of traumatic spinal injuries. Radiology 127:825–827, 1978.

Chapter 7

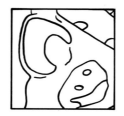

The
PELVIS

NORMAL STRUCTURE AND FUNCTION

Normal Anatomy

The two innominate bones form the greater part of the pelvis (Fig. 7–1). Each consists of ilium, ischium, and pubis, which are fused in the adult at the level of the acetabulum. The iliopectineal line divides the pelvis into an upper false pelvis and a lower true pelvis, which contains the reproductive organs and portions of the urinary tract, large bowel, major vessels, and nerves to the lower extremities. The bony pelvis protects the internal viscera, transmits body weight to the lower limbs, and provides attachment for trunk and lower limb musculature. In the upright position weight-bearing forces are transmitted from the spine to the sacrum, the sacroiliac joints, the ilia and the acetabula, and then to the upper femora. In the upright position these areas of force transmission are referred to as the femorosacral arch (Fig. 7–2).[1] A subsidiary, or tie, arch, made up of the bodies of the pubic bones and their horizontal rami, connects the ends of the femorosacral arch. In the sitting position weight is transmitted through the sacroiliac joints, into the ilia, and then to the ischial tuberosities, forming the ischiosacral arch. This arch is also augmented by a tie arch made up of the bodies of the pubic bones and the inferior pubic and ischial rami. When trauma occurs, the tie arches are the first to break.

Acetabulum

The acetabulum is the cavity on the lateral aspect of each innominate bone (Fig. 7–3). A

335

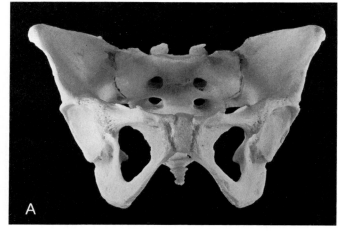

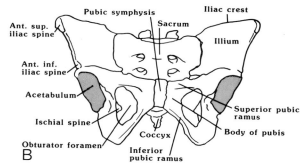

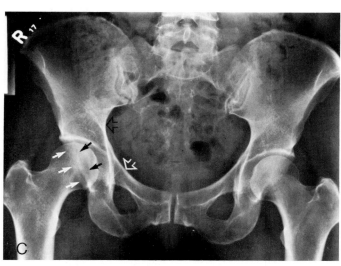

Figure 7–1. Normal Anatomy. Photographic, diagrammatic, and radiographic anatomy in the AP *(A, B, C)*, oblique *(D, E, F)*, and lateral *(G, H)* projections. The posterior (white arrows) and anterior (black arrows) acetabular rims are shown. Open arrow indicates the iliopectineal line. (The patient shown on the oblique view has pubic fractures.)

Illustration continued on opposite page

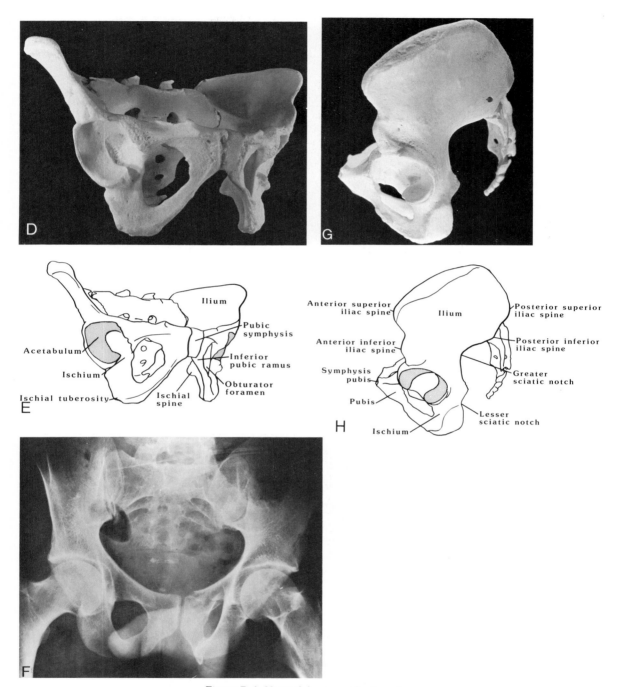

Figure 7–1. Normal Anatomy *Continued.*

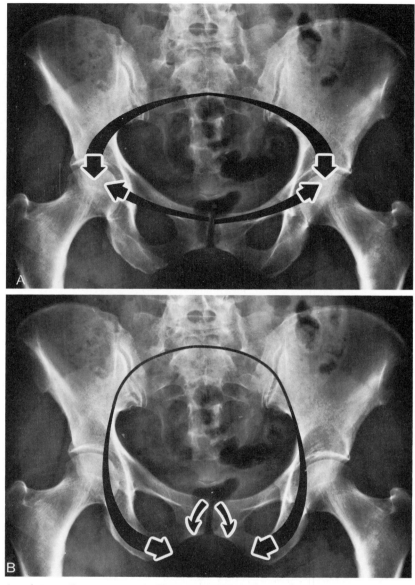

Figure 7–2. Paths of Force Transmission. *A,* The femorosacral arch. In the upright position weight-bearing forces are transmitted from the spine to the sacrum, the sacroiliac (SI) joints, the ilium, the acetabulum, and then to the upper femora. The tie arch is also shown. *B,* The ischiosacral arch. In the seated position weight is transmitted through the SI joints, the ilia, and the ischial tuberosities. The tie arch (small arrows) is shown. (After Kane, WJ: Fractures of the pelvis. *In* Rockwood CA Jr, Green DP, eds. Fractures. Philadelphia, JB Lippincott, 1975.)

bony rim projects from the superior, the anterior, and the posterior aspects of the acetabulum but is incomplete inferiorly, with the gap (the acetabular notch) bridged by the transverse ligament. The medial floor of the acetabulum, termed the acetabular fossa, is nonarticular, but its margins are bounded by the horseshoe-shaped articular surface.

The acetabulum is formed by union of iliac, pubic, and ischial components (see Fig. 7–30).

Judet and colleagues viewed the acetabulum as being within the concavity of an arch formed by two bony columns: an anterior (iliopubic) and a posterior (ilioischial) column (Fig. 7–4).[6] These columns fuse superiorly at the roof (or keystone) of the acetabulum. The anterior (iliopubic) column consists of a short segment of the ilium and pubis and extends superiorly to the anterior inferior iliac spine. The anterior portion of the articular surface of the acetabulum and the anterior acetabular rim are included in this column. The posterior (ilioischial) column is composed of the vertical portions of the ischium and of the ilium just above the ischium. The posterior part of the acetabular articular surface and the posterior acetabular rim are included in the anterolateral portion of this column. The flat surface of the ilium that forms the inner aspect of the acetabulum is known as its quadrilateral surface.

Pubic Symphysis

A symphysis is a fibrocartilaginous, nonsynovial articulation at which limited motion is possible by deformation of a connecting fibrocartilaginous disc.[1] At the pubic symphysis, each of the articular surfaces is covered by a thin hyaline cartilage layer and these are connected by the fibrocartilaginous interpubic disc (Fig. 7–5). A superior pubic ligament and an arcuate (inferior) pubic ligament connect the pubic bones.[1] The rectus muscles (rectus abdominis and pyramidalis) and the adductor muscles of the thigh insert on the pubis (Fig. 7–6). Conditions involving this area may therefore be associated with pain related to trunk or thigh motion.

Sacrum and Coccyx

The sacrum consists of five fused vertebrae that decrease in size distally (Fig. 7–7). The promontory of the first sacral vertebra projects anteriorly into the pelvis. On either side of the body of S1 arise the large triangular-shaped alae (the term *ala* [plural, *alae*] refers to a wing-like or expanded structure).[3] Four sets of sacral foramina are present anteriorly and posteriorly. Those easily visualized on sacral radiographs are the anterior sacral foramina, through which exit the ventral divisions of the sacral nerves and enter the lateral sacral arteries.[1]

The dorsal aspect of the sacrum displays a middle sacral crest with three or four tubercles, representing the rudimentary spinous processes of these sacral segments. The laminae of the fifth sacral segment are deficient, leaving an aperture termed the sacral hiatus. The dorsal foramina are less regular in size than the ventral ones and allow egress of the dorsal divisions of the sacral nerves.

The coccyx consists of four or five fused vertebral bodies that serve as the attachment for the gluteus maximus, the coccygeus, the sphincter ani, and the levator ani muscles.

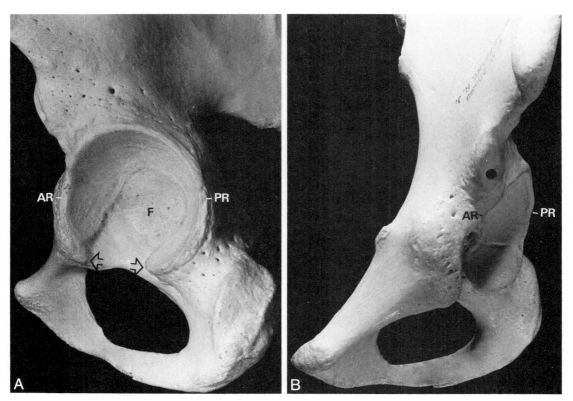

Figure 7–3. The Normal Acetabulum. *A,* This oblique view shows the acetabulum en face. The horseshoe-shaped articular surface and the anterior (AR) and posterior (PR) acetabular rims are well seen. The central acetabular fossa (F) is thin and nonarticular. In life the transverse ligament spans the gap (arrows) in the inferior acetabulum. *B,* View to correspond to an AP radiograph. The anterior (AR) and posterior (PR) acetabular rims are well seen.

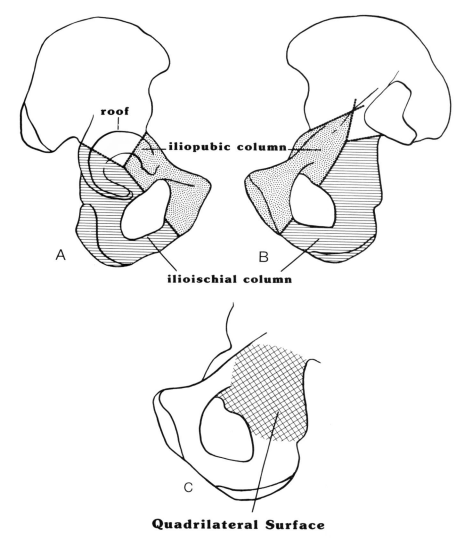

roof

iliopubic column

A

B

ilioischial column

C

Quadrilateral Surface

Figure 7–4. Acetabular Arches. *A,* The lateral view shows the anterior (iliopubic) and the posterior (ilioischial) columns (arches) that meet at the acetabular roof. *B,* Medial view. *C,* Medial view with quadrilateral surface crosshatched. (Redrawn from Judet R, Judet J, Letournel E. J Bone Joint Surg (Am) 64:1615, 1964.)

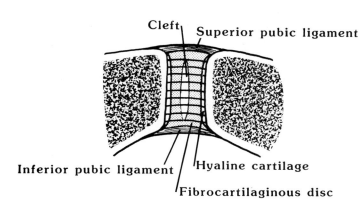

Cleft Superior pubic ligament

Inferior pubic ligament Hyaline cartilage

Fibrocartilaginous disc

Figure 7–5. The Pubic Symphysis. The articular surfaces are covered by thin layers of hyaline cartilage that are connected by a fibrocartilaginous interpubic disc. The superior pubic and the arcuate (inferior pubic) ligaments are indicated.

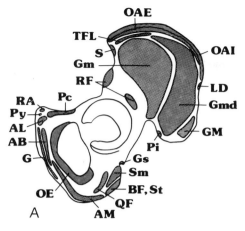

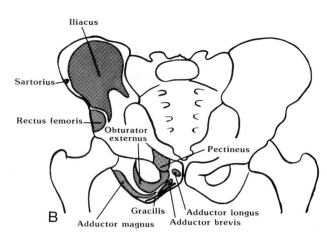

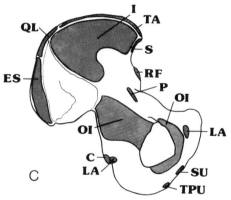

Figure 7–6. Muscle Attachments. *A*, Lateral, *B*, anterior pelvis. *C*, medial view. AB = adductor brevis; AL = adductor longus; AM = adductor magnus; BF, St = biceps femoris, semitendinosus; C = coccygeus; ES = erector spinae; G = gracilis; GM = gluteus maximus; Gm = gluteus minimus; Gmd = gluteus medius; Gs = gemellus superior; I = iliacus; LA = levator ani; LD = latissimus dorsi; OAE = obliquus externus abdominis; OAI = obliquus internus abdominis; OE = obturator externus; OI = obturator internus; P = psoas minor; Pc = pectineus; Pi = piriformis; Py = pyramidalis; QF = quadratus femoris; QL = quadratus lumborum; RA = rectus abdominis; RF = rectus femoris; S = sartorius; Sm = semimembranosus; SU = sphincter urethrae; TA = transversus abdominis; TFL = tensor fasciae latae; TPU = transversus perinei superficialis.

Body weight tends to rotate the upper end of the sacrum anteriorly and downward, and the coccyx posteriorly and upward. This rotation is prevented by the shape of the sacrum, the dorsal and interosseous sacroiliac ligaments, and the sacrotuberous and sacrospinous ligaments.[1]

Sacroiliac Joints

The sacroiliac joints are complex, each consisting of a posterior syndesmosis and an anterior inferior true joint (Fig. 7–8). The cartilaginous surface of the true joint is thicker on the sacral side than on the iliac side, a disparity that may account for the earlier and more severe erosion of the iliac side of the SI joints in patients with sacroiliitis.[2]

Normal Radiographic Anatomy

Pelvis

In cases of pelvic trauma or severe trauma with possible pelvic injury, standard examination of the pelvis consists of an anteroposterior view (see Fig. 7–1), followed by oblique views if abnormalities (such as a nondisplaced acetabular fracture) are suspected or if clarification is necessary (see Acetabular Fractures). Pennal and Sutherland suggest two additional views of the pelvis—the inlet projection (AP angled caudally) and the tangential projection (AP angled cranially)—when pelvic fractures are being evaluated.[38] Currently, however, CT scanning (if available) usually replaces these angled views and often the oblique views as well.

Acetabulum

The acetabulum is a particularly complex area to study on routine radiographs. On the anteroposterior radiograph six lines are of help in defining these structures and in understanding acetabular fractures and deformities (Figs. 7–9 and 7–10).[4, 6]

1. The *arcuate (iliopubic) line* begins at the superior edge of the greater sciatic notch and extends to the pubic tubercle. Discontinuity in this line indicates a fracture of the iliopubic column.

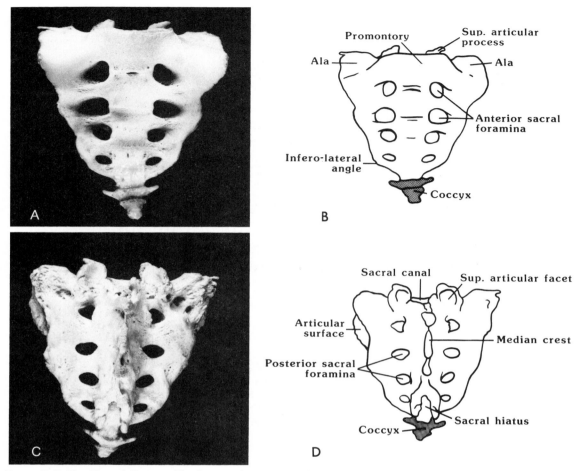

Figure 7–7. The Normal Sacrum. The five sacral segments and the coccyx are shown with four sacral foramina present anteriorly and posteriorly. The flared sacral alae are shown. *A,* Anterior view; *B,* diagram of anterior view; *C,* posterior view; *D,* diagram of posterior view.

2. The *ilioischial line* is formed by the quadrilateral surface of the ilium that is perpendicular to the x-ray beam. Discontinuity of this line indicates a fracture of the ilioischial column.

3. The U-shaped or *teardrop* shadow is a composite structure made up of the anterior

acetabular fossa laterally and the quadrilateral surface medially connected by the inferior margin of the acetabular notch. The position of this teardrop shadow with relation to the posterior ilioischial line depends upon patient positioning and rotation. Thus the moderate anterior

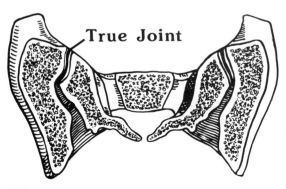

Figure 7–8. The Sacroiliac Joints. Transverse section at the level of S2 shows the anterior synovial joint (true joint) and the posterior fibrous articulation (syndesmosis). (Redrawn from Williams PL, Warwick R, eds. Gray's Anatomy, 36th Br. ed. Edinburgh, Churchill Livingstone, 1980, by permission.)

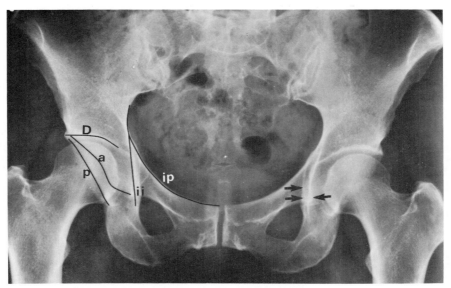

Figure 7–9. Pelvic Lines. The iliopubic (ip) and ilioischial (ii) lines help in assessing the anterior and posterior columns. The acetabular dome (D) and anterior (a) and posterior (p) lips (rims) of the acetabulum are seen. The teardrop figure (arrows) is a composite shadow made up laterally of the anterior aspect of the acetabular fossa and medially of the quadrilateral surface of the ilium. The more posterior aspect of the quadrilateral surface (represented by the ilioischial line) is superimposed on the teardrop in this nonrotated view.

oblique projection will position the teardrop medial to the ilioischial line, while a posterior oblique view will do the opposite.[4]

4. The *roof of the acetabulum,* also called the *acetabular dome,* corresponds to the major weight-bearing portion of the acetabulum.

5. The edge of the *anterior lip* of the acetabulum.

6. The margin of the *posterior lip* of the acetabulum.

Judet and associates advocated additional oblique views for evaluation of the acetabulum, particularly for the study of acetabular fractures. With the patient rotated 45 degrees away from the injured side (the anterior oblique view), the iliopubic column and the posterior lip of the acetabulum are well seen. Rotation 45 degrees toward the involved side (the posterior oblique projection) is suggested for evaluation of the ilioischial column and the anterior acetabular rim. Specimen radiography done by Armbuster and co-workers showed that the posterior ace-

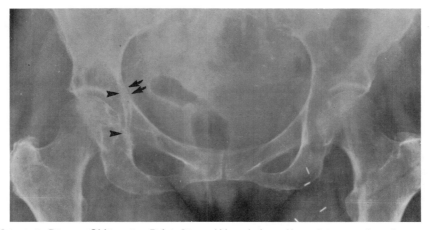

Figure 7–10. Metastatic Disease Obliterating Pelvic Lines. Although the radiograph is not technically optimal, the absence of portions of the right iliopubic (arrows) and ilioischial (arrowheads) lines in comparison with the normal left side makes it possible to detect bone destruction due to metastatic disease. The inferior margin of the right superior pubic ramus is also involved.

tabular rim is actually optimally visualized on 15 to 30 degrees anterior oblique projections, and the iliopubic column is best seen on 30 to 45 degrees anterior oblique projection.[4] They therefore advocate a single 30-degree anterior oblique projection for evaluation of both these structures. A 30 to 45 degree posterior oblique projection is suggested for evaluation of the ilioischial column and the anterior acetabular rim.

Computed tomography may be helpful in evaluating both the soft tissue and the bony structures of the pelvis and the acetabulum. Normal findings are shown in Figure 7–11.[5, 7, 8]

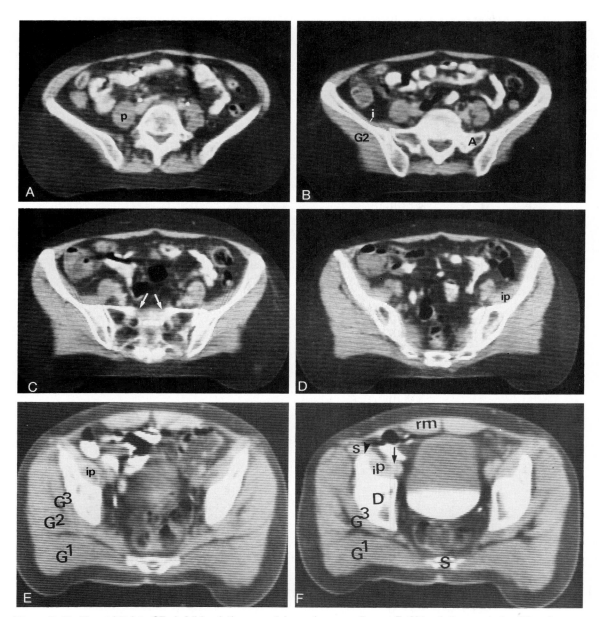

Figure 7–11. Normal Pelvic CT. *A,* L5 level: the psoas (p) muscles are well seen. *B,* SI level: the sacral alae (A) and upper portions of the SI joints are seen. *C,* S2 level: the anterior sacrum is in line with the adjacent ilia. The SI joints are sharply marginated, and normal bony condensation is present in the adjacent ilia. Arrows indicate the ventral foramina for the exiting S1 roots. *D,* Lower limit of SI joints: the psoas and iliacus muscles (ip) have merged. *E,* Junction of pubis, ilium, and ischium: the gluteal muscles (G1, G2, G3) are well seen. *F,* Acetabular dome: the acetabular dome (D) is well seen, with the anterior inferior iliac spine (arrowhead) protruding from it anteriorly. The arrow indicates the femoral nerve, artery, and vein.

Illustration continued on opposite page

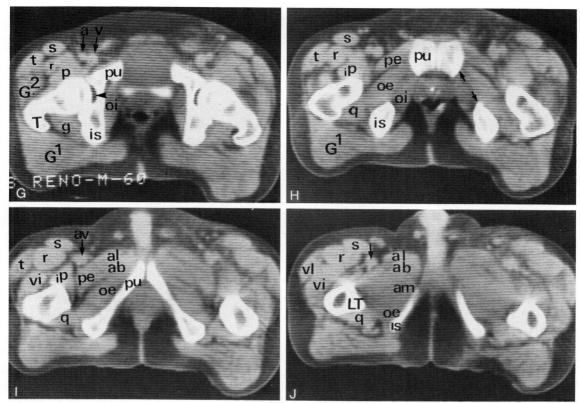

Figure 7–11. Normal pelvic CT *Continued. G,* Acetabulum: The acetabular fossa, with fat (arrowhead) filling the nonarticular portion, and various muscles are well seen. *H,* Obturator foramen: the anterior (pubic) and posterior (ischial) margins of the foramen are shown (arrows). *I,* Ischiopubic ramus. *J,* Ischial tuberosity. a = femoral artery; ab = adductor brevis; al = adductor longus; am = adductor magnus; D = acetabular dome; g = gemellus superior; G1 = gluteus maximus; G2 = gluteus medius; G3 = gluteus minimus; i = iliacus; ip = iliopsoas; LT = lesser trochanter; is = ischium; oe = obturator externus; oi = obturator internus; pe = pectineus; p = psoas; pu = pubis; q = quadratus femoris; r = rectus femoris; rm = rectus abdominis; s = sartorius; S = sacrum; t = tensor fascia lata; T = greater trochanter; v = femoral vein; vi = vastus intermedius; vl = vastus lateralis.

Pubic Symphysis

On radiologic examination the normal pubic symphysis usually, but not invariably, has a visible cortical margin with parallel or symmetrically convex margins. It is 5.9 ± 1.3 mm wide in males and about 1 mm narrower in females (4.9 ± 1.1 mm). Alignment of the pubic bones is best judged by evaluation of their inferior surfaces, since these are usually at the same level, particularly in males.[9] Stork views, taken with the patient standing first on one leg and then the other, may be useful in demonstrating instability in questionable cases. Gas within the pubic symphysis, widening of the pubic symphysis, and erosion and subsequent healing leading to an irregular, sclerotic articular surface have been noted accompanying pregnancy.

Sacrum and Coccyx

Angled oblique and lateral views may be used for evaluation of the sacrum, the coccyx, or both. On lateral views in the upright position the upper surface of S1 tilts anteriorly at an angle of 30 to 40 degrees.

On AP views dense curvilinear lines, corresponding to the superior aspects of the anterior foramina, are noted. The second foramen may appear as a continuation of the rim of the pelvis.[12] Lack of symmetry or absence of one of these lines should strongly suggest a destructive lesion in the area (Fig. 7–12) and should differentiate true bone destruction from overlying bowel gas.

CT shows the sacrum to advantage. Representative images are shown in Figure 7–11, but the interested reader is referred to the detailed evaluation by Whelan and Gold for additional information.[10]

Sacroiliac (SI) Joints

Because of the oblique orientation of the SI joints, questionably abnormal findings on an

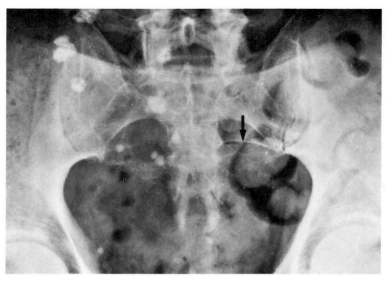

Figure 7–12. Sacral Tumor. There is absence of the cortical line above the right (S2) foramen as compared with the normal left (arrow). Angiography confirmed a vascular tumor mass (pheochromocytoma).

anteroposterior view of the pelvis should be confirmed by additional views. These consist of oblique views, with the patient supine and the side in question elevated 20 degrees, or an angled view, with the patient supine and the tube tilted 10 degrees cranially (Fig. 7–13). Generally, the angled view is of most help and shows the intact cortex on each side of the normal joint.

ABNORMAL CONDITIONS

Pelvic Fractures

Classification

Dunn and Morris.[14] Dunn and Morris classified pelvic fractures according to their stability (Table 7–1): (1) avulsion fractures, (2) stable fractures, and (3) unstable fractures. This classification is useful, since avulsion fractures and stable fractures are usually treated conservatively. Stability, however, applies only to the structure of the pelvic ring and associated soft tissue injuries, other fractures and retroperitoneal hemorrhage may place the patient in a precarious position.

Unstable fractures include the following:

Comminuted fractures of the tie arch (straddle fractures). These represented 30 percent of the group of unstable fractures.

Vertical shear injury. This was the next most frequent unstable fracture in this series. The posterior component of the injury occurs through the sacroiliac joints or the sacral or the iliac alae.

Pelvic dislocation due to anteroposterior compression. This force results in separation of the pubic symphysis and one or both of the sacroiliac joints. One half of the patients with this injury suffered damage to the bladder or the urethra.

Lateral compression injury. These are identified by the presence of fractures of both (ischio)pubic rami on the side of impact and by the disruption posteriorly of the sacral or the iliac ala or the sacroiliac joint on the same side. Bladder or urethral damage occurred in 3 of 4 patients with this injury.

Bucket handle injuries. This category refers to a combination of fractures involving the ischiopubic rami on the side opposite impact and the sacral or the iliac ala or the sacroiliac joint on the side of impact. The hemipelvis on the side of impact is displaced superiorly and inward and is rotated. Urinary tract disruption is uncommon, but retroperitoneal hemorrhage occurred in 2 of 4 patients in this group.

Total pelvic disruption. This injury involves dislocation in two planes of each hemipelvis as well as tie-arch fractures.

Tile and Pennal.[30, 38] Tile and Pennal classified fractures according to the underlying mechanism of injury and the subsequent radiographic

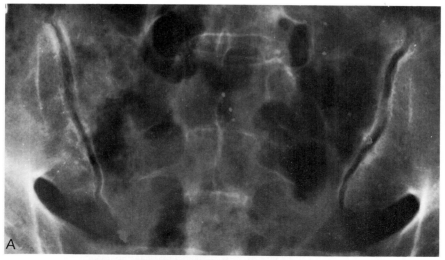

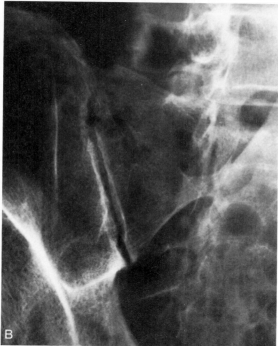

Figure 7–13. Normal SI Joints. The angled *(A)* and oblique *(B)* views show normally maintained cortices and cartilage spaces.

appearance (Fig. 7–14). This classification corresponds to the unstable fracture group in the Dunn and Morris scheme.

I. *Anterior Compression Injuries.*

   A. Symphysis disruption, open-book type. There is separation of the pubic symphysis and anterior sacroiliac ligaments. Genitourinary, rectal, or vascular injury may occur.

   B. Isolated bilateral anterior pubic rami

fractures (four-pillar type). Urethral rupture may be an associated injury.

II. *Lateral Compression.*

   A. Ipsilateral type. These injuries may be reduced in the supine position, leading to an innocuous radiographic appearance. The bladder may be pulled into the fracture site at the time of reduction.

   B. Contralateral type.

Table 7–1. Classifications of Pelvic Fractures

Dunn and Morris	Key and Conwell	Tile and Pennal	Mechanism	Associated Injuries	Comments
AVULSION (3.5%)[a] ASIS AIIS Ischial tuberosity	Type I: Fractures of individual bones without break in continuity of pelvic ring		Forceful muscular contraction		
STABLE (67%)[b] Ala of ilium Body of sacrum 1 to 3 pubic rami	Type II: Single break in pelvic ring				
UNSTABLE (30%) Straddle injury[c] (29.4%)[i]	Type III: Double break in pelvic ring	Anteroposterior compression, isolated bilateral anterior pubic rami fractures	Anterior or lateral compression	Urethral rupture Bladder injury Hemorrhage	
Vertical shear[d,j] (23.5%)[i]		Vertical shear	Vertical shear	Massive hemorrhage common Genitourinary or rectal	Most common unstable fracture
Pelvic dislocation[e,j] (17.6%)[i]		Anterior compression, symphysis disruption (open book type)	Anterior compression		
Lateral compression[f,j] (11.8%)[i]		Lateral compression, ipsilateral type	Lateral compression	Bladder and urethra	May reduce and appear innocuous on supine radiographs
Bucket handle[g,j] (11.8%)[i]		Lateral compression, contralateral type	Lateral compression or oblique AP compression	Urinary injury is rare	
Total disruption[h] (5.9%)[i]		? Lateral compression, posterior disruption plus bilateral pubic rami	Lateral compression	Hemorrhage, genitourinary injury	

See illustration T7–1: [a]Part A; [b]B; [c]C; [d]D; [e]E; [f]F; [g]G; [h]H. (Redrawn from Dunn, AW, Morris, HD: J Bone Joint Surg (Am) 50:1639, 1968.) [i]Percentage of unstable fractures. [j]Malgaigne's fracture.

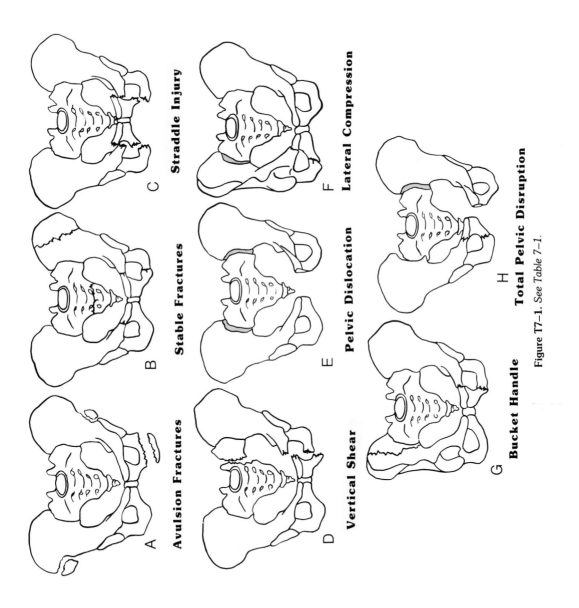

A Avulsion Fractures

B Stable Fractures

C Straddle Injury

D Vertical Shear

E Pelvic Dislocation

F Lateral Compression

G Bucket Handle

H Total Pelvic Disruption

Figure T7–1. See Table 7–1.

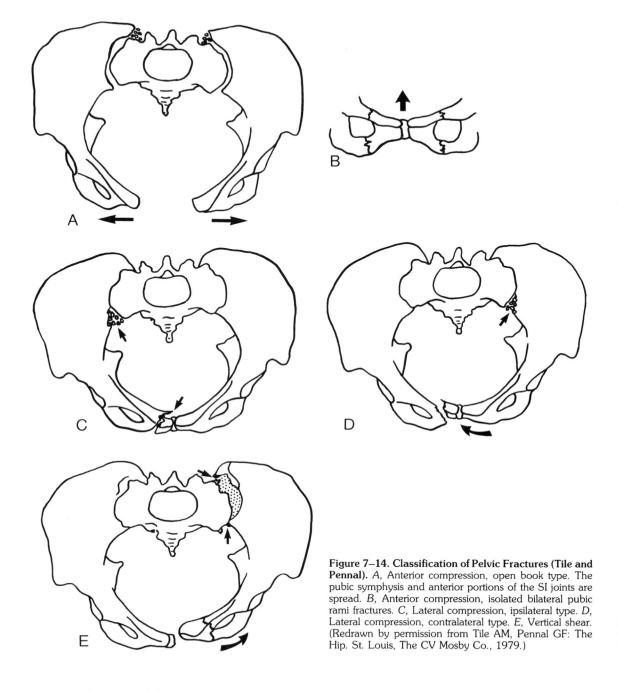

Figure 7–14. Classification of Pelvic Fractures (Tile and Pennal). *A,* Anterior compression, open book type. The pubic symphysis and anterior portions of the SI joints are spread. *B,* Anterior compression, isolated bilateral pubic rami fractures. *C,* Lateral compression, ipsilateral type. *D,* Lateral compression, contralateral type. *E,* Vertical shear. (Redrawn by permission from Tile AM, Pennal GF: The Hip. St. Louis, The CV Mosby Co., 1979.)

C. Fractures of both rami and posterior disruption. The sacrum, ilium, or sacroiliac joint may be involved.

III. *Vertical Shear.*

This is the most unstable type of pelvic disruption. According to Tile and Pennal, the radiographic demonstration of associated avulsion of the ischial spine is a sign of gross pelvic instability. Sciatic nerve lesions or avulsions of the fifth lumbar or

first sacral nerve roots may occur. Massive hemorrhage is common.[38]

Key and Conwell.[22, 23] The classification of Key and Conwell includes acetabular as well as pelvic fractures and is quite logical.

I. *Fractures of the individual bones without a break in the continuity of the pelvic ring*

A. Avulsion fractures
1. Anterior superior iliac spine
2. Anterior inferior iliac spine

Table 7–2. **Avulsion Fractures of the Pelvis**

Apophysis	Age at Union	Inserting Muscle	Activity Associated with Injury
Anterior superior iliac spine	16 to 20	Sartorius	Sprinting
Anterior inferior iliac spine	25	Rectus femoris	
Ischial tuberosity	20 to 25	Hamstrings	Hurdling, cheerleading
Pubic symphysis	20 to 25	Adductor longus Adductor brevis Gracilis	
Iliac crest apophysis	17–18 yrs.	Abdominal muscles	Abrupt directional change while running

Source: Urbaniak JR, Shaefer, WW, Stelling FH III: Clin Orthop 116:80, 1976.

3. Ischial tuberosity
   B. Fracture of the pubis or ischium
   C. Fracture of the wing of the ilium (Duverney)
   D. Fracture of the sacrum
   E. Fracture or dislocation of the coccyx
II. *Single break in the pelvic ring*
   A. Fracture of two ipsilateral rami
   B. Fracture near, or subluxation of, the pubic symphysis
   C. Fracture near, or subluxation of, the sacroiliac joint
III. *Double breaks in the pelvic ring*
   A. Double vertical fractures, dislocation of the pubis (straddle fractures), or both
   B. Double vertical fractures, dislocations (Malgaigne), or both
   C. Severe multiple fractures
IV. *Fractures of the acetabulum*
   A. Undisplaced
   B. Displaced

Description

The most frequent pelvic fractures, those involving the pubic rami, accounted for 69 percent of all fractures in Rankin's series of 449 patients.[31] Fractures of a single ramus were more frequent than were fractures of multiple rami. The next most frequent fractures were ilial, ischial, and acetabular. Sacral fractures occurred in 8 percent of cases and coccygeal fractures in 13 percent.

Avulsion Fractures. Avulsion fractures occur when fragments of bone are pulled from their original position by active muscular contraction. This is most likely to occur before the apophyses have fused (Table 7–2). Avulsion of the anterior superior iliac spine (ASIS), due to vigorous contraction of the sartorius muscle, is seen most often in athletes under age 16 or 17 (the age at which fusion of the iliac crest apophyses occurs;

Fig. 7–15).[22] Avulsion of the anterior inferior iliac spine by the forceful contraction of the rectus femoris occurs less commonly than does avulsion of the ASIS or of the ischial tuberosity.[19] The avulsed fragment is displaced inferiorly. Avulsion of the ischial tuberosity may occur during strenuous activities such as hurdling or acrobatics, when the strong pull of the hamstring muscles displaces the apophysis downward, forward, and laterally (Figs. 7–16 and 7–17).[22] This injury may occur in young adults, since the ischial apophysis does not unite until age 20 to 25.

Avulsion fractures are generally treated conservatively. Healing may result in bony overgrowth, with a large and sometimes painful bony mass at the site of an often forgotten injury producing a radiographic appearance that may suggest a primary bone tumor. The bone that is present, however, has a normal trabecular pat-

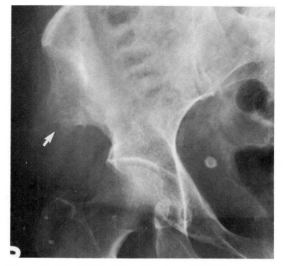

Figure 7–15. Old Avulsion Fracture ASIS. The irregular enlargement at the site of the anterior superior iliac spine suggests an old avulsion injury.

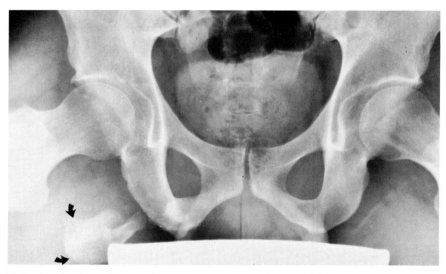

Figure 7–16. Old Ischial Avulsion Fracture. This young patient complained of left hip pain. A view of the pelvis and hips shows a well-corticated bony density and several smaller ossicles below the right ischium (arrows), indicating an old avulsion fracture. On questioning, a history of football injury many years before was obtained.

tern and an intact distal cortex. Barnes and Hinds noted that 68 percent of reported cases of ischial apophyseal avulsion did not unite, and a radiolucent zone therefore remained, separating the bony mass from the ischium.[11]

Stable Fractures. In the Key and Conwell classification, types I and II injuries are stable fractures of the pelvic rim.

Fractures of a *single* ramus of the pubis or ischium are frequent injuries and occur more commonly than do fractures of two or more rami.[31] Fractures of a single ramus are frequently seen in the elderly following a fall.

Stress fractures may occur in association with the last trimester of pregnancy, in runners, in military recruits, and following total hip replacement.[22] Treatment is conservative.

Iliac wing fractures (termed Duverney fractures) are due to direct trauma, usually lateral compression.[31] Little displacement of fragments occurs, and major hemorrhage is not usually a feature.

Sacral Fractures. Sacral fractures may result from direct trauma, such as a fall in the sitting position (Table 7–3). These fractures are usually horizontal and are occasionally displaced. Indi-

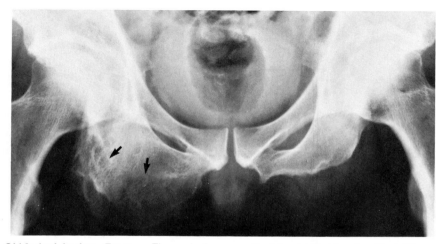

Figure 7–17. Old Ischial Avulsion Fracture. The marked overgrowth of the right ischium is evident. The normal trabecular pattern and the thin line demarcating the original cortex of the ischium (arrows) help distinguish this lesion from adjacent myositis ossificans or osteochondroma.

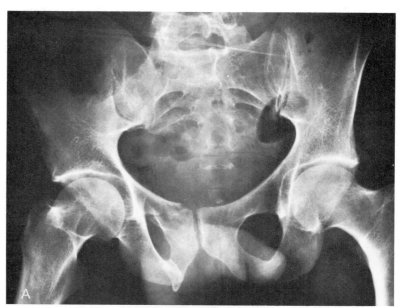

Figure 7–18. Subtle Sacral Fractures. *A,* An oblique view of the pelvis shows fractures of the right superior and inferior pubic rami. No definite sacral fracture is seen, although there is slight irregularity of the right second foramen in comparison with the left. *B,* A CT section clearly shows a fracture through the right side of the sacrum (arrow). *C,* Another patient with asymmetry of the sacral foramina, indicating sacral fracture (arrow).

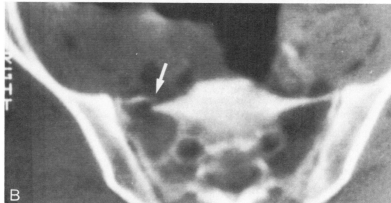

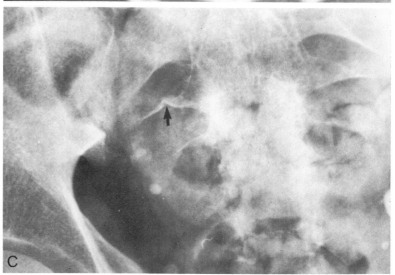

Table 7–3. **Etiological Classification of Sacral Fractures**

Direct injury
  Complex comminuted fractures from missiles
  Transverse fractures below the SI joints
  Compression fractures of the posterior arch
Indirect injury (force transmitted through SI joints)
  Juxtailiac marginal fractures
  Fractures through the first and second sacral foramina, with upward displacement of the lateral sacral mass
  Compressed and comminuted fractures of the first and second sacral foramina, with a loss of sacral pattern
  Fissure fractures through the first, second, third, and fourth sacral foramina, with little or no displacement
  Avulsion fractures at the insertion of the sacrotuberous ligament
  Transverse fractures at the level of the third sacral foramina (possibly due to direct trauma or avulsion injury)

Source: Modified from Bonnin JG: J Bone Joint Surg 27:113, 1945.

rect trauma more often results in nondisplaced vertical fractures.[37] Since the first and second foramina represent points of relative weakness in the femorosacral and ischiosacral arches, fractures of the sacrum that are due to transmitted forces (indirect fractures) tend to begin at these foramina.[12]

Sacral fractures are commonly seen in association with other pelvic fractures. A study by Medelman of 50 consecutive cases of pelvic fracture revealed sacral fractures in 22 patients (44 percent), and in only one instance was the fracture an isolated injury (Fig. 7–18).[28] The fractures are not usually displaced and may be longitudinal (most frequent), oblique, or horizontal. The fracture lines are rarely complete,

and detection, particularly in osteoporotic patients, is difficult. Medelman noted that sharp angulation of the upper margins of one foramen or of adjacent foramina may be the only evidence of fracture.[28] Northrop, Eto, and Loop also noted that the anterior, superior sacral foraminal lines are normally symmetrical and that disruption or lack of symmetry should suggest fracture.[29] They advocated tomography for confirmation. Laasonen noted that indirect soft tissue signs, such as the presence of a presacral soft tissue mass, would not have helped in detecting missed hairline fractures. Although this author noted: "Even small, non-dislocated hairline fractures can be combined with severe neural involvement," his analysis of 156 patients with pelvic fractures, including 12 patients in whom a sacral hairline fracture was missed, suggested that these missed fractures probably resulted from low-energy accidents and their "contribution to the prediction of or diagnosis of complications is minimal, or even nil. . . ."[24] Pelvic CT is likely to reveal an even higher incidence of sacral fracture than has been noted in previous studies (Fig. 7–18).

Linear fractures along the lower edge of the sacrum are due to traction by the sacrotuberous ligament (Fig. 7–19). These fractures provide evidence that there is motion of one side of the pelvis with consequent traction on the ligament.

Coccygeal fractures are more frequent in women and usually result from a fall in the sitting position. The diagnosis may be made on physical examination by the presence of pain and tenderness localized to the coccyx and by the demonstration of abnormal mobility of the coccyx on rectal examination.[22] Radiological ex-

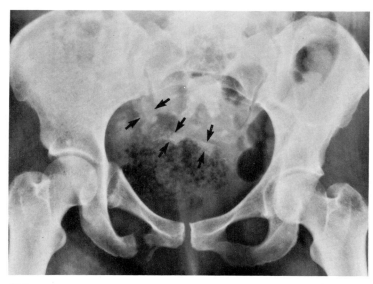

Figure 7–19. Pelvic Fractures (Vertical Shear) with Sacral Avulsion. Fractures of the right ischium and pubis and diastasis of the right SI joint are present. The right lateral margin of the sacrum has been avulsed (arrows) by the pull of the sacrotuberous ligament. This indicates instability.

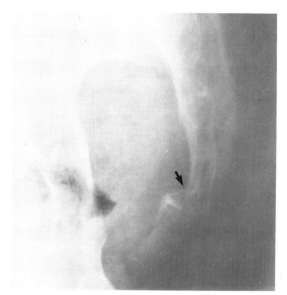

Figure 7–20. Sacral Fracture. The lateral view shows deformity (arrow) from a sacral fracture.

amination may show angular deformity of the fracture site on the lateral view (Fig. 7–20). Lateral angulation on the frontal view is said to be of little or no significance unless associated with dislocation at the sacrococcygeal articulation.[20]

Single Breaks in the Pelvic Ring: Type II Fractures (Key and Conwell). These fractures usually result from direct trauma and occur near the symphysis pubis or the SI joint since these

areas allow slight motion, and, therefore, a single (rather than double) fracture in the pelvic ring can occur. The concept that in a rigid ringlike structure two fractures must always occur when a displaced fracture is present is true; if minimal or no displacement occurs, however, an isolated fracture may be seen. Patients with only a single apparent fracture may demonstrate additional areas of injury on radionuclide bone scans.[17]

This category of injury includes fractures of two rami on one side, fractures near (or subluxation of) the pubic symphysis, and fractures near (or subluxation of) the sacroiliac joint (Fig. 7–21). Although these fractures are mechanically stable, severe soft tissue injuries may occur.[14] Kane notes that an isolated fracture near the symphysis or subluxation of the pubic symphysis is rare, but if this injury results from major trauma, genitourinary tract damage is present in a high percentage of cases.[22] More often, pubic symphysis separation is accompanied by sacroiliac separation. Widening of the symphysis to more than 1 cm in males or more than 8 mm in nonpregnant females or loss of alignment of the inferior pubic margins should suggest the possibility of traumatic disruption.[9]

An *isolated fracture near, or dislocation of, a sacroiliac joint* is a rare injury, since, more often, concomitant disruption of the pelvis occurs anteriorly.[22]

Double Breaks in the Pelvic Ring, Unstable Fractures (Figs. 7–22 to 7–26). Fractures in which there are two breaks in the pelvic ring

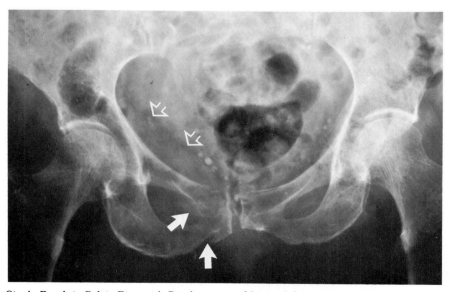

Figure 7–21. Single Break in Pelvic Ring with Displacement of Internal Obturator Fat Line. There are fractures of the right superior and inferior pubic rami (arrows). The right internal obturator fat line (open arrows) and the adjacent phleboliths are elevated in comparison with the normal side. This was an important finding, since it confirmed the acute nature of the injury in a patient who was unable to provide appropriate information.

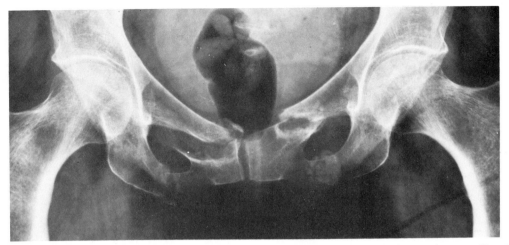

Figure 7–22. Straddle Fracture. There are healing bilateral fractures of the superior and inferior pubic rami. The absence of swelling at the time of this examination is demonstrated by the lack of displacement of the perivesical fat.

(type III, Key and Conwell) are unstable fractures. The presence of displacement of a major pelvic fragment is evidence that such a fracture falls into this category.[22] These injuries are half as frequent as stable fractures.[14]

Straddle Fractures. This category refers to a combination of bilateral fractures of the ischia and pubes (Fig. 7–22). A variant of the straddle fracture consists of fractures of the pubic rami on one side and disruption of the pubic symphysis. Straddle fractures represented almost 30 percent of the unstable fractures in the Dunn and Morris series.[14] Damage to the bladder or urethra or pelvic hemorrhage may occur.[14, 22]

Malgaigne Fractures. This term refers to a combination of two vertical fractures on one side of the pelvis, anterior and posterior to the acetabulum.[25] Anteriorly, the superior and inferior pubic rami are fractured, separating the pubis from the ilium and the ischium; posteriorly, there is a fracture behind the acetabulum involving the ilium, the SI joint, or the sacrum.[22] Kane notes that the term *Malgaigne fracture* has been expanded recently to include all fractures in which the anterior and posterior halves of the pelvis are simultaneously involved, including, for example, disruption of the symphysis accompanying a fracture through the ilium, SI joint, or sacrum.[22] Kane suggests the term be used to

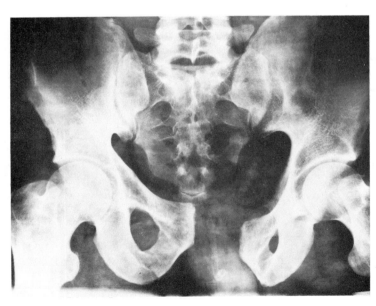

Figure 7–23. Pelvic Dislocation Due to Anteroposterior Compression. There is widening of the pubic symphysis and the left SI joint. One half of these patients have accompanying bladder or urethral damage.

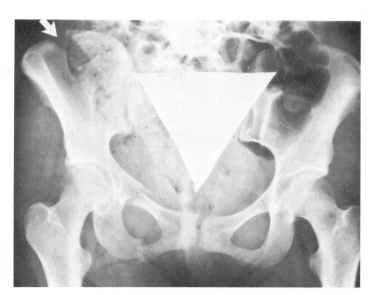

Figure 7–24. Lateral Compression Injury.
There are fractures of the right iliac wing (arrow), superior pubic ramus and ischium, and there is rotation medially of the separated fragment of the right hemipelvis. This is one type of Malgaigne fracture.

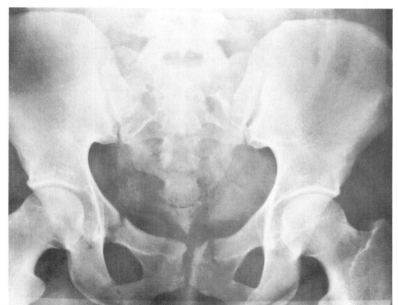

Figure 7–25. Bucket Handle Fracture. Fractures of the right superior and inferior pubic rami and diastasis of the left SI joint suggest a "bucket handle injury." The irregularity of the right first and second sacral foramina indicates a vertical sacral fracture.

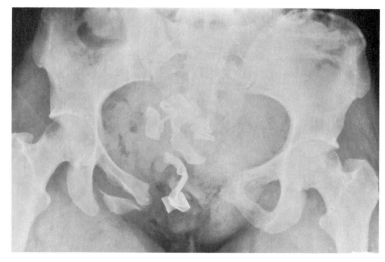

Figure 7–26. Total Pelvic Disruption.
Severe separation of the pubic symphysis and separation of the right sacroiliac joint can be seen. The right inferior pubic ramus is fractured. This was an open wound, and multiple dressings are noted.

signify disruption of the pelvis both anteriorly and posteriorly, with displacement of the intervening fragment.[22] Vertical shear, pelvic dislocation, and lateral compression fractures (Dunn and Morris) may then be classified as Malgaigne fractures.

Severe Pelvic Disruption. Severe pelvic disruption with multiple fractures is more frequently associated with hemorrhage and genitourinary complications than are other types of fractures.

Treatment

Most of these fractures, stable and unstable, are treated nonoperatively. With unstable fractures reduction of the displaced fragments is attempted by mechanical and postural means. Recently, external fixators of the Hoffmann type, attached to the pelvis via pins placed in the ilium, have been used to hold unstable fracture fragments (Fig. 7–27). This method of fixation has the advantages of pain relief,

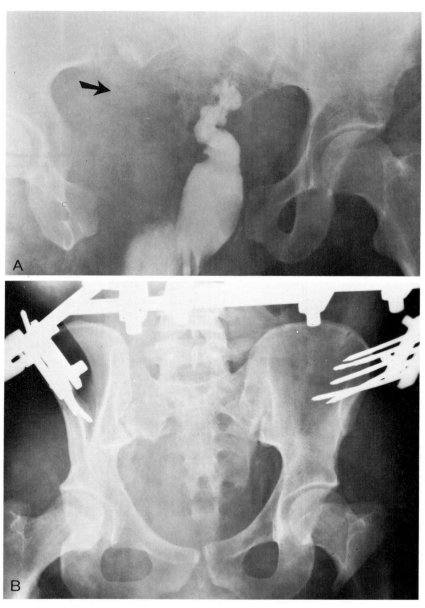

Figure 7–27. External Fixation. *A,* The initial AP view shows severe separation of the pubic symphysis and the right SI joint. There is avulsion of the right side of the sacrum as seen by the displacement of its lateral cortex (arrow). Contrast material instilled into the rectum did not demonstrate a tear. *B,* After external fixation there is marked improvement in pelvic alignment. The abnormal appearance of the lower right side of the sacrum is now obvious.

early ambulation, easier nursing care, and apparently reduced hemorrhage from the fracture sites.[21, 27, 34, 39]

Radiographically identifiable complications of pelvic fractures include loss of reduction, malunion, and post-traumatic osteoarthritis of the SI joints, characterized by the presence of subchondral sclerosis, irregular joint surfaces, hypertrophic lipping, and malalignment.[35] Partly as a result of the lack of knowledge regarding the time necessary for the healing of various pelvic fractures, the diagnosis of delayed union is unusual. Nonunion is also uncommon. When external fixators are used, bending or breakage of the fixation pins, pin tract infection, and fracture associated with pin placement are potential complications.

Hemorrhage. In addition to the fracture itself, attention must be directed toward accompanying injuries and to the identification and control of pelvic hemorrhage. The reported mortality rates of up to 26 percent in association with pelvic fractures are largely due to these factors.[47, 54] Hauser and Perry noted that patients with double breaks in the pelvic ring (Key and Conwell type III) more frequently required transfusions and needed more blood than did patients with other pelvic fractures.[22, 47] Several authors have noted recently that blood requirements appear to be lower in patients treated with external fixators, and this form of treatment may decrease the necessity for angiography and embolization (see the following paragraphs).[21, 39]

Arteriography and Venography in the Management of Associated Hemorrhage

In 1971 Athanasoulis, Duffield, and Shapiro introduced the concept that arteriography could be used to localize the source of hemorrhage in

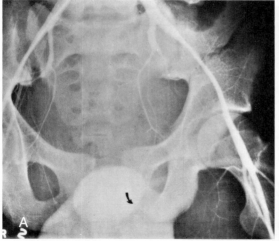

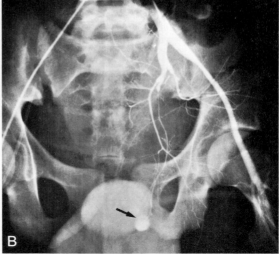

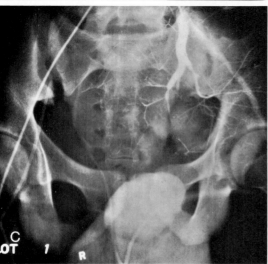

Figure 7–28. Arteriography for Pelvic Hemorrhage. *A,* There are diastases of the right SI joint and the pubic symphysis and an oblique fracture through the left ilium. An aortic injection shows a large pelvic mass (hematoma) and a faintly seen bleeding site (arrow). *B,* The internal iliac injection better demonstrates the bleeding site (arrow) and the marked vascular spasm proximal to it. *C,* After embolization of clot the bleeding has stopped. (Courtesy of Dr. Arthur Waltman, Massachusetts General Hospital, Boston, Mass.)

patients with pelvic fractures.[40] It was suggested that treatment might also be affected, and in 1972 Margolies and co-workers reported the control of hemorrhage occurring in such patients by selective embolization of autologous blood clots.[48]

Arteriography has subsequently been confirmed to be an effective method of localizing arterial bleeding sites in most patients with pelvic fractures and rapid blood loss,[49] and transcatheter embolization has been shown to be effective in reducing or stopping hemorrhage in almost all cases in which it is used (Fig. 7–28).[41, 49] In contrast with the experience in gastrointestinal bleeding, vasoconstrictor substances have not been of value in controlling pelvic bleeding.[41]

The method of examination consists of percutaneous catheterization of the femoral artery opposite the side of most severe trauma. A lumbar aortogram and a pelvic arteriogram, followed by bilateral selective internal iliac artery injections, are done, since according to Athanasoulis, aortography alone is an inadequate study for the exclusion of bleeding from the hypogastric arteries, the most frequent sites of hemorrhage.[40, 41] The source of bleeding is identified by extravasation of contrast medium outside the vessel lumen, although it has been shown experimentally that such extravasation requires bleeding at the rate of at least 0.5 ml per minute.[42] Lack of extravasation of contrast agent reliably excludes a major arterial source of bleeding.[54] After a bleeding site is identified, selective catheterization of the bleeding vessel and embolization (usually with surgical gelatin) is done, since the use of autologous clot may be associated with bleeding when lysis of the clot occurs.[41] Contrast material injection is repeated after embolization to confirm the lack of extravasation from the affected vessels. The contralateral hypogastric artery is also studied to evaluate the possibility of collateral supply to the bleeding site. The catheter is then removed and the femoral artery compressed until hemostasis is achieved.

Arteriography performed on patients with pelvic fracture and rapid blood loss early in the course of treatment may help to avoid the complications associated with multiple transfusions and large pelvic hematomas.[49] An additional advantage is the fact that the retroperitoneal hematoma itself need not be disturbed.

The major complication of transcatheter embolization is the reflux of embolized material into the arteries supplying the leg. The use of a balloon-tip catheter to occlude the vessel proximal to the point of embolization has apparently decreased the incidence of this complication;

however, in one series, embolization into the leg occurred in 1 of 18 patients undergoing the procedure.[49]

Reports prior to the introduction of arteriography for the study of post-traumatic hemorrhage suggested a role for venography.[51] Reynolds and Balsano performed bilateral simultaneous femoral venograms in 25 patients with pelvic fracture, and in one case a tear of an iliac vein was demonstrated. According to Athanasoulis, however, venography is generally unrewarding.[41] Patients with iliac vein transection have blood loss that is too rapid to allow angiographic evaluation, and the patients go directly to surgery without prior venography. Unfortunately, such major venous bleeding cannot be controlled by restricting arterial inflow.[41, 51] Reynolds and Balsano noted that major disruption of iliac veins is seen only after severe injury with sacroiliac joint displacement.[51]

Bleeding may also occur from the fracture margins, a finding supported in some patients by the cessation of bleeding after reduction and external fixation are accomplished.[39]

Acetabular Fractures

The problem of acetabular fractures is a complex one, beginning with differences in opinion as to the mode of production of these lesions and ending with multiple opinions regarding treatment.

Classification

Among the several classifications developed, that of Judet, Judet, and Letournel (1964) is probably the best known.[57] Acetabular fractures were classified into four "simple" types and one combined type. Because no two acetabular fractures are alike, the proposed classification actually represents isolated points along a spectrum of injury.[58] Most cases can, however, be classified into one of these groups.

Anatomical Classification, Judet, Judet and Letournel (173 patients;* Fig. 7–29),[57]

    I. *Posterior lip fracture*
        A. Fracture of posterior horn of the articular surface (1)
        B. Fracture of posterior lip (3)
        C. Fracture of posterior rim, posterior dislocation (45)
        D. Fracture of posterosuperior portion of the rim, posterosuperior dislocation (8)

---

*Numbers in parentheses are the numbers of patients afflicted.

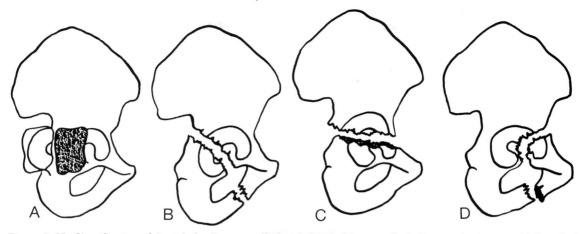

Figure 7–29. Classification of Acetabular Fractures (Judet, Judet, and Letournel). *A,* Posterior lip fractures. *B,* Ilioischial column fracture. *C,* Transverse fracture. *D,* Iliopubic column fracture. (Redrawn from Muller ME, Allgower M, Schneider R, et al.: Manual of Internal Fixation: Techniques Recommended by the AO Group. Heidelberg, Springer-Verlag, 1979.)

II. *Fracture of the ilioischial (posterior) column*

III. *Transverse fracture*
   A. Transverse fracture, posterior lip fracture, posterior dislocation (23)
   B. Transverse fracture, posterior lip, or posterosuperior fracture, central dislocation (10)
   C. Transverse fracture, central dislocation (25)
   D. T fracture, central dislocation (3)
   E. Transverse fracture, ilioischial column fracture (6)
   F. Transverse fracture, iliopubic column fracture (7)

IV. *Fracture of iliopubic (anterior) column*
   A. Anterior ridge fracture (4)
   B. Iliopubic column fracture (16)

V. *Associated fracture of both columns*

The simple types were most frequent and accounted for about 65 percent of patients (111 of 173). The most frequent combination lesions were T-shaped fractures, combined posterior wall and transverse fractures, and fractures involving both the anterior and the posterior columns.[58] Dislocation of the femoral head may accompany acetabular fractures and is the primary factor responsible for the development of avascular necrosis of the femoral head after acetabular fracture.[57]

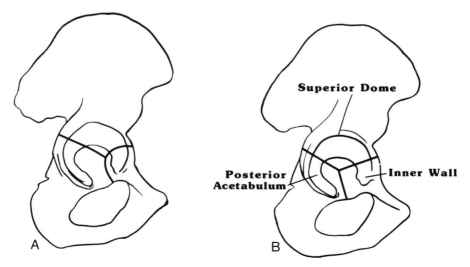

Epiphyseal Divisions

Figure 7–30. Classification of Acetabular Fractures (Rowe and Lowell). *A,* The epiphyseal divisions of the acetabulum in childhood are shown. *B,* The classification of acetabular fractures corresponds to the epiphyseal divisions shown in *A.* (Redrawn from Lowell JD: AAOS Instructional Course Lectures 22:145, 1973.)

361

Rowe and Lowell proposed a classification based again on anatomical location of the fracture lines (Fig. 7–30).[61, 68] They noted that the acetabulum, when viewed from the lateral side, can be divided into three segments that roughly correspond to the epiphyseal divisions present in childhood. The divisions are designated as the anterior third, or inner wall; the superior third, or superior dome; and the posterior wall. The term *bursting fracture* is applied when two or more of these segments are involved.

Anatomical Classification, Rowe and Lowell[61, 62, 63, 68]

I. *Linear or undisplaced acetabular fractures*
II. *Inner wall fractures (dome intact)*
   A. With normal head-dome relationship
   B. With central dislocation of the head
III. *Posterior fractures and fracture dislocations*
   A. Minor rim fracture
   B. Large single rim fracture
   C. Comminuted with or without major fragment
   D. Fractures of the rim and floor
   E. Fracture of the head with or without other fractures
IV. *Fractures of the superior dome*
   A. With normal head-dome relationship
   B. With head-dome incongruity or loss of normal relationship
V. *Bursting fractures*
   A. With good head-dome relationship
   B. With loss of normal head-dome relationship
VI. *Anterior fracture dislocations*

The basis for classifying fractures in this system is the area maximally involved. Thus superior dome fractures are commonly associated with fractures in all segments of the acetabulum, but the primary area of involvement and displacement is in the superior dome.

Radiographic Findings

Despite the fact that radiography plays a critical and ongoing role in the evaluation and treatment of acetabular fractures, the difficulty in understanding the radiological anatomy in three dimensions and in using this information for classification and evaluation of the results of treatment is considerable. The burden was eased by the classic work of Judet, Judet, and Letournel, who described a series of radiographically identifiable lines that correspond to structures important in understanding and classifying acetabular fractures.[57] On the anteroposterior view of the pelvis or hip six contours should be evaluated (see Fig. 7–9): the *arcuate, or iliopubic line* along the inner margin of the ilium and the superior aspect of the pubis (representing part of the anterior column); the *ilioischial line,* representing the posterior four fifths of the quadrilateral surface of the ilium (and therefore documenting the status of the posterior column); the *teardrop, or U,* representing laterally the inferior anterior part of the acetabular fossa and medially the quadrilateral surface of the ilium; the *anterior lip of the acetabulum;* the *posterior lip of the acetabulum;* and the *acetabular roof.* The ana-

Table 7–4. Radiographic Findings in Acetabular Fractures

	Anatomical Structure	Posterior Rim Fracture	Fracture of Ilioischial Column	Simple Transverse Fracture	Simple Iliopubic Fractures
Arcuate (iliopubic) line	Inner margin of ilium, which is continuous with inner superior aspect of pubis			+	+
Ilioischial line	Posterior four-fifths of quadrilateral surface of ilium		+	+	
Teardrop (U)	Laterally: inferior, anterior part of acetabular fossa Medially: quadrilateral surface of ilium				Displaced with ilio-pubic line
Anterior lip of acetabulum	Anterior rim			+	−
Posterior lip of acetabulum	Posterior rim	+		+	
Acetabular roof		±			
Dislocation		Posterior	Central	Central	Central

Sources: Judet R, Judet J, Le Tournel E: J Bone Joint Surg (Am) 46:1615, 1964; Armbuster TG, Guerra J Jr, Resnick D, et al: Radiology 128:1, 1978

+ = discontinuity; − = continuity.

tomical structures responsible for producing these lines and the areas involved in each of the basic fracture types described by Judet and associates are summarized in Table 7–4. The interested reader is referred to the original article for additional details.

In addition to standard anteroposterior views, oblique views of the hip have been recommended (see section on normal anatomy), since nondisplaced fractures of the acetabulum may be incompletely evaluated or inapparent on the anteroposterior view. In fact, Pearson and Har-

gadon noted that in 29 percent of 80 patients with acetabular fractures the fracture line through the acetabulum could not be seen on the initial examination. They noted that the presence of a fracture through the inferior pubic ramus and another through the superior pubic ramus at its junction with the ilium virtually assures the presence of an acetabular fracture. Rogers, Novy, and Harris emphasized the value of the 35 degree to 45 degree posterior oblique projection in demonstrating nondisplaced acetabular fractures (involving the quadrilateral sur-

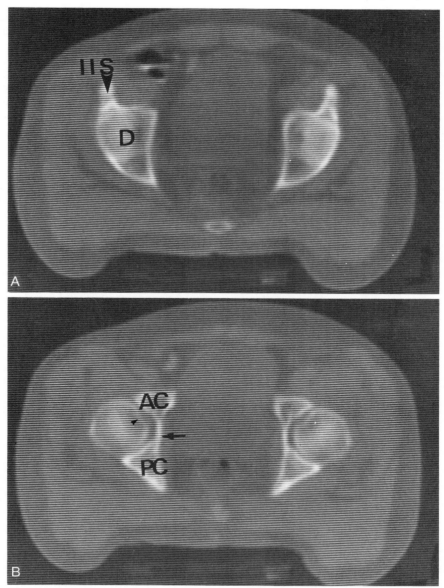

Figure 7–31. CT Demonstration of the Bony Anatomy of the Acetabulum and Lower Pelvis. *A,* At the level of the anterior inferior iliac spine (IIS), the acetabular dome (D) is seen. The bony hiatus between the acetabulum and the sacrum at this level is the lesser sciatic notch. *B,* A lower CT scan shows the femoral heads within the acetabula. The anterior (AC) and posterior (PC) columns are well seen. The arrow indicates the flat, quadrilateral surface of the ilium. An arrowhead marks the fovea of the femoral head.

face) not seen on anteroposterior or true lateral views.[67] In 2 of their 4 cases the obturator internus muscle was displaced on the affected side, emphasizing the need to search for this swelling in patients with pelvic trauma (see Fig. 7–21).

Preliminary study of patients with known acetabular fractures indicates that computed tomography is extremely helpful in demonstrating the location of fracture lines, the extent of soft tissue injury, and the presence of bony fragments within the joint space (Figs. 7–31 to 7–34).[64, 69] Of the 10 patients with acetabular fractures studied by Shirkhoda and co-workers, 6 had loose bodies within the joint demonstrable on CT scan but not revealed by conventional radiographs.[70] Postoperative healing and/or complications may also be evaluated with this technique.

Treatment

It is essential that a stable, congruous relationship be preserved or established between the femoral head and the acetabular roof and that this relationship be maintained until union of the fracture fragments occurs. In other words, radiographs should show the femoral head to be under the acetabular dome, the joint space should be of normal and uniform width, and no step-off should be present in the subchondral bone of the acetabular roof or femur.

Methods of treatment vary from surgery in all cases with displacement[57–59] to the more conservative approach advocated by Lowell.[63] In the latter linear or *undisplaced fractures* are treated symptomatically with bedrest and traction and later with crutch support until union is solid, at about 6 to 8 weeks. *Inner-wall fractures* without dislocation are treated conservatively with bedrest in balanced suspension, then with exercise and ambulation with crutches until bony union is present, at about 3 months. If medial displacement of the femoral head is present, manipulation is done to reposition the head under the acetabular dome, and the reduction is maintained with traction. *Posterior fractures* and fracture-dislocations are treated by closed reduction, with later surgery performed through a posterior approach if the obtained reduction is unstable in less than 60 degrees of flexion, if there are fragments of bone within the joint, if there is a significantly displaced femoral head fragment, if sciatic nerve palsy develops, or if sciatic pain persists after reduction. Fractures of the *superior dome* are treated conservatively if the femoral head is under the acetabular dome. If this relationship is abnormal, the fracture is reduced by closed or open means. *Bursting fractures* have the poorest prognosis. They are usually reduced by closed methods and maintained with traction (Fig. 7–35).[62] *Anterior fracture-dislocations* are uncommon. These injuries are unstable, and surgical reconstruction is necessary.[63]

Complications[58]

Osteoarthritis. Post-traumatic osteoarthritis may result if the joint surfaces of the femoral head and acetabular roof are incongruous. Unfortunately, osteoarthritis may also follow mild acetabular fractures without radiographically apparent incongruity, or it may follow surgical intervention with "perfect" surgical reduction. Letournel, for example, found significant osteoarthritis in 5.4 percent of perfect operative reductions and in 30.7 percent of imperfect reductions.[58] Osteophytic lipping around the femoral head occurred in about one quarter of surgically corrected acetabular fractures, but in most cases the clinical result remained good.[58] In addition to osteophytes, another 12 percent of patients developed other evidence of osteoarthritis, and in slightly more than half of these

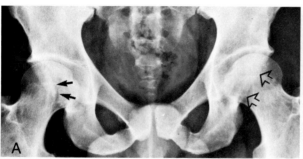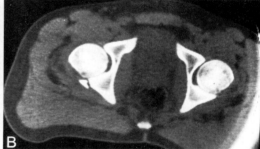

Figure 7–32. Posterior Lip Fracture. *A,* There is a fracture (small arrows) through the posterior rim of the right acetabulum. The normal posterior rim on the left is well seen (open arrows). *B,* The CT scan confirms the localization of the fracture to the posterior rim of the acetabulum and shows no subluxation of the femoral head.

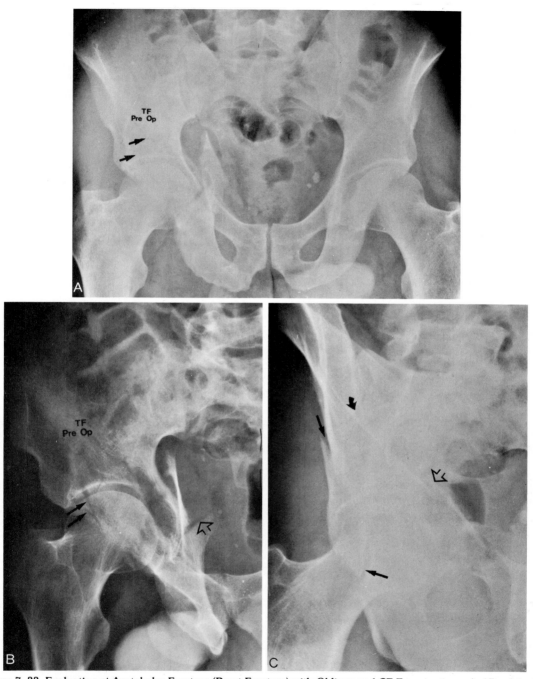

Figure 7–33. Evaluation of Acetabular Fracture (Burst Fracture) with Oblique and CT Examinations. *A,* AP pelvic view shows disruption of the right ilioischial line, with displacement of the quadrilateral surface of the ilium (and the adjacent fat lines) medially. Thin fracture lines (arrows) are faintly seen through the ilium and acetabular dome. *B,* The posterior oblique view shows fractures extending into the anterior rim (arrows). In addition to the posterior column fracture, the ischial spine is noted to be split (open arrow). *C,* An underpenetrated anterior oblique view shows posterior lip and posterior column fractures (arrows) and documents an anterior column fracture (open arrow) as well. A proximal ilial fracture is suggested (curved arrow).

Illustration continued on following page

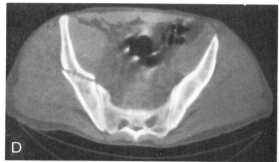

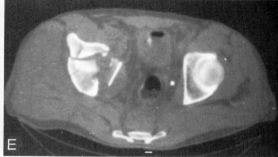

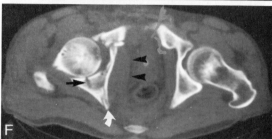

Figure 7–33. Evaluation of Acetabular Fracture (Burst Fracture) with Oblique and CT Examinations *Continued. D,* CT section through the ilia shows a right ilial fracture oriented along the frontal plane. This would understandably be difficult to see on AP views. *E,* There is a comminuted fracture of the acetabular dome and medial displacement of the quadrilateral surface. *F,* CT section at the level of the joint confirms the presence of a comminuted fracture of the anterior column and fractures of the posterior lip (arrow) and the ischial spine (white arrow). The adjacent soft tissue swelling, including displacement of the obturator internus (arrowheads), is better seen on CT than on conventional radiography.

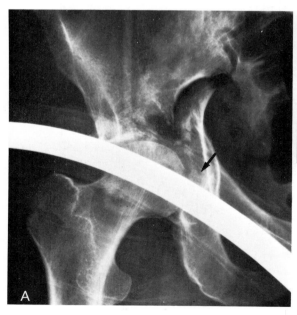

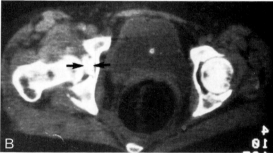

Figure 7–34. Acetabular Fracture with Intraarticular Loose Body. *A,* An AP view in traction apparatus shows displaced fractures of the anterior and posterior columns and the medial aspect of the weight-bearing dome. Several small, bony fragments are seen and, in retrospect, there may be a large density overlying the medial joint space (arrow). *B,* A CT scan through the joint shows a large intraarticular loose body (arrows).

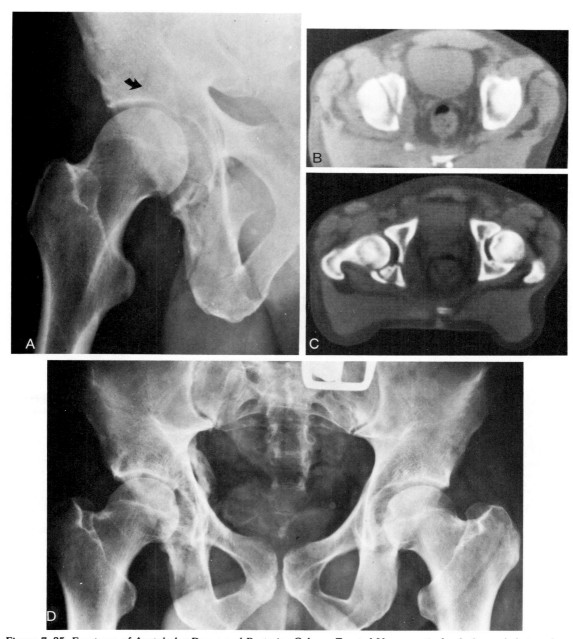

Figure 7–35. Fractures of Acetabular Dome and Posterior Column Treated Nonoperatively. *A,* An angled view shows questionable lucencies through the acetabular dome (arrow) and fractures of the posterior column and the ischium. *B,* There is a minimally displaced fracture of the acetabular dome. *C,* Posterior column and lip fractures are present, but there are no intraarticular loose bodies. The slight widening of the right hip-joint space suggests subluxation of the femoral head laterally and posteriorly. *D,* After conservative therapy, healing has occurred. There is mild cartilage-space narrowing (osteoarthritis).

patients the clinical outcome was adversely affected.

Pseudarthrosis. This complication is rare, noted in less than 1 percent of postoperative cases.[58]

Avascular Necrosis (Osteonecrosis). Avascular necrosis may involve the femoral head if dislocation is also present. Avascular necrosis involving the acetabulum and isolated cartilage necrosis have also been reported.

Ectopic Calcification. Radiographic evidence of ectopic calcification is not uncommon, and in one series 18 percent of patients with calcification following surgery developed some limitation of motion (Fig. 7–36).[58]

Hip Dislocation

The key to the successful management of hip dislocation is early recognition and reduction. These lesions may, however, be overlooked clinically in the presence of other serious injuries, fractures near the hip, or fractures of the ipsilateral femur. For this reason Epstein recommends that radiographs of the pelvis be obtained in all patients who sustain severe trauma. Even with the appropriate films, however, radiographic diagnosis may be difficult, and attention to detail is critical.

Dislocations may be classified by the final position of the femoral head as posterior, anterior, or central.[72]

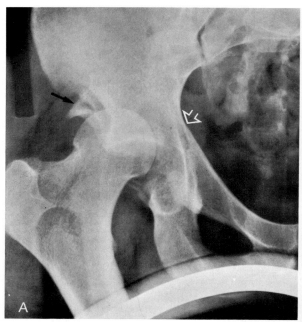

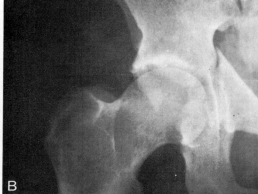

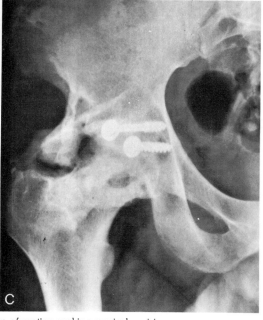

Figure 7–36. Ectopic Bone Complicating Reduction of Posterior Fracture Dislocation. *A,* The initial AP view shows superior and lateral displacement of the femoral head, with overlap of the femoral head and the ilium. Oblique views confirmed posterior dislocation of the femoral head. There is apparent disruption of the posterior acetabular rim, and a fracture fragment (arrow) is noted posteriorly. A fracture is seen disrupting the iliopubic line (open arrow), indicating an anterior column fracture, but the ilioischial line (posterior column) is intact. *B,* Closed reduction was done on the day of admission. The postreduction radiograph shows complete reduction of the femoral head into the acetabulum. The posterior rim and the anterior column and rim fractures are more apparent. *C,* At surgery a large posterior lip fragment was present and the hip was unstable in flexion and adduction. Several osteocartilaginous loose bodies were present, and there was a cartilage defect in the femoral head. Following internal fixation, extensive ectopic bone developed, with limitation of motion making surgical excision necessary.

Posterior Dislocations

These injuries occur when the hip and knee are in flexion and force is applied to the knee, a situation that most commonly results from the knee hitting the dashboard of a car during a head-on collision. The degree of abduction or adduction determines which type of posterior dislocation results. If the hip is in neutral position or is adducted at the time of injury, a simple dislocation is most often the result. If the hip is slightly abducted, a fracture of the postero-superior portion of the acetabulum may occur. The greater the degree of hip flexion, the more likely it is that a simple dislocation will be produced.[72]

Classification. Posterior dislocations have been divided into five types by Thompson and Epstein, and this is the most frequently used classification:[88]

type I—with or without a minor fracture

type II—with a large single fracture of the posterior acetabular rim

type III—with a comminuted fracture of the rim of the acetabulum

type IV—with fracture of the acetabular rim and the floor

type V—with fracture of the femoral head.

Clawson and Melcher include types III and IV in one category.[72] In general, type I dislocations do not have a significant fracture associated with them and are usually considered separately, whereas the other categories include a significant fracture.

Clinical Examination. Typically, the leg is shortened, internally rotated, adducted, and flexed. The sciatic nerve should be evaluated, since nerve injury occurs in 10 to 13 percent of these patients.[72]

Radiological Examination. Problems in radiographic examination may occur during the entire patient course, from the time of initial diagnosis to follow-up after treatment. Since hip dislocations are usually the result of a severe accident, other soft tissue and bony injuries that overshadow the hip problem may be present. It is because of this circumstance that views of the pelvis, including the hips, have been suggested as routine procedure in all patients with severe trauma.[76] Ipsilateral femoral fractures were noted in 22.5 percent of one series of patients with posterior dislocation, and the most frequent of these is a fracture involving the inferomedial aspect of the femoral head. Rarely, the presence of a femoral shaft fracture may obscure a coincident hip dislocation, but a film of the pelvis will eliminate this error. If such a film is not obtained, hip dislocation should be suspected

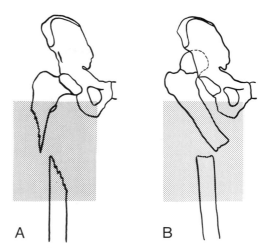

Figure 7–37. Posterior Hip Dislocation and Femoral Fracture. Dislocation should be suspected on the AP view of the femur if there is a short transverse fracture of the shaft and the proximal fragment is adducted rather than abducted. The crosshatched area only may be included on the radiograph. *A,* Femoral fracture, no hip dislocation. *B,* Femoral fracture and hip dislocation. (Redrawn from Gregory CF: AAOS Instructional Course Lectures 22:105, 1973.)

on the AP view of the femoral shaft if a short transverse fracture of the shaft is present and the proximal fragment is adducted rather than in the usual abducted position (Fig. 7–37).[77] Other femoral fractures, including a compression fracture of the femoral head, intertrochanteric fracture, femoral neck fracture (occasionally created during attempted reduction), and distal femoral fracture may also occur. In addition to these coincident femoral fractures, fractures or dislocations and significant soft tissue injury outside the hip area are frequent accompanying findings. These findings include injuries to the pelvis, knee, face and head, and abdomen.

In patients with posterior hip dislocation the standard anteroposterior radiograph typically shows the femoral head to overlie the iliac wing, above and lateral to the acetabular roof (Figs. 7–38 and 7–39). Oblique views should be routine. A lateral view, tomography, or computed tomography may be helpful.

Gregory noted several radiographic signs that may help avoid missing subtle cases of dislocation on a nonrotated AP radiograph.[77] These include the following:

1. *Disturbance in Shenton's line.* The superior edge of the obturator foramen and the medial aspect of the femoral neck normally form a smooth arch (Shenton's line). Superior displacement of the dislocated femoral head will disrupt this line.

2. *Loss of the normal uniform thickness of*

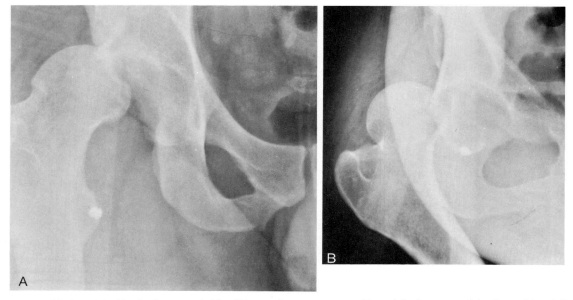

Figure 7–38. Posterior Hip Dislocation. *A,* The AP view shows superior and lateral displacement of the femoral head. *B,* The anterior oblique view confirms the posterior position of the femoral head. No acetabular fracture is present.

the cartilage space. In the absence of preceding osteoarthritis or other known joint disease, alteration in the dimension of the cartilage space on the affected side as compared with the normal side raises the possibility of dislocation. The abnormal joint space may be due to an abnormal relationship between the femoral head and the articular surface of the acetabulum or to interposition of loose bodies. Thus either *narrowing* or *widening* of the cartilage space on the affected side is suspicious.

3. *Disparity in size of the femoral heads.* Since objects closest to the film appear less magnified than objects farther from the film, disparity in the dimensions of the two femoral heads suggests that they are at different distances from the film, and in the absence of patient rotation this occurrence raises the possibility of hip dislocation. Thus in the anteroposterior view a femoral head that is posteriorly dislocated appears smaller than the normally positioned contralateral one.

Once the diagnosis is made, categorization into the previously listed Thompson-Epstein classification is in order. However, Smith and Loop found that in 10 of 14 cases of posterior hip dislocation the final Thompson-Epstein classification differed from the initial radiographic classification, and in 2 of the 7 patients who underwent surgery the operative diagnosis differed from the final preoperative radiographic diagnosis.[85] These authors point out several failures of the radiographic examination, including

difficulty in identifying the presence of associated fractures (particularly those of the femoral head) and osteochondral fragments, even if tomography is done. It is suggested that tomography in additional planes might be helpful and that the presence of a persistently widened hip joint should not be ignored but should suggest the possibility of intraarticular osteochondral fragments or femoral head fragments, even if tomography and plain films are negative for fracture.[85] Computed tomography has been shown to be of considerable value in the identification of intraarticular loose bodies and in the definition of fracture lines. This examination should improve the preoperative assessment.

Treatment. The treatment of posterior dislocation without associated fracture consists of early reduction, followed by skeletal traction and, later, protected weight bearing with crutches until pain and limp are absent.[72] Closed reduction is usually attempted, but if this procedure is difficult or unsuccessful, open reduction is performed. In Epstein's series of 117 adults with posterior dislocation and no significant acetabular fracture (posterior type I dislocation), 70 percent had good or excellent clinical results.[76] Early reduction is apparently critical, and Epstein found no good or excellent results in adults with type I posterior dislocations who had had reduction after 48 hours.

The treatment of posterior dislocations with a major acetabular fragment is more controversial.[76] Usually, closed reduction is done as soon

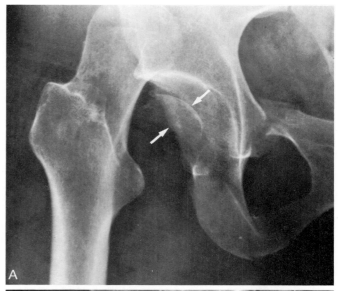

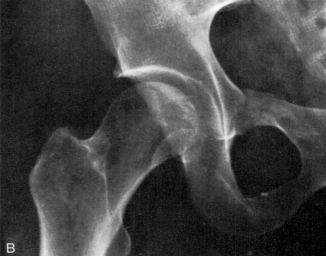

Figure 7–39. Posterior Hip Dislocation with Femoral Head Fracture. *A,* The femoral head is dislocated superiorly (and posteriorly). A bony fragment (arrows) overlies the joint. Pubic and ischial fractures are present. *B,* Postreduction view. The bony fragment remains in the joint. Although its site of origin is not seen, its shape strongly suggests that it originated from the femoral head.

as possible, and the hip is checked for stability in flexion. If the reduction is unstable, operative intervention and internal fixation of the fracture fragments are done (see Fig. 7–36).[72] The object is to obtain stability and congruous articular surfaces.

Epstein, in contrast, recommends primary surgical, rather than primary closed, reduction. This recommendation is based on his comparison study of closed and open reductions, in which the incidence of good results in all categories of posterior dislocation with associated fractures was highest in patients who had primary open reductions.[75] In patients treated with primary open reduction the incidence of traumatic osteoarthritis was 17 percent in comparison with 30 percent in patients treated with all methods,

and the incidence of avascular necrosis dropped to 8 percent in comparison with the 22 percent incidence noted in the total group. Epstein feels that primary open reduction decreases some of the factors that lead to the development of avascular necrosis and traumatic arthritis. These factors include intraarticular bone fragments and debris, which he feels are virtually always present and which are removed at the time of open reduction. There is also less trauma to the hip that undergoes primary operative reduction in comparison with the trauma to a hip that first undergoes closed reduction and redislocation for joint inspection at the time of surgery.

It is generally agreed that open reduction is necessary when closed reduction is not possible or when the reduction is unstable, when multiple fragments are present within the joint (particularly in the weight-bearing area), and when an associated femoral neck fracture is present.[79] Optimal demonstration of the nature of a fracture and the presence of intraarticular loose bodies before any reduction is done may therefore significantly alter therapy. Computed tomography can play a significant role in this regard.

It has been stressed repeatedly that internal fixation should be carried out through a posterior approach, to avoid injury to any remaining anterior blood supply.[75]

Postoperative Radiographic Examination. Ideally, postreduction radiographs should be taken in two projections to confirm the adequacy of reduction. The cartilage space should appear normal in width and uniform in size. Too wide a cartilage space raises the possibility of either incomplete reduction or retained intraarticular (osteo-) cartilaginous fragments.[74] Postoperative traction, however, may produce apparent widening of the joint space. Epstein notes that failure to see the lesser trochanter because of persistent internal rotation should suggest the possibility that dislocation remains.[74]

Complications. The most frequent complications of posterior dislocation are post-traumatic osteoarthritis (OA), osteonecrosis (ON), and sciatic nerve damage. In a series of 368 posterior fracture-dislocations treated by all methods, post-traumatic OA occurred in 30 percent, ON in 22 percent, nerve injuries in 12 percent, and infection in 5 percent.[75] Despite the fact that most or all of the blood supply to the femoral head is damaged at the time of posterior dislocation, osteonecrosis is detectable radiologically in only 10 to 26 percent of patients, usually 1½ to 2 years after injury.[72] The incidence of ON seems to increase dramatically if reduction is delayed.

Following posterior (or central) dislocations, damage to the sciatic nerve or its peroneal branch may result from pressure on it by posterior fracture fragments or by the dislocated femoral head.

Anterior Dislocations

Anterior dislocations make up about 11 percent of all dislocations and result from forced abduction of the thigh, usually resulting from an automobile accident.[75] The final position of the head depends on the degree of flexion at the time of injury. If the hip was flexed, dislocation into the area of the obturator foramen occurs; if extended, pubic or iliac dislocation results. Thus there are three anatomic subdivisions of anterior

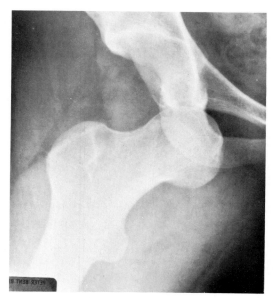

Figure 7–40. Anterior Hip Dislocation. The femoral head is displaced inferiorly and medially.

dislocation: obturator, pubic, and iliac. A fourth subcategory includes cases in which a fracture of the femoral head occurs when the head impacts on the acetabulum during dislocation.

Physical Examination. In obturator dislocations the hip is abducted, externally rotated, and flexed. In iliac or pubic dislocations the hip is extended.[72] Often the dislocated femoral head is palpable.

Radiographic Examination. Anterior dislocations are often obvious radiographically, the femoral head usually being displaced inferiorly and medially (Fig. 7–40). In iliac dislocations, however, the head may be displaced superiorly and laterally, mimicking the findings of a posterior dislocation. Not as obvious, but of considerable importance in treatment planning, is the identification of associated fractures of the acetabulum or the femoral head. This assessment is most easily done using computed tomography.

Treatment. Closed reduction within 48 hours is the treatment of choice. If this is unsuccessful, open reduction is done as soon as possible, since early reduction is an important factor in achieving a satisfactory result.[73, 76]

Complications. In children the results following early reduction of anterior dislocations are uniformly good or excellent.[76] In adults, however, post-traumatic osteoarthritis and avascular necrosis may alter this favorable outcome. The incidence of osteonecrosis and osteoarthritis is, however, less than is seen following posterior dislocations. Damage to the sciatic nerve may occur. Overall, Epstein noted that 75 percent of adults had good or excellent results.[76]

Central Acetabular Fracture-Dislocations

Central acetabular fracture-dislocations usually result from a force applied laterally to the trochanter and pelvis, such as might occur when a pedestrian is struck by an oncoming car.[72, 78] Occasionally, a force applied along the long axis of the femur with the hip in abduction also produces this injury.

Clawson and Melcher classify central fracture dislocations in the following manner:[72]

Type I—central displacement fractures, intact superior dome

Type II—fracture-dislocations with partial dome fracture

Type III—comminuted fractures with central displacement.

Radiological Examination. Central fracture-dislocations may be associated with other severe injuries of the ipsilateral leg, head, chest, or abdomen. In addition, hemorrhage into the pelvis may be massive, and both arteriographic localization of the bleeding site and embolization may be required (see previous section on pelvic fractures, arteriography, and embolization).

Treatment. As discussed in the section dealing with treatment of acetabular fractures, the

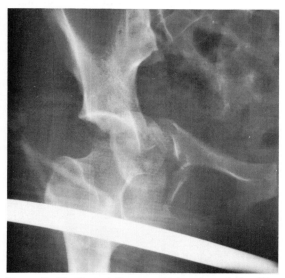

Figure 7–41. Central Fracture-Dislocation of the Hip. There is a complex acetabular fracture involving anterior and posterior columns, but with the weight-bearing dome intact. Other pelvic injuries (including the visible right SI joint and inferior pubic ramus fractures), extremity fractures, sciatic nerve palsy, and a severe head injury were present. The patient was treated with traction to relocate the femoral head under the acetabular dome.

integrity of the weight-bearing superior acetabular dome and a congruous relationship between it and the femoral head are of major importance in defining treatment and prognosis (Fig. 7–41). Irregularities of the inner wall are apparently not critical.

When the dome is partially involved, surgical reconstruction may be used if an anatomical reduction is possible. Conservative treatment is often recommended for severely comminuted acetabular fractures when such a reduction would be impossible. (See section on acetabular fractures, treatment, and complications.)

Pelvic Lesions Due to Bone Marrow Aspiration or Biopsy

Gilsanz and Grunebaum noted small, circular, lucent defects in the posterior superior iliac spines of patients who had undergone bone marrow biopsy.[91] A smooth sclerotic rim was noted around these defects immediately after biopsy, and this sclerosis became more prominent in the next several weeks. The lesions gradually became less well defined, but they may persist for years.

Similar changes have been noted following marrow aspiration with a 14-gauge needle (Fig. 7–42).[92] The series of patients studied by Kagan underwent 50 to 60 needle aspirations in each posterior superior iliac crest, and multiple, poorly defined, 0.2- to 0.3-cm lucencies were noted immediately thereafter. Subsequently, these areas developed surrounding sclerosis.

Open biopsies of the anterior superior iliac spine (such as may be done during staging laparotomy for Hodgkin's disease) may result in a poorly defined lucent defect in the left hemipelvis that could be mistaken for lymphomatous involvement.[90]

Exostoses may occur at former biopsy sites. These may be distinguished from myositis ossificans or dystrophic calcification by the presence of a central lucency in the biopsy-induced cases.[93]

Obviously, considering the possibility that these lesions represent biopsy sequelae and obtaining appropriate information will prevent serious misinterpretations.

Sacroiliitis

Spondyloarthritides

The changes involving the SI joints in a number of spondyloarthritides are similar, differing primarily in the symmetry and severity of damage.

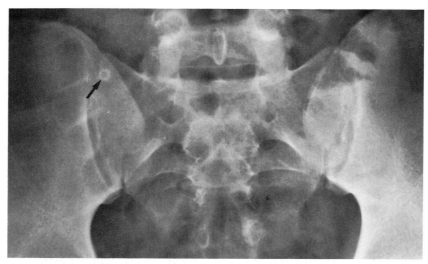

Figure 7–42. Bone Biopsy Defect. The small lucency (in the ilium) with well-defined sclerotic margins (arrow), is typical of a defect from a prior bone-marrow biopsy. This patient has chronic myelogenous leukemia.

Initial radiographic abnormalities consist of loss of definition of the subchondral cortex, particularly in its mid- and lower portions (stage I of Forestier).[100] The iliac side of the joint is involved earliest on radiographs, since the articular cartilage on that side is thinner than on the sacral side. With increasing erosion along the joint margins an apparent widening of the joint space that has been termed *pseudowidening* occurs. Progressive erosion is accompanied by areas of sclerosis (stage II of Forestier) that may be so prominent that osteitis condensans ilii is suggested (Figs. 7–43 and 7–46). Late changes of ankylosing spondylitis consist of gradual decrease in sclerosis and development of bony ankylosis across the sacroiliac joints (stage III of

Forestier; Fig. 7–44). Since involvement is not uniform, areas of retained articular cartilage occur, and in those areas the subchondral cortices remain visible.

In ankylosing spondylitis (AS) involvement is always bilateral and usually symmetrical.[99, 103] Unilateral involvement, in fact, makes a diagnosis of ankylosing spondylitis extremely unlikely. In contrast with ankylosing spondylitis, the sacroiliac involvement in Reiter's syndrome is likely to be unilateral or asymmetrical, and bony ankylosis is uncommon (Fig. 7–45). Of 48 patients with Reiter's syndrome studied by Sholkoff 20 (42 percent) had evidence of sacroiliitis.[107] Abnormalities were unilateral in 9 patients, bilateral but markedly asymmetrical in 7, and

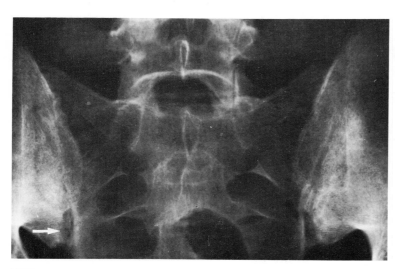

Figure 7–43. Ankylosing Spondylitis (Grade 2, Forestier). Erosion of the SI joints is particularly well shown inferiorly on the right, where the subchondral bone is absent (arrow). There is accompanying sclerosis. The changes are bilateral and symmetrical.

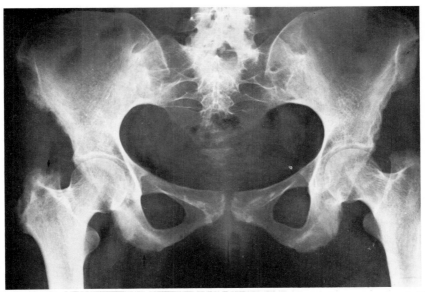

Figure 7–44. Late Ankylosing Spondylitis. The inferior (synovial) portions of each SI joint are fused. There is irregular bone proliferation from the greater trochanters and the ischia (arrows).

bilateral and symmetrical in 4. Patients with unilateral involvement usually have had the disease less than 1 year. Sacroiliitis is much more common in HLA-B27 positive than in HLA-B27 negative patients.

Sacroiliitis is noted in one quarter to one third of patients with psoriatic arthritis. Damage is usually bilateral and symmetrical, but, again in contrast with ankylosing spondylitis, damage may be asymmetrical or unilateral. Radiographic findings of the sacroiliitis accompanying inflammatory bowel disease are identical to those seen in ankylosing spondylitis.

Pyogenic infections of the SI joints are uncommon. A delay of up to 2 weeks may be noted between the clinical presentation and the pres-

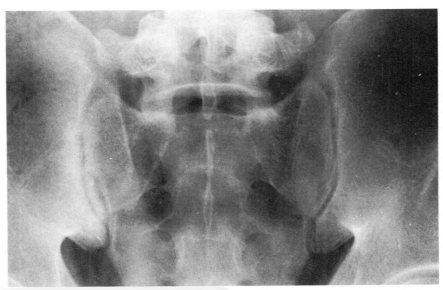

Figure 7–45. Reiter's Syndrome with Unilateral Sacroiliitis. The left SI joint is normal. On the right there is loss of sharp cortical definition, particularly on the iliac side, with accompanying subchondral sclerosis. (From HLA B27 Arthritis. *In* Feldman F: The Radiology, Pathology and Immunology of Bones and Joints. New York, Appleton-Century-Crofts, 1978.)

ence of radiographic abnormalities.[98] Blurring of the margins of the SI joint with pseudowidening of the joint space are the earliest radiographic findings. Features that distinguish AS from infection are the bilateral involvement in AS and the occurrence of ankylosis in both the lower two thirds (the synovial portion) and the proximal one third (the site of the interosseous ligaments) of the SI joints in AS. This contrasts with the findings in septic arthritis, in which involvement is unilateral and only the synovial joint is involved.

Computed Tomography (Fig. 7–46). The role of CT in the evaluation of inflammatory conditions of the SI joints is not yet defined. Martel and colleagues noted in a study of patients with Reiter's disease that asymmetrical involvement was more often apparent on CT examination than on conventional film and that the sites of erosion and sclerosis were more clearly seen on the CT study. There were no cases, however, in which evidence of SI arthritis was present on the CT study and not on conventional films.[102] But Carrera and associates have demonstrated increased sensitivity of the CT examination in the detection of inflammatory disease as compared with conventional radiographs.[97]

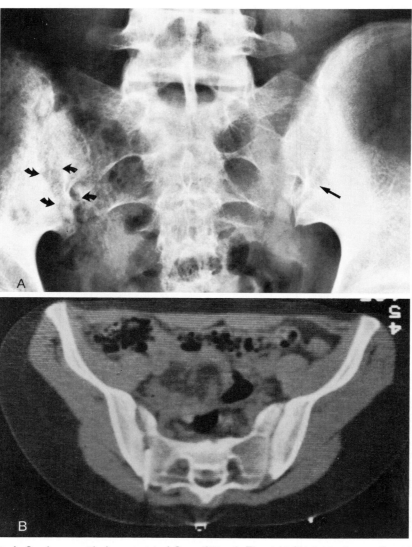

Figure 7–46. Reiter's Syndrome with Asymmetrical Sacroiliitis. *A,* The right SI joint is abnormally wide in appearance (curved arrows), owing to erosion of subchondral bone. There is questionable focal erosion of the left SI joint (arrow) as well. *B,* A CT scan was obtained to facilitate biopsy (done to exclude infection). The biopsy needle is seen within the right SI joint, which is irregular and widened.

Radionuclide Scintigraphy. Increased uptake is normally seen in the SI joint areas with the new technetium-99m phosphate compounds. Quantitative methods to assess SI joint uptake have been suggested as being preferable to a purely visual evaluation. The quantitative method usually involves comparing the peak isotopic uptake of each SI joint with the sacral uptake. The ratios thus obtained have been evaluated in control patients and in patients with early, moderate, and advanced sacroiliitis with mixed results. Several studies have shown increased activity ratios in patients with erosive sacroiliitis in comparison with controls and decreased uptake ratios in late-stage disease with ankylosis.[109-112] In the study by Lentle and coworkers patients showing strong clinical evidence of ankylosing spondylitis but with normal or questionable findings on sacroiliac radiographs had mean uptake ratios higher than those of the control group (Fig. 7-47). Some overlap between normal and affected individuals did occur. Increased uptake ratios have also been noted in patients with metabolic bone disease (such as renal osteodystrophy) and in patients with structural abnormalities in the low back, in patients with rheumatoid arthritis, and in males as compared with females.[109, 110, 114] In contrast

with the above findings, Dequeker and associates noted that, as a group, patients with sacroiliitis had *lower* uptake ratios than the control group and that early sacroiliitis could not be detected using the isotope method.[108] Spencer and colleagues noted marked overlap between the uptake ratios of control patients and those with ankylosing spondylitis and concluded: "It is unlikely that scintigraphy will be of diagnostic value in the absence of improved methodology."[113] Thus the role of quantitative sacroiliac joint scintigraphy remains controversial.

Osteitis Condensans Ilii

In contrast with male predominance in ankylosing spondylitis, osteitis condensans ilii usually affects women. Involvement is most often bilateral, with sharply marginated sclerosis occurring in the ilia adjacent to the SI joints (Fig. 7-48).[104] Cartilage-space narrowing and erosion are not features of this condition. Resolution of the radiological abnormalities may occur.

Abnormalities of the Pubic Symphysis

Congenital widening of the pubic symphysis may be the result of true separation of the

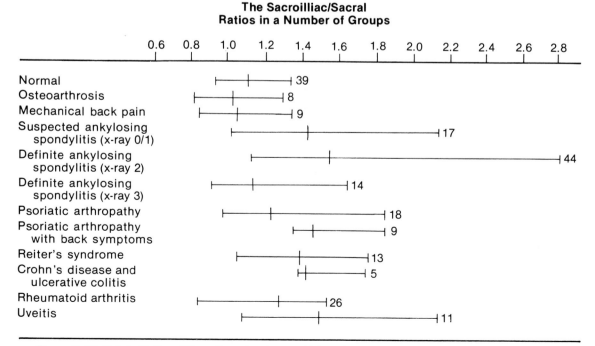

Figure 7-47. Uptake Ratios of Bone Scanning Agents. (Adapted from Lentle, et al. J Nucl Med 18:529, 1977.)

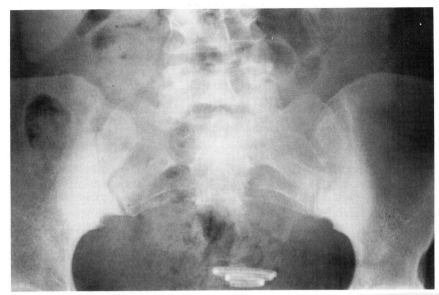

Figure 7–48. Osteitis Condensans Ilii. There is sclerosis along the inferior portions of each SI joint, involving only the iiac sides of the joint. The absence of erosion helps to exclude other disorders associated with sacroiliitis. (From HLA B27 Arthritis, *In* Feldman F: The Radiology, Pathology and Immunology of Bones and Joints. New York, Appleton-Century-Crofts, 1978.)

symphysis (as seen in association with exstrophy of the bladder or with epispadias) or may be apparent only because of delayed mineralization around the symphysis (such as occurs in cleidocranial dysostosis).[117] *Calcification* (of fibrocartilage) may be seen in calcium pyrophosphate dihydrate (CPPD) deposition disease (Fig. 7–49)[118, 120] The pubic symphysis is, in fact, the second most frequent site for calcification in patients with CPPD disease and this was noted in 69 percent of patients with radiologically identified calcification anywhere, as compared with the 79 percent incidence in the knees.

Evaluation by Resnick and co-workers of patients with CPPD disease and joint calcification showed that radiographs of the knees alone would have detected calcification in 89 percent of patients; radiographs of the knees and pubic symphysis would have detected calcification in 98 percent of patients; and films of the knees, symphysis, and wrists would have increased the detection of calcification to 100 percent. Irregularity of the articular surfaces, cartilage-space narrowing, sclerosis, "cyst formation" and fragmentation may also occur in association with CPPD disease.[118]

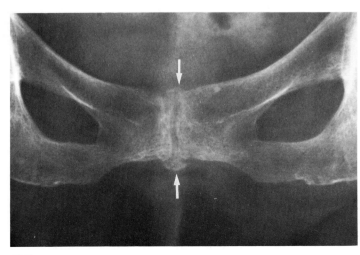

Figure 7–49. Chondrocalcinosis. Calcification of the pubic symphysis (arrows) is present.

Osteitis pubis refers to a "distinct clinical entity characterized by a self-limiting, non-suppurative osteonecrosis which usually begins at the symphysis."[115] It has most often occurred as a complication of urologic surgery but has become distinctly uncommon in recent years.[121] After a latent period of 4 to 12 weeks following the surgical procedure, 1 to 7 weeks following the onset of pain, bone destruction begins at the symphysis and extends into the pubic rami and the ischia. Healing occurs after 2 to 8 months. The final appearances are usually marked narrowing or bony ankylosis of the symphysis and sclerosis and spurring at the sites of muscle attachments, especially the inferior pubic rami and the ischial tuberosities.[115] In contrast with osteomyelitis (the most likely differential diagnostic possibility), fever and sequestration apparently do not occur.

A number of *rheumatological disorders* may also be associated with changes in the pubic symphysis. Ankylosing spondylitis in particular is associated with erosion, sclerosis, and eventual bony ankylosis of the symphysis. Almost three quarters of the patients with ankylosing spondylitis studied by McEwan and colleagues had involvement of the pubic symphysis, and after 15 years of disease involvement was severe in almost 50 percent.[116] Patients with inflammatory bowel disease, psoriatic arthritis, and Reiter's syndrome may have similar involvement, although severe changes are not usually seen in patients with Reiter's syndrome (Fig. 7–50).

Erosion is also seen in metabolic disorders such as *hyperparathyroidism*. The involvement is always associated with bone changes elsewhere in the skeleton, including the sacroiliac joints.

Traumatic avulsion by the adductor muscles of the thigh at their origins near the pubic symphysis produces characteristic *unilateral* irregularity of the pubic symphysis and often of the adjacent inferior pubic ramus (Fig. 7–51).[119] A typical clinical picture, consisting of pain on active adduction of the leg against resistance and on forceful passive abduction, develops.

Trauma may also result in widening of the symphysis (to greater than 1 cm in males, 8 mm in nonpregnant females) or in abnormal alignment of the two pubic bones. Even a slight offset of the inferior pubic margins should suggest the possibility of traumatic disruption, given the ap-

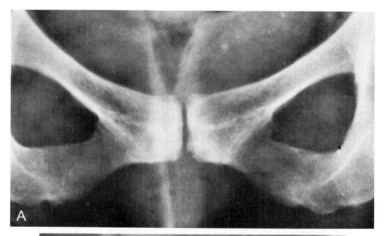

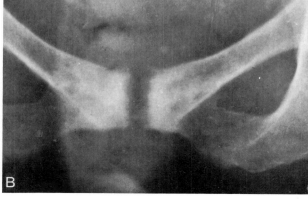

Figure 7–50. Psoriatic Arthritis with Erosion of the Pubic Symphysis. *A,* There is mild erosion and moderate sclerosis of the pubic symphysis. Also, the hip cartilage spaces were narrowed, and there was mild sclerosis along the left SI joint. *B,* Eleven years later erosion has progressed.

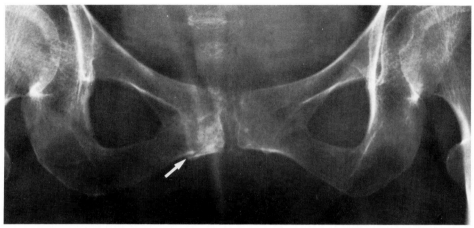

Figure 7–51. Avulsion Fracture of the Pubic Symphysis. A fracture (arrow) involving the inferior portion of the pubic symphysis at the site of insertion of the gracilis is noted. Incidentally noted is chondrocalcinosis of the pubic symphysis.

propriate clinical setting.[121] Careful scrutiny for associated separation of the SI joints is then warranted.

References

Normal Structure and Function

1. Goss CM, ed.: Gray's Anatomy: Anatomy of the Human Body, 29th ed. Philadelphia, Lea & Febiger, 1973.
2. Kane WJ: Fractures of the pelvis. In Rockwood CA Jr, Green DP, eds. Fractures. Philadelphia, JB Lippincott, 1975.
3. Stedman's Medical Dictionary, 24th ed. Baltimore, Williams & Wilkins, 1982.

Normal Radiographic Anatomy

4. Armbuster TG, Guerra J Jr, Resnick D, Goergen TG, Feingold ML, Niwayama G, Danzig LA: The adult hip: an anatomic study. Part I: The bony landmarks. Radiology 128:1–10, 1978.
4a. Bowerman JW, Sena JM, Chang R: The teardrop shadow of the pelvis: anatomy and clinical significance. Radiology 143:659–662, 1982.
5. Gilula LA, Murphy WA, Tailor CC, Patel RB: Computed tomography of the osseous pelvis. Radiology 132:107–114, 1979.
6. Judet R, Judet J, Letournel E: Fractures of the acetabulum: Classification and surgical approaches for open reduction. J Bone Joint Surg (Am) 46:1615–1646, 1964.
7. Naidich DP, Freedman MT, Bowerman JW, Siegelman SS: Ten section approach to computed tomography of the pelvis. Skeletal Radiol 5:213–214, 1980.
8. Redman HC: Computed tomography of the pelvis. Radiol Clin North Am 15:441–448, 1977.
9. Vix VA, Ryu CY: The adult symphysis pubis: Normal and abnormal. AJR 112:517–525, 1971.
10. Whelan MA, Gold RP: Computed tomography of the sacrum: 1. Normal anatomy. AJR 139:1183–1190, 1982.

Pelvic Fractures

11. Barnes ST, Hinds, RB: Pseudotumor of the ischium: a late manifestation of avulsion of the ischial epiphysis. J Bone Joint Surg (Am) 54:645–647, 1962.
12. Bonnin JG: Sacral fractures and injuries to the cauda equina. J Bone Joint Surg (Am) 27:113–127, 1945.
13. Borlaza GS, Seigel RS, Kuhns LR, Good AE, Rapp R, Martel W: CT in the evaluation of sacroiliac arthritis. J Comput Assist Tomogr 2:519–520, 1978 (abs).
14. Dunn AW, Morris HD: Fractures and dislocations of the pelvis. J Bone Joint Surg (Am) 50:1639–1648, 1968.
15. Fountain SS, Hamilton RD, Jameson RM: Transverse fractures of the sacrum: A report of six cases. J Bone Joint Surg (Am) 59:486–489, 1977.
16. Furey WW: Fractures of the pelvis: with special reference to associated fractures of the sacrum. AJR 47:89–96, 1942.
17. Gertzbein SD, Chenoweth DR: Occult injuries of the pelvic ring. Clin Orthop 128:202–207, 1977.
18. Gilchrist MR, Peterson DH: Pelvic fracture and associated soft-tissue trauma. Radiology 88:278–280, 1967.
19. Irving MH: Exostosis formation after traumatic avulsion of the anterior inferior iliac spine. Report of two cases. J Bone Joint Surg (Br) 46:720–722, 1964.
20. Johnson HF: Derangements of the coccyx. Nebr Med J 21:451–457, 1936.
21. Johnston R: Stabilization of pelvic fractures with Hoffmann external fixation: the Colorado experience. In Brooker AF, Edwards CC, eds. External Fixation. The Current State of the Art. Proceedings of the Sixth International Conference on Hoffmann External Fixation. Baltimore, Williams & Wilkins, 1979: 133–159.
22. Kane WJ: Fracture of the pelvis. In Rockwood CA Jr, Green DP, eds. Fractures. Philadelphia, JB Lippincott, 1975.
23. Key JA, Conwell HE: Management of Fractures, Dislocations and Sprains. St. Louis, CV Mosby, 1951.
24. Laasonen EM: Missed sacral fractures. Ann Clin Res 9:84–87, 1977.
25. Malgaigne JF: Double vertical fractures of the pelvis. Clin Orthop 151:8–11, 1980.
26. Mears DC, Fu FH: External fixation in pelvic fractures. Orthop Clin North Am 11:465–479, 1980.
27. Mears DC, Fu FH: Modern concepts of external skeletal fixation of the pelvis. Clin Orthop 151:65–72, 1980.
28. Medelman JP: Fractures of the sacrum: their incidence in fracture of the pelvis. AJR 42:100–103, 1939.
29. Northrop CH, Eto RT, Loop JW: Vertical fracture of

the sacral ala: significance of non-continuity of the anterior superior sacral foraminal line. AJR 124: 102–106, 1975.

30. Pennal GF, Tile M, Waddell JP, Garside H: Pelvic disruption: assessment and classification. Clin Orthop 151:12–21, 1980.
31. Rankin LM: Fractures of the pelvis: A review of four hundred forty-nine cases. Ann Surg 106:266–277, 1937.
32. Rowe CR, Lowell JD: Prognosis of fractures of the acetabulum. J Bone Joint Surg (Am) 43:30–59, 1961.
33. Sauser DD, Billimoria PE, Rouse GA, Mudge K: CT evaluation of hip trauma AJR 135:269–274, 1980.
34. Slatis P, Karaharju EO: External fixation of unstable pelvic fractures: experiences in 22 patients treated with a trapezoid compression frame. Clin Orthop 151:73–80, 1980.
35. Smith-Peterson MN, Rogers WA: End-result study for arthrodesis of the sacro-iliac joint for arthritis—traumatic and non-traumatic. J Bone Joint Surg 8:118–136, 1926.
36. Stayton CA Jr: Ischial epiphysiolysis. AJR 76: 1161–1162, 1956.
37. Thaggard A III, Harle TS, Carlson V: Bony pelvis and hip. In Felson B, ed. Roentgenology of Fractures and Dislocations. New York, Grune & Stratton, 1978: 111–120.
38. Tile M, Pennal GF: Fractures of the pelvis. In The Hip. Proceedings of the Seventh Open Scientific Meeting of the Hip Society. St. Louis, CV Mosby, 1979.
39. Wild JJ Jr, Hanson GW, Tullos HS: Unstable fractures of the pelvis treated by external fixation. J Bone Joint Surg (Am) 64:1010–1019, 1982.

Arteriography in Pelvic Fractures

40. Athanasoulis CA, Duffield R, Shapiro JH: Angiography to assess pelvic vascular injury. N Engl J Med 284:1329, 1971.
41. Athanasoulis CA, Harris WH, Stock RJ, Waltman AC: Arterial embolization to control pelvic hemorrhage. In The Hip. Proceedings of the Seventh Open Scientific Meeting of the Hip Society. St. Louis, CV Mosby, 1979: 247–259.
42. Baum S, Nusbaum M, Blakemore WS, Finkelstein AK: The preoperative radiographic demonstration of intra-abdominal bleeding from undetermined sites by percutaneous selective celiac and superior mesenteric arteriography. Surgery 58:797–805, 1965.
43. Bree RL, Goldstein HM, Wallace S: Transcatheter embolization of the internal iliac artery in the management of neoplasms of the pelvis. Surg Gynecol Obstet 143:597–601, 1976.
44. Carey LS, Grace DM: The brisk bleed: control by arterial catheterization and gel foam plug. J Can Assoc Radiol 25:113–115, 1974.
45. Fleming WH, Bowen JC III: Control of hemorrhage in pelvic crush injuries. J Trauma 13:567–570, 1973.
46. Gerlock AJ: Hemorrhage following pelvic fracture controlled by embolization: Case report. J Trauma 15:740–742, 1975.
47. Hauser CW, Perry JF Jr: Massive hemorrhage from pelvic fractures. Minn Med 49:285–290, 1966.
48. Margolies MN, Ring EJ, Waltman AC, Kerr WS Jr, Baum S: Arteriography in the management of hemorrhage from pelvic fractures. N Engl J Med 287:317–321, 1972.
49. Matalon TSA, Athanasoulis CA, Margolies MN, Waltman AC, Novelline RA, Greenfield AJ, Miller SE: Hemorrhage with pelvic fractures: efficacy of transcatheter embolization. AJR 133:859–864, 1979.
50. Patel D, Crothers O, Harris WH, Waltman A, Fahmy N, Carey R: Arterial embolization for radical tumor resection. Acta Orthop Scand 48:353–355, 1977.
51. Reynolds BM, Balsano NA: Venography in pelvic fractures. A clinical evaluation. Ann Surg 173: 104–106, 1971.
52. Ring EJ, Athanasoulis C, Waltman AC, Margolies MN, Baum S: Arteriographic management of hemorrhage following pelvic fracture. Radiology 109:65–70, 1973.
53. Saletta JD, Freeark RJ: Vascular injuries associated with fractures. Orthop Clin North Am 1:93–102, 1970.
54. Stock, JR, Harris WH, Athanasoulis CA: The role of diagnostic and therapeutic angiography in trauma to the pelvis. Clin Orthop 151:31–40, 1980.
55. Wittenberg J, Athanasoulis CA, Shapiro JH, Williams LF Jr: Mesenteric angiography. N Engl J Med 285:1539–1540, 1971.

Acetabular Fractures

56. Brooker AF Jr, Edwards CC, eds: External Fixation. The Current State of the Art. Proceedings of the Sixth International Conference on Hoffmann External Fixation. Baltimore, Williams & Wilkins, 1979: 113–121.
57. Judet R, Judet J, Letournel E: Fractures of the acetabulum: Classification and surgical approaches for open reduction. J Bone Joint Surg (Am) 46: 1615–1646, 1964.
58. Letournel E: The results of acetabular fractures treated surgically: 21 years' experience. In The Hip. Proceedings of the Seventh Open Scientific Meeting of the Hip Society. St. Louis, CV Mosby, 1979.
59. Letournel E: Acetabulum fractures: Classification and Management. Clin Orthop 151:81–106, 1980.
60. Lipscomb PR: Closed management of fractures of the acetabulum. In The Hip. Proceedings of the Seventh Open Scientific Meeting of the Hip Society. St. Louis, CV Mosby, 1979.
61. Lowell JD: Bursting fractures of the acetabulum, involving the inner wall and superior dome. AAOS Instructional Course Lectures 22:145–158, 1973.
62. Lowell JD: Fractures of the acetabulum. Syllabus of the Post-Graduate Course in Orthopedic Radiology. Harvard Medical School and the Peter Bent Brigham Hospital, Cambridge, 1978.
63. Lowell JD: Methods of treatment and clinical results in major pelvic and acetabular injuries. In Brooker AF, Edwards CC, eds. External Fixation. The Current State of the Art. Proceedings of the Sixth International Conference on Hoffman External Fixation. Baltimore, Williams & Wilkins, 1979:113–122.
64. Mack LA, Harley JD, Winquist RA: CT of acetabular fractures: analysis of fracture patterns. AJR 138:407–412, 1982.
65. Naidich DP, Freedman MT, Bowerman JW, Siegelman SS: Computerized tomography in the evaluation of the soft tissue component of bony lesions of the pelvis. Skeletal Radiol 3:144–148, 1978.
66. Pearson JR, Hargadon EJ: Fractures of the pelvis involving the floor of the acetabulum. J Bone Joint Surg (Br) 44:550–561, 1962.
67. Rogers LF, Novy SB, Harris NF: Occult central fractures of the acetabulum. AJR 124:96–101, 1975.
68. Rowe CR, Lowell JD: Prognosis of fractures of the acetabulum. J Bone Joint Surg (Am) 43:30–59, 1961.
69. Sauser DD, Billimoria PE, Rouse GA, Mudge K: Computed tomography evaluation of hip trauma. AJR 135:269–274, 1980.
70. Shirkhoda A, Brashear HR, Staab EV: Computed tomography of acetabular fractures. Radiology 134:683–688, 1980.

Hip Dislocations

71. Browne PS: Central dislocation of the hip with complications. Injury 8:70–71, 1976.
72. Clawson DK, Melcher PJ: Fractures and dislocations of the hip. In Rockwood CA Jr, Green DP, eds. Fractures. Philadelphia, JB Lippincott, 1975.
73. Duncan CP, Shim S-S: Blood supply of the head of the femur in traumatic hip dislocation. Surg Gynecol Obstet 144:185–191, 1977.
74. Epstein HC: Traumatic dislocations of the hip. Clin Orthop 92:116–142, 1973.
75. Epstein HC: Open management of fractures of the acetabulum. In The Hip. Proceedings of the Seventh Open Scientific Meeting of the Hip Society. St. Louis, CV Mosby, 1979: 17–42.
76. Epstein HC: Fractures and dislocations of the hip and fractures of the acetabulum. Part II. Traumatic anterior and simple posterior dislocations of the hip in adults and children. AAOS Instructional Course Lectures 22:115–158, 1973.
77. Gregory CF: Fractures and dislocations of the hip and fractures of the acetabulum. Part I. Early complications of dislocation and fracture-dislocations of the hip joint. AAOS Instructional Course Lectures 22:105–115, 1973.
78. Heppenstall RB: Fractures and dislocations of the hip. In Heppenstall RB, ed. Fracture Treatment and Healing. Philadelphia, WB Saunders, 1980: 666–668.
79. Jazayeri M: Resident Review #6. Posterior fracture-dislocations of the hip joint with emphasis on the importance of hip tomography in their management. Orthop Rev 7:59–64, 1978.
80. Hirasawa Y, Oda R, Nakatani K: Sciatic nerve paralysis in posterior dislocation of the hip. A case report. Clin Orthop 126:172–175, 1977.
81. Mack LA, Harley JD, Winquist RA: CT of acetabular fractures: analysis of fracture patterns. AJR 138:407–412, 1982.
82. Rogers LF, Novy SB, Harris NF: Occult central fractures of the acetabulum. AJR 124:96–101, 1975.
83. Sauser DD, Billimoria PE, Rouse GA, Mudge K: CT evaluation of hip trauma. AJR 135:269–274, 1980.
84. Schoenecker PL, Manske PR, Serti GO: Traumatic hip dislocation with ipsilateral femoral shaft fractures. Clin Orthop 130:233–238, 1978.
85. Smith GR, Loop JW: Radiologic classification of posterior dislocations of the hip: refinements and pitfalls. Radiology 119:569–574, 1976.
86. Stein MG, Barmeir E, Levin J, Dubowitz B, Roffman M: The medial acetabular wall: normal measurements in different population groups. Invest Radiol 17:476–478, 1982.
87. Thaggard A III, Harle TS, Carlson V: Fractures and dislocations of bony pelvis and hip. Semin Roentgenol 13:117–134, 1978.
88. Thompson VP, Epstein HC: Traumatic dislocations of the hip. A survey of 204 cases covering a period of 21 years. J Bone Joint Surg (Am) 33:746–778, 1951.
89. Whitehouse GH: Radiological aspects of posterior dislocation of the hip. Clin Radiol 29:431–441, 1978.

Bone Biopsy Sequelae

90. Braunstein EM: Iliac biopsy defects mimicking Hodgkin's disease. AJR 135:289–290, 1980.
91. Gilsanz V, Grunebaum M: Radiographic appearance of iliac marrow biopsy sites. AJR 128:597–598, 1977.
92. Kagan C, Graze P, Collins JD, Mink J: Radiographic changes in the posterior-superior iliac crests following bone marrow aspiration. Radiology 124:658, 1977.

93. Murphy WA: Exostosis after iliac bone marrow biopsy. AJR 129:1114–1115, 1977.
94. O'Gara CM, Cigtay OS: Iliac marrow biopsy sites in adults. J Can Assoc Radiol 30:230, 1979.

Sacroiliitis

95. Baker H, Golding DN, Thompson M: Psoriasis and arthritis. Ann Intern Med 58:909–925, 1963.
96. Barraclough D, Russel AS, Percy JS: Psoriatic spondylitis: A clinical, radiological, and scintiscan survey. J Rheumatol 4:282–287, 1977.
97. Carrera GH, Foley WD, Kozin F, Ryan L, Lawson TL: CT of sacroiliitis. AJR 136:41–46, 1981.
98. Delbarre F, Rondier J, Delrieu F, Evrard J, Cayla J, Menkes CJ, Amor B: Pyogenic infection of the sacroiliac joint: reprint of thirteen cases. J Bone Joint Surg (Am) 57:819–825, 1975.
99. Edeiken J, Hodes PJ: Roentgen Diagnosis of Diseases of Bone. Baltimore, Williams & Wilkins, 1973: 735.
100. Forestier J: The importance of sacro-iliac changes in the early diagnosis of ankylosing spondylarthritis. Radiology 33:389–402, 1939.
101. Jajic I: Radiological changes in the sacro-iliac joints and spine of patients with psoriatic arthritis and psoriasis. Ann Rheum Dis 27:1–6, 1968.
102. Martel W, Braunstein EM, Borlaza G, Good AE, Griffin PE Jr: Radiologic features of Reiter disease. Radiology 132:1–10, 1979.
103. McEwen C, DiTata D, Lingg C, et al: Ankylosing spondylitis and spondylitis accompanying ulcerative colitis, regional enteritis, psoriasis and Reiter's disease: a comparative study. Arthritis Rheum 14:291–318, 1971.
104. Numaguchi Y: Osteitis condensans ilii, including its resolution. Radiology 98:1–8, 1971.
105. Peterson CC Jr, Silbiger ML: Reiter's syndrome and psoriatic arthritis. Their roentgen spectra and some interesting similarities. AJR 101:860–871, 1967.
106. Romanus R, Yden S: Pelvo-Spondylitis Ossificans. Chicago, Year Book, 1955.
107. Sholkoff SD, Glickman MG, Steinbach HL: Roentgenology of Reiter's syndrome. Radiology 97:497–503, 1970.

Sacroiliac Joint Scintigraphy

108. Dequeker J, Goddeeris T, Walravens M, De Roo M: Evaluation of sacro-iliitis: Comparison of radiological and radionuclide techniques. Radiology 128:687–689, 1978.
109. Goldberg RP, Genant HK, Shimshak R, Shames D: Applications and limitations of quantitative sacroiliac joint scintigraphy. Radiology 128:683–686, 1978.
110. Ho G Jr, Sadovnikoff N, Malhotra CM, Clauch BC: Quantitative sacroiliac joint scintigraphy: a critical assessment. Arthritis Rheum 22:837–844, 1979.
111. Lentle BC, Russell AS, Percy JS, Jackson FL: Scintigraphic findings in ankylosing spondylitis. J Nucl Med 18:524–528, 1977.
112. Lentle BC, Russell AS, Percy JS, Jackson FL: The scintigraphic investigation of sacroiliac disease. J Nucl Med 18:529–533, 1977.
113. Spencer DG, Adams FG, Horton PW, Buchanan WW: Scintiscanning in ankylosing spondylitis: A clinical, radiological and quantitative radioisotopic study. J Rheumatol 6:426–431, 1979.
114. Vyas K, Eklem M, Seto H, Bobba VR, Brown P, Haines J, Krishnamurthy GT: Quantitative scintigraphy of sacroiliac joints: effect of age, gender, and laterality. AJR 136:589–592, 1981.

Pubic Symphysis

115. Leucutia T: Osteitis pubis and its treatment by roentgen irradiation. AJR 66:385–404, 1951.
116. McEwen C, DiTata D, Lingg C, et al: Ankylosing spondylitis and spondylitis accompanying ulcerative colitis, regional enteritis, psoriasis and Reiter's disease: A comparative study. Arthritis Rheum 14:291–318, 1971.
117. Muecke EC, Currarino G: Congenital widening of the pubic symphysis. Associated clinical disorders and roentgen anatomy of affected bony pelvis. AJR 103:179–185, 1968.
118. Resnick D, Niwayama G, Goergen TG, et al: Clinical, radiographic and pathologic abnormalities in calcium pyrophosphate dihydrate deposition disease (CPPD): pseudogout. Radiology 122:1–15, 1977.
119. Schneider R, Kaye JJ, Ghelman B: Adductor avulsive injuries near the symphysis pubis. Radiology 120:567–569, 1976.
120. Vix VA: Articular and fibrocartilage calcification in hyperparathyroidism: associated hyperuricemia. Radiology 83:468–471, 1964.
121. Vix VA, Ryu CY: The adult symphysis pubis: Normal and abnormal. AJR 112:517–525, 1971.

Chapter 8

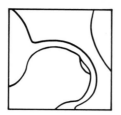

The
HIP

NORMAL STRUCTURE AND FUNCTION

Essential Anatomy

The ball-and-socket configuration of the hip joint allows considerable motion, with flexion averaging 120 degrees, extension 9.5 degrees, internal rotation 35.5 degrees, external rotation 33.6 degrees, abduction 38.5 degrees, and adduction 30.5 degrees.[6] The anterior tilt of the acetabulum explains the greater potential for flexion as compared with extension. The hip has inherent

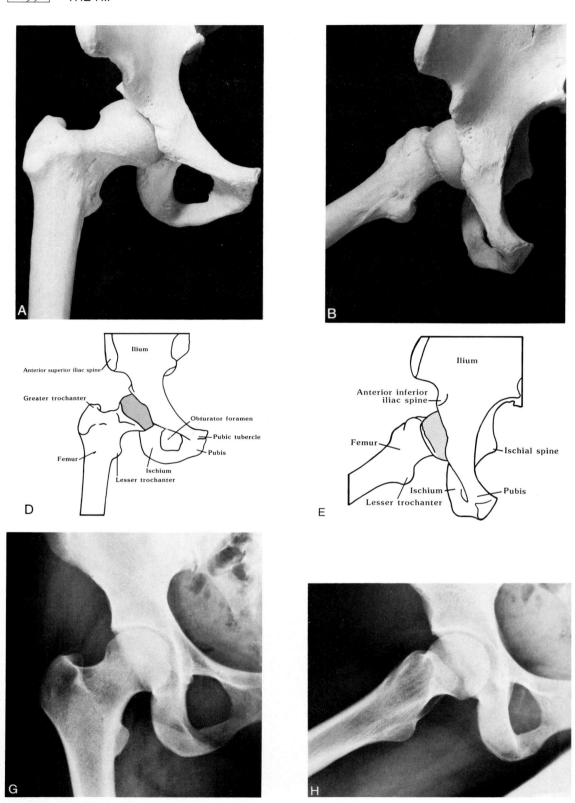

Figure 8–1. The Normal Hip. Photographic, diagrammatic, and radiographic anatomy of the hip in the AP *(A, D, G)*, frog lateral *(B, E, H)*, and true lateral *(C, F, I)* projections.

Illustration continued on opposite page

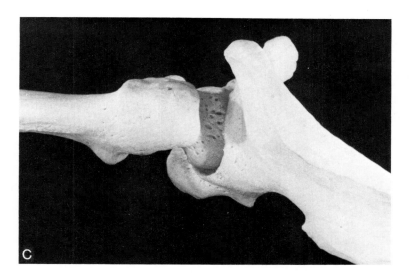

C

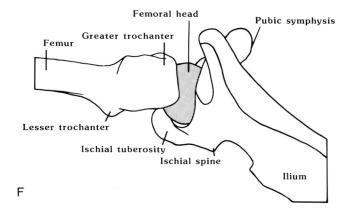

Femoral head

Greater trochanter

Femur

Pubic symphysis

Lesser trochanter

Ischial tuberosity

Ischial spine

Ilium

F

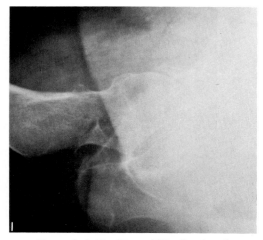

I

Figure 8–1. The Normal Hip *Continued.*

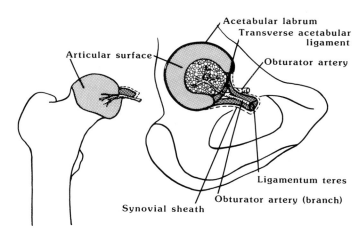

Figure 8–2. The Articular Cartilage of the Hip and the Ligamentum Teres. The horseshoe-shaped articular surface of the acetabulum is shown. The acetabular fossa is filled with fat, and the subjacent vessels are shown. The branch of the obturator artery located in the ligamentum teres is usually a minor source of blood supply to the femoral head.

bony stability owing to the concave shape of the acetabulum, which is deepened by a bony rim around its anterior, superior, and posterior portions (Fig. 8–1). A fibrocartilaginous labrum extends from the acetabular margins and is inferiorly continuous with the transverse ligament, across the acetabular notch. The labrum encircles the femoral head and increases joint stability.

The femoral head is spherical in shape but is slightly flattened both anteriorly and posteriorly. With the exception of the fovea it is covered by articular cartilage that ends approximately at the level of the epiphyseal plate (Fig. 8–2). On the acetabular side the articular cartilage covers a horseshoe-shaped peripheral region, while the more central deep acetabular fossa is nonarticulating and filled with fat, synovial membrane, and the ligamentum teres.

The joint capsule inserts proximally on the rim of the acetabulum and distally on the femur, in which it inserts anteriorly along the intertrochanteric line and posteriorly halfway down the neck (Fig. 8–3). The dense fibrous tissue of the capsule is anteriorly and inferiorly reinforced but minimally so posteriorly. One area of thickening, the zona orbicularis, encircles the femoral head and reinforces the function of the labrum. The retinacula are fibrous extensions of the capsule that are reflected onto the femoral neck. The vessels that ascend along these structures provide the major blood supply to the femoral head.

Blood Supply to the Femoral Head[1, 2, 4, 8]

The blood supply to the femoral head is derived from three sources (Fig. 8–4):

1. *Retinacular (capsular) vessels.* These are branches of the circumflex artery (predominantly the medial femoral circumflex) that course within the joint in synovial reflections along the femoral neck. It is generally agreed that the superior retinacular arteries and their intraosseous lateral epiphyseal branches are the most important vessels supplying the femoral head and that through these vessels the entire femoral head can be nourished when all other vessels are

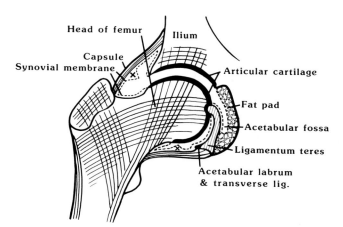

Figure 8–3. The Joint Capsule. A diagrammatic cross section of the hip shows the joint capsule and the synovial lining (dashed lines). The area of thickening of the capsule, termed the zona orbicularis (x), produces an indentation in the synovial contour that is visible on arthrograms. (After Grant JCB: Atlas of Anatomy. Baltimore, Williams & Wilkins, 1962.)

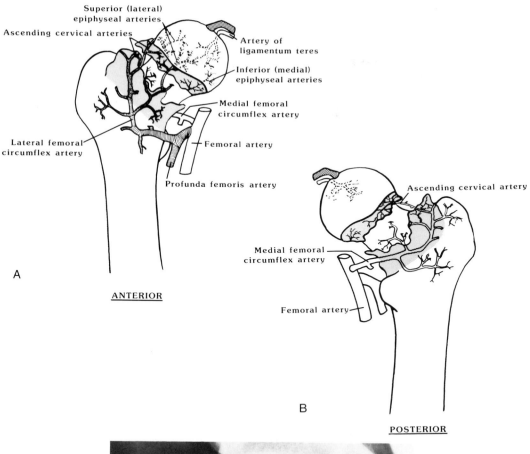

A

Superior (lateral)
epiphyseal arteries

Ascending cervical arteries

Artery of
ligamentum teres

Inferior (medial)
epiphyseal arteries

Medial femoral
circumflex artery

Lateral femoral
circumflex artery

Femoral artery

Profunda femoris artery

__ANTERIOR__

B

Ascending cervical artery

Medial femoral
circumflex artery

Femoral artery

__POSTERIOR__

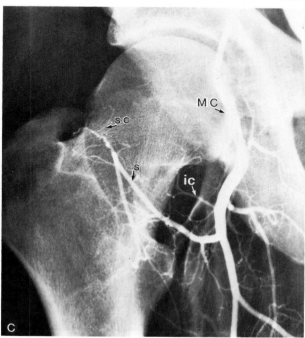

Figure 8–4. Blood Supply to the Femoral Head. The anterior *(A)* and the posterior *(B)* views of the femur show the normal blood supply to the femoral head. *C,* After injection of the medial femoral circumflex artery, an arteriogram shows filling of its branches. MC = medial femoral circumflex artery, ic = inferior capsular, sc = superior capsular, and s = superior branch of medial circumflex.

389

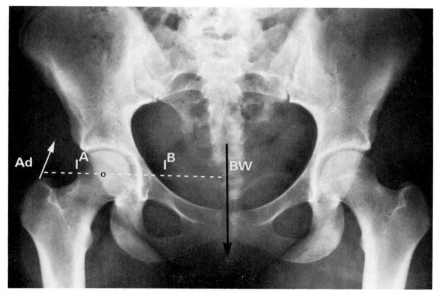

Figure 8–5. Moment Arms. Normally, there is a balance between the resultants of body weight (BW) and force of the adductors (Ad) and their respective distances (l^B and l^A) to the center of the femoral head (o).

experimentally severed. The inferior retinacular vessels are of less importance but can supply the inferior portion of the femoral head. Anterior and posterior retinacular vessels are usually small or absent. The retinacular vessels are often torn when displaced intracapsular fractures occur. In addition, since these vessels lie under the joint capsule, they may be occluded by elevations in intraarticular pressure that may follow hemorrhage or effusion into the joint.[90]

2. *Arteries in the ligamentum teres.* These vessels are branches of the obturator artery or the medial circumflex artery. They are absent or of little importance in most cases, but in occasional instances they supply blood to the entire femoral head.

3. *Vessels within the femoral neck.* These vessels are branches of the medullary artery of the femoral shaft. Sevitt and Thompson found that they supplied none of or only the lateral

portion of the normal femoral head when the retinacular vessels and the vessels of the ligamentum teres were severed.[8] They concluded that, although anastomoses exist between the nutrient arteries in the diaphysis and the vessels of the normal femoral head, the nutrient artery cannot supply the entire femoral head when other sources of blood supply are absent. In osteoarthritic hips, however, the anastomoses may become extensive enough to provide nutrition to the femoral head.

Biomechanical Adaptations

Normally, the forces acting across the hip are balanced so that the product (moment) of body weight (acting anterior to the sacrum) and the distance from the midline to the center of the femoral head is equal to the product of the pull of the abductor muscles and the distance from their insertion on the greater trochanter to

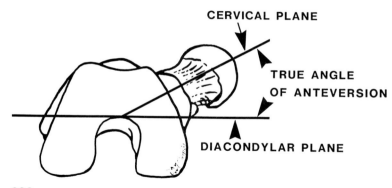

Figure 8–6. Femoral Anteversion. The femoral neck projects anterior to the plane of the femoral condyles (the diacondylar plane).

the center of the femoral head (Fig. 8–5). The structure of the proximal femur reflects these forces. The valgus neck-shaft angle seen in neonates (non–weight-bearing) is gradually replaced by the more varus adult neck-shaft angle of 113 to 136 degrees,[3] which places the abductors farther from the center of the femoral head and, therefore, in a more mechanically advantageous position.

In addition to the neck-shaft angle, the femoral neck is deviated away from the coronal plane of the femur; this deviation is termed femoral torsion (twisting), or version (inclination). In the adult 8 to 15 degrees of anteversion (anterior version) is normal (Fig. 8–6). This increases the lever arm of the gluteus maximus so that less work must be expended to maintain hip extension when standing.[5]

Muscle Groups

In the thigh and gluteal region four muscle groups that affect hip motion can be identified. The anterior femoral muscles—including the tensor fascia lata, the sartorius, and the rectus femoris—flex, abduct, and externally rotate the thigh.[10] A medial group–including the gracilis, the pectineus, the adductor longus, the adductor brevis, and the adductor magnus—act as ad-

ductors but also internally rotate and flex the hip. A gluteal group consisting of the gluteus maximus, medius, and minimus extend and abduct the hip; the piriformis, the obturator internus and externus, the gemelli superior and inferior and the quadratus femoris produce external rotation. A posterior femoral group consisting of the hamstring muscles (the biceps femoris, the semimembranosus, and the semitendinosus) integrate hip extension and knee flexion. The origins and insertions of these muscles are shown in Figure 8–7. In addition, the iliopsoas (the compound muscle consisting of iliacus and psoas major and minor) flexes the hip and externally rotates the thigh.

Normal Radiographic Findings

Soft Tissues

Fat Planes. There are four fat lines visible near the hip: the obturator line along the pelvic inlet, the iliopsoas line along the medial femoral neck, and the capsular and the gluteal lines lateral to the femoral neck (Table 8–1; Fig. 8–8).

Obturator Line. In 1942 Hefke and Turner showed by anatomical studies that the soft-tissue densities paralleling the inner aspect of the pelvis were the obturator internus muscles and that

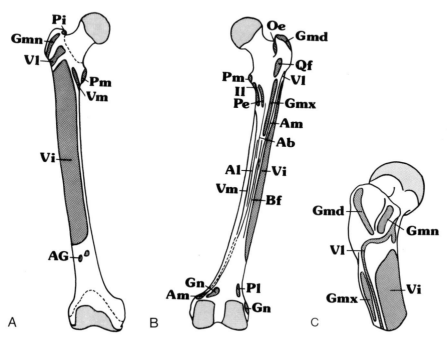

Figure 8–7. Muscular Attachments. Anterior *(A)* and posterior *(B)* views of the femur. *C*, Lateral view of the proximal femur. Ab = adductor brevis; AG = articular muscle; Al = adductor longus; Am = adductor magnus; Bf = biceps femoris; Gmd = gluteus medius; Gmn = gluteus minimus; Gmx = gluteus maximus; Gn = gastrocnemius; Il = iliacus; Oe = obturator externus; Pe = pectineus; Pi = piriformis; Pl = plantaris; Pm = psoas major; Qf = quadratus femoris; Vi = vastus intermedius; Vl = vastus lateralis; Vm = vastus medialis. (Redrawn from Williams P, Warwick R: Gray's Anatomy, 36th Br. ed. Edinburgh, Churchill Livingstone, 1980.)

Table 8–1. **Fat Lines About the Hip**

% in which fat plane visible	Obturator Line*		Iliopsoas Line†		"Capsular" Line†		Gluteal Line†	
	Male	Female	Male	Female	Male	Female	Male	Female
% in which fat plane visible	18	23	84	73	85	65	27	28
Average width (mm)	7	8	14	12	13	12	31	29
Range (mm)	1–21	4–14	5–30	8–19	5–25	7–18	21–51	14–42
Anatomical location	Above obturator internus		Medial to iliopsoas tendon		Between rectus femoris and tensor faciae latae		Between gluteus minimus and gluteus medius	
Relation to joint capsule	Proximal		Anterior		Anterior		Lateral	

Source: Guerra J et al. Radiology 128:11–20, 1978.
*Measured to pelvic brim.
†Measured to femoral neck.

the adjacent fat line might be displaced, bowed, or obliterated in children with septic arthritis.[15] In fact, 50 percent of the children with septic arthritis studied had abnormalities in the obturator line (the obturator sign) during the first week of symptoms. By the end of the second week, 94 percent showed these changes, whereas only 19 percent showed bone damage and 25 percent showed joint changes. The obturator sign was of less importance in patients with tuberculous arthritis because they presented after weeks or months of disease and the vast majority already had bone changes on the initial radiographic examination.

The application of this obturator sign to adults is limited, since a recent study has demonstrated that these fat planes were visible in less than 25 percent of normal patients.[14] When present, however, the appearances on each side tend to be similar, the contours infrequently bulging and the average thickness from pelvis to fat plane 7 mm in males and 8 mm in females.[14]

Iliopsoas Line. The fat line seen along the medial femoral neck on AP radiographs represents the widest portion of the collection of fat medial to the iliopsoas tendon. This is actually anterior to the hip joint and can be expected to be an insensitive indicator of intraarticular effu-

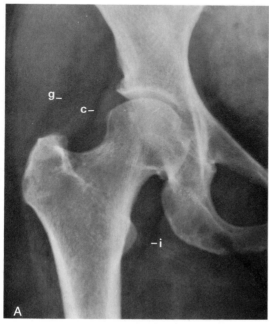
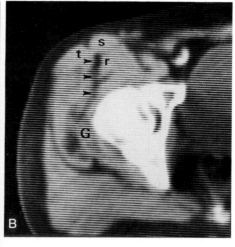

Figure 8–8. Normal Fat Lines. *A,* The iliopsoas (i), the capsular (c), and the gluteal (g) fat lines are well seen. The gluteal line lies between the gluteus minimus and the gluteus medius. The psoas line lies along the medial aspect of the iliopsoas. *B,* The capsular line (arrowheads) begins vertically between the rectus femoris and the tensor fasciae latae and extends posteriorly between the gluteus minimus and the joint capsule. r = rectus femoris; s = sartorius; t = tensor fasciae latae; g = gluteus minimus.

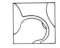

sion. A posterior extension of the iliopsoas fat line is adjacent to the medial aspect of the joint capsule, but this portion is not radiographically identifiable. Therefore, the iliopsoas fat line seen on radiographs is not displaced when small to moderate amounts of intraarticular fluid are present in the adult.[14] However, when large amounts of fluid are present, the fluid may decompress into the iliopsoas bursa and produce displacement of the adjacent fat line.

Unlike the obturator line, the iliopsoas line is seen in more than 70 percent of normal hips (Fig. 8–8). Asymmetry in the appearance of the iliopsoas fat lines however is frequent, with poor definition of the line on one side occurring commonly and unilateral bulging occurring in about 10 percent of cases.[14]

Capsular Line. The more medial of the lateral fat lines (the capsular line) is actually the result of fat between the rectus femoris muscle and the tensor fascia lata anterior to the joint proper (Fig. 8–8).[17] A thin projection of this fat plane extends posteriorly and superiorly and becomes adjacent to the superolateral aspect of the joint capsule. However, this juxtaarticular portion of the fat plane is not visible on routine AP or oblique radiographs.[17] Even if this fat line were seen, the joint capsule in this area is reinforced by ligaments, and it is doubtful that much displacement of adjacent structures could occur.

Gluteal Line. The more lateral of the two lateral fat lines is at the level of the hip joint, but lateral to it, between the gluteus medius and the gluteus minimus muscles. It is visible in about one fourth of normal hips. Thus, particularly in adults, the configuration of fat lines adjacent to the hip is of little value in suggesting or excluding the presence of joint distension.

Cartilage Spaces. Analysis of the normal adult hip joint on AP radiographs has demonstrated no difference in the average measurements among various age groups.[13, 14] The width of the superior and axial (in line with the axis of the femoral neck) joint space primarily reflects the combined thickness of the femoral and the acetabular articular cartilages and averages 4 mm (Fig. 8–9).[13, 14] The medial joint space, measured at the level of the center of the femoral head, is usually about twice the superior or axial joint space measurements, averaging 8 mm (in women) to 9 mm (in men). The articular cartilage of the femoral head and the fat, synovial lining, and ligamentum teres present within the acetabular fossa fill this soft-tissue space. No acetabular cartilage is present at this site (see Fig. 8–2). Inferior to the acetabular fossa, the inferomedial articular surface of the joint is not

well seen on the frontal view but can be seen in profile on externally rotated projections (Fig. 8–9). It is in this latter view that articular cartilage narrowing in osteoarthritis with inferomedial cartilage loss can be detected.[63]

Arthrosonography

Arthrosonography (ultrasound) examination of the hip joint allows detection of intraarticular effusion as well as paraarticular fluid collections. Normally, scans obtained along the axis of the femoral neck show close apposition of the echoes produced by the joint capsule and those produced by the femoral head and neck.[18] Effusion produces an anechoic region separating the capsule and the bone (Fig. 8–10). Wilson and co-workers suggested that differences of more than 3 mm in the measured distances between capsule and bone on each side strongly suggest joint effusion.[20]

Arthrography

Traction Arthrography. One relatively simple method of demonstrating articular surfaces makes use of the gas that is released into a joint when traction is applied and no effusion is present. Martel and Poznanski applied traction to the lower extremities of normal children and adults, and in most of these joint distraction was produced and gas was seen outlining the articular cartilage.[26] In a few patients no distraction of the joint was possible, and no gas arthrogram was obtained. In contrast, several patients with abnormal hips had no gas visible within the joint, despite adequate joint distraction (defined as separation of articular surfaces by more than 1 mm). This failure to obtain a gas arthrogram when adequate joint separation is achieved indicates the presence of joint effusion—a fact confirmed by studies that show disappearance of the gas following injection of fluid into the joint.

Traction arthrography is of particular value in areas such as the hip, where joint effusion is difficult to detect on physical examination or on standard radiographs. Abnormal hips without joint effusion may demonstrate a gas arthrogram, and in those cases the contour and thickness of articular cartilage can be examined. It has been emphasized by Martel and Poznanski that no conclusions regarding the presence of joint disease can be made if there is no measurable increase in the joint space with applied traction.[26]

Contrast Arthrography

Indications. Hip arthrography is primarily performed to confirm intraarticular needle placement during joint aspiration for suspected infec-

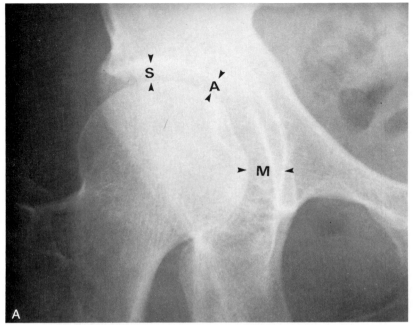

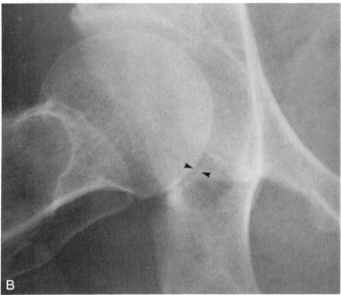

Figure 8–9. Normal Cartilage Space. *A,* The AP view shows the superior (S) and the axial (A) cartilage spaces. The medial joint space (M) is wider, since it includes the area of the acetabular fossa. *B,* This slightly externally rotated frog lateral view shows the inferomedial (arrowheads) cartilage space.

tion. Other indications include the evaluation of painful hips without specific radiographic findings and of painful joint prostheses.

Method. One method used at Brigham and Women's Hospital is described, although numerous variations have been successfully applied. The patient is positioned supine on the fluoroscopic table with the hip in neutral rotation and a sponge under the knee to flex the hip and to relax the joint capsule. The femoral artery is palpated and its course noted and marked with an indelible pen. The groin is prepared and

draped, and a sterile clamp is then positioned under fluoroscopic guidance until its tip overlies the femoral neck just below the head-neck junction and slightly medial to the midline. At this site after local anesthesia is administered, a 20-gauge spinal needle is directed vertically downward until bone (or metal) is felt. Variations in this needle-placement technique include needle entry slightly below, lateral, or medial to the suggested point so that the needle can be angled toward its final entry site into the capsule. This method helps ensure that the bevel of the needle

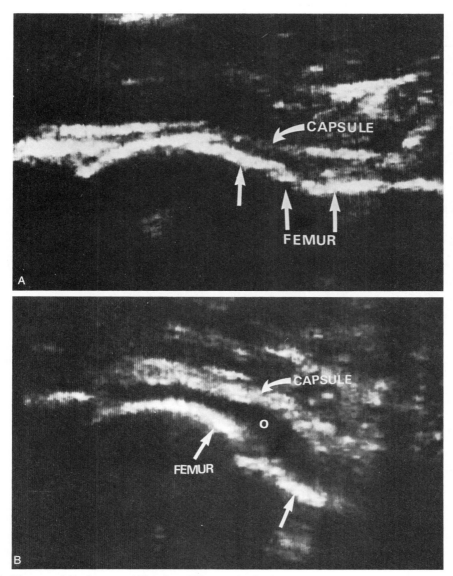

Figure 8–10. Ultrasound Evaluation of Hip Joint Effusion. *A,* On the normal side the sagittal ultrasound examination shows minimal separation between the joint capsule and the femur. *B,* On the side of the joint effusion (due to septic arthritis), an anechoic region (o), representing fluid within the joint, separates the femur and the capsule. (With permission, from Seltzer SE, Finberg HJ, Weissman BN: Invest Radiol 15:19, 1980.)

is entirely within the joint capsule; it is also helpful when the femoral head is unusually high or medial in position (as may occur in severe rheumatoid arthritis). When a prosthesis is present, the oblique approach allows the hub of the needle to be seen during fluoroscopy.

After brief fluoroscopy to confirm needle location, an attempt is made to aspirate joint fluid. If successful, specimens are sent for aerobic and anaerobic cultures, Gram stain, and cell count. If no fluid is obtained, contrast agent may be injected and reaspirated for culture, since the agent does not significantly interfere with bac-

terial growth. However, lidocaine (Xylocaine) inhibits bacterial growth and cannot be used for joint lavage.[30] Whether or not fluid is obtained, contrast material is always injected to confirm correct intraarticular needle placement and to define joint anatomy. The joint is usually adequately filled after injection of 5 to 15 ml through an extension tubing; injection is stopped after fluoroscopic confirmation of adequate filling or development of patient discomfort. The needle is removed, and AP and frog lateral views before and after exercise are obtained. Occasionally, complex motion tomography is used to show

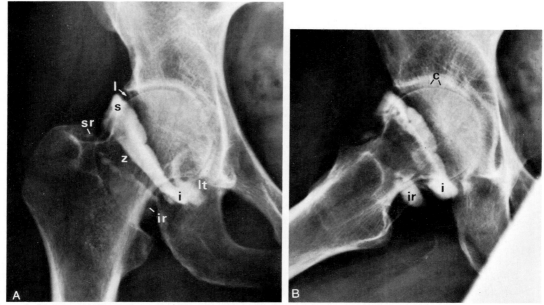

Figure 8–11. Normal Hip Arthrogram. Normal examination after intraarticular injection of about 6 ml of contrast medium. AP *(A)* and frog lateral *(B)* views. c = contrast agent outlining articular cartilage (recess capitus); i = inferior articular recess; ir = recess colli inferior; l = acetabular labrum; lt = defect in contrast from transverse ligament; s = superior articular recess; sr = recess colli superior; z = zona orbicularis (the impression on the intraarticular contrast by the iliofemoral and ischiofemoral ligaments of the hip joint capsule).

the labrum or articular cartilage to advantage. In these cases, a small amount (0.1 to 0.3 ml) of 1:1000 epinephrine is added to the injected contrast medium to maintain sharp definition of structures throughout the period of filming.

Normal Arthrogram. A normal arthrogram is shown in Figure 8–11. The joint capsule is seen to insert proximally just superior to the acetabular labrum; anteriorly, along the distal intertrochanteric line of the femur; and posteriorly, halfway down the femoral neck. A thin layer of contrast material outlines the normally smooth articular surface, but traction or exercise may be necessary to demonstrate this. Normal capsular constriction, due to the zona orbicularis, with recesses proximal and distal to this area is noted. The ligamentum teres extends from the fovea of the femoral head to the inferior acetabulum at the level of the acetabular notch and is not usually seen. Communication with the overlying iliopsoas bursa has been noted in 14 percent of cadavers but is an unusual finding on arthrography.[31]

Bony Structures

Acetabular Roof. Bony condensation in the roof of the acetabulum, called the acetabular sourcil (eyebrow), reflects bone apposition in response to applied stress. In normal hips under normal stress, this zone of acetabular sclerosis is

thin and of equal width over the weight-bearing surface (see Fig. 8–1). Abnormalities in the amount or the distribution of stress are reflected by changes in the shape and the distribution of this sclerotic zone.[38] For example, in subluxation of the femoral head the area of sclerosis be-

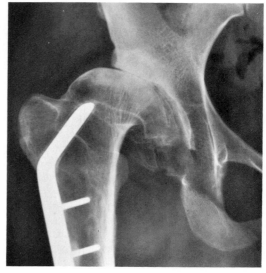

Figure 8–12. Congenital Hip Dislocation with Secondary Osteoarthritis. Increased stress on the lateral acetabulum, associated with the subluxation of the femoral head, has led to the formation of a prominent zone of acetabular sclerosis. A femoral osteotomy has been done.

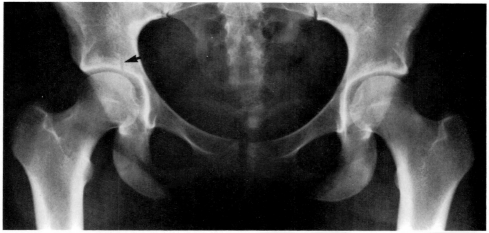

Figure 8–13. Normal Acetabular Notch Defect. A normal accessory fossa (arrow) is present on the right.

comes triangular and is located at the edge of the acetabulum, corresponding to the concentration of stress on this area (Fig. 8–12).[135] Pauwels noted that a convex sourcil is the shape expected when only one layer of articular cartilage is present and that the appearance of such an area is the "very first sign of primary osteoarthritis" (see Fig. 8–23).[38] A notched defect in the medial acetabular roof that interrupts this normal zone of sclerosis is sometimes present. An accessory fossa, not a vascular channel, has been shown to produce this defect (Fig. 8–13).[35]

Trabecular Architecture of the Proximal Femur. The proximal femur is largely composed of cancellous bone, the trabecular pattern of which has traditionally been ascribed to the bones' response to applied force. Because the force on the proximal femur can be resolved into a bending force perpendicular to the axis of the femoral neck and a compressive force along the axis of the femoral neck, two major groups of trabeculae (tensile and compression) are present. These have further been classified as follows (Fig. 8–14):[39, 40]

1. *Principal compressive trabeculae.* These trabeculae course from the femoral head toward the medial cortex of the femoral neck, following the direction of the resultant compressive force.[38] Distally, they form an angle of 160° with the medial femoral cortex; proximally, they are in line with similar trabeculae in the pelvis.

2. *Principal tensile trabeculae.* These trabeculae arch from the lateral to the medial cortices in the direction of tensile (bending) forces.

3. *Secondary compressive trabeculae.* These trabeculae arise from the medial cortex, distal to the principal compressive trabeculae; they fan out laterally toward the greater trochanter. Normally, they are thin and widely spaced.

4. *Secondary tensile trabeculae.* These trabeculae lie below and parallel to the principal tensile trabeculae; they end irregularly near the midline.

The central area bounded by these trabecular groups contains thin, sparse trabeculae and is known as Ward's triangle.

The trabecular structure just described is seen in patients whose weight-bearing is normal and who have normal neck-shaft angles. Individuals with varus deformity have accentuation of the tensile trabecular arches; conversely, individuals with valgus deformity have lower tensile forces, and the trabeculae in the neck course downward along the path of the resultant compressive force, with Ward's triangle obscured.[38]

Calcar Femorale.[3, 33, 34] The calcar femorale is a lamellated vertical bony plate deep to the lesser trochanter, continuous with the medial femoral cortex. The compression trabeculae end here (Fig. 8–15). In common usage, however, the lower portion of the femoral neck above the lesser trochanter may (erroneously) be referred

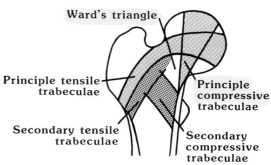

Figure 8–14. The Normal Trabecular Pattern. The trabecular pattern reflects the compressive and bending (tensile) forces on the proximal femur.

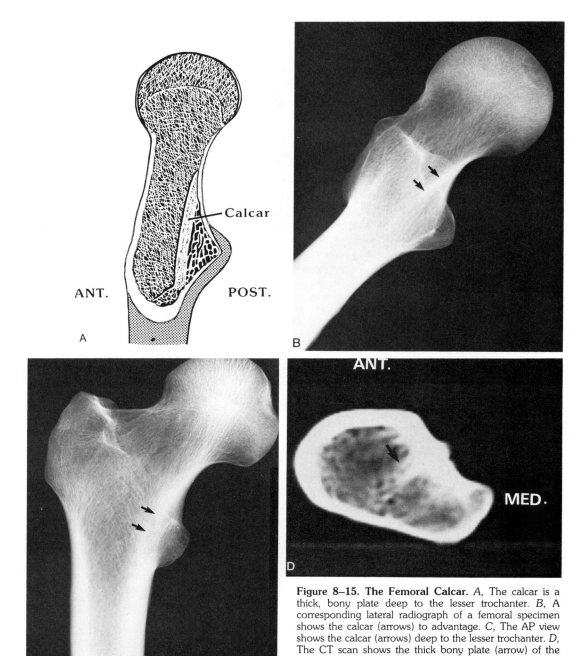

Figure 8–15. The Femoral Calcar. *A,* The calcar is a thick, bony plate deep to the lesser trochanter. *B,* A corresponding lateral radiograph of a femoral specimen shows the calcar (arrows) to advantage. *C,* The AP view shows the calcar (arrows) deep to the lesser trochanter. *D,* The CT scan shows the thick bony plate (arrow) of the calcar. ANT. = anterior; MED. = medial. (*A,* redrawn from Williams PL, Warwick R: Gray's Anatomy, 36th Br. ed. Edinburgh, Churchill Livingstone, 1980, by permission.)

to as the calcar. The importance of the calcar femorale is its strength to resist compression and to prevent collapse of the femoral neck, which may occur when this area is violated by tumor or trauma.

Femoral Anteversion. Although the concept of femoral anteversion is not difficult, variations in nomenclature and the plethora of radiological techniques available for its assessment have led to some confusion.

The femoral neck is usually anteriorly angled from the coronal plane of the femur, and it is this deviation that is termed femoral torsion, or version. The amount of torsion is measured as the angle between the central axis of the femoral neck and the coronal plane of the femur (the diacondylar, or transcondylar, plane) (Fig. 8–6). If the femoral neck is inclined anterior to this plane, then anteversion, antetorsion, or anterior twist is present, and the measured angle is given a plus sign. Conversely, posterior inclination is termed retroversion, retrotorsion, or posterior twist, and the angle is designated by a minus sign. The angle of version is sometimes referred to as the angle of declination to differentiate it from the neck-shaft angle (the angle of inclination).[44]

During childhood the angle of anteversion decreases. Adult measurements of 8 to 15 degrees are reported as normal.[44, 52, 53]

Direct Measurement of the Angle of Anteversion

Radiography. Femoral version can be measured directly from the radiograph when the central ray is directed along the transcondylar plane of the femur. These projections can be obtained in children in the seated or the supine position, with the hips and knees flexed to 90 degrees (Fig. 8–16).[46, 47] Axial tomography has been used to improve the visibility of the femoral neck and to extend the use of the technique to older children.[48] Because of the large amounts of soft tissue in the thigh, radiation exposure is high, and the procedure (without tomography) is generally not applicable to children over 6 years old or to adults. In addition, the axial radiograph that results is of little additional clinical use. Such direct methods do appear to be quite accurate, however, since comparison with

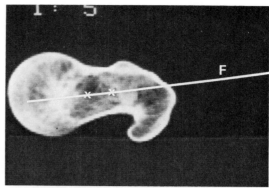

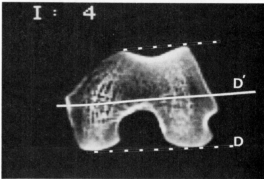

Figure 8–17. CT For Determining Femoral Anteversion (Using a Femoral Specimen). The diacondylar line (D) is drawn along the condyles, although Hernandez and coworkers construct it (D′) midway between the anterior and posterior femoral sufaces (dashed lines). The axis of the femoral neck (F) is shown. The angle between the femoral neck axis (F) and the diacondylar line is the angle of anteversion. In this case there is 2 degrees of retroversion.

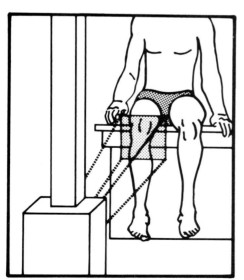

Figure 8–16. Direct Measurement of Femoral Anteversion. This method provides a true axial projection of the femur. The angle between the femoral neck and the diacondylar plane (which is perpendicular to the tibia) can be measured directly. The film is placed behind the hip. (After Budin E, Chandler E: Radiology 69:209, 1957.)

measurements made on dried femora show differences averaging only 2 degrees.[48]

Computed Tomography. Computed tomographic images through the femoral necks with the femoral shafts parallel to the radiographic table and in neutral rotation also directly show the degree of femoral torsion. Recent studies measure the angle of anteversion by constructing the axis of the neck on the CT scan of the proximal femur, constructing the diacondylar plane on the CT scan of the distal femur, and determining the angle between these lines (Fig. 8–17).[47, 60] Hernandez and colleagues use palpation of the pubic symphysis to determine the approximate location of the femoral necks, and they emphasize that scans taken just at the top of the greater trochanter are ideal, although the trochanter itself is not used in determining the neck angle.[47] The distal femoral sections are taken just below the upper poles of the patellae. These authors determine the transcondylar (diacondylar) plane by bisecting the angle formed by tangents to the anterior femur and the posterior femoral condyles.

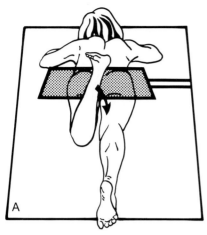 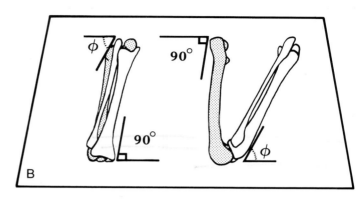

Figure 8–18. Fluoroscopic Method of Determining Femoral Anteversion. As described by Rogers (1931), the patient lies prone on the fluoroscopic table; the knee on the side to be studied is flexed to 90 degrees, and the tibia is rotated medially (the femur therefore being externally rotated) until the head and neck of the femur are in line with the femoral shaft. At that point the angle between the table and the medial aspect of the flexed leg is equal to the angle of anteversion. *A,* Diagram of patient position. *B,* Diagram of bony structures before and after the leg is rotated (ϕ is the angle of anteversion). (Redrawn from Rogers SP: J Bone Joint Surg 13:82, 1931.)

Indirect Measurement of the Angle of Anteversion. These techniques can broadly be classified into two groups, fluoroscopic and trigonometric.

Fluoroscopic Techniques. There are several fluoroscopic methods described for measuring femoral torsion, but they all offer the same disadvantages—namely, limited reproducibility and the lack of a permanent record.[55, 58]

In the method described by Stewart and Karshner, the patient lies prone on the fluoroscopic table with the knee of the leg to be examined flexed to 90 degrees.[58] While the femoral neck is being observed fluoroscopically, the leg is rotated medially (the femur therefore being rotated externally) until the femoral neck and shaft form a straight line (the shortest neck).[56] The angle of the leg to the table is measured with the fulcrum of the goniometer at the level of the centers of the femoral condyles (Fig. 8–18). According to the authors, this determination is within 2 to 5 degrees of the actual value. Any rotation of the pelvis necessary to bring the femoral neck in line with the shaft apparently does not affect the measured result. Significant error may occur, however, when instability of the knee is present, since the position of the leg may then not accurately reflect that of the femur.

A modification of the Stewart technique was proposed by Rogers. It uses the relationship of the femoral head to the femoral neck to define the fluoroscopic end point (Fig. 8–18).[54] This is of questionable validity, particularly since the definition of femoral torsion specifically refers to the angle between the femoral neck and the transcondylar plane of the femur, not to any relationship between the femoral head and the femoral neck.

Trigonometric Methods. The angle of anteversion can be calculated by using trigonometric principles from the measured neck-shaft angles obtained from two different projections of the upper femur. Variations in technique are based largely on the projections that are used.[49–51, 57] Each of these methods offers the advantages of being applicable to all age groups, having a relatively small amount of intraobserver error (about 5 degrees), and using radiographic projections that provide a permanent record and that are generally clinically relevant.

The disadvantages of these methods relate to the difficulty in defining the necessary reference lines, the relative complexity of the final calculations, and, in some, the necessity for using specially constructed devices for patient positioning.

The method described by Magilligan uses standard AP and true lateral projections to obtain neck-shaft angles from which the true angle of anteversion is derived (Fig. 8–19).[50] The AP view is obtained with the femur parallel to the table and in neutral rotation (patella facing straight up). According to Ozonoff, this is best done by having the patient flex his legs over the end of the table so that they are perpendicular to the femora.[52] Ideally, the x-ray tube should be centered over the hip to be studied, although a single exposure that includes both hips probably produces very little distortion. The medial-lateral roentgenogram is obtained without moving the patient and with the cassette at right angles to the table top and parallel to the long

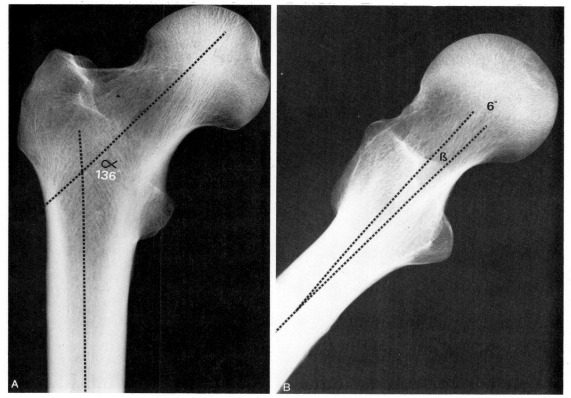

Figure 8–19. Calculation of Angle of Anteversion Using AP and Lateral Views (Method of Magilligan). *A,* The AP view is obtained with the tube centered over the hip joint and the leg in neutral rotation. The neck-shaft angle, α, (136 degrees in this example) is determined. *B,* For the lateral view the cassette is perpendicular to the table top and parallel to the femoral neck. The projected angle of anteversion (β) is determined and the true angle of anteversion calculated or derived from the table (see Fig. 8–20). In this specimen (same as in Fig. 8–17) the angle of anteversion is ≤14 degrees.

axis of the femoral neck, the position of the femoral neck having been determined from the AP view. Slight degrees of abduction or adduction, flexion or extension will not affect the results. However, the parallelism of the cassette to the femoral neck is of importance. Lines are then constructed along the axes of the femoral neck and the femoral shaft, and the observed neck-shaft angle is measured on the AP and the lateral views. The position of the center of the

Table 8–2. Table for the Determination of the Angle of Anteversion (β′)*

β	α	100 (80)	110 (70)	120 (60)	130 (50)	135 (45)	140 (40)	150 (30)	160 (20)	170 (10)
10		10	11	12	13	14	15	19	27	46
20		20	21	23	25	27	29	36	47	64
25		25	26	27	31	33	36	43	53	69
30		30	31	34	37	39	42	49	60	73
35		35	36	39	42	45	48	55	64	76
40		41	42	44	48	50	52	59	68	78
45		46	47	49	52	55	57	64	71	80
50		51	52	54	57	59	62	67	74	82
55		55	56	59	62	63	66	70	76	83
60		60	61	64	66	68	69	73	78	84
70		70	71	73	74	76	77	79	82	86
80		80	81	82	83	83	83	84	86	88

Source: Magilligan DJ: J Bone Joint Surg (Am) 38:1231, 1956, by permission.
*From the projected angle of anteversion (β) on horizontal lateral view and from the projected cervicofemoral angle (α) on anteroposterior view.

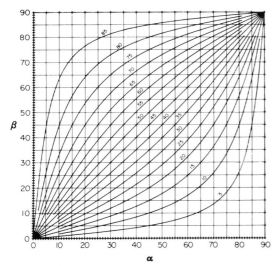

Figure 8–20. Chart for Determining Femoral Anteversion from Measurements Derived from AP (α) and Lateral (β) Radiographs. (From Ogata K, Goldsand EM: J Bone Joint Surg (Am) 61:846, 1979, by permission).

femoral head should not be used as a guide to the central axis of the femoral neck, since the head is eccentrically located in up to two thirds of adults.[44, 48, 52] The axis of the femoral shaft on either the AP or the lateral view can be constructed by connecting a point midway between the cortices and just below the lesser trochanter to a midpoint 10 cm distal to the first.[48] The true angle of anteversion is obtained by comparison with the published graph or table of observed values of α and β (Fig. 8–19; Table 8–2). The true angle of anteversion is never less than the observed angle. As valgus deformity increases, the discrepancy between the observed angle and the true angle of anteversion increases.

Another modification of the biplanar technique for determining femoral anteversion has been developed by Ogata and Goldsand.[51] An AP film is paired with a lateral view taken with the patient lying on the table with the hip and knee of the side to be studied flexed to 90 degrees and the entire lateral aspect of the leg in contact with the table top. The measured neck-shaft angle on each film is inserted into the prepared graph to determine the true angle of anteversion (Fig. 8–20). The true neck-shaft angle can also be determined.

Comparison of Methods. Ruby and associates compared a fluoroscopic technique (the Rogers technique, but measuring the shortest and longest neck-shaft angles), a biplanar method (Ryder-Crane), and a direct method (Dunn) for measuring the anteversion of a dried femur and the femora of patients.[56] There was little difference in the accuracy or reproducibility

Table 8–3. Radiation Dose from Various Methods of Determining Femoral Anteversion

Method	Exposure
Direct x-ray	1.5R
CT	? < 1.7R
Fluoroscopy	1R/minute
Biplanar method	0.12R (per exposure)

Sources: Ruby L et al. J Bone Joint Surg (Am) 61:46, 1979; Hernandez RJ et al. AJR 137:97, 1981.

of these methods, although the direct axial technique was slightly less accurate. All methods had an average error of less than ± 5 degrees and a range of reproducibility of 13 degrees with a maximum error of 9 degrees. The radiation dose to the midpelvis was highest with the direct technique (1.5R), intermediate with the fluoroscopic technique (1R for 1 minute of fluoroscopy time), and lowest with the biplanar technique (0.12R per exposure). The CT methods were not evaluated in this report. The radiation dose delivered in CT scanning is only to the area of the scans, and Hernandez and colleagues noted the dose on their scanner to be less than 1.7R (Table 8–3).[47] The choice of a method to be used clinically should be based on the radiation dose, the ease of performance, the general utility of the films obtained, and the reliability of the examination. The biplanar (geometric) and the fluoroscopic methods are therefore favored.

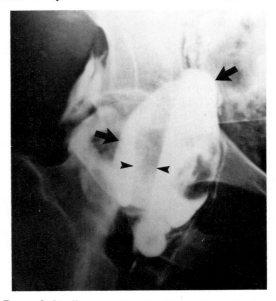

Figure 8–21. Iliopsoas Bursitis. This patient with rheumatoid arthritis had an increasing mass in the groin. Contrast medium injected into the hip joint filled a large circular area (arrows) that represents a distended iliopsoas bursa. The impression of the iliopsoas tendon (arrowheads) is seen. Polypoid filling defects and prominent lymphatic opacification are due to the rheumatoid process.

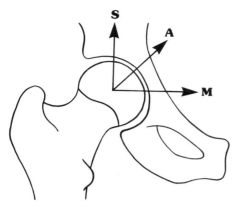

Figure 8–22. Patterns of Migration of the Femoral Head. With osteoarthritis cartilage loss and migration of the femoral head are usually superior (S) and occasionally medial (M). With rheumatoid arthritis the femoral head usually migrates axially (A), eventually producing a protrusio deformity.

ABNORMAL CONDITIONS

Soft-Tissue Abnormalities

Effusion

Injection of fluid into cadaver hips has confirmed the inaccuracy of the iliopsoas and the capsular fat planes in the detection of joint effusion. In addition, lateral rotation and abduction of the leg, a posture frequently assumed when hip pain is present, produce lateral displacement and blurring of the capsular shadow.[11]

Iliopsoas Bursitis

The iliopsoas bursa, located between the iliopsoas tendon and the pubis and the hip joint capsule, has been shown to communicate with the hip in 14 percent of cadavers studied.[23, 31] Bursal distension due to rheumatoid arthritis or other causes may result in a palpable groin mass and in displacement of the iliopsoas fat line on hip radiographs. Hip arthrography usually confirms the diagnosis by showing communication with the distended bursa (Fig. 8–21). The fluid-filled bursa can also be shown on CT or ultrasound.

Cartilage-Space Narrowing in Arthritis

Osteoarthritis. Loss of articular cartilage in the hip often occurs in typical patterns and, when taken in concert with other radiological findings, may imply a specific diagnosis (Fig. 8–22). Thus in approximately 80 percent of patients with primary osteoarthritis, Resnick noted cartilage loss in the superior aspect of the joint (15 percent in the superolateral direction, 48 percent in a superomedial direction, and 15 percent in an intermediate location).[63] In the

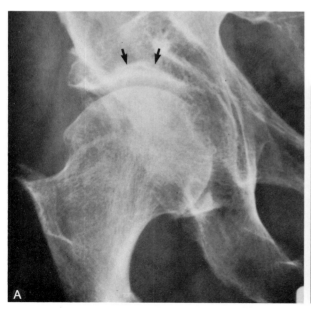

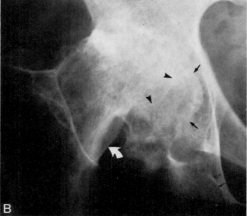

Figure 8–23. Osteoarthritis. *A,* Early osteoarthritis. There is mild hypertrophic lipping from the femoral head. A zone of focal acetabular sclerosis (arrows) attests to the abnormal stress distribution across the joint. *B,* Severe osteoarthritis. Superiorly, there is complete loss of articular cartilage. Very large medial osteophytes are present, projecting from the medial femoral head (arrows) and the acetabulum. The medial femoral cortex (arrowheads) remains visible, deep to the medial osteophytes. The presence of this cortical line helps differentiate the tilt deformity of the femoral head occurring in osteoarthritis from that occurring with other conditions, such as old Legg-Calvé-Perthes disease. The curved arrow indicates new bone formation (buttressing bone) along the medial femoral neck.

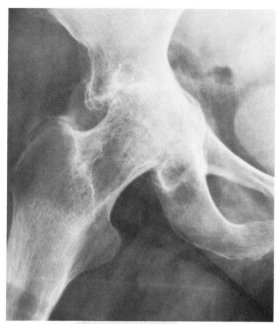

Figure 8–24. Rheumatoid Arthritis. There is complete cartilage loss with protrusio deformity. Despite the severe destruction, no osteophytes are present.

remaining 20 percent of patients, cartilage loss in the inferior aspect of the joint, with medial "migration" of the femoral head and mild protrusio deformity, was noted. Such inferior cartilage-space narrowing is best appreciated on frog lateral, external oblique views. In the patients with cartilage-space narrowing caused by osteoarthritis, other radiographic findings that support the diagnosis are usually present, including

osteophytes, buttressing bone (periosteal reaction along the medial femoral neck), and subchondral sclerosis (Fig. 8–23).[62]

Rheumatoid Arthritis (RA). In contrast with the more focal cartilage narrowing noted in osteoarthritis, cartilage loss in RA is diffuse, and femoral head migration occurs most often in an axial direction (along the axis of the femoral neck) and less frequently in the superior direction (Fig. 8–24). Isolated medial cartilage loss and buttressing bone along the femoral neck are not seen. Sclerosis and osteophytes are minimal or absent, but protrusio deformity may be present.

Ankylosing Spondylitis. Patients with ankylosing spondylitis and cartilage-space narrowing in the hips frequently have a characteristic pattern of damage consisting of concentric narrowing of the joint space and axial migration of the femoral head (similar to rheumatoid arthritis), but, in addition, osteophytes form a collar around the base of the femoral head (Fig. 8–25).[61] In the minority of patients with hip cartilage loss associated with ankylosing spondylitis, there is narrowing in the superior aspect of the joint with superior migration of the femoral head.

Bony Abnormalities

Osteoporosis and the Singh Index
The constancy of the normal trabecular pattern is of practical importance in the assessment of

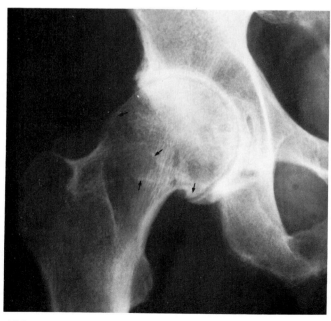

Figure 8–25. Ankylosing Spondylitis. There is diffuse cartilage loss similar to that occurring in rheumatoid arthritis but with a ring of osteophytes present (arrows). The SI joints were fused.

Table 8–4. **Singh Index for Osteoporosis**

Singh Grade	Penciling of Cortex	Trabeculae in Ward's Triangle	2° Compressive Trabeculae	2° Tensile Trabeculae	Principal Tensile Trabeculae	Principal Compressive Trabeculae
VII	0	Minor trabeculae as dense as major trabeculae	Normal	Normal	Obscured	Obscured
VI	0	Less dense inner trabeculae	Normal	Normal	Barely perceptible	Barely perceptible
V	0	No trabeculae	Mottled	Normal	Accentuated	Accentuated
IV	+	No trabeculae	Absent	Absent or don't reach midfemur	Intact	Intact
III	+	No trabeculae	Absent	Absent	Interrupted near greater trochanter	Intact
II	+	No trabeculae	Absent	Absent	Also lost in upper femoral neck	Intact
I	+	No trabeculae	Absent	Absent	Absent even laterally	Decreased

osteoporosis. Singh and co-workers compared the trabecular architecture of the proximal femur with clinical and histological data and noted that as bone loss develops the trabecular groups disappear in a definite sequence, with the least stressed areas resorbed earliest.[39, 40] Seven radiological grades have been defined according to this trabecular pattern and the presence or absence of cortical thinning (Table 8–4; Fig. 8–26). In grade VII all trabeculae are present,

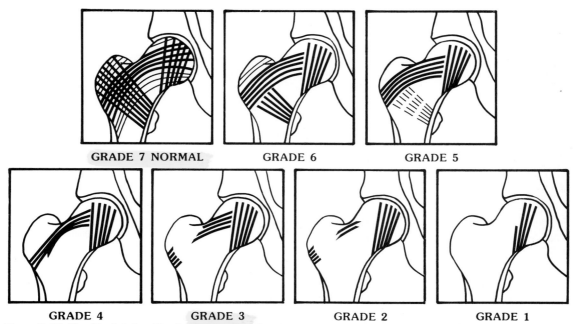

Figure 8–26. The Singh Index. The Singh index describes the trabecular groups that are present. As osteoporosis develops, trabeculae disappear in sequence, the least stressed areas disappearing earliest. Patients with grade IV or less are considered to have abnormally reduced amounts of bone (osteoporosis). (Redrawn from Jowsey J: Metabolic Diseases of Bone. Philadelphia, WB Saunders, 1977:99–101.)

obscuring the principal trabecular groups. Grade VI is similar, but the trabeculae in Ward's triangle are less dense than in adjacent areas, and the principal trabecular pattern is just perceptible. If bone loss continues, there is a reduction in the number of trabeculae in Ward's triangle (grade V), thinning (called penciling) of the femoral cortex and loss of secondary compressive trabeculae (grade IV), absence of the secondary tensile trabeculae and beginning interruption of the principal tensile trabeculae (grade III), further loss of the principal tensile trabeculae (grade II), and thinning of the principal compressive trabeculae (grade I).

All normal ambulatory individuals less than 20 years of age have a Singh grade of VII.[36] There is a negative correlation between the Singh index and clinical and radiological evidence of osteoporosis,[36] and individuals with grade IV or less are considered to have an abnormal degree of bone loss and a higher risk of developing the clinical complications of osteoporosis.

Fractures

Intracapsular Fractures

Femoral fractures are usually subdivided by their location into intra- and extracapsular groups, apparently a worthwhile effort since the two groups differ in terms of patient age, incidence, mechanism of injury, treatment, mortality, potential for healing, and development of complications.[90]

Intracapsular femoral neck fractures are further subdivided by their location into (1) subcapital fractures, involving the base of the head or the high neck area; (2) transcervical fractures, involving the midportion of the neck; and (3) basicervical fractures, involving the lower portion of the neck. In common usage, however, all intracapsular fractures are collectively referred to as subcapital.

Radiological Examination. In the event of suspected intracapsular fracture, AP and true lateral radiographs of the hip are usually sufficient for diagnosis. In questionable cases tomography may define an otherwise imperceptible fracture. A thin rim of osteophytes around the femoral head may mimic an impacted fracture on standard views, but tomography will confirm the peripheral location of these densities and exclude a fracture (Fig. 8–27).

In patients with fractures rotation of the femoral head may produce a deceptively ominous radiographic appearance, suggesting a lytic lesion of the femoral neck, although postoperative views show no such lytic area. Similarly, external

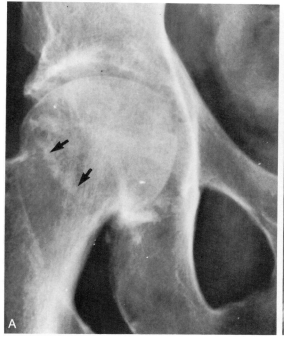 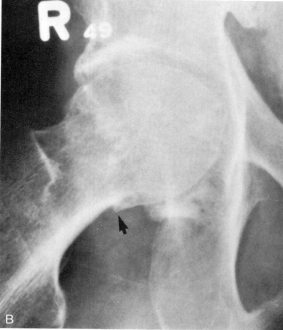

Figure 8–27. Osteophytic Lipping Mimicking an Impacted Fracture. *A,* The AP view shows an irregular zone of sclerosis (arrows) overlying the femoral neck. *B,* The frog lateral view shows a medial osteophyte (arrow) joining the sclerotic line, confirming a diagnosis of osteoarthritic hypertrophic lipping rather than a diagnosis of impacted fracture. In questionable cases tomography will show the osteophytes to be located peripherally, whereas the density caused by an impacted fracture is more central, within the substance of the femur.

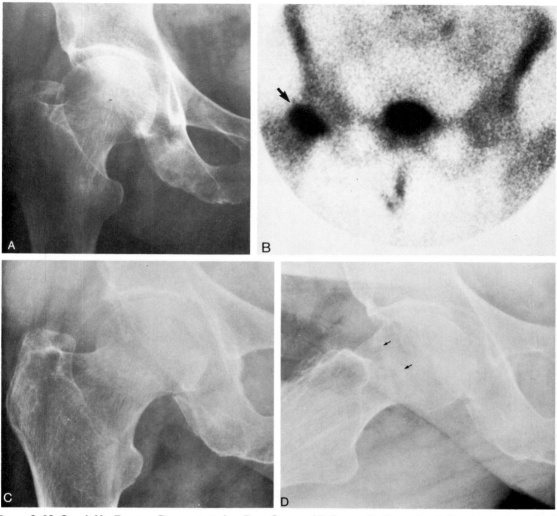

Figure 8–28. Occult Hip Fracture Demonstrated on Bone Scan and Follow-up Radiographs. *A,* Examination immediately after injury shows the femur to be held in external rotation. No fracture line was identified. *B,* A bone scan 2 weeks later shows marked focal increase in isotope uptake in the subcapital region (arrow). AP *(C)* and frog lateral *(D)* radiographs 2 weeks later (1 month after the initial injury) show mild sclerosis along the fracture line (arrows).

rotation of the leg may produce a diffuse increase in the apparent density of the femoral shaft that may be confused with metastatic disease.[80]

Bone Scintigraphy. Bone scanning may be used in patients with clinically suspected but radiologically occult subcapital fracture (Fig. 8–28). Studies of various fractures by Matin showed that within 24 hours of fracture 16 of 20 patients (80 percent) had abnormal bone scans.[100] Of the false negative scans one was a suboptimal study and three were in patients over age 65. Thus a technically adequate negative scan at 24 hours in a younger patient essentially excludes an acute fracture. At 3 days

after fracture all patients under age 65 and 95 percent of older patients had abnormal studies.

Classifications

Pauwels. Pauwels classified subcapital fractures by the angle of the fracture line in relation to the horizontal (as seen on the postreduction radiograph; Fig. 8–29).[113] He postulated that the more horizontal the fracture line (class 1 fractures), the more stable the fracture would be with weight-bearing. Conversely, the more vertically oriented the fracture line, the more unstable it would be.

Garden notes, however, that the direction of the fracture line is actually the same in most subcapital fractures and, as seen on the AP

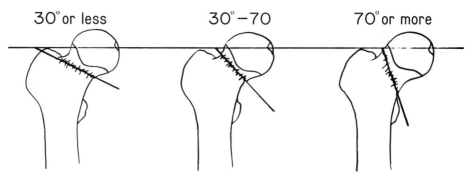

30° or less   30° – 70   70° or more

Figure 8–29. Pauwels's Classification of Fractures. This classification is based on the obliquity of the fracture line in relation to the horizontal.

radiograph, is oriented at an angle of 50 degrees with the horizontal. The apparent differences in obliquity that underlie Pauwel's classification are thought to be the result of varying degrees of rotation rather than true differences in fracture orientation.

Garden. Currently, the most frequently used method for preoperatively classifying subcapital fractures is that proposed by Garden in 1961, based on the degree of displacement of the fracture fragments (Fig. 8–30).[86] In stage 1 the fracture is "incomplete" and the femoral head is tipped posterolaterally (Fig. 8–31). Although it appears on radiographs to be an impacted

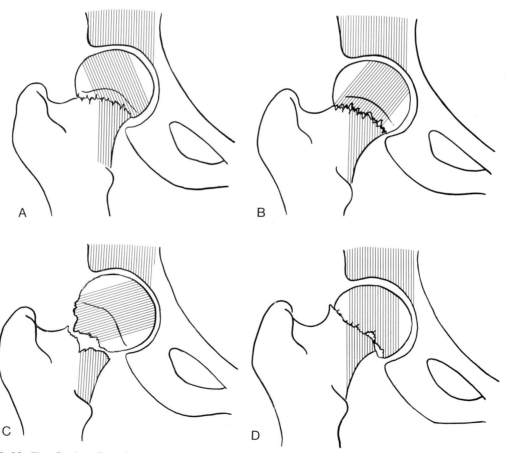

Figure 8–30. The Garden Classification of Fractures. *A,* Stage 1: There is an impacted femoral fracture with valgus deviation of the femoral-head trabeculae. *B,* Stage 2: The fracture is complete but nondisplaced, and there is varus deviation of the femoral head. *C,* Stage 3: The fracture is displaced, and the femoral-head trabeculae are deviated medially. *D,* Stage 4: The fracture is displaced. The femoral-head trabeculae are aligned with those in the pelvis.

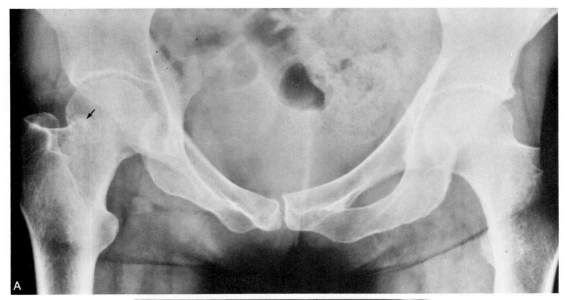

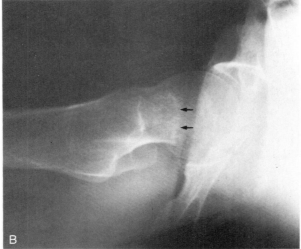

Figure 8–31. Subtle Garden 1 Fractures. *A,* AP pelvis. The right hip is flexed, accounting for the closed appearance of the obturator foramen, and the patient is slightly rotated. The head-neck junction on the right laterally has an angular appearance in contrast with the smooth contour noted on the left. A small zone of sclerosis (arrow) is noted, suggesting impaction of fracture fragments. *B,* The true lateral view documents a sclerotic zone of impaction (arrows) and disruption of the posterior cortex. There is slight posterior rotation of the femoral head.

fracture, no true impaction occurs.[89] Stage 2 fractures are complete fractures without associated displacement (Fig. 8–32). Stage 3 fractures are also complete but are partially displaced. Stage 4 fractures are displaced. Rotation of the proximal fragment is determined by noting the direction of the medial (compressive) trabeculae of the femoral head in relation to the analogous trabeculae in the pelvis. In stage 3 fractures the head is tilted into varus, and the trabeculae of the head and the corresponding trabeculae in the pelvis are no longer aligned (Fig. 8–33). The posterior superior retinaculum (containing the ascending branch of the lateral femoral circumflex artery) remains intact and tethers the head in the varus position.[79] In stage 4 lesions the posterior retinaculum is torn and no longer holds the femoral head in varus. The distal fragment is completely separated from the proximal one, and the femoral head remains in its normal position, with the compression trabeculae aligned with the corresponding acetabular trabeculae (Figs. 8–34 and 8–35). The distal fragment is displaced proximally and rotated laterally.

It should be noted that the term *stage* is used

409

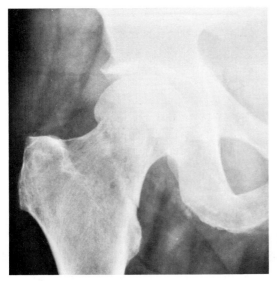

Figure 8–32. Garden 1–2 Fracture. There is a complete fracture through the femoral neck, with slight valgus deformity.

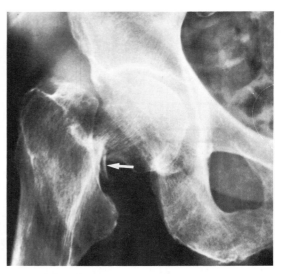

Figure 8–34. Posterior Comminution. A Garden 3–4 fracture is present. The medial bony fragment (arrow) attests to the presence of posterior comminution.

to imply that all these fractures represent gradations of response to a similar displacing force.[89]

Posterior Comminution. The normal configuration of the femoral neck is convex, and the femoral head sits eccentrically on it, overhanging the neck posteriorly and inferiorly.[87] The head-neck junction at this posterior location is quite thin, particularly in the elderly, osteoporotic women who are the most likely to sustain subcapital fractures. Lateral rotation of the distal fragment produces compression in this area,

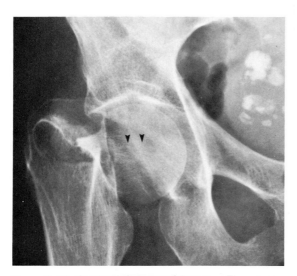

Figure 8–33. Garden 3 Subcapital Fracture. The primary compression trabeculae (arrowheads) are no longer aligned with their counterparts in the pelvis but are directed medially.

resulting in a comminuted fracture termed posterior comminution.[87] In general, posterior comminution accompanies all displaced femoral neck fractures.

Posterior comminution of the femoral neck is an important radiological observation, since the degree of comminution affects the stability of the fracture and the likelihood of its healing. The presence, as well as the degree, of comminution is difficult to evaluate on prereduction radiographs but can usually be seen on postreduction lateral views as a posterior triangular fragment at the head-neck junction (Figs. 8–34 and 8–35). Comminution of the posterior femoral neck is often more severe than is apparent on radiographs.[79]

Acceptable Reduction. When anatomical alignment is achieved, an AP radiograph shows the medial trabeculae of the femoral head to be in line with the corresponding trabeculae of the acetabulum and to form an angle of 160 degrees with the medial cortex of the femoral shaft. In addition, the true lateral view shows that the central axes of the head and neck form an angle of 180 degrees when anatomical positioning is achieved. This optimal reduction on AP and lateral views is abbreviated as an alignment index of 160/180 (Fig. 8–36).[88] Union following such ideal reduction results in the lowest incidence of avascular necrosis (Table 8–5). In Garden's series of patients with subcapital fractures, those with an alignment index of 160/180 who were followed had no evidence of segmental collapse of the femoral head (an indicator of

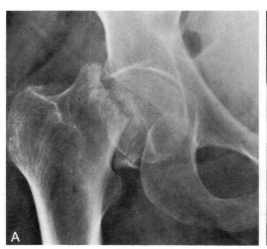

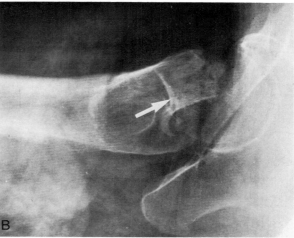

Figure 8–35. Garden 3 Fracture with Posterior Comminution. *A,* AP view shows a subcapital fracture with the primary compression trabeculae aligned with those in the pelvis, indicating a Garden 4 fracture. Medially, there is a separate bony fragment. *B,* The true lateral view shows posterior rotation of the femoral head and separate bony fragments (arrow), again indicating posterior comminution.

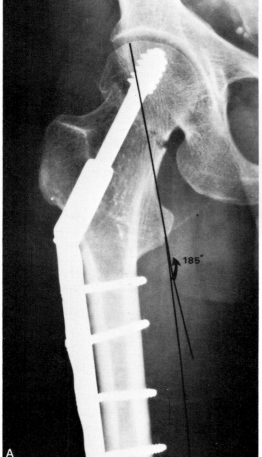

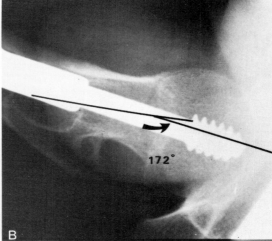

Figure 8–36. Measuring Reduction. *A,* The angle between the compression trabeculae and the medial femoral cortex of the femoral shaft is measured. Anatomical reduction is 160 degrees. In this case 185 degrees of valgus reduction is present. *B,* The angle between the femoral neck and the femoral head is measured. Anatomical position is 180 degrees. In this case 172 degrees of reduction has been obtained. The examples differ from the ideal numbers stated.

Table 8–5. **Incidence of Segmental Collapse of the Femoral Head Following Reduction of Subcapital Fractures**

Reduction	Position in Which Fracture United*	Superior Segmental Collapse (%)
Good		0
Acceptable	155 to 180 (AP and lateral)	7.3
Poor	<155 or >180 (AP or lateral)	53.8
Frank malreduction	<150 or >185 AP view	86.3

Source: Garden RS: Orthop Clin North Am 5:683, 1974.

$$*\text{Alignment index} = \frac{\text{angle of medial trabeculae to medial femoral cortex (AP)}}{\text{angle of axes of head and neck (lateral)}}$$

avascular necrosis). With alignment values on the AP and lateral views of 155 to 180, superior segmental collapse occurred in 7.3 percent of patients. With values above or below this on either the AP or the lateral view, the incidence of osteonecrosis was far greater, and when angles of less than 150 or more than 185 degrees were noted on the postoperative AP view alone, 86.3 percent of patients developed superior segmental collapse.[88] Slight valgus reduction is acceptable, however, and Barnes and colleagues noted the rate of union of displaced fractures in women to be greatest when a valgus reduction of 170 to 179 degrees was present.[70] A reduction of 155 to 180 degrees on *both* anteroposterior and lateral views is therefore considered acceptable.

Malreduction. Malreduction is recognized on the AP view by a trabecular angle of less than 150 or more than 185 degrees.[88] Within this range the appearance on lateral view will help predict the incidence of avascular necrosis. If the alignment on the lateral view is 180 degrees, then the incidence of superior segmental collapse is relatively low (5.4 percent), whereas it is much higher when the angle on the lateral view deviates from 180 degrees (30.1 percent).

Valgus Reduction. Valgus position of the femoral head is said to restore stability and promote union. This is in concert with the conclusions arrived at by Pauwels and underlies his fracture classification. Since the reduction is not anatomical, however, incongruity of the articular surfaces always results and is documented by the asymmetrical width of the cartilage space that may be seen postoperatively (Fig. 8–37). In addition to this incongruity, the possibility of subsequent avascular necrosis is increased with "over-valgus" reduction. Excessive (over-) valgus of the femoral head may be defined as an alignment angle of greater than 180 degrees between the compressive trabeculae of the femoral head and the medial femoral cortex.[88]

Varus Reduction. "Over-varus" reduction is present if the angle between the medial trabeculae and the medial femoral cortex on the

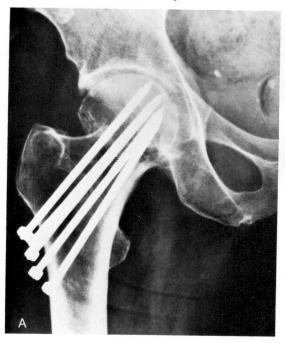

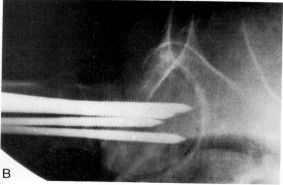

Figure 8–37. Valgus Reduction and Pinning (Knowles Pins). This patient had a fracture with valgus deformity. *A,* The AP postreduction film shows valgus alignment. *B,* There is no malalignment on lateral view (180-degree Garden angle). Healing was uneventful.

anteroposterior view is less than 150 degrees. This type of reduction frequently leads to nonunion or to avascular necrosis following union.

Achieving Reduction. Stage 1 (valgus "impacted") and stage 2 (nondisplaced) fractures are inherently stable; therefore, no manipulation is necessary.

Stages 3 and 4 fractures may be reduced by closed manipulation or, if this fails, by open (surgical) reduction. Obtaining excellent reduction is apparently quite difficult; it was achieved, for example, in only 65 of 427 patients with subcapital fractures reviewed by Garden.[88] In another series acceptable reduction (defined for this study as 160 to 180 degrees on AP and 160 to 200 degrees on lateral radiographs) was achieved in 81 percent of the stages 3 and 4 fractures studied.

Radiographs at the time of reduction should include a lateral view, since according to Garden, "when the central axis of the head and the central axis of the neck lie in a truly straight line, and the wide circular sweep of the posterior cervical cortex has been restored . . . the fracture—if it is transfixed and held in this position—is almost certain to unite irrespective of the appearance in the frontal radiograph; the age, weight, or sex of the patient; the time of weight-bearing; the delay in reduction and fixation; or the presence of osteomalacia or osteoporosis."[88, 89]

Internal Fixation. Internal fixation is used to resist the forces of gravity and muscular pull that tend to produce upward displacement of the distal fragment, medial rotation of the proximal fragment, and displacement of the fracture. Stable fractures can be held by any fixation device that crosses the fracture site and is securely fixed to each fragment. The fixation of unstable fractures also requires that the fixation device maintain the achieved reduction. The brunt of the weight-bearing force should be taken up by the femur itself rather than by the hardware.[89]

Numerous methods are available for fixation of subcapital fractures. The radiographic features of some of these will be discussed in the following sequence (after Muckle):[106] (1) The trifin nail, (2) multiple pins or screws, (3) pin and plate or fixed-angle nail-plate, and (4) sliding or telescoping nail-plate.

Trifin Nail. The trifin nail (i.e., Smith-Petersen) is little used now since the advent of newer methods of fixation (see Fig. 8–57). It is unsuitable for displaced fractures and is associated with a higher incidence of nonunion and avascular necrosis than are other methods of fixation.[70, 106] Furthermore, in nondisplaced, impacted fractures the fragments may be disimpacted during insertion of the nail. When it is used, the Smith-Petersen nail should be as close as possible to the center of the femoral head and to the central articular surface.[68]

Multiple Pins or Crossed Screws. Fixation with three to five pins (e.g., Knowles or Moore) is commonly used in patients with nondisplaced fractures.[106] Knowles advocated that after optimal reduction multiple threaded pins be placed in the femoral head in parallel and as far apart as possible (Fig. 8–37).[96, 122] Deyerle developed a method in which multiple, peripherally placed pins are inserted in a parallel arrangement through a side plate fixed to the femoral shaft.[77, 78a, 79]

Muscle-Pedicle Graft. Meyers and associates have suggested that the large defect in the posterior femur caused by posterior comminution might be filled with autogenous iliac bone chips to increase the likelihood of bony union and that the placement of an autogenous muscle-pedicle bone graft into the femoral head might restore femoral head circulation and prevent later superior segmental collapse.[103–105] The fracture itself is fixed with pins, which should traverse the posterior inferior portion of the neck and extend into the head, terminating no less than 3 mm from the subchondral bone. One or two screws are used to secure the muscle pedicle bone graft to the posterior aspect of the femoral head and neck.

Pin and Plate or Fixed-Angle Nail Plate (e.g., Jewett). A pin and plate or a fixed-angle nail plate with additional screw fixation may be used for both subcapital and intertrochanteric fractures (see section on intertrochanteric fractures). However, the sliding nail is usually preferred in subcapital fractures because a nontelescoping pin may protrude into the hip joint should collapse of the femoral head occur.

Sliding-Nail Plate (Pugh, Massie, or Richards). These devices consist of a single screw and a lateral plate. The screw can telescope (slide) into the barrel of the side plate as compression occurs at the fracture site. Rotation of the screw within the barrel is prevented in some designs by flattening of one side of the screw and the barrel. The Richards compression screw has a small screw that, when inserted through the barrel of the side plate into the larger lag screw and tightened, provides additional impaction (compression) at the fracture site (Fig. 8–38).

Radiographic Evaluation of Internal Fixation Devices

Pin Position. It is usually assumed that the position of intramedullary nails or screws can be established by obtaining two radiographic projections at right angles to each other. However,

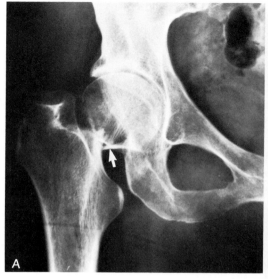

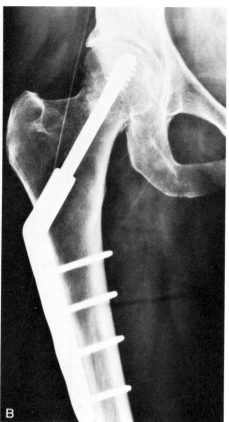

Figure 8–38. Garden IV Fracture. *A,* The AP view shows a displaced subcapital fracture with the medial compression trabeculae of the femoral head almost realigned to those in the pelvis, indicating a Garden 4 injury. A separate cortical fragment (arrow) indicates comminution of the medial cortex (posterior comminution). *B,* After reduction and internal fixation, normal alignment is restored. The hardware is optimally positioned on the AP view, with the tip of the screw centrally located in the femoral head, a few millimeters from the cortex. A lateral view is also necessary to define pin position.

it has been documented that this reasoning is faulty because of the curved bony surface involved. Thus a screw across a femoral fracture site may appear to be within the bone on both AP and lateral projections but may actually lie outside the cortex. Volz and Martin suggest two clinically useful methods of confirming that the shaft of the fixation device is actually within the

bone.[119] In the first method two radiographs, such as an AP and a lateral taken at right angles to each other, are superimposed, the smaller image centered within the larger (Fig. 8–39). If all pins fall within the cortex by at least one pin diameter, the pin is probably within the bone; if a pin is less than one pins diameter from the cortex, it may lie outside the bone (Fig. 8–40).

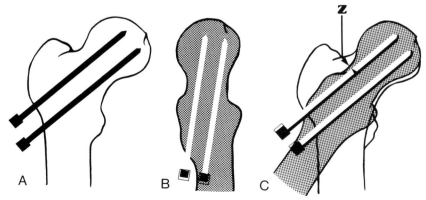

Figure 8–39. Screw Position. *A,* AP view. *B,* Lateral view. *C,* When the views are superimposed, all the pins or screws should fall within the narrowest diameter of bone by at least the width of the pin (z). In the illustrated case the lateral screw should be considered to be outside the cortex. (Redrawn from Volz RG, Martin MD: Radiology 122:695, 1977.)

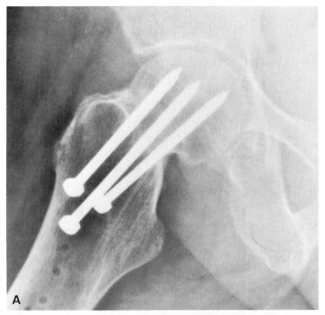

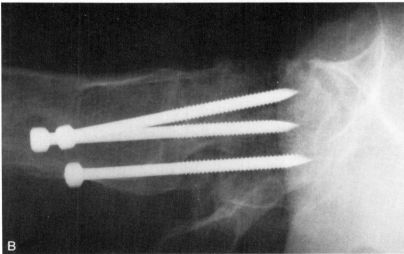

Figure 8–40. Malposition of Knowles's Pin. *A,* The frog lateral view shows three pins overlying the femoral neck and head. *B,* The true lateral view shows that one of the pins (the most medial and posterior) actually lies outside the femoral neck, although its tip is within the femoral head.

This technique is applicable if the diameter of the pin is no more than one eighth of the diameter of the bone.

The second method is to measure the distance from the pin to the peripheral cortex. This distance should be no less than 15 percent of the overall diameter of the bone in order to ensure the internal location of the pin. Neither of these rules is necessary if fluoroscopy with a portable C-arm unit is available or if an additional radiograph is obtained in a position midway between the first two.

It has also been shown that the tip of an internal fixation device such as a compression screw, which appears to be within the femoral head on both AP and lateral views, may actually protrude through the subchondral plate of the femoral head (Fig. 8–41).[114, 120] The discrepancy between the actual position of the tip of the screw with relation to the femoral subchondral plate and the apparent position of the screw on radiographs is a result of the inability to see the tip of the screw and the adjacent cortex in an exactly tangential projection. The difference between the actual distance of the pin to the femoral cortex and the measured distance is

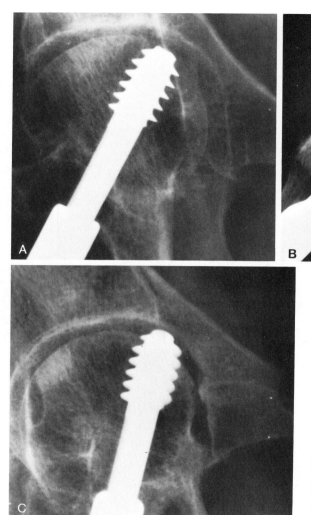

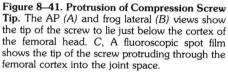

Figure 8–41. Protrusion of Compression Screw Tip. The AP *(A)* and frog lateral *(B)* views show the tip of the screw to lie just below the cortex of the femoral head. *C,* A fluoroscopic spot film shows the tip of the screw protruding through the femoral cortex into the joint space.

minimal when the pin is exactly central in location but may be significant with more peripheral pin locations (Fig. 8–42).

Following Changes in Screw-Tip Position.

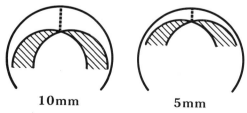

Figure 8–42. Screw Tip Position. The safety margin for the screw tip is shown in two examples. In one the screw is 10 mm from the cortex, and in the other it is 5 mm from the cortex. The difference between the actual and the measured distance of the pin to the femoral cortex is very little when the pin is central in location but may be more marked with peripheral pin positions. (Redrawn from Walters R, Simon SR: *In* Hip Society: The Hip, Vol 8. St. Louis, CV Mosby, 1980.)

Doppelt emphasizes that the distance from the screw tip to the cortex of the femoral head cannot be measured along the axis of the screw because this measurement changes with rotation.[131] Instead, he proposes that the vertical distance between the screw tip and the subchondral bone be measured between parallel lines drawn perpendicular to a line paralleling the side plate or the lateral femoral cortex.

Following Changes in Screw Length Due to Telescoping. As the femur is externally rotated, the apparent lengths of the barrel and the screw decrease; thus corrections for variations in rotation on follow-up radiographs are useful. The following correction factor has been developed:[131]

$$\text{Correction factor} \atop \text{(screw length)} = \frac{\text{Barrel length on first postoperative radiograph}}{\text{Barrel length on the given radiograph}}$$

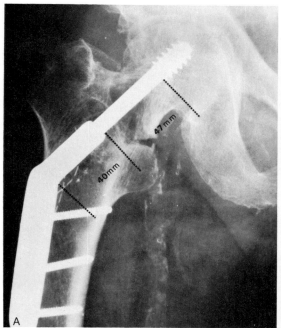
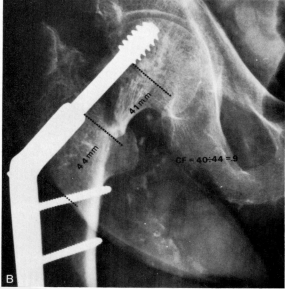

Figure 8–43. Correction for Rotation When Judging the Telescoping of the Femoral Screw. *A,* The initial view, with measurements of the length of the barrel and of the screw. *B,* Follow-up view with more internal rotation than in *A.* The correction factor is calculated to correct for differences in positioning. The amount of telescoping is 47 − [41 × 0.9] = 10.1 mm. CF = correction factor.

This correction factor (CF) is then multiplied by the apparent screw length on the second film to yield the corrected length. The amount of telescoping of the screw is the difference between the screw length on the first examination and the corrected length on the follow-up examination (Fig. 8–43).

Detecting Changes in the Neck-Shaft Angle. Comparison of the neck-shaft angles on follow-up radiographs is facilitated by a correction factor derived from the barrel-plate angle of the device. This correction factor is necessary because increased external rotation will increase the apparent neck-shaft angle. The correction factor that can be used to compare two postoperative radiographs is derived as follows:[131]

$$\text{Correction factor (neck-shaft angle)} = \frac{\text{Screw-plate angle on first postoperative radiograph}}{\text{Screw-plate angle on given radiograph}}$$

The corrected neck-shaft angle is equal to the measured angle multiplied by the correction factor. This determination is of particular value in the follow-up of intertrochanteric fractures after compression plating.

Healing. Femoral neck fractures, like other intraarticular fractures, heal by endosteal repair. Since no periosteal reaction occurs, there is no evidence of periosteal new bone visible on radiographs, and this circumstance makes the evaluation of healing difficult. Banks noted new bone formation resembling fiber-bone at the fracture site by 10 days after injury, and by 3 weeks this was well developed.[68, 69] This internal callus extends from both sides of the fracture site if the femoral head is viable but only from the distal fragment if the femoral head is avascular.

Fractures are generally considered to be healed when on radiographs the fracture line is obliterated and trabeculae cross the fracture site.[68] The judgment as to whether or not trabecular continuity is present may be difficult, however, since excellent apposition of fracture fragments may result in the spurious appearance of trabeculae crossing the fracture site even before healing has occurred. Healing of treated displaced fractures occurred in 3 to 12 months in Banks's series, whereas most impacted fractures healed by 5 months.[68]

Complications. The two major late complications of subcapital fractures are nonunion and avascular necrosis. Although several factors are implicated in the development of each of these complications, the quality of reduction appears to be one of the most significant.

Nonunion. Impacted or nondisplaced fractures are associated with a nonunion incidence

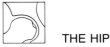

Table 8–6. **Factors Affecting Union and the Development of ON After Subcapital Fracture**

	Nonunion	ON
Incidence	Female 73% Male 77%	Female 24% (after union) Male 15%
Stage of fracture	I and II heal faster than III and IV	Female 1–16% Female III and IV 27.6%
Age	↓ speed and % of union with ↑ age	More frequent if female <75
Patient's weight	No effect	More frequent if heavy
Patient's activity	Greater in active patients	
Delay before surgery (≤ 1 week)	No effect	No effect
Type of fixation	All similar, except higher nonunion in displaced fractures treated with Smith-Petersen nail	No difference
Location of fracture	> in high subcapital fractures	
Quality of reduction	Lowest union rate if > 20° varus* or angulation of > 20° on lateral view	Highest incidence if marked valgus
Position of nail or screw (displaced fractures)	Best if nail central on AP and lateral and tip within ½ cm of articular cortex	No effect

Source: Barnes R et al.: J Bone Joint Surg (Br) 58:2, 1976.
*< 160-degree Garden angle.

of less than 1 percent, whereas displaced fractures have a significantly higher incidence, approaching 30 percent in one series, although usually about 10 percent.[68, 99, 103, 104, 121]

Several factors have been implicated in the development of nonunion after subcapital fracture (Table 8–6).

1. *Posterior comminution.* It has been suggested that the presence of posterior comminution alone plays a role in the development of nonunion.[68, 97]

2. *Multiple insertions of a nail.* Multiple attempts to position a nail, particularly in osteoporotic bone, may lead to poor fixation of fracture fragments and subsequently to nonunion.[68]

3. *Fixation devices.* When screws are used for internal fixation, the threads should not cross the fracture line, because they may hold the fracture fragments apart when resorption occurs at the fracture surfaces. Fixed-angle nails may also prevent apposition of fracture surfaces when bone resorption occurs.

Fixation devices should be centrally located (as shown on both the AP and the lateral radiographs), since union rates are the highest (76.6 percent) when this position is achieved. In Barnes's series a low, posterior screw position resulted in union in 65.4 percent of patients. A high, anterior screw position seemed the least desirable, since union under this circumstance occurred in 63 percent of stage 3 and only 47 percent of stage 4 fractures.[70, 97]

4. *Reduction.* The position of fracture fragments is critically important in the development of nonunion.[88] For example, conservative treatment of impacted varus fractures resulted in nonunion in all patients in one series.[97] Similarly, after nailing, varus angulation with a Garden angle of <160 degrees is associated with eventual nonunion in over 50 percent of patients with displaced fractures.[70] Anteroposterior angulation of greater than 20 degrees as seen on the lateral view resulted in nonunion in half the patients in one series.[70, 97] Garden, who relies heavily on the appearance of the reduction on the lateral film, noted nonunion in less than 10 percent of cases when perfect alignment was indicated on the lateral view but noted higher incidences of nonunion with less than perfect reductions (Fig. 8–44).[85]

The diagnosis of nonunion is based on radiological findings. Banks considered nonunion to be present if (1) the fracture had not healed 1 year or more after surgery or (2) the fracture line was grossly visible and reduction had been lost less than 1 year after treatment (Fig. 8–45). Sclerosis of the bone ends and separation between fracture fragments also indicate nonunion.

Post-traumatic Osteonecrosis Incidence (AVN). Partial or complete osteonecrosis (ON) was noted histologically in two thirds of unselected femoral heads examined by Sevitt after intracapsular fracture.[217] Radiographic evidence of ON is considerably less frequent, however, being seen in about 20 percent of patients

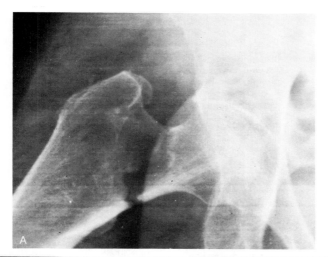

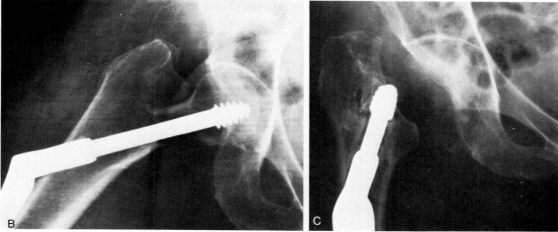

Figure 8–44. Malreduction of Intracapsular Fracture. *A,* An intraoperative radiograph after reduction shows realignment of the medial femoral cortex. *B,* During insertion of the compression screw, the femoral head rotated so that the medial femoral cortex is in a lateral position. *C,* Nonunion followed. (Courtesy of Dr. James Polga.)

studied by Bayliss and Davidson.[183] The incidence of post-traumatic osteonecrosis is highest following displaced fractures and higher in Garden stage 4 than in stage 3 fractures. For example, using a modified Garden classification, Bayliss and Davidson found radiographic evidence of osteonecrosis in 8 percent of stage 1, 4 percent of stage 2, 21 percent of stage 3, and 30 percent of stage 4 fractures.[183] Although marked proximal displacement of the distal fragment is often associated with partial or total avascularity of the femoral head, in an individual case development of ON and later collapse of the femoral head cannot be predicted.

Osteonecrosis is most often detected during the second or third year after injury, and its onset after that time is unusual.[88] Thus Jacobs noted that in 90 percent of patients osteonecrosis was radiographically apparent within 2 years after fracture. Linton, however, noted radiological changes of ON in 30 percent of patients followed 2 to 3 years and in 56 percent of those followed 3 to 7 years.[217]

The finding of osteonecrosis on radiographs is not always associated with clinical symptoms. Dead bone per se is not painful, although pain may occur later as a result of secondary osteoarthritis.[207] Barnes and associates found osteonecrosis to be clinically disabling in 29.2 percent of patients, functionally acceptable in 46.1 percent, and asymptomatic in 24.3 percent.[70]

Predisposing Factors. The development of osteonecrosis is said to be related to several factors, including the following (Table 8–6):

1. *Fracture type:* The incidence of osteonecrosis is lower in nondisplaced than in displaced fractures.

2. *Reduction:* Garden emphasized the relationship between postoperative reduction and subsequent development of osteonecrosis.[88, 89]

419

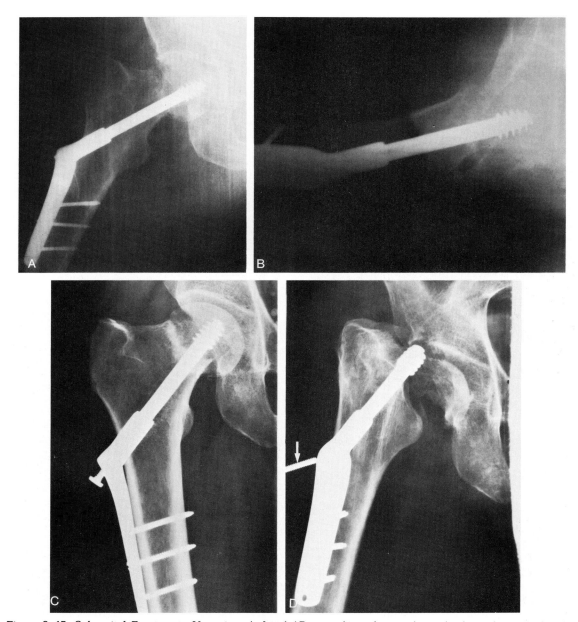

Figure 8–45. Subcapital Fracture to Nonunion. *A,* Initial AP view after reduction shows the femoral screw inferiorly positioned in the head and neck. *B,* The lateral view shows a slightly posterior position of the compression screw. The femoral head is posteriorly rotated. *C,* The femoral head has rotated farther posteriorly creating a zone of increased density at the head-neck junction. *D,* This film shows loss of reduction and nonunion. The side screw (arrow) has become disengaged.

Thus in 402 united subcapital fractures followed for at least 3 years, patients with an alignment index of 160 to 180 did not develop late superior segmental collapse (an indicator of osteonecrosis). With increasingly poor reductions, the incidence of osteonecrosis increased, and in those with "frank malreduction" on the frontal view, 86.3 percent developed this complication.[89]

3. *Time to reduction:* It has been reported

that osteonecrosis is less common if reduction is achieved within 12 hours after fracture.[99] However, Barnes and co-workers found no significant change in the incidence of this complication with delays in surgery of up to 7 days.[70]

4. *Fixation devices:* With regard to the currently used fixation devices, Jacobs has judged that there is no conclusive evidence to indicate the superiority of one device over another in reducing the incidence of this complication.

5. *Fracture union:* The incidence of osteonecrosis is thought to be higher in patients with nonunion.[92] This is controversial, however.

Etiology. The major mechanism in the production of osteonecrosis appears to be damage to the retinacular vessels, particularly the superior ones.[92] The vessels in the ligamentum teres are usually of secondary importance. An additional mechanism may be the increase in intraarticular pressure that is produced following fracture with intracapsular hemorrhage. This pressure may obstruct the flow of blood through the retinacular vessels that run along the joint capsule.

Radiographic Findings. The radiographic findings in post-traumatic osteonecrosis are similar to those in idiopathic osteonecrosis, described with that entity in a following section (Figs. 8–46 and 8–47).

Results. Although dead bone cannot repair itself or remodel in response to changing stress, dead bone per se is not weak. Presumably, if healing of the avascular bone were complete or did not occur at all, clinical sequelae of osteonecrosis would be minimal. It is postulated that in cases of idiopathic ON repair is often incomplete and that the repair process itself is respon-

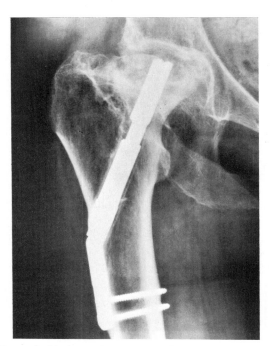

Figure 8–46. Avascular Necrosis After Internal Fixation of an Intracapsular Fracture. The fracture has healed, and there is a Massie nail in place. The femoral head has collapsed, with a central area of lucency and a more peripheral area of sclerosis attesting to the presence of avascular necrosis.

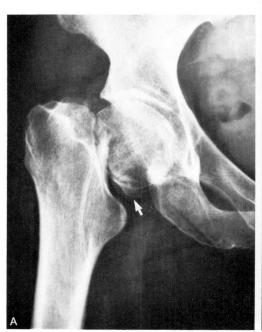

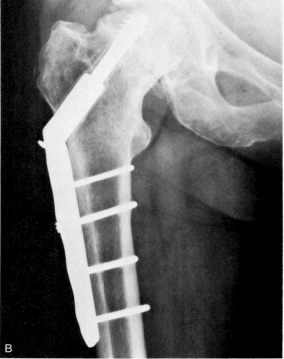

Figure 8–47. Avascular Necrosis Following Subcapital Fracture. *A,* The initial AP view shows a Garden 3–4 fracture with posterior comminution (arrow) and external rotation of the femoral shaft, as evidenced by the profile view of the lesser trochanter. Avascular necrosis was evident on radiographs 1½ years after reduction. *B,* Examination 2½ years after reduction shows collapse of the femoral head without cartilage-space narrowing.

sible for the intracapital fractures and the eventual collapse of the femoral head.[197–200] So, too, in patients with osteonecrosis as a consequence of intracapsular fracture, healing of the avascular femoral head is usually incomplete, despite the fact that the femoral fracture unites.[206]

Repair of the avascular femoral head occurs via vessels in the ligamentum teres, any retinacular vessels that remain intact, and vessels that cross the fracture site as it heals. Vascularized repair tissue grows between the involved trabeculae. Undifferentiated mesenchymal cells differentiate into osteoblasts that form new bone on the surfaces of dead trabeculae.[197–199] Repair tissue extends across the fracture line into the femoral head but is then blocked by the intracapital fractures that have occurred between the necrotic and the newly formed bone. The differentiation of mesenchymal cells is then redirected to the formation of chondroblasts and fibroblasts rather than osteoblasts, and a dense layer of fibrous tissue and fibrocartilage occurs at the margin of the intracapital fracture site. The net result is a halting of the healing process, extensive resorption of dead trabeculae, and their replacement with fibrous tissue and fibrocartilage.

Extracapsular Fractures

Extracapsular fractures include fractures in and below the region of the trochanters.

There are multiple classifications of trochanteric and subtrochanteric fractures—based on the anatomical location of the fracture, the fracture configuration, the number of fracture fragments, the difficulty in obtaining or maintaining reduction, and/or the prognosis, or all these last three.

Anatomical Classifications. *Heppenstall* advocates classification of extracapsular fractures by their location.[90] *Intertrochanteric fractures* involve the intertrochanteric line (between the greater and lesser trochanters); simple fractures in this area do not involve the trochanters per se. These fractures are not very common.

Pertrochanteric fractures are the most frequent extracapsular fractures and include the four-part intertrochanteric fracture. These lesions involve the intertrochanteric area but extend into the greater trochanter or both trochanters. Comminution is usually present.

Confusion arises when the term *trochanteric*

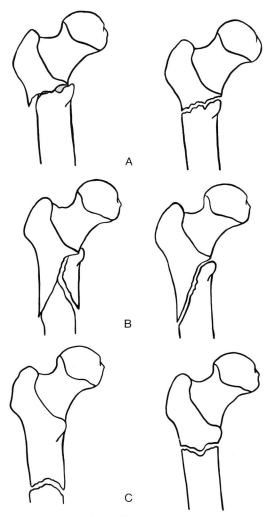

Figure 8–49. Zickel Classification of Subtrochanteric Fractures. *A, Type I:* Short, oblique fractures with or without comminution. *B, Type II:* Long, oblique fractures with or without comminution. *C, Type III:* High (right) and low (left) transverse fractures. (Redrawn from Zickel RE: J Bone Joint Surg (Am) 59:866, 1976.)

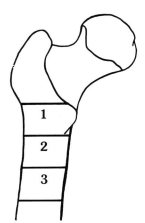

Figure 8–48. Classification of Subtrochanteric Fractures (Fielding and Magliato). Type 1 fractures are at the level of the lesser trochanter, type 2 occur within 1 inch below the lesser trochanter, and type 3 occur 1 to 2 inches below the lesser trochanter. (Redrawn from Fielding JW, Magliato HJ: Surg Gynecol Obstet 122:555, 1966.)

fracture is used in a general way to refer to both pertrochanteric and intertrochanteric fractures as well as to subtrochanteric fractures that extend into the intertrochanteric region. In addition, confusion is compounded by the need to identify the subtrochanteric region, an area that is not clearly delineated anatomically. The most frequently used definition is that of *Fielding and Magliato,* in which a 3-inch bony segment extending from the proximal border of the lesser trochanter to 2 inches distal to the lesser trochanter is defined as the subtrochanteric area.[134] Fractures in this region are further subdivided into three types: type I, at the level of the lesser trochanter; type II, within 1 inch below the lesser trochanter; and type III, from 1 to 2 inches below the lesser trochanter (Fig. 8–48). Type I fractures are most frequent; type III, least frequent.

Zickel noted difficulties in using the preceding classification because of the obliquity of the fracture lines he observed. He therefore developed another classification of subtrochanteric fractures based on the fracture configuration, including the obliquity of the fracture line, the presence of comminution, and the level of the fracture (Fig. 8–49).[168] Type I fractures are short and oblique, with or without comminution; type II, long and oblique, with or without comminu-

tion; and type III, transverse, either in a high or a low position. The low fractures are well below the subtrochanteric area as defined by Fielding and Magliato.

Seinsheimer defined the subtrochanteric region as including the area from the inferior aspect of the lesser trochanter to a level 5 cm distal to the lesser trochanter. He then classified subtrochanteric fractures according to the degree of displacement and the amount of comminution present (Fig. 8–50).[160] Three-part spiral fractures that included a lesser trochanteric fracture with a long inferior spike of cortex had the highest risk of failure after internal fixation.

Clinical Classifications. *Boyd and Griffin* (1949) proposed a classification of trochanteric fractures based on prognosis and difficulty in establishing and maintaining reduction.[127] This is the most frequently used classification; it includes intertrochanteric, pertrochanteric, and subtrochanteric fractures (Fig. 8–51). Type I fractures are almost linear in configuration and extend along the intertrochanteric line; comminution is not present. Obtaining and maintaining reduction is least difficult in this type. Type II fractures also involve the intertrochanteric line but have additional breaks in the cortex. The comminution that is present can be appreciated only on the true lateral view. Reduction is more

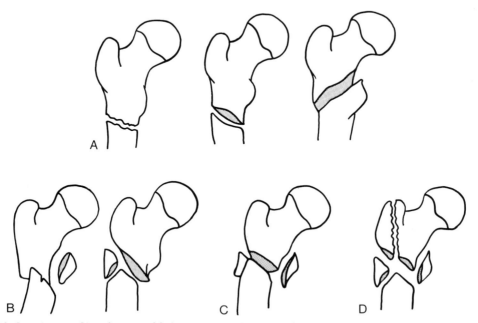

Figure 8–50. Seinsheimer Classification of Subtrochanteric Fractures. Classification is based on the number of fragments ≥ 1 cm in size and the location and shape of the fracture line. In type I no displacement or < 2 mm of displacement is present. *A,* Type II. Two-part fractures: transverse, spiral with lesser trochanter attached to proximal fragment, and spiral with lesser trochanter attached to the distal fragment. *B,* Type III. Three-part fractures: spiral fracture with butterfly fragment and spiral fracture with the lesser trochanter a part of the third fragment and with an attached inferior spike of cortex. *C,* Type IV. Four or more fragments. *D,* Type V. Subtrochanteric, intertrochanteric fractures. (Redrawn from Seinsheimer F: J Bone Joint Surg (Am) 60:300, 1978.)

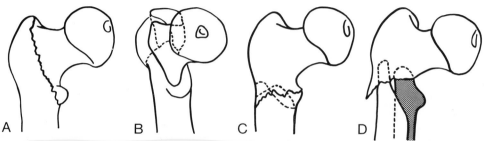

Figure 8–51. Boyd and Griffin Classification of Trochanteric Fractures. This classification is based on the difficulty in obtaining and maintaining reduction. *A,* Type I. Linear fracture along the intertrochanteric line. *B,* Type II. Comminuted fracture along the intertrochanteric line. *C,* Type III. Subtrochanteric fracture. *D,* Type IV. Comminuted fracture that extends through the trochanteric region and usually extends into the shaft, with fracture lines in two planes. (Redrawn from Boyd HB, Griffin LL: Arch Surg 58:84. Copyright 1949, American Medical Association.)

difficult than with type I fractures. Type III fractures have subtrochanteric fracture lines that may coexist with fractures of types I and II. Type III fractures are even more difficult to treat, with coxa vara, medial migration of the distal fragment, nonunion, and nail protrusion more frequent after these injuries. Type IV fractures are comminuted, with trochanteric components and, usually, with fractures extending into the shaft. The fracture lines are in at least two planes; therefore, internal fixation, if done, requires fixation in two planes.

Evans (1949) attempted to simplify matters by categorizing fractures as stable or unstable (Fig. 8–52).[133] He emphasized the importance of the femoral calcar in determining stability and noted that when there is cortical overlap or cortical destruction in the region of the calcar the fracture is unstable and varus deformity should be expected. Some fractures become stable on reduction, others do not. Unstable fractures in which stability is not achieved with reduction represent 25[130] to 40 percent[152] of intertrochanteric fractures.

Radiographic Evaluation. The location of the fracture, the degree of comminution, and the resulting deformity are noted.

Stability. Stability is assessed on good-quality AP and true lateral views. An unstable intertrochanteric fracture results from comminution of the medial aspect of the femoral neck in the region of the femoral calcar or from posterior discontinuity, identified as a large posterior trochanteric fragment (Table 8–7). Either of these abnormalities leaves a bony defect between the opposing surfaces of the proximal and distal fragments that makes the reduction unstable after anatomical reduction.[130] The frequent four-part intertrochanteric fracture, consisting of a head and neck component, a femoral shaft component, and separate greater and lesser trochantric fragments, is a classic example of an unstable fracture. The femoral calcar is also

critical in maintaining stability in *subtrochanteric* fractures, and Seinsheimer noted an increased risk of failure of internal fixation in patients with three-part subtrochanteric fractures in which the lesser trochanter (containing much of the femoral calcar) is separated.[160] Overlap of the cortices in the anteroposterior or lateral projections suggests instability,[133] as does the presence of a subtrochanteric component or vertical fracture lines.[126, 158]

Treatment. The average age of individuals with intertrochanteric fractures is older than that of patients with intracapsular fractures. Because of their advanced age, these patients are subject to the numerous complications of prolonged recumbency, and operation with internal fixation and early ambulation therefore is currently preferred.

Subtrochanteric fractures are uncommon (5 to 7 percent of all hip fractures), but in general, achieving and maintaining reduction and fixation are difficult because these fractures are frequently comminuted, slow in healing, and subject to strong deforming (muscular) forces.[134, 161] The more distal fractures have a higher incidence of varus deformity and nonunion as compared with the more proximal (Fielding type I) fractures.

Reduction. The method used to reduce these fractures depends on the prereduction deform-

Table 8–7. Radiographic Findings Indicating Instability of Intertrochanteric Fractures

Disruption of medial keystone arch of the femoral neck.
  More than one fracture line crossing the medial cortex in the region of the calcar (comminution)
  Separation of a large lesser trochanter fragment with associated cortex
Presence of a large posterior fragment on lateral view (i.e., a four-part fracture)
Overlap of fragments
Presence of a subtrochanteric component
Vertical fracture lines

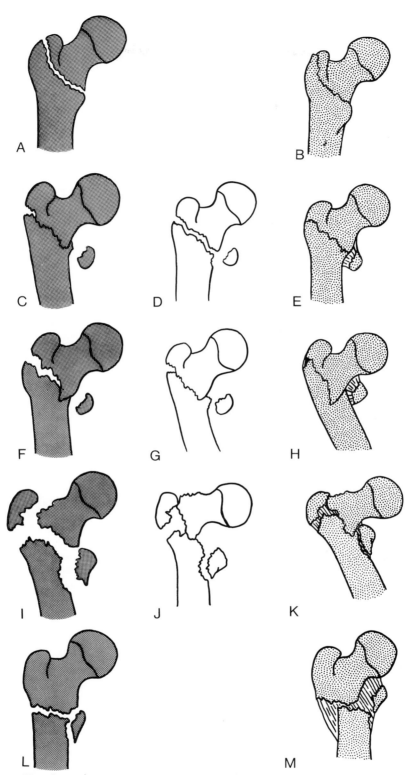

Figure 8–52. Evans Classification of Trochanteric Fractures. In type I the fracture line runs upward and outward from the lesser trochanter. *A–B,* group 1: cortical buttress not disturbed. *C–E,* group 2: overlap of medial cortical buttress (can occur with manipulation). *F–K,* groups 3, 4: irreducible overlap or destruction of medial cortical buttress is present.

In type II *(L,M)* the fracture lines are almost the reverse of those of type I. Groups 1 and 2 in type I are stable fractures; all others are unstable. Heavily stippled figures = initial appearance; nonstippled = position after reduction; lightly stippled = position of healing. (Redrawn from Evans EM: J Bone Joint Surg (Br) 31:190–203, 1949.)

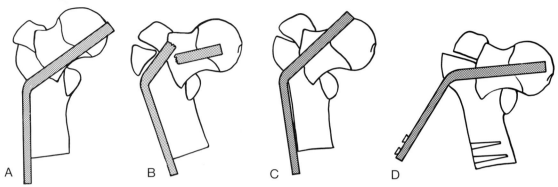

Figure 8–53. Possible Complications After Fixation of Unstable Intertrochanteric Fractures. *A,* Penetration of the nail through the femoral head. *B,* The nail bends or breaks. *C,* The nail "cuts out" of the head and neck. *D,* The plate separates from the femoral shaft. (Redrawn from Dimon JH III, Hughston JC: J Bone Joint Surg (Am) 49:440, 1967.)

ity. Fractures proximal to the external rotators (that insert posteriorly on the greater trochanter) are associated with marked external rotation of the shaft and trochanters, but the proximal head and neck remain in neutral position.[151] With fractures distal to the external rotators, the proximal fragment with the attached trochanters is externally rotated, and the lesser trochanter is seen in profile.

A stable reduction is achieved when there is apposition of cortical margins on each side of the fracture site, particularly when the medial cortices of the proximal and distal fragments are aligned.[156, 157] Fractures in which there is comminution of the medial femoral neck and calcar or a large posterior fragment represent a particular problem because anatomical reduction will not make these fractures stable. These fractures have a tendency to develop varus deformity after fixation, subsequent penetration of the femoral head by the nail, bending or breaking of the nail, or breakage of the screws holding the side plate to the femur (Figs. 8–53 and 8–54).[130] Attempts to improve the outcome of unstable intertrochanteric fractures include the development of stronger fixation devices (e.g., the Holt nail), sliding compression screws that allow impaction at the fracture site during healing, and techniques that realign the fragments in an effort to establish stability prior to internal fixation. These latter techniques may result in radiological appearances that are far from anatomical; therefore, it is of particular importance that radiologists have some familiarity with them. The *Dimon-Hughston* technique (1966) is the most popular of these.[130] In this procedure an attempt is made to achieve stability by doing an osteotomy through the distal fragment, displacing the distal fragment (femoral shaft) medially under the spike of the head and neck fragment and impacting the proximal fragment into the

distal one (Figs. 8–55 and 8–56). A nail or compression screw may be used for fixation. Disadvantages of the reduction include shortening of the extremity and the requirement for crutches instead of full weight-bearing until healing occurs.[148]

Sarmiento and Williams have introduced a *valgus osteotomy* technique for the treatment of unstable intertrochanteric fractures (Fig. 8–55). An oblique osteotomy of the distal fragment is done, changing the vertical orientation of the fracture to a more horizontal, therefore more stable, one. The fragments are then positioned so that the medial cortices proximally and distally are aligned—a critical factor in maintaining stability, according to Sarmiento.

The method used at the *Wayne County General Hospital* produces stability by medially displacing the proximal fragment so that the calcar impinges on the medial cortex of the shaft fragment (Fig. 8–55).[162]

Thus, depending on the procedure used, the proximal medial femoral cortex may be placed lateral to, medial to, or in line with the corresponding distal cortex.

Internal Fixation. The proper placement of internal fixation devices is determined by several factors, including the distribution of good bone within the proximal fragment, the net forces acting on the proximal fragment, and the particular characteristics of the implant itself.[145] It is theoretically best to place the tip of the fixation device in the posterior inferior quadrant of the head so that it must go through the maximum amount of bone before it "cuts out" of the femoral head. However, Mulholland noted best results after central nail placement.[152] The depth of nail insertion also depends on bone structure and the characteristics of the internal fixation devices. Placing the tip deep in the femoral head, in the subchondral bone, provides maxi-

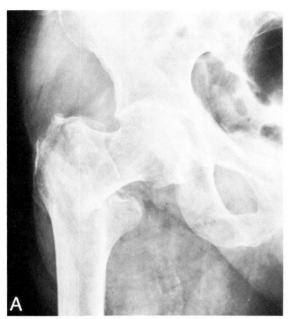

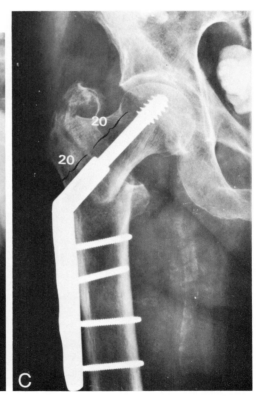

Figure 8–54. Intertrochanteric Fracture with Loss of Reduction. *A*, AP view shows an intertrochanteric fracture without separation of the lesser trochanter. This should be a stable fracture (see the Evans classification). *B*, Anatomical reduction has been obtained. The tip of the compression screw is in good position. *C*, Follow-up study shows impaction at the fracture site, with development of varus deformity. Healing continued in this position. The telescoping of the compression screw is documented by the 6-mm decrease in the barrel-screw threads measurement from *B* to *C*. The absence of change in the apparent length of the barrel and the unchanged appearance of the lateral screws attest to the similar positioning and magnification on the two films.

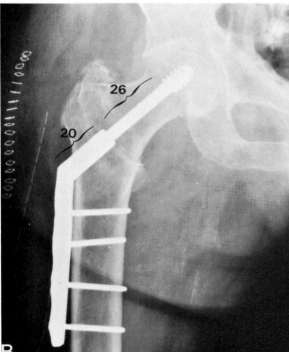

mum control of the proximal fragment and helps protect against varus deformity. But if a varus deformity occurs, a nail placed nearer the subchondral bone is more likely to penetrate into the joint. Also, devices with sharp tips are more likely to penetrate the femoral head than are those with blunt ends. Telescoping devices are least likely to penetrate and may therefore be

inserted more deeply into the femoral head. According to Kaufer, Matthews, and Sonstegard, the best compromise is to position the tip of the device in the femoral head 1 to 2 cm from the subchondral cortex.[145] The tip of the nail will then be in the area where the principal tensile and compressive trabeculae cross.

Nail-Plate and Fixed–Angle Nail-Plate Devices

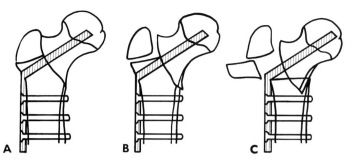

Figure 8–55. Methods of Reduction of Intertrochanteric Fractures. *A, Anatomic:* The medial cortex is aligned proximally and distally at the fracture site. *B, Wayne County:* The proximal fragment is displaced medially, so that the calcar impacts against the medial cortex of the shaft. *C, Hughston-Dimon:* Osteotomy of the distal fragment is followed by medial displacement of the distal fragment and impaction of the proximal fragment into the distal one.

(e.g., Jewett). Several different nails have been used.[151] In general, the shaft of the nail should be centrally located within the femoral neck, parallel to the weight-bearing trabeculae, with the tip reaching well into the femoral head. Femoral neck fracture may occur if the nail is too short (Fig. 8–57).[124] The side plate should be flush with the femoral shaft, and the screws holding the side plate should extend past the medial cortex a few millimeters.[151]

The use of these devices has largely been eclipsed by the development of compression screws.

Compression Screws (e.g., Richards). These devices allow impaction at the fracture site without motion of the screw within the femoral head.

Instead, the screw telescopes into the barrel of the side plate. Optimal position of the screw is achieved when its tip is in the subarticular bone and its shaft parallels the medial compressive trabeculae.[152, 163]

Mulholland and Gunn evaluated just how critical screw placement is in 80 patients with unstable intertrochanteric fractures fixed with compression screws.[152] The central position of the screw within the femoral head on frontal and lateral views was classified as follows (Fig. 8–58):

Position 1: The center of the screw tip lay in the center of or within half the screw diameter from the center of the femoral head.

Position 2. The center of the screw tip lay

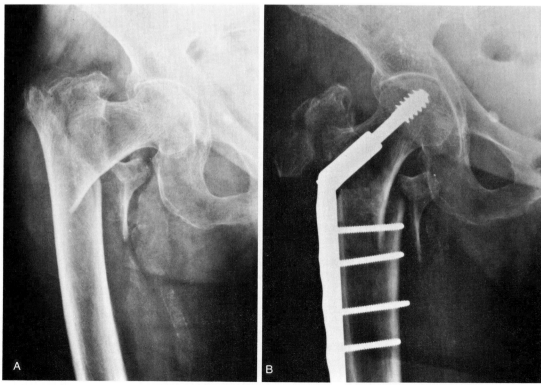

Figure 8–56. Hughston-Dimon Osteotomy. *A,* There is a four-part intertrochanteric fracture with displacement of the lesser trochanter and a large segment of the medial cortex. *B,* There has been impaction of the proximal fragment into the distal fragment. The fracture healed.

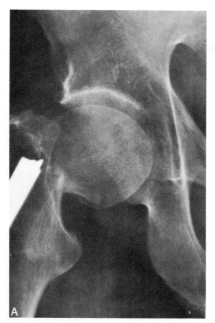

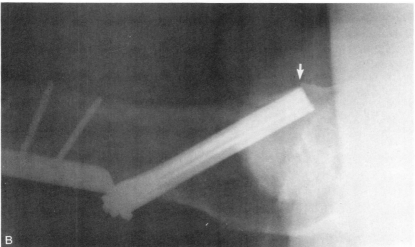

Figure 8–57. Subcapital Fracture Years After Pinning an Intertrochanteric Fracture. *A,* The tip of a Smith-Petersen nail is seen at the base of the femoral neck, where a recent intracapsular fracture has occurred. *B,* The lateral view confirms the location of the new fracture (arrow) at the level of the tip of the nail.

between a half and one screw diameter from the center of the head.

Position 3. The center of the screw tip was more than one screw diameter from the center of the femoral head.

It was shown that screw placement was indeed critical. The poorest position, position 3 in both AP and lateral views, was associated with movement of the screw within the femoral head in all cases. Positions 3 on the AP and 2 on the lateral view may have allowed some motion, but the screw did not "cut out." The best placement, with the screw position 1 or 2 and penetration to within ½ inch of the subchondral bone,

produced the best results, with no evidence of loosening of the nail.

Intramedullary Nailing (Ender's Nailing, Condylocephalic Nailing). Küntscher (1966) developed a rigid curved intramedullary nail with a cloverleaf cross section (condylocephalic nail) that could be introduced from the medial femoral condyle and advanced proximally across an intertrochanteric or subtrochanteric fracture site.[176] Ender modified this technique by using multiple prebent nails, 4.5 mm round and semielastic, rather than the single condylocephalic nail. This was advantageous because the divergent tips of Ender nails improve rotational sta-

429

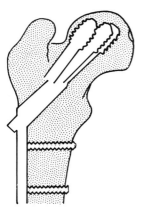

Figure 8–58. Screw Position. The position of the head of the screw on either the lateral or the AP view has been described as follows: (1) The center of the screw tip is in or within half a screw diameter from the central axis of the femoral head. (2) The center of the screw tip is between one-half and one screw diameter from the central axis of the head. (3) The center of the screw tip is more than one screw diameter from the central line of the femoral head. Central placement (position 1 or 2 on both AP and lateral views) and penetration of the screw to within ½ inch of the articular surface is ideal. (Redrawn from Mulholland RC, Gunn DR: J Trauma 12:581, 1972.)

bility and in addition do not injure the medial collateral ligament and are associated with a lower incidence of postoperative knee discomfort.[170]

Indications. Fixation of intertrochanteric fractures using prebent intramedullary nails is gain-

ing in popularity. Most trochanteric fractures are suitable for this type of fixation.[179] The integrity of the medial and posterior portions of the femoral neck is not as important a consideration when using this type of fixation; therefore, both stable and unstable fractures can be treated with

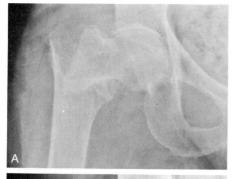

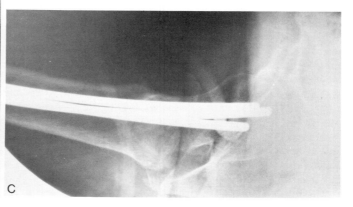

Figure 8–59. Intertrochanteric Fracture Fixed with Ender's Rods. *A,* A stable intertrochanteric fracture is noted in varus position. AP *(B)* and lateral *(C)* views after reduction and the placement of Ender's rods show good positioning of the fracture fragments. The rods, however, do not fill the femoral shaft. The lesser trochanter is now seen to be fractured. Healing was uneventful.

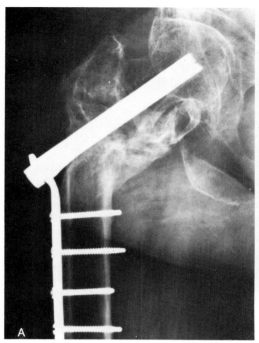
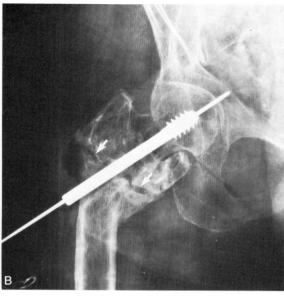

Figure 8–60. Nonunion of an Intertrochanteric Fracture. *A,* The intertrochanteric fracture had been reduced and a Smith-Petersen nail and a side plate used for fixation. The fracture line remains visible months after surgery, despite considerable medial callus. *B,* An intraoperative view during placement of a compression screw shows the site of nonunion (arrows) more clearly. The screw is threaded over the guide wire, which in this case was driven into the acetabulum but more often is positioned within the femoral head. A second guide wire is usually inserted into the greater trochanter to help control rotation of the proximal fragment. If this second guide wire is not used, rotation of the femoral head, as seen in Figure 8–44, may occur.

this method. Subtrochanteric fractures, including those caused by metastatic disease, can also be treated in this way.

From both clinical and mechanical standpoints intramedullary nailing has advantages over other forms of internal fixation. Operating time is shorter than for the insertion of a nail-plate system. Minimal blood loss and low rates of infection are noted, and immediate weight-bearing is possible in many cases.[171, 175] The intramedullary location of these nails makes them load-sharing (rather than load-bearing) devices and therefore less subject to bending stress.

Surgical Procedure. The surgical technique requires the use of image intensification. Closed reduction is usually sufficient and anatomic reduction is not essential, as long as there is good surface contact between the fragments.[172] The pins are inserted through the medial femoral condyle; the correct pin length is determined by laying a pin over the surface of the thigh so that its distal end is a few millimeters distal to the insertion site and the proximal point projects just over the articular space. This will provide for the increased length necessary because of anteversion of the femoral neck. The number of nails used is determined by the diameter of the medullary canal, which should be filled as completely as possible. The position of the nails is checked

fluoroscopically. In treating subtrochanteric fractures, nails may be inserted from the lateral condyle as well.

Radiographic Assessment. Usually three, four, or five nails are inserted; these should approximately fill the medullary canal. When optimally positioned, the proximal ends of the nails should fan out and reach to within 5 to 10 mm of the subchondral cortex (Fig. 8–59).[172, 177] Distally, the ends of the nails should protrude about 1 cm from their point of insertion in the femur, and their flat ends should be stacked against the femoral condyle. They should be positioned so that they can be extruded distally for a few millimeters (a common finding) without producing knee discomfort.

Healing. Callus formation is first seen between 6 and 8 weeks. The fracture gap is closed by callus at 10 to 12 weeks, and the fracture line disappears after 16 to 18 weeks.[171, 175]

Complications of Intramedullary Nailing. Radiographically demonstrable complications include nonunion, proximal or distal migration of the pins, and fracture of the distal femoral metaphysis or diaphysis. Poigenfurst and Schnabl noted that even with correct positioning of the nails 1 in 4 patients had some fragmentation at the site of nail insertion. In addition, follow-up radiographic studies showed there was a ten-

431

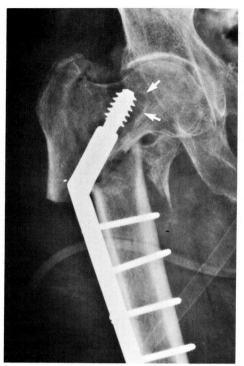

Figure 8–61. An Intertrochanteric Fracture That Collapsed into Varus After Internal Fixation. AP examination after attempted reduction and internal fixation with a compression screw and a plate shows the tip of the screw to be located in the femoral neck. The femur has collapsed into a varus position, leaving a lucent zone with adjacent sclerosis (arrows) marking the former location of the screw tip.

dency to develop varus and bowing deformities. In fact, a change of the fracture fragments position in comparison with the immediate postoperative position was noted in one series in 29 of 80 followed cases.[177] However, all fractures had healed or were healing.

Complications of Extracapsular Fractures. The complications of extracapsular fractures are quite different from those of intracapsular fractures. The blood supply to the femoral head is not jeopardized as it is in intracapsular fractures; therefore, avascular necrosis and nonunion are very infrequent (Fig. 8–60). Complications are generally less frequent in stable fractures as opposed to unstable ones. As summarized by Dimon and Hughston, local complications associated with unstable intertrochanteric fractures result from the adductor pull, which tends to displace the femoral shaft medially, coupled with longitudinal stress, which tends to collapse the fracture into a varus position.[130] Following this collapse the nail may break, or it may "cut out" through the head and neck and enter the ace-

tabulum, or the screws fixing the plate to the femoral shaft may break (Fig. 8–61).

Isolated Fractures of the Trochanters
These fractures are usually of the avulsion type and most often occur in the young (Fig. 8–62). According to Heppenstall, displacement of the greater trochanter by more than 1 cm or of the lesser trochanter by more than 2 cm should be treated operatively with a compression screw; otherwise patients are treated nonoperatively.[90]

Osteonecrosis
Osteonecrosis (ON), avascular necrosis (AVN), and ischemic necrosis are all terms used to describe the same syndrome of clinical, radiographic, and histopathological findings.

Etiology
The causes of ON can be grouped into traumatic and nontraumatic categories (Table 8–8). Traumatic ON in the hip is usually the result of intracapsular femoral neck fracture or femoral head dislocation.[188] Nontraumatic ON may be associated with intravascular obstruction, damage to vessel walls, or vascular compression.

ON of every etiology is believed to be initiated by ischemia within the affected bone, which according to Hungerford then results in bone-marrow edema and fibrosis that increase intramedullary pressure (IMP). The elevated intramedullary pressure further decreases bone blood flow. In traumatic osteonecrosis the direct

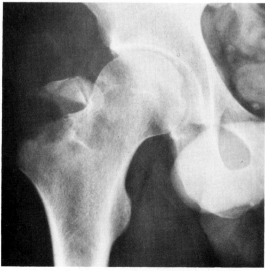

Figure 8–62. Greater Trochanter Fracture. The AP view shows a mildly comminuted transverse greater trochanter fracture with proximal displacement of the trochanter, a result of direct injury to the area.

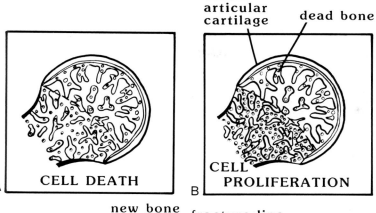

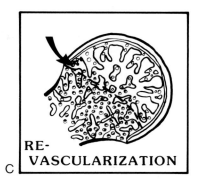

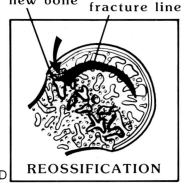

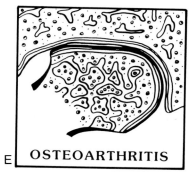

Figure 8–63. Histological Stages of Idiopathic Osteonecrosis. *A,* Cell death. Death of bone and marrow cells has occurred. *B,* Cell proliferation. *C,* Revascularization. Proliferating cells and capillaries invade the marrow spaces between the dead trabeculae. Bone resorption (at arrow) leads to structural weakening and eventually to the development of a fracture. *D,* Reossification. New bone (heavy black lines) is being deposited on the surface of dead trabeculae. A fracture has developed (the crescent sign), beginning at the area of bone resorption (arrow). *E,* Osteoarthritis. There is collapse of the femoral head that eventually leads to osteoarthritis. (Redrawn from Glimcher MJ, Kenzora JE: Clin Orthop 140:273, 1979, by permission.)

tearing of vessels, the formation of an intramedullary hematoma (which elevates the intramedullary pressure), and the presence of intracapsular hemorrhage lead to bone ischemia.

Clinical Features

Nontraumatic ON occurs more commonly in males, particularly between the ages of 30 and 50. It is bilateral in 33 to 80 percent of patients, although the initial clinical presentation is often unilateral.[196]

Pain resulting from osteonecrosis in the hip may be acute or gradual in onset and may affect the groin, the proximal thigh, and the buttocks. The pain may be aching and throbbing, and motion, particularly forced internal rotation, is limited.[203]

Radiographic Changes

Radiographic changes are the result of the repair process rather than of the bone death itself. The hallmark of this repair process is the ingrowth of fibrous tissue and capillary buds into the necrotic areas of bone and the formation of new living

bone on the surfaces of dead trabeculae (Fig. 8–63). Bone resorption leads to the formation of a fracture line (the crescent sign) that propagates under the subchondral cortex in nontraumatic cases or more centrally in post-traumatic cases. The intrafemoral fractures eventually re-

Table 8–8. **Causes of Osteonecrosis**

Traumatic
  Intracapsular fracture
  Hip dislocation

Nontraumatic
  Excess glucocorticoids
    Corticosteroid therapy
    Cushing's syndrome
  Systemic lupus erythematosus
  Hemoglobinopathies, such as sickle cell and sickle
    cell–hemoglobin C diseases
  Metabolic disorders
    Gout
    Gaucher's disease
    Alcoholism
    Pancreatitis
  Dysbarism
  Idiopathic

433

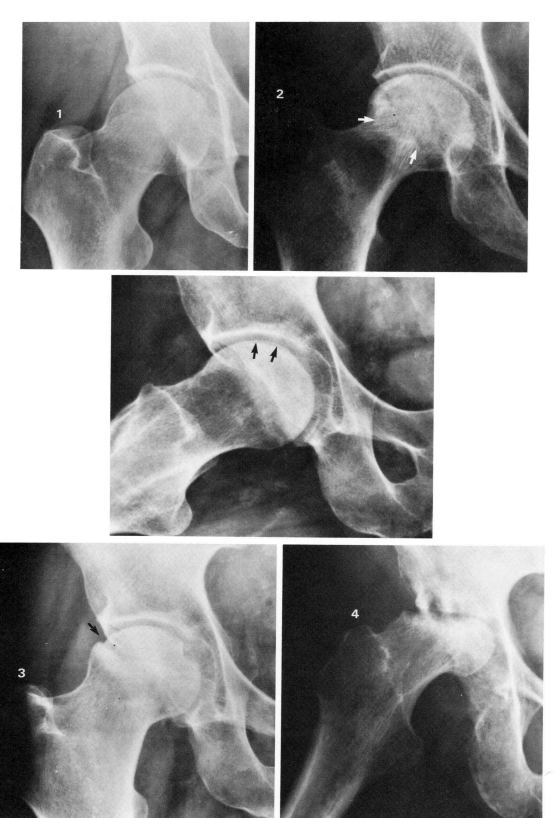

Figure 8–64. *See legend on opposite page*

sult in collapse of the femoral head, joint incongruity, and secondary osteoarthritis.

The sequence of events in osteonecrosis secondary to subcapital fracture and in osteonecrosis that is idiopathic or is associated with other disorders is similar.[199] The rate and extent of repair may differ, however, depending on the underlying disorder, the amount of the femoral head that is involved, and the administration of drugs, such as cortisone.

The earliest radiographs of a partially or completely avascular femoral head show no abnormality, despite the histologically apparent death of marrow cells and osteoblasts. Later findings include the following (Fig. 8–64):

Increased Bone Density. An increase in radiodensity of the femoral head is thought to be the first observable radiographic finding.[206] It had been suggested by Phemister that following subcapital fractures with avascularity of the femoral head, the bone resorption normally accompanying disuse does not occur in the affected portion of the femoral head; therefore, the avascular bone appears relatively denser than does the adjacent viable bone.[215] Glimcher and Kenzora suggest that this is not a reliable or reproducible early sign of osteonecrosis.[199] It is perhaps less relevant now, since internal fixation of fractures and early ambulation often preclude the development of disuse osteoporosis.

Later, the radiographically identifiable increase in density that occurs in the femoral head prior to its collapse largely results from the deposition of additional living bone on and between dead trabeculae.[184, 199, 206] Bayliss and Davidson noted such an increase in density in about half of the patients they studied who had osteonecrosis of the femoral head following intracapsular fractures.[183] The increased density appeared as early as 3 months or as late as 36 months following fracture. After collapse, compression of trabeculae will account for some absolute increase in radiographic density. Thus increased bone density in patients with ON results from (1) the inability to develop osteoporosis in the necrotic segment when disuse osteoporosis occurs elsewhere, (2) the laying down of new bone on dead trabeculae, and (3) compression of trabeculae.

Crescent Sign. The appearance of a radiolucent crescent under the subchondral cortex as

an "early" sign of avascular necrosis in adults was first noted by Norman and Bullough.[213] It is generally agreed that the visualized radiolucency is caused by a fracture through dead bone, and Glimcher and Kenzora have shown that these fractures begin in areas of local weakness produced by bone resorption occurring as part of the repair process.[198–200] In idiopathic osteonecrosis the fracture extends through the dead subchondral bone owing to differences in the elastic properties of the subchondral plate and the underlying cancellous bone. In osteonecrosis following subcapital fracture, the fracture begins in the same location but typically propagates more distally along the junction between the dead and repairing bone, although subchondral fractures may also occur.

The subchondral crescent sign is usually best seen on the frog lateral view, since this projection brings the affected anterolateral aspect of the femoral head into profile. Distraction of the hip, either by traction or by abduction (as in the frog lateral view), may result in the production of a vacuum phenomenon, with gas filling the crescentic fracture site. Interestingly, no gas will be seen within the joint itself, presumably because a joint effusion is present.

V-Shaped Lucency and Adjacent Density. The ingrowth of granulation tissue from the femoral neck (or across the fracture site) and consequent bone resorption may produce a V-shaped lucency, the distal margin of which is often delimited by a thin sclerotic zone that is usually attributed to healing with new bone deposition on dead trabeculae.[206, 213]

"Cysts." Subchondral lucencies ("cysts") occurring in association with osteonecrosis actually represent localized areas of bone resorption and replacement by fibrous tissue and fibrocartilage. They are surrounded by areas of sclerosis resulting from new bone formation.

Buttressing New Bone. Periosteal reaction along the femoral neck, particularly medially, may be noted in cases of ON or osteoarthritis or both; it is apparently caused by alterations in weight-bearing stress. Parenthetically, this finding is not a feature of rheumatoid arthritis and therefore may be used in differentiating these conditions.[210]

Deformity of the Femoral Head. Following the development of subchondral fractures,

---

Figure 8–64. Stages of Osteonecrosis. Stage 1. The radiographic appearances are normal. Stage 2. There is a thin sclerotic rim (arrows) defining the area of osteonecrosis. *Transition* (center illustration). A crescent sign is present (arrows). Stage 3. Collapse, with a lateral step-off (arrow), has occurred. Stage 4. There is marked collapse of and bone loss from the femoral head, with complete cartilage loss from the hip joint. Subchondral cysts are present in the acetabulum.

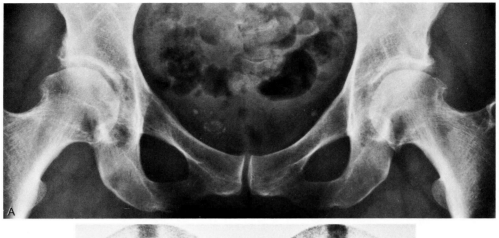

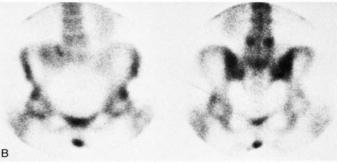

Figure 8–65. Stage 1 Osteonecrosis with Abnormal Bone Scan. *A,* There are hypertrophic changes at each hip, but there is no evidence of avascular necrosis. *B,* The bone scan shows decreased isotope uptake in each femoral head, consistent with avascular necrosis. There is increased uptake in the lateral acetabula bilaterally and in the lower lumbar spine.

radiographs may reveal a loss of the usual round contour of the femoral head, seen either as a flattening of a portion of the femoral head or as a discrete step-off in the continuity of the subchondral cortex. The end result of this process is marked flattening of the femoral head with depression of the articular surface or separation of a superior fragment and its overlying articular cartilage.

Late Segmental Collapse

Compression of the superior aspect of the femoral head following intracapsular fractures (termed late segmental collapse or superior segmental collapse) is viewed by most authors as a consequence of osteonecrosis. This conclusion was substantiated by Catto, who found histological evidence of osteonecrosis essentially involving the whole femoral head in each of the cases of late segmental collapse reviewed.[187] However, there is still some room for controversy regarding the etiology of superior segmental collapse because this collapse occurs long after the presumed onset of avascularity (the time of fracture or internal fixation), and patients with both nonunion and osteonecrosis of the femoral head do not develop such collapse.

Bayliss and Davidson noted superior segmen-

tal collapse as the first feature indicative of traumatic osteonecrosis in 11 of 24 patients with this complication following intracapsular fracture.[183] The sign was initially seen at 5 months after injury, and the mean time to its occurrence was 13 months.

Loss of Reduction. Loss of reduction at the fracture site is not necessarily indicative of osteonecrosis.

Secondary Osteoarthritis. The cartilage space remains normal in width, even when extensive bone involvement is noted. Eventually, however, secondary osteoarthritis develops, largely because of joint incongruity produced by collapse of the femoral head.

Staging. Attention has recently been directed toward staging the clinical and radiographic findings of osteonecrosis so that newer treatment modalities, such as core decompression, can be evaluated.[194, 196] The classification proposed by Arlet and Ficat is most often used (Fig. 8–64):[196]

Stage 1—Clinical signs are present, but the radiographic appearance is normal except possibly for spotty osteopenia.

Stage 2—Osteopenia as well as sclerotic and "cystic" changes are present. The cartilage space and the shape of the femoral head are normal.

436

Transition—A crescent sign is present.

Stage 3—Partial collapse or flattening of the articular surface is present. The entire sequestrum of necrotic bone may impact into the femoral head, resulting in flattening of its superior margin.

Stage 4—The loss of sphericity of the femoral head is marked. The hallmark of stage 4 disease, secondary osteoarthritis, with cartilage-space narrowing and acetabular changes, has developed.

The transition between stage 2 and stage 3 disease, marked by the appearance of a subchondral fracture, is apparently critical, since stage 3 disease is considered irreversible, and core decompression is no longer recommended by most surgeons.[194]

Scintigraphy

Bone Scanning. Bone scanning is useful in the early diagnosis of ON and is often abnormal before any changes are apparent on radiographs. A scan obtained only a few days after vascular compromise shows decreased isotopic uptake in the affected area because of the inability of the radiopharmaceutical to reach this region (Fig. 8–65).[190] In established osteonecrosis there is increased isotopic uptake on bone scans obtained hours after isotopic injection, although the radiographs may remain normal. It is believed that this increased uptake results from chronic vascular stasis, from the repair and revascularization process, or from both conditions. Dynamic scanning with images obtained minutes after isotope injection may help assess regional blood flow, and in one series all patients with osteonecrosis showed significantly decreased flow to the affected area on these early scans.[192]

Marrow Scanning. Technetium Tc-99m- sulphur colloid is generally used for liver scanning; 85 to 90 percent of an intravenously injected dose is removed from circulation by phagocytes in the liver and spleen. The remaining portion of the injected dose is picked up by phagocytes in the bone marrow, and this provides adequate isotope accumulation for assessment of bone marrow distribution. Meyers and associates studied patients after femoral neck fracture and correlated scan findings with histological and clinical data.[211] The scans were correct in predicting the findings in 95 percent of histologically examined displaced fractures. All patients with scans showing activity in the femoral head were later proved not to have ON on biopsy, and all those with decreased uptake had histologically confirmed ON. Equivocal scans showed a variable extent of bone death on histological examination.

Arteriography

Arteriography with selective injection of the femoral or the medial femoral circumflex vessels has been used to study patients with ON. The vessels that can be studied by supraselective contrast agent injection are shown in Figure 8–4. Abnormalities identified on arteriography include stenosis or occlusion of small vessels, diffuse arterial narrowing, delay in appearance of the medial circumflex artery in its retrocervical course, and hypertrophy of small collateral vessels around an area of necrosis.[200]

Intraosseous Venography

One of the most useful clinical advances in the diagnosis of osteonecrosis has been intraosseous venography (phlebography). *Intertrochanteric phlebography* is usually done in the operating room at the time of a decompression procedure. A trocar is introduced into the intertrochanteric region, and 8 ml of contrast material is injected into the bone marrow. Radiographs are obtained immediately and at 5 minutes after injection, and delayed films are obtained as necessary.[203] Normally, contrast is drained by efferent veins almost immediately, and there should be no remaining contrast (indicative of metaphyseal stasis) at the end of 5 minutes. Other findings that indicate venous stasis include engorgement of intramedullary vessels, irregular accumulation of intraosseous contrast material, and reflux into diaphyseal veins, with slow drainage (Table 8–9; Fig. 8–66). Theoretically, venous return presupposes arterial supply, and if contrast agent drains immediately via the venous system, arterial circulation is assured.[214] In one large series phlebography correctly identified 95 percent of cases of ON.[196]

Intramedullary venography involves contrast injection into the femoral head itself. While similar to intertrochanteric phlebography, this

Table 8–9. Findings on Intraosseous Venography Indicating Osteonecrosis

Absence of filling of major efferent extraosseous veins
Engorgement of intramedullary vessels
Slow flow through metaphyseal veins, with intramedullary stasis
Reflux into the diaphyseal system and the nutrient vein, with slow elimination
Globular, irregular intraosseous contrast medium accumulation

Source: Ficat RP, Arlet J: Ischemia and Necroses of Bone. Baltimore, Williams & Wilkins, 1980.

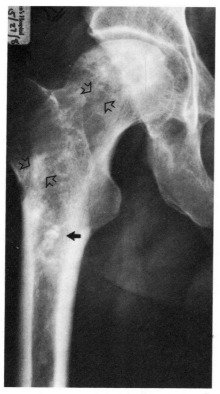

Figure 8–66. Abnormal Osseous Phlebography. Contrast medium was injected into the medullary cavity of the intertrochanteric region via a trocar. Long after injection, reflux of the contrast medium into diaphyseal veins and intramedullary stasis of the medium (arrow) are seen. The defect from the trocar (open arrows) and the increase in density of the femoral head are also apparent.

procedure often results in better radiographic images and is superior for demonstrating the vein of the ligamentum teres.[196]

Intramedullary Pressure Measurement. To obtain intramedullary pressure (IMP) measure-

ments, a trocar is placed in the bone marrow in the area of interest, and a manometer is connected to it.[196] The average pressure in the normal adult femoral neck is about 17 mm Hg, and measurements of greater than 30 mm Hg are abnormal.[204] In doubtful cases a stress test can be performed by injecting 5 ml of saline solution into the trocar over 15 to 30 seconds and recording pressure over the next 5 minutes. A rise of more than 10 mm Hg sustained for more than 5 minutes is abnormal.[203] It has been found that such an increased IMP often correlates with early (stage 1) ON. In one series an elevated IMP was found in 72 percent of cases of ON, and with the addition of a stress test, 85 percent of cases could be detected.[196] Only 1 of 38 hips with ON studied by Hungerford and Zizic had both normal pressure and normal stress-test values.[204]

Treatment[195, 203, 233]

Before collapse of the femoral head has occurred, treatment by non–weight-bearing may be tried, although nontraumatic ON rarely heals spontaneously.[188] Therefore, a number of surgical alternatives have been developed.

Core Decompression. Core decompression involves the removal of an 11 mm core of cancellous bone from the femoral neck and the involved segment of femoral head via a drill hole below the greater trochanter. This procedure reduces elevated intramedullary pressure and, according to Hungerford, is of lasting benefit in patients with stage 1 (preradiological) or stage 2 (precollapse) disease. Complications of the procedure are shown in Figures 8–67 and 8–68.

Following collapse of the femoral head, bone grafting, rotational osteotomy, prosthetic replacement of the femoral head, or total joint

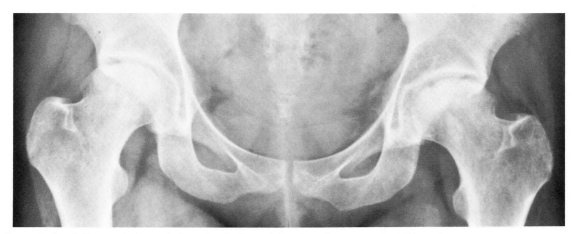

Figure 8–67. Collapse of Femoral Articular Surfaces After Core Decompression. Bilateral core decompressions were done for Stage 2 osteonecrosis. Follow-up examination shows bilateral irregular collapse of the femoral heads.

438

Another method of grafting has been described for patients with stage 3 disease. The infarcted bone and the overlying cartilage and subchondral bone are removed down to bleeding bone. The defect is packed with autogenous cancellous bone graft and resurfaced with an allograft of articular cartilage and subchondral bone.[211]

Osteotomy. Because ON typically involves the anterosuperior aspect of the femoral head, osteotomies have been used to rotate the affected area to a non–weight-bearing position. Particularly for early cases (stages 1 and 2 disease), Sugioka recommends a rotational osteotomy in which the osteotomy line is in the intertrochanteric region, perpendicular to the long axis of the femoral neck but angled slightly cephalad (apex posterior) (Fig. 8–69).[233] The femoral head is internally and anteriorly rotated, shifting weight-bearing onto the posterolateral portion of the femoral head.

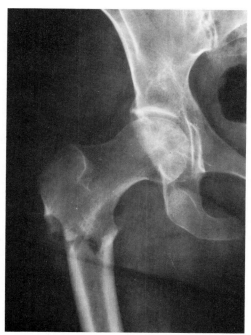

Figure 8–68. Fracture After Core Decompression. As the result of a fall, fracture has occurred through the level at which the trocar had been inserted for core decompression.

replacement (if the acetabulum is secondarily affected) will be necessary.

Bone Grafting. Bone graft inserted through a tunnel into the area of infarction has been used to treat early cases of ON. In addition to the possibility that the tunnel itself decompresses the marrow, bony union has been shown to take place between the graft and the trabeculae at the site of infarct, and this may help prevent subsequent collapse of the femoral head.

Proximal Femoral Osteotomy for Osteoarthritis

The use of osteotomy of the proximal femur has been cyclical, declining with the success of total joint replacement and then increasing as the complications of total joint replacement became more evident, particularly in young individuals.[279] Osteotomies are now performed particularly in younger adults with post-traumatic or congenital deformities, slipped capital femoral epiphyses, or osteoarthritis and also in older individuals with delayed union or nonunion of femoral neck fractures and in some cases with osteoarthritis (Table 8–10).

In the mid 1930s, osteotomy techniques were

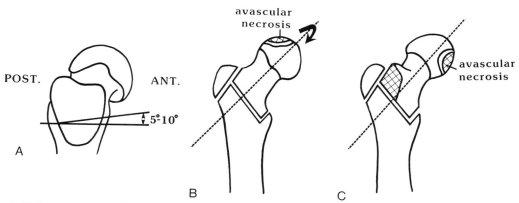

Figure 8–69. Intertrochanteric Rotational Osteotomy. A lateral view (A) showing the anterior wedge of bone that is to be removed. The preosteotomy location of the area of avascular necrosis (osteonecrosis) (B) is shown. The femoral head will be rotated (arrow) around the long axis of the femoral neck. The postoperative (non–weight-bearing) position of the avascular area (C) is shown. (Redrawn from Braunstein, et al.: Skeletal Radiol 10:258, 1983; Sugioka Y: Clin Orthop 130:191, 1978.)

applied to the treatment of osteoarthritis of the hip, with more than 80 percent of patients experiencing pain relief following the procedure. The mechanisms for clinical improvement following osteotomy are uncertain, but hypotheses include (1) transferring the body weight to the distal fragment through the pelvis when medial displacement osteotomy is done; (2) changing the area of the femoral head that contacts the acetabular surface; (3) altering the blood supply to the femoral head as a consequence of the operation; and (4) altering biomechanical factors (due to enlargement of the weight-bearing surface and decrease of muscular forces across the joint).[230]

McMurray Oblique Osteotomy

This osteotomy was one of the earliest osteotomy techniques applied to patients with osteoarthritis. In this procedure the upper shaft of the femur was obliquely transected across the lesser trochanter and the distal fragment medially displaced until it was just under the acetabulum.[229] The object of the procedure was twofold, to transfer some of the body weight from the pelvis directly to the femoral shaft and to rotate the femoral head to allow a new portion of the articular surface to be weight-bearing. Review of 58 such osteotomies by Adams and Spence, showed, however, that the amount of medial displacement of the distal fragment did not correlate with the surgical outcome and, furthermore, that in 26 hips in which the relationship of the femoral head to the acetabulum could be ascertained preoperatively and postoperatively, 21 (81 percent) demonstrated no change in this relationship.[223] Despite the inability to explain the underlying mechanism, the pain relief that follows osteotomy is often immediate and striking and, in many cases, long-lasting. Adams and Spence noted that 78 percent of patients treated with osteotomy and external fixation had pain preoperatively, whereas only 6 percent had pain postoperatively.[223] In those patients in whom

internal fixation was used, the improvement was even more striking.

Ferguson Rotational Osteotomy

Ferguson (1964) noted clinically and experimentally that patients with osteoarthritis often had limited internal rotation of the hip and tended to walk with the limb externally rotated.[227] He introduced an intertrochanteric osteotomy, based on these findings, in which the *proximal* fragment is externally rotated 20 to 30 degrees in relation to the distal femur. No internal fixation was used. Only 8 of 57 patients so treated did not achieve relief of pain.

Varus and Valgus Osteotomies

According to Pauwels, joint incongruity (such as is seen in osteoarthritis) reduces the joint surface available for weight bearing.[230] This weight-bearing surface can be increased by rotating the femoral head inward (varus, or adduction, osteotomy) or outward (valgus, or abduction, osteotomy), depending on the configuration of the joint (Fig. 8–70). In addition to increasing the

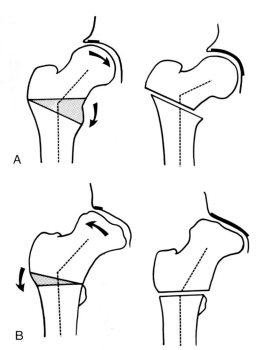

Figure 8–70. Osteotomy. *A,* Varus osteotomy. A wedge of bone wider medially is removed, and the femoral head is rotated medially, increasing the congruity of the joint. *B,* Valgus osteotomy. The excised wedge of bone is wider laterally. The femoral head is rotated laterally, increasing the congruity of the joint. (Redrawn from Pauwels F: Biomechanics of the Normal and Diseased Hip. Theoretical Foundation, Technique and Results of Treatment. An Atlas. Heidelberg, Springer-Verlag, 1976:146.)

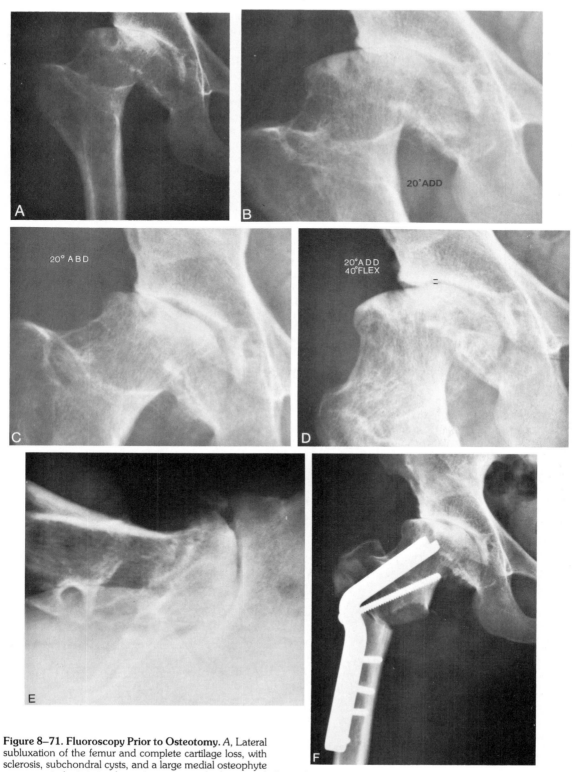

Figure 8–71. Fluoroscopy Prior to Osteotomy. *A*, Lateral subluxation of the femur and complete cartilage loss, with sclerosis, subchondral cysts, and a large medial osteophyte are present. An intertrochanteric osteotomy had previously been done. Fluoroscopy with the leg in 20 degrees of adduction *(B)* and in 20 degrees of abduction *(C)*. *D*, Twenty degrees of adduction and 40 degrees of flexion show the best cartilage space (lines). *E*, A true lateral view, also taken with the leg in 20 degrees of adduction and 40 degrees of flexion, shows the femoral head to be completely covered. *F*, A valgus, extension osteotomy was done.

441

surface area, these operations are thought to relax appropriate muscle groups, resulting in a decrease in the compressive force on the joint.

Procedure. Varus osteotomy involves excising a wedge of bone (the base of the wedge medially directed) and medially rotating and displacing the femoral head until the articular surfaces become congruent. The adductor muscles are released, and the abductor and iliopsoas muscles are relaxed because of the more proximal final position of the trochanters. The distal fragment is displaced medially about 1 cm (Fig. 8–70).

In valgus osteotomies the wedge of bone removed is wider laterally. The lower border of the wedge is perpendicular to the femoral shaft and at the level of the lesser trochanter. The femoral head is laterally rotated a little in excess of what is required to make the joint surfaces congruent, resulting in the lateral aspect of the joint appearing about 2 mm wider than the central portion. Muscle relaxation is produced by tenotomy of the adductor and iliopsoas muscles and by proximal displacement of the greater trochanter or by detachment of the abductors. The distal femoral fragment is displaced laterally to decrease the valgus forces at the knee. The medial shift of the femoral shaft with the varus osteotomy and the lateral shift with the valgus osteotomy realign the mechanical axis of the leg so that it passes through the center of the knee.[231] In patients with acetabular dysplasia, the anterior as well as the lateral portion of the acetabulum is deficient, and correction is then done in two planes, that is, valgus and extension, to better cover the femoral head.

Radiographic Evaluation

Preoperative Evaluation. The diagnosis of osteoarthritis due to mechanical overload is confirmed by the presence of localized sclerosis, cartilage-space narrowing, and subchondral cyst formation on radiographs. In patients with osteoarthritis the choice of whether to do a valgus or a varus osteotomy depends on which procedure will most increase the weight-bearing area of the joint.[230] This determination is made by obtaining radiographic or fluoroscopic studies of the involved hip with the leg in adduction and abduction with and without flexion and noting when the articular surfaces are congruent (Fig. 8–71). Varus osteotomy is considered when the femoral head is essentially spherical, the joint is most congruent on abduction, and cartilage-space narrowing is superolateral. Valgus osteotomy is considered when the femoral head is not spherical and joint congruity is best on adduction or when there is medial osteoarthritis.[231]

Postoperative Evaluation. Both healing of the operative site and changes in the cartilage space and subchondral bone should be evaluated. The presence of callus at the osteotomy site is the most frequently used guide to assess the progress of healing.[228] Nonunion is suggested by loosening of the hardware and by separation and sclerosis at the osteotomy site.

Immediate postoperative radiographs may show widening of the cartilage space, probably caused by change in position of the femoral head with interposition of preserved cartilage into the weight-bearing area. Within 6 to 12 months reconstitution of the cartilage space (as

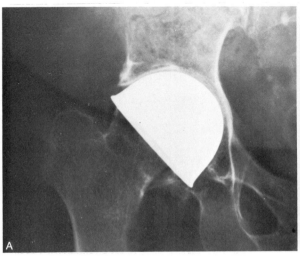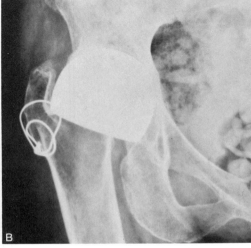

Figure 8–72. Mold Arthroplasty. *A,* The flared edges of the base of the cup are characteristic of this early type of mold arthroplasty; they were designed to keep the prosthesis from rotating into the acetabulum. *B,* A later model cobalt-chromium alloy (Vitallium) cup. The thin lucency between the cup and the acetabulum may represent fibrocartilage.

a result of the formation of fibrocartilage) may occur. There may be an associated marked improvement in the subchondral bone, with filling in of subchondral cysts and reduction in sclerosis. This radiographic improvement usually correlates well with clinical improvement.[223, 230] When osteotomy is successful, there should be no progression in the radiographic findings of osteoarthritis.

Mold Arthroplasty

The term *mold (cup) arthroplasty* refers to the insertion of a mold of inert material between the reshaped surfaces of the femoral head and the acetabulum (Fig. 8–72). The mold stays in place by virtue of its shape, its position between the acetabulum and the femoral head, and muscular forces. Smith-Petersen postulated that such a mold would guide the repair process so that when the interposed material was removed, a newly formed joint with smooth congruent surfaces would remain.[240] Autopsy specimens after mold arthroplasty have indeed shown that fibrous tissue or fibrocartilage may form over the newly created joint surfaces.[234, 236] Several different materials were unsuccessfully used in creating these molds—including glass, Pyrex glass, and Bakelite—until the relatively successful cobalt-chromium alloy (Vitallium) mold was developed in 1938.[240]

The Vitallium-mold arthroplasty was developed before Austin Moore and Thompson hemiarthroplasties were available. Mold arthroplasty continued to be used, even after the development of femoral-head endoprostheses, particularly for young or active patients. Currently, however, this technique is rarely used, and its significance is limited to its place in the history of hip reconstruction and to the fact that patients with prior mold arthroplasties are returning for revision.

Hemiarthroplasty

Indications

Prosthetic replacement of the femoral head is largely used in cases of femoral neck fracture that are complicated by avascular necrosis or by nonunion when the acetabulum is relatively spared. Replacement of the femoral head as a primary treatment for femoral neck fractures is controversial and is used most often in elderly or debilitated patients, in individuals with neurological diseases such as parkinsonism, and for the treatment of fractures with a high incidence

Table 8–11. Indications for Primary Femoral Head Replacement After Femoral Neck Fracture
Probable Indications
Fractures that cannot be adequately reduced or nailed
Fractures that lose fixation several weeks after surgery
The presence of underlying hip disease, such as arthritis
Malignancy
Uncontrolled seizures or parkinsonism
Nonimpacted, nontreated, nonreduced fractures more than 3 weeks old
The presence of associated hip dislocation
Poor general patient condition
Psychosis or mental deterioration
Relative Indications
Advanced age
Pauwels's type 3, or acute oblique fracture
Fracture-dislocation
Osteoporosis of the femoral head
Invalidism

Source: Sisk TD. *In* Edmonson AS, Crenshaw AH, eds. Campbell's Operative Orthopedics. St. Louis, CV Mosby, 1980.

of complication (Table 8–11).[241] In some institutions bipolar endoprostheses are being used instead (see Bipolar Endoprostheses).

Moore and Thompson Prostheses

Moore and Bohlman inserted the first Vitallium proximal femoral prosthesis in 1940.[247] In 1950 a redesigned intramedullary prosthesis was developed by Austin T. Moore, and a modified version of this prosthesis is in use today (Fig. 8–73). The modified prosthesis has a fenestrated stem to allow packing of cancellous bone around it to facilitate fixation (hence the term *self-locking prosthesis*) and to improve the blood supply to the upper femur.[249]

The optimal size of the prosthetic femoral head should be equal to the combined size of the normal femoral head and its articular cartilage.[245] Replacement by a prosthetic head that is too small may result in painful pressure erosion in the center of the acetabulum, whereas the use of a femoral head that is too large may erode the edges of the acetabulum, predispose to repeated subluxation or dislocation, and produce a sticking sensation with motion.[241, 245, 247]

As in the normal hip, the center of the prosthetic femoral head should be at the level of the tip of the greater trochanter to maintain normal abductor length. With the Moore prosthesis the femoral neck is removed to a level of ½ to ¾ inch above the lesser trochanter, and the flange of the prosthesis is inserted so that it rests on the medial femoral cortex on both the frontal

443

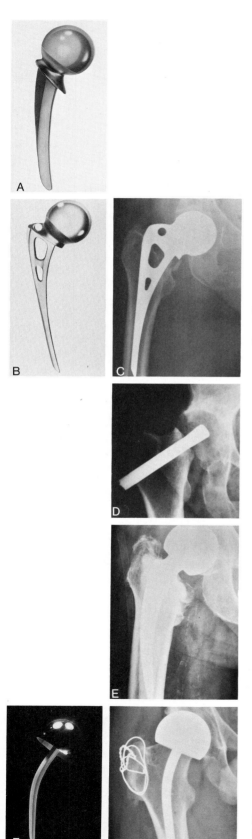

Figure 8–73. Joint Prostheses, Hemiarthroplasty. *A*, Thompson (Howmedica); *B* and *C*, Moore (Howmedica); *D*, Judet; *E*, De Puy; *F* and *G*, TARA.

and the lateral views.[245, 247] The femoral neck is placed in a neutral or slightly anteverted position. As summarized by Freedman, the length of the prosthetic femoral neck may be determined preoperatively in several ways, the most straightforward being comparison with the uninvolved side.[245] Correction for radiographic magnification can be estimated by assuming a 20 percent magnification (when the films are taken at the standard 40-inch tube-film distance) or by placing a ruler alongside the hip at the same level as the joint at the time of radiography.

The stem of the prosthesis should abut the lateral cortex, and the prosthesis should fill the medullary canal.[248] The bone plugs placed within the fenestrations of the femoral stem eventually form a hard cortical bridge between the anterior and posterior aspects of the femur. However, the bone does not fill the entire area of each fenestration. Methylmethacrylate fixation may be used.

The Thompson prosthesis (Figs. 8–73 and 8–77) is made for insertion at the base of the femoral neck.[249] This may be a consideration when the femoral neck is deficient owing to fracture or to bone resorption, which may follow nonunion of a prior fracture. The stem of this prosthesis is not fenestrated and may be inserted with or without methylmethacrylate fixation. The acetabulum may be reamed and reshaped or left intact.

Normal Radiographic Appearances of Uncemented Prostheses (Table 8–12)

Position. As noted in the preceding paragraphs, the center of the femoral head should be level with the tip of the greater trochanter. The lateral aspect of the stem should abut the lateral cortex, and the flange of the prosthetic femoral neck should rest on cortical bone.

Periosteal Reaction and Cortical Thickening. A small amount of periosteal reaction along the lateral aspect of the femur may be seen in the early postoperative period. Later, cortical thickening may be seen even in asymptomatic patients in areas of increased stress, particularly along the lateral femur at the level of the tip of the prosthesis and for several centimeters proximal to the tip.[245, 249] Medial cortical thickening may also be seen.

Sclerosis Around the Prosthesis. Sclerosis frequently occurs in areas of stress adjacent to the prosthesis—near the tip, along the fenestrations, and under the flange.[247] According to Sarmiento this sclerosis reflects motion of the prosthesis within the bone, and apparently such minimal motion is expected to occur in most instances after prolonged use of the extremity.[248] The concept that this "loosening" occurs in most patients is supported by the demonstration of motion between the prosthesis and the bone in all 24 post-mortem femoral specimens examined 5 months to 8 years following the insertion of a Moore prosthesis.[248] Use of a femoral stem that incompletely fills the femoral canal or of a large prosthetic femoral head with a resulting increase in frictional torque predisposes to *excessive* motion.

Sclerosis or Resorption of the Proximal Medial Femoral Cortex. Increased density along the medial femoral cortex adjacent to the flange of the prosthesis may be noted. Resorption of the medial femoral cortex, occasionally amounting to 5 to 10 mm, may also occur without associated symptoms.[245]

Table 8–12. Significance of Radiographic Findings Associated with Moore and Thompson Prostheses

Finding	Incidence	Clinical Significance
Sclerosis at tip	Very frequent	None
Sclerosis of "calcar"	Very frequent	None
Resorption of calcar (Moore prosthesis)	Mild degrees common	None
Radiolucency <2 mm	One third of cases	Occasionally painful or loose
Radiolucency >2 mm		High incidence of loosening
Cartilage-space narrowing Early		Consider infection Infection, especially if groin pain or loss of subchondral cortex
Late		Exacerbation or development of OA or other arthritis
Acetabular sclerosis	Frequent if mild	Mild—asymptomatic Severe—may be symptomatic

Source: Freedman MT: Radiol Clin North Am 13:45, 1975.

Thin Lucency Around the Prosthesis. A thin zone of radiolucency, defined on one side by the metallic prosthesis and on the other side by a thin sclerotic line, is seen in about one third of patients.[245] When this lucency is less than 2 mm in diameter, it is not usually associated with pain.

Acetabular Sclerosis. Thompson noted that in patients in whom cartilage-space narrowing was present at the time of surgery there was a tendency to develop sclerosis of the acetabulum on follow-up radiographs.[249] In fact, mild sclerosis was present in the majority of cases followed by Thompson and was not associated with symptoms. However, greater amounts of sclerosis may be associated with pain.

Abnormal Radiographic Findings

Lucency Greater Than 2 mm Around the Prosthesis or Widening of the Lucent Zone. Motion of the prosthesis within the bone is a frequent occurrence after hemiarthroplasty, and it increases in incidence with time.[245] As in total

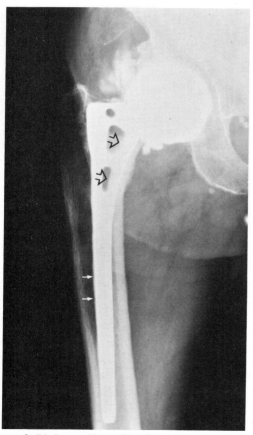

Figure 8–74. Loose Moore Prosthesis Demonstrated by Arthrography. The loosening of this Moore prosthesis is documented by the contrast medium along the tang (arrows). Contrast material around the bone plugs (open arrows) does not indicate prosthetic loosening.

joint replacement, loosening may or may not be the result of infection, and when infection is present, its only sign may be loosening.

Progressive widening of a lucent zone around an uncemented prosthesis or a lucent zone of 2 mm or more suggests loosening, as does sinking of the prosthesis into the femoral shaft. As in total hip replacement, loosening may not be associated with pain severe enough to warrant surgical revision. Arthrographic confirmation of loosening can be made at the time of joint aspiration by noting tracking of contrast around the prosthetic stem (Figs. 8–74 and 8–75).

Sinking of Prosthesis into Femur. Settling of the prosthesis into the femur farther than 1/4 inch was noted in 27.2 percent of patients with uncemented Thompson prostheses and in 17 percent of patients with Moore prostheses.[241] It has been suggested that if the femoral neck was preoperatively normal, sinking of the prosthesis is a consequence of poor surgical technique, with inadequate seating of the flange of the prosthesis on the femoral neck, excessive rasping of the medullary canal, or the use of a prosthesis that is too small and does not fill the medullary canal.[248]

Marked Femoral Sclerosis. Mild sclerosis is frequently seen in areas of increased stress, but marked sclerosis past the tip of the prosthesis raises the possibility of low-grade infection.[249]

Cartilage-Space Narrowing. Progressive cartilage-space narrowing in the early postoperative period should suggest infection, particularly if there is associated groin pain. Radiographic diagnosis of infection is virtually assured when loss of the subchondral cortex of the acetabulum develops (Fig. 8–76). Later cartilage loss is more likely to be the result of osteoarthritic damage of the acetabular cartilage than of infection.

Protrusion into the Pelvis. Migration of the prosthesis into the acetabulum is said to occur most often in patients with rheumatoid arthritis or Paget's disease and in patients in whom the acetabulum is surgically reamed or deepened. Anderson noted this finding in 14.7 percent of patients with Moore prostheses and in 16.2 percent of those with Thompson prostheses. Acetabular protrusion seems to be associated with pain and a poor result in most patients, although some with this finding maintain good or even excellent results.[241, 243]

Ectopic Bone. Ectopic bone in the soft tissues adjacent to the femoral head is quite common but has been related by some authors to infection. Sarmiento believes that groin pain with narrowing of the cartilage space and ectopic calcification is diagnostic of infection.[248]

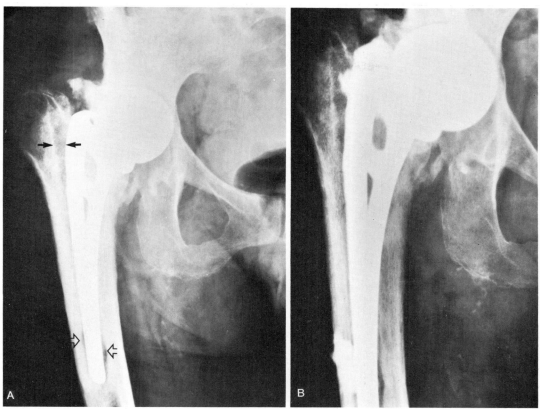

Figure 8–75. Infection Around a Moore Prosthesis. *A,* There has been distal and medial settling of the Moore prosthesis, leaving a lateral, wide metal-bone lucent zone (arrows). A distal focal area of bone resorption is noted (open arrows). Periosteal reaction is noted along the lateral femoral shaft. There is a protrusio deformity. *B,* Arthrography shows contrast agent tracking along the lateral margin of the prosthesis, filling the distal area of bone loss. Infection with *Staphylococcus epidermidis* was found.

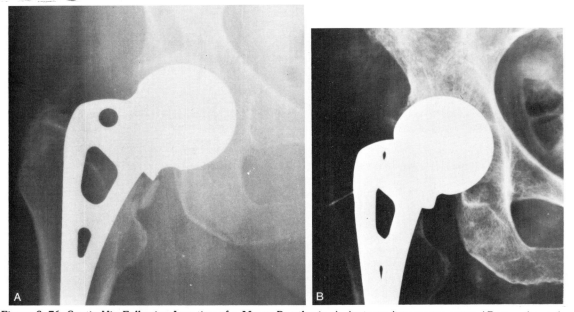

Figure 8–76. Septic Hip Following Insertion of a Moore Prosthesis. *A,* An immediate postoperative AP view shows the acetabular cartilage space and subchondral bone to be normal. *B,* Examination immediately prior to arthrography shows cartilage loss and diffuse erosion of subchondral bone, virtually diagnostic of infection.

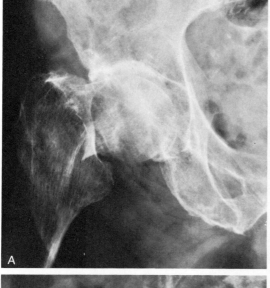

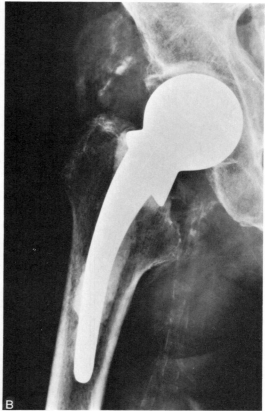

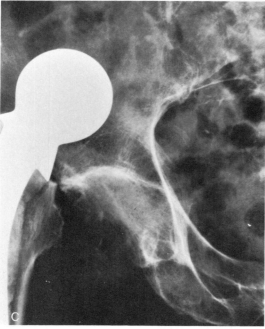

Figure 8–77. Dislocated Thompson Prosthesis. *A,* A Garden 3 femoral neck fracture is present. *B,* A Thompson prosthesis was inserted, and methylmethacrylate cement was used for fixation. There is a moderate amount of ectopic bone. *C,* The prosthesis has dislocated.

Dislocation. As with conventional total hip replacement, dislocation may occur early or late in the postoperative course (Fig. 8–77). This complication occurred in 5.4 percent of 256 patients with Moore prostheses reviewed by Sarmiento.[248]

Fracture. Fracture of the femoral shaft may occur during insertion of the prosthesis or at the time the inserted prosthesis is being reduced into the acetabulum. Nondisplaced fractures may be very difficult to see on the immediate postoperative films, but their detection prior to weight bearing is of obvious importance.

Judet Prosthesis

The Judet prosthesis was introduced in the late 1940s and consisted of an acrylic (methylmethacrylate) head and a steel-reinforced acrylic stem (Fig. 8–73).[246]

Despite the fact that Judet and Judet felt that their prostheses were firmly secured within the femur, subsequent radiological studies have demonstrated almost invariable loosening of the femoral stem, recognized by widening of the lucency around the steel core in comparison with the known dimension of the acrylic sleeve, by extension of contrast around the stem on arthrography, or by gradual sinking of the prosthesis toward the medial femoral cortex. In addition, breakage of the prosthesis and development of an inflammatory reaction to the acrylic material of the femoral head occur.[241] Because of its high complication rate, this prosthesis is no longer used.

Bipolar Endoprostheses

Bipolar endoprostheses (e.g., Giliberty and Bateman) are used in some institutions instead of Thompson or Moore hemiarthroplasty for the treatment of conditions associated with minimal or no acetabular damage, such as displaced subcapital fractures, avascular necrosis of the femoral head, or osteoarthritis with minimal acetabular involvement. The prostheses consist of a metallic femoral head, neck, and stem component and an acetabular component in which a high-density polyethylene liner is enclosed within a metallic cup (Fig. 8–78). The acetabular component is not fixed to the pelvis and can move within the acetabular socket. The advantage of bipolar endoprostheses over conventional hemiarthroplasties is that, with the former, motion occurs preferentially between the femoral and acetabular components rather than between the metallic cup and the acetabulum, and degenerative changes in the acetabulum therefore should be minimized. If acetabular changes do occur, the acetabular component can be replaced with a cemented acetabular socket.

Postoperative radiographic examination should show most motion occurring between the femoral component and the acetabular liner, although some motion does occur at the outer articulation, particularly at the extremes of motion (Fig. 8–79).[251] Because the metallic cup obscures the nonopaque liner, no radiographic assessment of its integrity can be made except by indirect evaluation of femoral-acetabular motion.

Dislocation of the acetabular component, with or without separation of the femoral component from the acetabular liner, has been reported (Figs. 8–80 and 8–81).[250] A radiographically apparent precursor to dislocation is the use of a prosthesis that is too large or too small.

Articular changes, such as acetabular sclerosis and cartilage-space narrowing, signify the onset of osteoarthritic damage and should be noted. Loosening of the femoral component is evaluated in the same way as is loosening of the femoral component of a cemented total-hip replacement (Fig. 8–82). (See Total Hip Joint Replacement, section on arthrography.)

Surface Replacement Arthroplasty

Rationale

The concept of resurfacing the acetabular and femoral sides of the joint stemmed from an effort to save femoral head and neck bone stock that is routinely lost during conventional total hip replacement. Surface replacement could therefore be a temporizing procedure in young patients and in patients with good bone stock, buying time until conventional total hip replacement may be necessary. Other theoretical advantages of surface replacement over conventional total hip replacement include absence of complications related to the femoral stem (such as stem breakage), more limited infection (should it occur), and easier revision should complications develop.

Types of Prostheses

These prostheses are still in a period of evolution and evaluation. Most prostheses consist of ultra–high-molecular weight polyethylene acetabular components and metal femoral cups fixed to bone with methylmethacrylate cement (Table 8–13; Fig. 8–83). The femoral component is cemented on the reshaped femoral head, which—depending on the prosthesis used—is reamed into a hemispherical, cylindrical, or chamfered (the corners removed) cylindrical shape. Care is taken neither to notch the cortex of the femoral neck nor to leave exposed areas of cancellous bone distal to the femoral component, since these factors predispose to later femoral neck fracture.

The acetabular components are generally hemispherical or less than hemispherical in order to decrease the possibility of impingement of the femoral on the acetabular component at the extremes of motion. Acetabular components may be superiorly thicker in the weight-bearing area. Proximal femoral osteotomy and acetabular bone grafting may be necessary in selected cases.

Indications

Whereas surface replacement was thought to be particularly valuable in young, active patients with disabling concentric hip joint disease and no significant deformity, indications for the procedure are changing because of the high failure rate.[263]

Contraindications

Contraindications to surface replacement arthroplasty include severe osteoporosis, osteonecrosis

Text continued on page 456

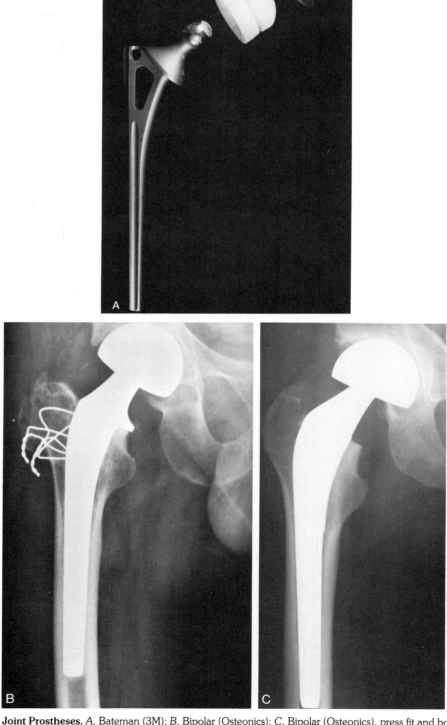

Figure 8–78. Joint Prostheses. *A,* Bateman (3M); *B,* Bipolar (Osteonics); *C,* Bipolar (Osteonics), press fit and bone ingrowth.

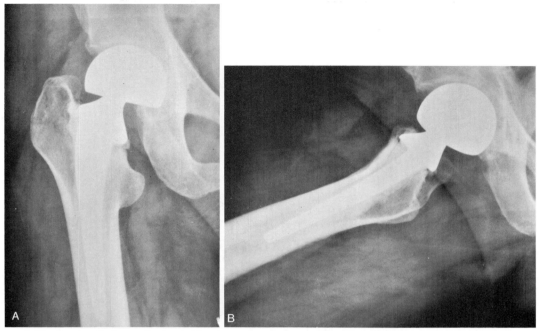

Figure 8–79. Bipolar Endoprosthesis. *A,* The femoral component is fixed with methylmethacrylate cement. *B,* Motion occurs primarily between the femoral and acetabular components and secondarily between the acetabular component and the acetabulum.

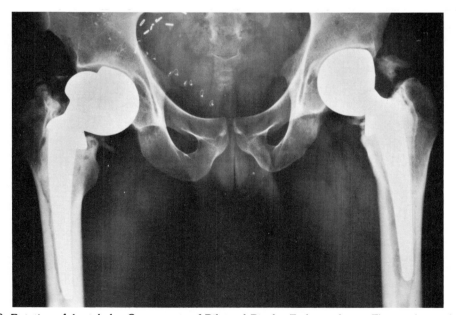

Figure 8–80. Rotation of Acetabular Components of Bilateral Bipolar Endoprostheses. This renal transplant recipient had osteonecrosis of the femoral heads, for which he underwent bilateral hip replacement with bipolar endoprostheses. This follow-up examination shows bilateral rotation of the acetabular components, with the right femoral head partially uncovered. Also noted is loosening of both femoral components.

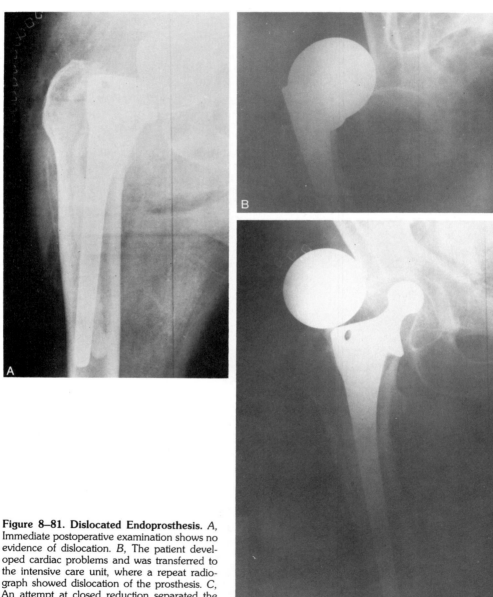

Figure 8–81. Dislocated Endoprosthesis. *A,* Immediate postoperative examination shows no evidence of dislocation. *B,* The patient developed cardiac problems and was transferred to the intensive care unit, where a repeat radiograph showed dislocation of the prosthesis. *C,* An attempt at closed reduction separated the femoral and the acetabular components. (Courtesy of Dr. David Freeman, Boston, Mass.)

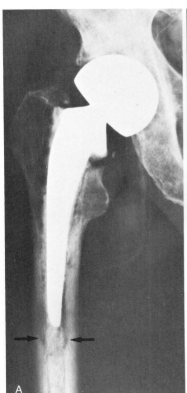

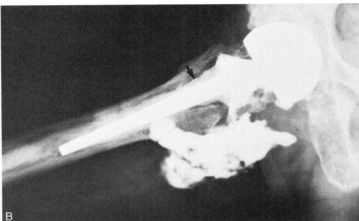

Figure 8–82. Infected Bipolar Endoprosthesis. *A,* The AP examination prior to injection of contrast agent shows proximal loosening of the femoral component with a wide cement-bone lucent zone. The distal, irregular bone destruction (arrows) suggests infection. *B,* Injection of contrast agent into the joint documented loosening of the femoral component (arrow indicates contrast agent at the cement-bone interface). Filling of an irregular posterior cavity strongly suggests infection.

Table 8–13. Characteristics of Some Surface Replacements

Surface Replacement	Acetabular Component	Femoral Component	PMM Cement	Failure (Overall)	Complications		
					Loosening	Ectopic Bone	Femoral Fracture
Wagner	Polyethylene (also fits conventional total hip femoral component)	Cobalt-chromium-molybdenum alloy Rough inside Central aperture to expel excess cement and debris at time of insertion Also aluminum-oxide component	Yes	16/41 (39%)	Femoral 7/41 (17%) (4 AVN) (2 trauma)		
KLH double-cup (Freeman)	1975–79 polyethylene (168°; not full hemisphere) 1980 thicker and 140°; not full hemisphere	Metal (neck reamed to cylinder shape) Non-metallic	Yes No	21% (most aseptic loosening)			2/204 (0.4%)
Tharies (total hip articular replacement with internally eccentric shells; Amstutz)	Polyethylene eccentric	Eccentric cobalt-chromium alloy (chamfer remaining femoral neck)	Yes	14/150 (9%) at 3–6 yrs.	4.4% loosening at 1½–3 yrs. 8.6% at 3–6 yrs.		1/150 (0.7%)
Indiana conservative (Capello)	Polyethylene metal-backed subchondral bone preserved 45° angle of inclination	Cobalt-chromium hemispherical porous inner lining	Yes	17/115 (15%) (11% due to loosening)	Femoral 10/115 (9%) Acetabular 10/115 (9%)		
Paltrinieri-Trentani	Polyethylene	Stainless steel with collar should be in 15–20° valgus Ends at midfemoral	Yes		Femoral 28/114 (25%) Acetabular 12/114 (11%)	16/114 (14%)	2/114 (2%) (Trauma)
TARA (total articular replacement; arthroplasty, Townley)	Polyethylene thicker laterally and superiorly Lateral brim with hole for screw 45° inclination	Spherical outer cup with inner flat topped cylinder Thin intramedullary stem to guide placement; does not normally bear stress	Yes		6/222 (3%) Symptomatically loose acetabula No femoral loosening		

Sources: Black J, Sholtes V.: Orthop Clin North Am 13:709, 1982; Steinberg ME: Orthop Clin North Am 13:661, 1982; Trentani C, Vaccarino F: Clin Orthop 134:36, 1978; Wagner H: Clin Orthop 134:104, 1978.

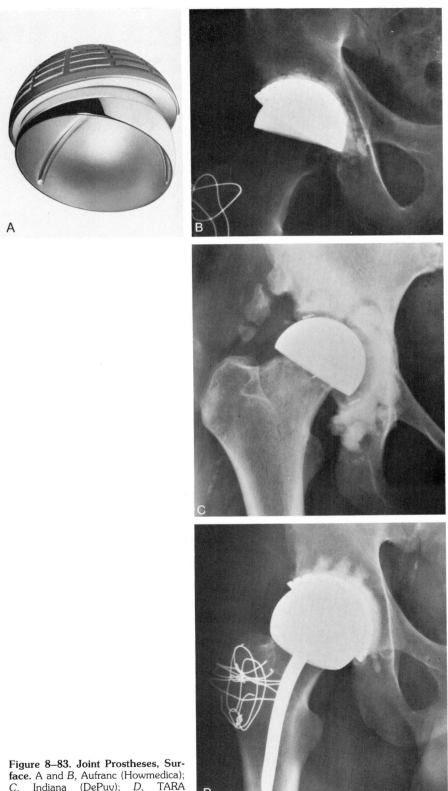

Figure 8–83. Joint Prostheses, Surface. A and B, Aufranc (Howmedica); C, Indiana (DePuy); D, TARA (DePuy).

involving more than one third of the femoral head, congenital hip dislocation with marked deformity, and bilateral disease.[264] Because of the inflammatory nature of the processes occurring in rheumatoid arthritis and ankylosing spondylitis, some authors consider these conditions relative contraindications to the procedure. Active sepsis is an absolute contraindication, but prior infection is not.[263]

Radiographic Evaluation

Component Position. The optimal orientation for each prosthesis varies slightly. In general, the acetabular component is directed between 45 and 53 degrees from the horizontal and is anteverted in accordance with the tilt of the natural acetabulum. The lateral margin of the acetabular component should be aligned with the lateral margin of the acetabulum, since lateral offset of the acetabular component by more than 20 percent of the component diameter predisposes to loosening.[258] Femoral component position is described by noting the angle formed between a line perpendicular to the surface of the femoral cup and a line along the axis of the femoral shaft. The femoral component is generally positioned in slight valgus, varus positioning increasing the chance of fracture at the junction between the femoral neck and the femoral component.[260]

Cement-Bone Interface. The femoral cement-bone interface cannot be evaluated on radiographs because of the opacity of the femoral component. A thin rim of cement should be seen around the acetabular component and extending into small notches (made to improve fixation) in the acetabulum.[265] Sclerotic bone in the superior articular surface of the acetabulum may be left to improve anchoring of the prosthesis. On the acetabular side, guidelines for cement-bone lucencies developed by observation of conventional total hip prostheses are assumed to be applicable to surface replacement arthroplasty. Thus radiolucent lines should remain less than 2 mm wide and should not widen progressively on follow-up examination. Amstutz noted that 96 percent of patients followed for 2 or more years had cement-bone lucencies and in 60 percent these were circumferential.[254]

Complications

As summarized by Black and Sholtes, surface replacement prostheses generally differ from conventional total hip replacements by having (1) thinner acetabular components, (2) larger bearing surfaces, (3) bearing surfaces closer to the areas of cement fixation, (4) thinner layers of cement, and (5) less intrinsic femoral-component stability.[263]

Among the implications of these differences is the greater likelihood of producing thin cement fragments (debris) that are prone to become entrapped in the joint, leading to accelerated wear, inflammatory changes, and component loosening. Deformity of the thin acetabular component and the increased torque resulting from the large component size also increase the possibility of component loosening.

Loosening. In general, loosening of either the femoral or the acetabular component is the major cause of failure. Freeman and Bradley noted, "The rate of aseptic loosening is far in excess of that reported for conventional total hip arthroplasty and is unacceptable if surface replacement arthroplasty of the hip is to be considered as a viable alternative to conventional total hip arthroplasty."[263] Wagner, however, noted clinical loosening in only 6 of 426 patients (1.4 percent) followed up to 4 years after surface replacement.[263] Three of these instances involved the femoral component only, and three involved both femoral and acetabular components. He noted that loosening occurred only in patients with a particular subtype of osteoarthritis (inflammatory osteoarthrosis) that is characterized by rapid onset and progression of damage. Trentani and Vaccarino noted femoral component loosening in 5 of 70 patients (7.1 percent)

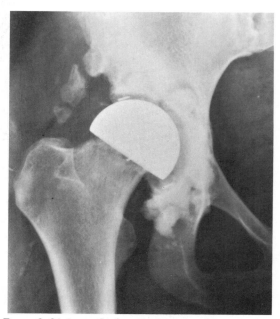

Figure 8–84. Loose Surface Replacement. There is a thick lucent zone indicative of loosening around the acetabular cement. The femoral cement-bone interface cannot be evaluated.

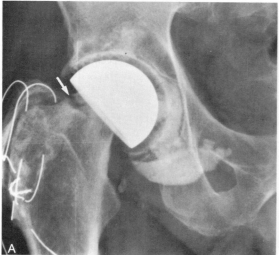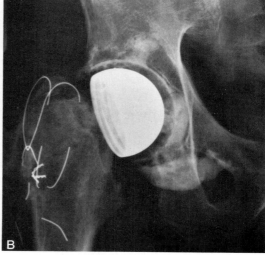

Figure 8–85. Femoral Fracture After Surface Replacement. *A,* There is an incomplete fracture (arrow) near the base of the femoral component. A 1-mm lucent zone around the acetabular cement, fragmentation of the trochanter wires, and probable fibrous union of the greater trochanter are also noted. *B,* A follow-up view shows a change in the position of the femoral component resulting from the now complete femoral fracture.

reviewed 2 to 6 years postoperatively.[264] The incidence of loosening is shown in Table 8–13.

Loosening of the acetabular component is documented radiographically by a wide or widening cement-bone lucent zone (Fig. 8–84). In one series all patients with loose acetabular components had such abnormalities at the cement-bone interface.[263] Femoral component loosening is much more difficult to detect and is demonstrable only by a change in component position (Fig. 8–85). Therefore, this should carefully be evaluated on serial examinations.

Bone scans may show increased isotope uptake around a loose femoral or acetabular component, although false-negative studies occur. A normal bone scan at 13 to 18 months after surgery suggests that the femoral head is viable and that no loosening or infection is present.[257]

Osteonecrosis. Despite early concerns regarding the loss of femoral head viability as a consequence of the surgical procedure, the femoral head apparently remains viable in most cases. This is supported by sequential bone scans in which increased isotopic uptake was noted immediately after surgery that returned to normal by 1 year in uncomplicated cases.[257] Experimental surface replacement in dogs showed no histological evidence of osteonecrosis when the surgery was done after epiphyseal closure.[262] Head, however, noted osteonecrosis with subsequent loosening of the femoral component to be the leading cause of prosthetic failure.[263]

Femoral Neck Fracture. The incidence of this complication varies greatly, depending on the series, with 1 fracture in 426 cases reported by Wagner but 8 fractures in 65 cases noted by Capello.[255] The fracture line usually occurs either at the superolateral aspect of the femoral neck or under the cup and extends inferiorly and medially to the midportion of the femoral neck (Fig. 8–85).

Factors that predispose to femoral neck fracture include notching of the femoral neck at the time of surgery, varus placement of the femoral component (less than 140 degrees), and intracapsular trochanteric osteotomy.[255]

Ectopic Bone. Ectopic bone occurs in up to 43 percent of patients, and although it is not often clinically significant, the larger components of the surface replacement, in comparison with the components of conventional total hip prostheses, provide less room for ectopic bone and make this problem potentially more serious. Of 62 resurfacing procedures reviewed by Bierbaum, ectopic bone was present in 44 percent but was severe in only 5.5 percent.[255] The amount of ectopic bone may be related to the surgical procedure, being seen more commonly with an anterior approach.

Dislocation. Following surface replacement the incidence of dislocation is considerably lower than after conventional total hip replacement. Component malposition, particularly an acetabular component that is too vertical, predisposes to dislocation.

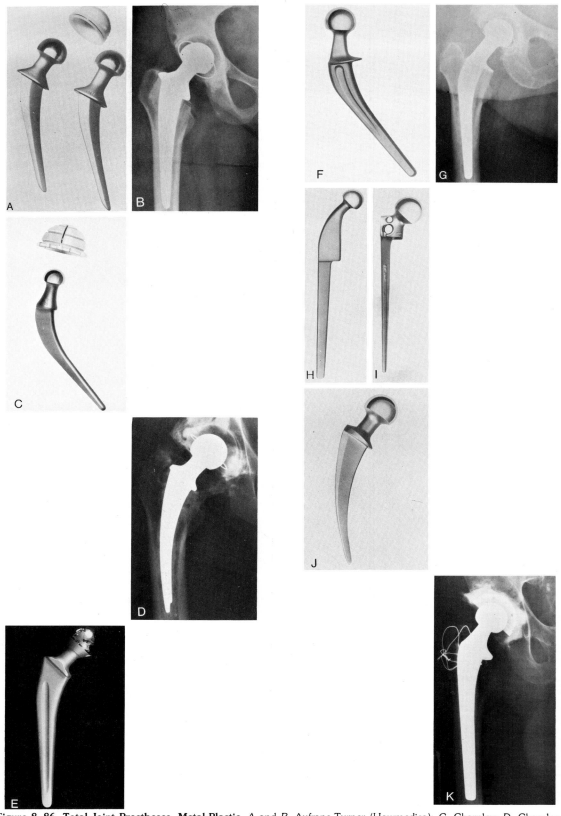

Figure 8–86. Total-Joint Prostheses, Metal-Plastic. *A* and *B*, Aufranc-Turner (Howmedica); *C*, Charnley; *D*, Charnley-Muller; *E*, Muller (Protek); *F* and *G*, Harris (HD2) (Howmedica); *H*, Harris Calcar (Howmedica); *I*, Leinbach (Howmedica); *J*, Muller (Howmedica); *K*, Osteonics (Biomet acetabulum).

Illustration continued on opposite page

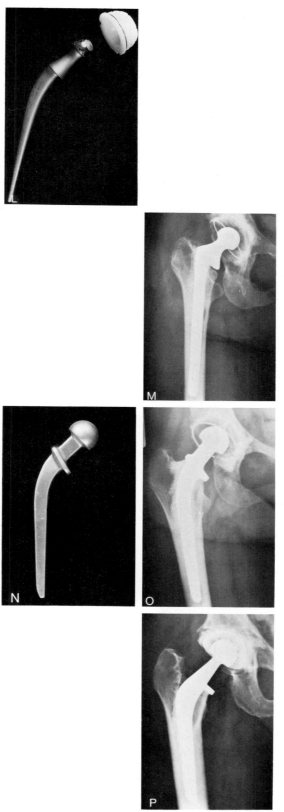

Figure 8–86. Total-Joint Prostheses, Metal-Plastic *Continued.* L, Richards; M, SST (Howmedica); N and O, T-28 (Zimmer); P, Triad (Johnson & Johnson) (Biomet acetabulum).

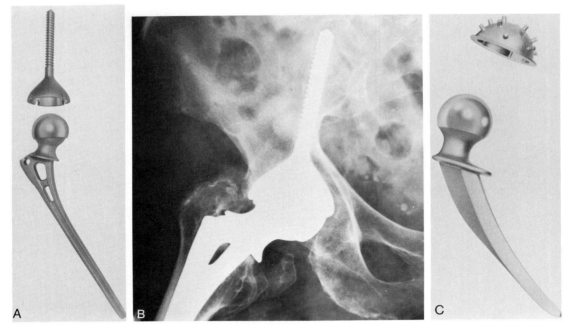

Figure 8–87. Total-Joint Prostheses, Metal-Metal. *A* and *B*, Ring-Moore (Howmedica); *C*, McKee-Farrar (Howmedica).

Infection. The rates of infection are low after surface replacement, with 1 case in 200 procedures noted by Amstutz. The lack of an intramedullary femoral stem is an advantage should infection develop.

Total Hip Joint Replacement*

Types of Prostheses, Normal Appearances

Total-hip prostheses can be categorized by the composition of the acetabular and the femoral components.

In the *metal-plastic type* the acetabular component is made of ultra–high-density polyethylene plastic and the femoral component of stainless steel, a chromium-cobalt-molybdenum

---

*Portions of this section have been previously published in Weissman BNW: Evaluation of Total Joint Replacement. *In* Kelley WN, Harris ED Jr, Ruddy S, Sledge CB, eds.: Textbook of Rheumatology. Philadelphia, WB Saunders, 1981.

alloy, or titanium. The Charnley, the Charnley-Muller, the Trapezoidal-28 (T-28), and the Aufranc-Turner prostheses are of this type (Fig. 8–86). Metal backing of the acetabular component is a recent modification.

Metal-metal prostheses consist of metal acetabular and femoral components and include the McKee-Farrar, the Ring and the Stanmore prostheses. The acetabular component may be fixed to the acetabulum with methylmethacrylate, screws, or spikes (Fig. 8–87).

Positioning of Components

Postoperative radiographs allow assessment of the positions of the acetabular and the femoral components.

Acetabular Component. Frontal and lateral views centered over the acetabulum are necessary for accurate evaluation of acetabular component position.

Acetabular Inclination. In each of these prostheses, the acetabular component is placed so that the base of the cup is at a particular

---

Figure 8–88. Evaluating Component Position. *A*, The tilt of the acetabular component (arrow) with relation to the horizontal is determined by using a baseline drawn along the ischia (the ischial tuberosity or biischial line) and a line alone the long axis of the acetabular marker wire. *B*, The degree of anteversion (flexion) or retroversion of the acetabular component is best determined from the true lateral view. *C*, Example of measuring acetabular component horizontal tilt (curved arrow) on the AP view. Comparison of the distances (D) from the lesser trochanters to the biischial line allows relative leg lengths to be evaluated. *D*, True lateral view. The angle of acetabular anteversion (arrow) is shown. It may also be measured to the horizontal (as in *B*). Dashed line = plane of the acetabular orifice. Solid lines = horizontal plane and the perpendicular to this plane. (*C* is from Weissman BNW: *In* Kelley WN, et al., eds.: Textbook of Rheumatology. Philadelphia, WB Saunders, 1981:2022, by permission.)

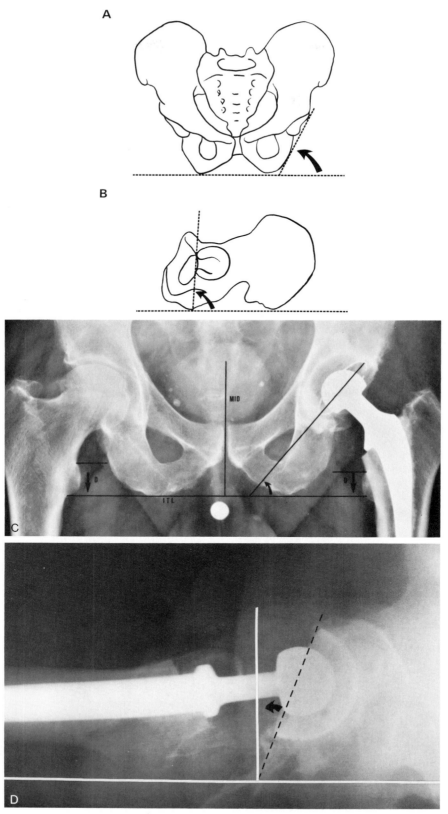

Figure 8–88. *See legend on opposite page.*

angle to the horizontal (e.g., 45 degrees for the Charnley and the Charnley-Muller prostheses, 42 degrees for the Trapezoidal-28, and 30 degrees for the Aufranc-Turner prosthesis) in an effort to provide as much motion as possible without too great a hazard of dislocation.[268, 303] The acetabular inclination is the measured angle between a line through the medial and lateral poles of the equatorial marker wire and the biischial line, through the most inferior aspect of each ischial tuberosity (Fig. 8–88).

Acetabular Anteversion. The orifice of the acetabular component is placed in slight anteversion (tipped anteriorly) or in neutral position. The degree of acetabular anteversion is measured on a true lateral film (Fig. 8–88). When only frontal views are available, however, the equatorial marker wires should form a thin ellipse if the prosthesis is in slight anteversion. With increasing anteversion (or retroversion) the wire marker assumes a more circular shape. Quantitation of the degree of acetabular version from frontal views can be done by dividing the maximum diameter of the acetabular ring by the minimum diameter and comparing this quotient with an available reference table (Table 8–14).[327]

The change in acetabular appearance with differences in centering of the x-ray beam can be used to determine the degree and direction of acetabular version. Two AP views are taken; in one the x-ray beam is centered on the pubic symphysis, and in the other it is centered on the acetabulum.[296, 337] When the ring appears wider (more circular) on the film centered on the acetabulum than on that centered on the pubic

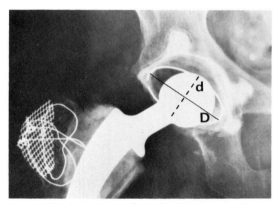

Figure 8–89. **Calculating the Angle of Acetabular Version (β) from an AP View.** On this view, centered over the acetabulum, the angle of version may be derived from the formula $\sin \beta = d/D$ when d is the short and D the long diameter of the acetabular marker wire. The d measurement is estimated because the density of the femoral head obscures most of the acetabular marker wire. (After Fackler CD, Poss R: Clin Orthop 151:169, 1980.)

symphysis, the component is anteverted. When it is more circular in appearance on the film centered on the symphysis, the component is retroverted. The angle of version (β) can then be derived from the formula $\sin \beta = d/D$ where d is the short diameter and D the long diameter of the acetabular marker wire as projected on the film centered over the acetabulum (Fig. 8–89), or the previously mentioned chart may be used as described.

The "portable" postoperative film may suggest that the acetabular cup is in too much anteversion (or retroversion), but the appearances often result from the flexed postoperative position that is assumed. Subsequent films centered on the acetabulum demonstrate the true tilt of the acetabular component.

Two points should be emphasized when determining the degree of acetabular anteversion from frontal views alone. The first is that although anteversion is usually assumed, retroversion cannot be excluded. The second is that the apparent degree of acetabular anteversion varies considerably, depending on the location of the central ray of the x-ray beam.

Fluoroscopy has also been used to determine the angle of anteversion.[301] As the fluoroscopic tube is angled either toward the feet or toward the head, the degree and the direction of angulation at which the anterior and posterior rims of the acetabular marker wire are superimposed are noted. The component is anteverted if the superimposition occurs with the tube angled toward the head and retroverted if it is directed toward the feet. Using a reference table, correction can be made for the degree of inclination

Table 8–14. **Quotient of Maximum and Minimum Prosthesis Diameters and Its Relationship to the Angle of Anteversion**

Quotient	Angle of Anteversion
11.47	5°
9.56	6°
8.20	7°
7.18	8°
6.39	9°
5.75	10°
5.24	11°
4.81	12°
4.44	13°
4.13	14°
3.86	15°
3.62	16°
3.42	17°
3.23	18°
3.07	19°
2.92	20°

Source: McLaren RH: Radiology 107:705, 1973, by permission.

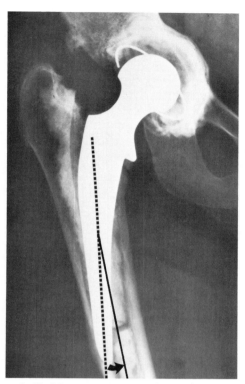

Figure 8–90. Measuring Femoral Component Position. The axes of the femur (solid line) and the femoral component (dashed line) are shown. The prosthesis is loose and in varus position. The degree of varus (arrow) can be measured as the angle formed by the axes.

of the component because this influences the observed angle of anteversion.

Femoral Component. On the frontal view the prosthetic femoral stem should be in the center of the medullary cavity or in slight valgus position.[268] Valgus or varus position of the stem refers to the angle between the long axis of the stem and the long axis of the femoral shaft.[345] When the tip of the stem is near the lateral femoral cortex, the prosthesis is in varus; when near the medial cortex, it is in valgus (Fig. 8–90). On true lateral views the femoral head should be in about 10 degrees of anteversion or in neutral position.[268]

Leg Length. A view of the pelvis with the hips in neutral position can be used to determine differences in limb length by comparison of the distances on each side from the proximal end of the lesser trochanter to a line through the most inferior portions of each ischial tuberosity (Fig. 8–88).[307]

Cement Fixation

The surgical procedure of total hip arthroplasty includes cleaning the acetabulum of cartilage and eburnated bone, enlarging the acetabulum

if necessary, and drilling holes ¼ to ½ inch in diameter into the ischium, the ilium, and the pubis. The methylmethacrylate is prepared, and when it reaches a doughy consistency is pressed into the acetabulum and the prepared holes. The acetabular component is then inserted and held in position. Methylmethacrylate is also placed into the medullary canal of the femur after the cancellous bone is removed. Because Beckenbaugh and Ilstrup found loosening of the femoral component to be inversely related to the degree of extension of cement past the prosthetic tip, cement should fill the medial and lateral medullary cavity along the distal two thirds of the shaft and should extend 2 cm distal to the tip of the prosthesis.[270] According to Amstutz and colleagues, inadequate cement fixation is suggested by radiolucent zones at the cement-bone or the cement-metal junction, or by the presence of voids and laminations within the cement.[266] Filling of the femoral canal by cement is facilitated by the use of a plastic or cement plug (cement restrictor) that obstructs the femoral canal distal to the tip of the femoral stem (Fig. 8–91).[313]

Cement-Bone Lucencies. Radiological evaluation of the cement-bone interface can be accomplished only when the methylmethacrylate is made opaque, usually by the addition of barium sulfate. If a radiolucent zone is present

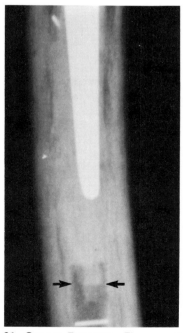

Figure 8–91. Cement Restrictor. The cement restrictor (arrows) limits the distal flow of cement, allowing higher injection pressure and better filling of the proximal canal to be achieved.

463

Table 8–15. Cement-Bone Lucency

	DeLee and Charnley, 1976	Bergstrom et al., 1973	Beckenbaugh and Ilstrup, 1978	Salvati et al., 1976	Amstutz et al., 1976
Acetabular component					
Number of hips with lucent zones	98/141 (70%) (13 loose)	15/15 (100%) control patients	252/255 (99%) without symptoms of loosening	93/93 (100%)	300/389 (77%)
Percentage of circumference involved	—	—	87.5% incomplete	Widest and most frequent laterally	13% completely around acetabular cement
Thickness	>1.5 mm in 3/85 without motion and in 9/13 with motion	<1 mm lucency in 100% of controls	≤1 mm in 87.5%; >1 mm in 6.5%	≤1 mm in 63/93 (68%); 1–2 mm in 29/93 (31%)	—
Time to appearance	17% immediate; 71% within first year; 5.3% after 3 years postoperative	100% before 6 months	—	—	—
Femoral component					
Number of hips involved	—	10/15 (67%) of control patients	—	55/93 (59%)	43/389 (11%)
Thickness	—	<1.5 mm in controls	—	≤1 mm in 36/55; 1–2 mm in 19/55	Most frequent proximally and medially

Source: from Weissman BNW: Radiographic evaluation of total joint replacement. In Kelley WN, et al., eds. Textbook of Rheumatology. Philadelphia, WB Saunders, 1981: 2023, by permission.

at the cement-bone interface, it will be apparent on radiographs by its contrast with the adjacent opaque cement on one side and a thin sclerotic line on the other. When such a radiolucent line is present in the immediate postoperative period, it may represent residual cartilage, soft tissue, or blood within the prosthetic bed. Later, the lucency may correspond to a layer of fibrous tissue (see Chapter 1).

Radiolucent zones at the cement-bone interface are very frequent around the acetabular component and less frequent around the femoral component. A summary of the data relating to this lucency is shown in Table 8–15. These zones are usually established by 6 months postoperatively but may occasionally begin later.[287] Lucencies of more than 2 mm suggest the possibility of loosening or infection and correlate on histological examination with the presence of a synovial-like lining capable of producing substances that stimulate bone resorption.[305]

Trochanteric Osteotomy

Trochanteric osteotomy may be done to facilitate surgical exposure. The trochanter is reattached, using heavy wire sutures or a specially constructed device, to the anatomical position or to a more distal location, depending on mechanical considerations. In more than 95 percent of patients, bony union between the trochanter and the femur is evident on radiographic examination within 6 to 12 weeks.[268, 345] If bony union is not seen at 3 months but the trochanter remains unchanged in position, it is likely that fibrous union has occurred, especially if the wire sutures remain intact. Clinical results appear to be equally satisfactory with fibrous or with bony union, and fibrous union may progress to bony union.[280, 294] Separation of the greater trochanter may be of clinical significance since this is occasionally associated with pain, a limp, and a tendency to develop an adduction contracture.[289] Separation of the greater trochanter was present in 2.7 percent of hips followed for 9 to 10 years by Charnley, and all these patients were classified as having excellent clinical results.[280] Bergstrom and co-workers noted that displacement of the greater trochanter 5 to 20 mm (44 hips) did not impair the functional result, whereas 2 of 4 patients with more than 2 cm of displacement required reoperation.[271]

Fracture of the wires holding the greater trochanter occurs in up to one third of hips and is of very little significance unless it is associated with proximal migration of the trochanter. Wire breakage can occur as a result of metal fatigue, even after there is solid bony union between the trochanter and femur. Occasionally, symptoms result from irritation of the overlying soft tissues. Rarely, a metal fragment can migrate into an intraarticular location.

Wire Mesh Reinforcement

Chrome-cobalt alloy (Vitallium) mesh or a metal shell may be used to reinforce the medial acetabular wall in cases in which this area is deficient (e.g., protrusio acetabuli or excessive removal of bone at the time of surgery). According to Harris and Jones, half of the methacrylate is inserted into the prepared acetabulum; then the wire mesh is pressed into the methacrylate.[312] The remaining cement is then added on top of the mesh and the acetabular component positioned as usual. The wire mesh projections are bent around the edges of the acetabular rim before insertion to control acetabular component position.

These authors also describe the use of wire mesh to cap an osteoporotic greater trochanter at the time of initial surgery or at the time of repair of a migrated osteoporotic trochanter. The trochanteric wires are brought through the mesh and tied over it to distribute the load across the trochanter.

Bone Graft

Bone graft is readily incorporated into the acetabulum. Large grafts (such as a femoral head) may be used to replace deficient areas of acetabular bone. The graft is held in place by screws (Fig. 8–92). In some patients with acetabular component loosening and marked bone loss, graft may be placed into the acetabulum followed by insertion of a bipolar endoprosthesis (see Fig. 8–97). Presumably, after the graft becomes incorporated into the acetabulum, a cemented acetabular component can be inserted should it become necessary.

Measuring Wear

Theoretically, wear can be assessed by measuring changes in the distance from the metallic femoral head to the metallic wire on the surface of the acetabular cup. Two methods have been used to assess wear.[280, 281] In the first the width of the narrowest part of the socket in the weight-bearing area is subtracted from the width of the widest part in a non–weight-bearing area and the result halved. In the second method the thickness of the acetabular component in the latest radiograph is compared with the thickness determined on the immediate postoperative radiograph. Correction for magnification is done by comparison with the known diameter of the

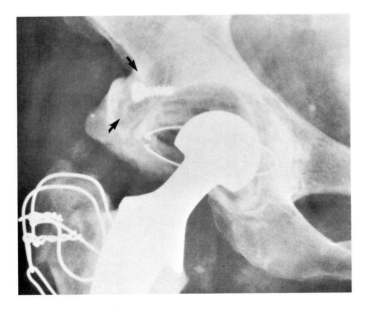

Figure 8–92. Bone Graft. Posterolaterally, where insufficient bone had been present, a screw holds a bone graft (arrows) in place. The junction between the graft and the underlying bone is not shown in this view.

femoral head. Using the second method, in 72 hips with 9- to 10-year follow-up, total wear ranged from 0.0 to 4.5 mm and averaged 1.5 mm. Patient weight and physical activity did not seem to influence the rate of wear, and the rate of wear appeared to decrease with time.

Clarke and associates assessed both methods of measuring wear in vitro using a total hip prosthesis mounted on a Plexiglas orientation apparatus.[282] Although the technique of comparison of early and later films at first seemed more accurate, assessment of wear by clinicians, even when shown the approximate area of wear, yielded errors so large that it was "impossible to make any valid wear assessments . . . it was concluded that wear measurements could not be made from clinical radiographs."[282]

Resorption of the Medial Femoral Neck

When the femoral prosthesis is fixed with cement, 3 or 4 mm of resorption of the femoral neck (apparently resulting from ischemic necrosis or from stress shielding) occurs in almost 20 percent of patients.[280, 324] Resorption does not usually occur in the absence of cement fixation.[324] Generally, this bone loss is of no clinical consequence and does not indicate loosening.[348] Bechtol, however, has suggested that this represents an early stage in a sequence of findings that eventually leads to bending or fracture of the femoral stem.[269] (Also see Development or Widening of a Metal-Cement Lucency and Femoral Stem Fractures, under Complications, following.)

Complications

Dislocation. Dislocation is most frequent in the immediate postoperative period, presumably as a consequence of laxity of paraarticular soft tissues combined with improper handling of the patient during transfer from the operating room or with poor positioning of the leg in bed.[308, 331] Improper positioning or selection of the prosthesis may also be responsible for early dislocation.[332]

Dislocation occurring later than 3 months postoperatively is most often the result of component malposition but may also be the result of failure to develop adequate muscle control, of a range of motion that exceeds the tolerance of the prosthesis, or of trauma.[332]

Radiographic examination confirms the presence of dislocation, helps define any associated component malposition, and aids in the identification of associated complications (Fig. 8–93). Anteroposterior and true lateral radiographs best define the type of dislocation present. Daffner and associates described the Saturn-ring sign, useful in detecting subtle dislocation when only a frontal radiograph is available.[286] This sign is based on the observation that when the femoral head is in the center of the acetabular component, distances measured medially and laterally from the femoral head to the poles of the acetabular wire are equal (Fig. 8–94). When the femoral head is dislocated, these measurements are unequal.

This sign is of value only for prostheses in which the femoral head is centrally located (e.g., the Charnley and the Charnley-Muller

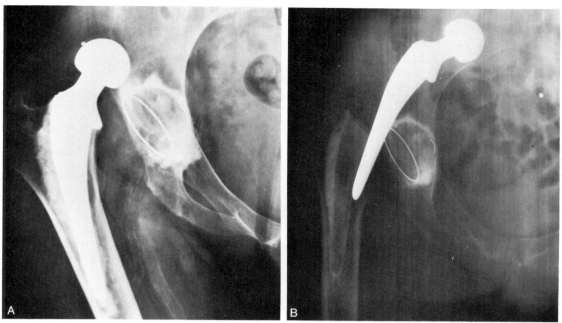

Figure 8–93. Complication After Attempted Reduction of Dislocated Total Hip Prosthesis. *A,* The femoral component is superiorly (and posteriorly) dislocated. *B,* After attempted manual reduction, the femoral component has become dislodged from its cement sleeve.

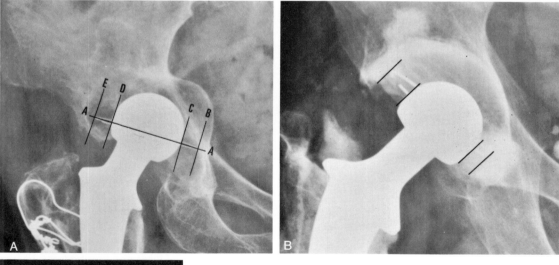

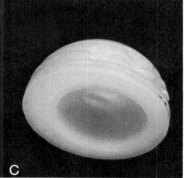

Figure 8–94. The Saturn-Ring Sign. *A,* In early prostheses, such as this Charnley-Muller design, the femoral head is centrally located within the acetabular component, and distances B–C and E–D are equal. *B,* More recent prostheses are superolaterally thicker; therefore, medial and lateral distances (lines) are normally unequal. *C,* The acetabular component of an Aufranc-Turner prosthesis such as shown in *B* has a thicker superolateral wall. (From Weissman BNW: *In* Kelley WN, et al., eds.: Textbook of Rheumatology. Philadelphia, WB Saunders, 1981: 2025, by permission.)

467

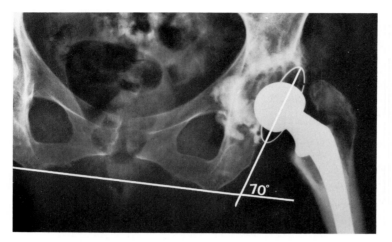

Figure 8–95. Excessively Vertical Orientation of the Acetabular Component Associated with Recurrent Dislocation. Measurement of the angle of the acetabular component with relation to the biischial line shows that the acetabular component is more vertically oriented than usual. The degree of anteversion or retroversion is difficult to assess, owing to centering of the x-ray beam on the pelvis (instead of the acetabulum) and rotation of the patient toward the left. Two dislocations occurred in the first 2 postoperative weeks and were attributed to the acetabular malposition. Revision surgery was necessary. (From Weissman BNW: Orthop Clin North Am 14:171–191, 1983, by permission.)

prostheses). With others, such as the Aufranc-Turner prosthesis, the acetabular component is thicker along the superolateral aspect to provide extra durability in the weight-bearing area. The femoral component of these prostheses will normally appear eccentrically located, with the lateral measurement about twice the medial one. In fact, equal measurement may indicate dislocation in these cases.[306, 317]

Malposition of the acetabular or the femoral component, or both facilitates dislocation (Fig. 8–95). Fackler and Poss, for example, noted component malposition (defined as acetabular or femoral component retroversion or acetabular anteversion of more than 25 degrees) to be present in 44 percent of patients with dislocated prostheses as compared with only 6 percent of control patients.[296] Excessive anteversion of the acetabular component favors anterior dislocation with the hip in extension; retroversion may lead to posterior dislocation with the hip in flexion; and excessive vertical tilt favors dislocation with adduction of the leg. Excess bone or cement around the acetabular rim may lever the femoral head out of the acetabulum. Eleven of 13 dislocations in a series studied by Beckenbaugh and Ilstrup occurred with the hip in flexion with internal rotation or adduction or both.[270]

Detachment of the greater trochanter may accompany posterior dislocations. Rarely, displacement of a fragment of cement or wire into the joint blocks attempts at successful closed reduction of a dislocated total hip prosthesis.[275] These intraarticular foreign bodies may be visible on plain films or on arthrography.

Loosening and Infection. Two of the most frequent postoperative complications leading to failure of total hip replacement are loosening and infection. Loosening may involve one or both components and may be caused by inadequate fixation at the time of surgery or by infection.[266] Recent improvements in surgical technique, including better filling of the medullary canal with cement and the use of large femoral stems with rounded medial margins, have markedly decreased the incidence of femoral component loosening.[313]

Plain Film Findings. Plain film findings that suggest loosening or infection or both include a wide cement-bone interface, widening of the cement-bone interface, development of a metal-cement lucency, migration of prosthetic components, cement fractures, periosteal reaction,

Table 8–16. **Radiographic Findings Suggesting Loosening and/or Infection of Total Hip Prostheses**

Plain Film Findings
1. Cement-bone lucency of 2 mm or more
2. Widening of the cement-bone lucency
3. Migration of prosthetic components
4. Development or widening of metal-cement lucency
5. Cement fracture
6. Periosteal reaction
7. Motion of components demonstrable on stress views or fluoroscopy
8. Bone destruction

Arthrographic Findings
1. Extension of contrast between cement and bone or between prosthesis and bone
2. Filling of irregular paraarticular cavities or fistulous tracts
3. Lymphatic opacification

Scintigraphic Findings
Increased activity in acetabular and/or femoral shaft regions after the sixth month postoperatively

Source: from Weissman BNW: Radiographic evaluation of total joint replacement. *In* Kelley WN et al., eds. Textbook of Rheumatology. Philadelphia, WB Saunders, 1981; 2026, by permission.

motion demonstrated on stress views, evidence of osteomyelitis, and gas within the joint (Table 8–16).

Cement-Bone Lucency Greater Than 2 mm or Widening of the Cement-Bone Lucent Zone. A lucency of 2 mm or more at the cement-bone interface suggests loosening (Figs. 8–96 and 8–97). This finding correlated with motion of

prosthetic components with manual stress at surgical exploration in 16 of the 18 patients in whom it was observed.[293] Lucency around both the femoral and the acetabular components was associated with an increased incidence of infection. Similarly, progressive widening of the cement-bone lucency suggests loosening, infection, or both. The significance of wide or

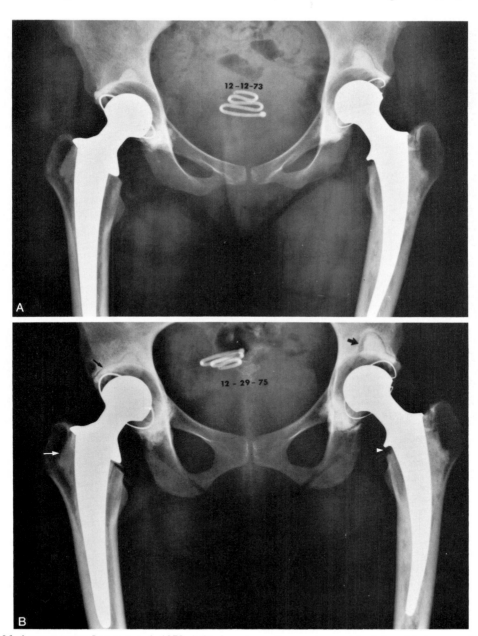

Figure 8–96. Asymptomatic Loosening. *A,* 1973: A thin lucent zone is present around the left acetabular cement. The right total hip prosthesis had just been inserted and no lucent zone is apparent. *B,* 1975: The left acetabular lucency has widened (heavy arrow) and is more than 2 mm in its greatest diameter, indicating loosening. The patient was asymptomatic. Also noted are thin lucencies along the right cement-bone interface (arrows) and resorption of the medial femoral cortex bilaterally (arrowhead). (From Weissman BNW: *In* Kelley WN, et al., eds.: Textbook of Rheumatology. Philadelphia, WB Saunders, 1981:2028, by permission.)

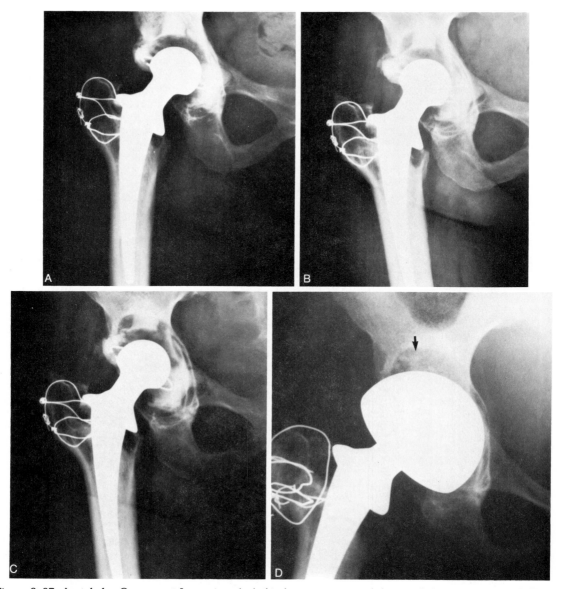

Figure 8–97. Acetabular Component Loosening. *A,* A thin lucent zone around the acetabular cement is noted. This is within the expected range and does not indicate component loosening. There is marked medial femoral neck resorption but no loosening of the femoral component. *B,* Three years later marked widening of the acetabular cement-bone lucent zone, indicating loosening, has occurred. *C,* Two years after *B,* acetabular loosening (with wider cement-bone lucent zones) has progressed, and increased protrusio deformity of the acetabulum is evident. There is no loosening of the femoral component. *D,* The acetabular component was removed and bone graft (arrow) inserted. An uncemented bipolar acetabular component was used. After incorporation of the bone graft, the acetabular bone stock will be improved, making further revision with a cemented acetabular component less difficult.

increasing cement-bone lucent zones is more certain if they occur on the femoral, rather than on the acetabular, side. In one study of the efficacy of the plain film in the diagnosis of loosening, no false-positive or false-negative results were found on the femoral side (using the criteria of a wide cement-bone or metal-cement lucency; a change in component position; and the presence of an irregular, wide zone of bone resorption as evidence of loosening). In contrast, of 50 acetabular components embedded in

opaque cement, there were 5 false-positive and 1 false-negative cases.[253]

Patients with clear radiographic evidence of loosening may be asymptomatic. In these cases, however, careful follow-up is suggested because radiographic evidence of loosening may precede clinical symptoms (Figs. 8–96 and 8–98). It is noteworthy that the diagnosis of infection cannot be reliably excluded using standard radiographs.

Development or Widening of a Metal-Cement Lucency. Separation between the femoral com-

470

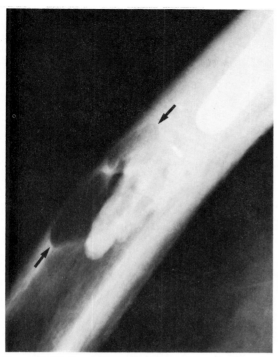

Figure 8–98. Focal Bone Resorption Near the Tip of a Femoral Stem. A localized area of bone resorption (arrows), which in all likelihood is the site of a macrophage response to methylmethacrylate, has developed distally. In this patient the resorption was unassociated with pain or evidence of loosening elsewhere. (Courtesy of Dr. Stanley Foster, Mt. Auburn Hospital, Cambridge, Mass.)

ponent and the cement is most frequently seen along the proximal lateral aspect of the femoral stem (Fig. 8–99). Although Beabout states that there should be "intimate" contact between the acrylic cement and the femoral prosthesis,[268] lucencies in this area are noted in the immediate postoperative period and on follow-up examination in 3.6[334] to 24 percent[270] of patients. When seen early in the postoperative period, it is likely that the cement did not remain in contact with that portion of the femoral component (because of motion of the component while the cement was setting)[266] or that the cement was eccentrically placed along a portion of the stem. In these cases loosening should not be suggested. Some cases of stable 1 to 2 mm lucent zones at the cement-metal interface have been shown to result from the Mach effect,[298] a visual phenomenon in which accentuation of high-contrast borders of objects occurs because of lateral inhibition produced by the neural networks in the eye.[318] Later development of lucency between the femoral component and the adjacent cement or between the cement and the bone with distal migration of the component has been referred to as subsidence.[354] The prosthesis

sinks distally and sometimes medially and at last, according to Charnley, a new point of stability is reached.[270, 354] This view is in concert with the findings of DeSmet and Martel in which a metal-cement lucency was present along the lateral aspect of 23 of 101 Charnley-Muller total hip prostheses, but only 4 of these hips had clinical evidence of infection or loosening.[288] Similarly, Weber and Charnley noted that patients with subsidence of up to 3.5 mm generally had good or excellent clinical results.[354] Even progressive widening of a metal-cement lucency may be seen in patients without clinical evidence of loosening.[288] However, Beckenbaugh and Ilstrup noted a higher incidence of pain in patients with more than 2 mm of drift, and the long-term effects of this finding are unknown.[270]

Subsidence may be associated with radiographically demonstrable cement fracture (seen in 20 of 61 patients with subsidence studied by Beckenbaugh and Ilstrup), but presumably all cases have cement fracture or breakdown as the underlying mechanism.[270] Beckenbaugh and Ilstrup noted that subsidence occurs least often when all the cancellous bone is removed medially at the level of the lesser trochanter and more than 0.5 cm of cement is inserted, when the cancellous bone is removed along the lateral aspect of the distal two thirds of the shaft, and when the canal is filled with cement to a level extending more than 2 cm past the tip of the femoral component.[270]

Change in Position of Prosthetic Components. Motion resulting in a change in component position between the cement and bone or between the prosthesis and the cement may occur. Four patterns of femoral component loosening have been described (Fig. 8–100).[310] In the first and most common pattern there is pistoning of either the prosthesis within the cement or the prosthesis and cement within the bone. Loosening of the stem within the cement may result from weak support at the proximal medial femoral neck and is seen as medial migration of the prosthesis with lucency at the cement-metal interface, usually along the lateral aspect. A crack in the cement at the tip of the prosthesis may be seen. When the loosening occurs between the cement and the bone, a lucency wider than 2 mm or an increasing zone of lucency may be noted.

The second mode of failure, termed the medial midstem pivot mode, results from poor medial as well as distal support at the calcar and is seen as medial migration of the proximal stem, lateral migration of the distal stem, and a cement fracture in the midstem region.

The third category of femoral loosening con-

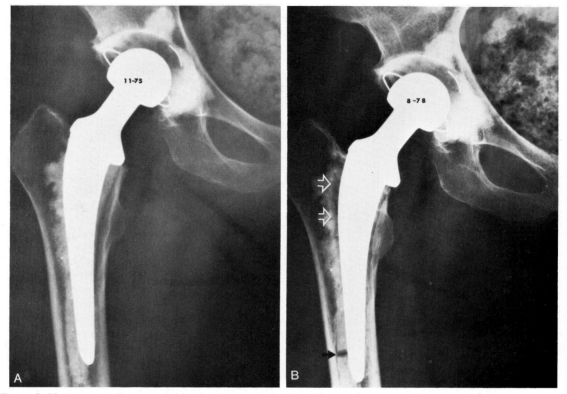

Figure 8–99. Loosening Documented by Development of a Metal-Cement Lucency, a Change in Component Position, and a Cement Fracture. *A,* 1975: There is no evidence of acetabular or femoral component loosening. *B,* 1978: The prosthesis has shifted medially (into varus) as a result of proximal loosening. Lateral separation between the femoral stem and the cement (open arrows) is seen, and a distal cement fracture (arrow) is present. (From Weissman BNW: *In* Kelley WN, et al., eds.: Textbook of Rheumatology. Philadelphia, WB Saunders, 1981:2030, by permission.)

sists of pivoting of the distal stem on the calcar, owing to poor distal fixation. This is uncommon.

The fourth type results from poor medial and proximal support but good fixation of the distal stem. Medial migration of the proximal stem, followed by fracture of the stem, may occur in some cases (see Fig. 8–110).

Acetabular component loosening may occur at the cement-bone or component-cement in-terface. On serial examinations a change in orientation of the acetabular component may be noted (Fig. 8–101).

Cement Fracture. Review of 6649 total hip replacements documented a transverse fracture through the opaque cement near the tip of the femoral component in 1.5 percent of hips (Fig. 8–98).[354] In most instances, the fracture was demonstrable within the first postoperative year.

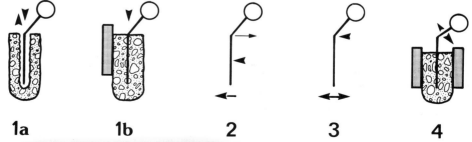

Figure 8–100. Patterns of Femoral Component Loosening. *(1a)* There is pistoning of either the prosthesis within the cement or *(1b)* the prosthesis and cement within the bone. *(2)* The prosthesis pivots with medial migration of the proximal stem, with lateral migration of the distal stem, and with cement fracture in the midstem region. *(3)* Poor distal fixation allows the stem to pivot on the calcar. *(4)* There is poor medial and proximal support but good distal fixation. Medial migration of the proximal stem, with bending of the prosthesis, is seen. Fracture of the prosthesis may also occur. (After Gruen TA, McNeice GM, Amstutz HC: Clin Orthop 14:17, 1979.)

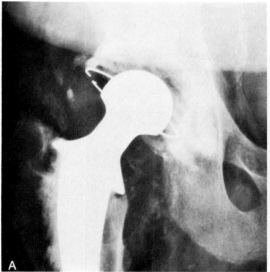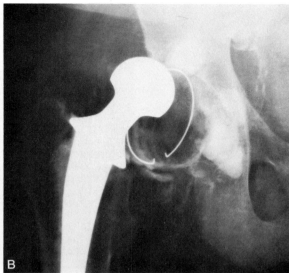

Figure 8–101. Loosening (and Infection) of Acetabular Component, Documented by a Change in Component Position. *A,* Initial position of acetabular component, without apparent loosening. *B,* The acetabular component has rotated, allowing the femoral component to dislocate superiorly.

Most patients with distal cement fracture show medial migration of the proximal femoral stem, thought to result from weak proximal and medial cement support (see the preceding section). Cement fracture may also occur in the midstem region when there is poor distal as well as proximal support. As with other findings indicative of loosening, the majority of patients with cement fracture are asymptomatic.[354]

Periosteal Reaction. Cortical thickening and periosteal reaction may occur with or without infection or loosening. Salvati and co-workers noted that in 4 hips with periosteal reaction near the tip of the femoral component cortical thickening occurred laterally when the stem was in varus and both medially and laterally when the stem was in neutral position.[345] Dussault and associates suggest that periosteal reaction tends to be thicker and more uniform in cases of loosening alone and more lamellar when associated with infection.[293]

Visible Motion of Components. Stress views (push, pull, adduction, or abduction) or fluoroscopy may demonstrate motion of one or both components (Fig. 8–102). Usually, such examination is done at the time of fluoroscopy for joint aspiration and arthrography.

Osteomyelitis. Radiographic evidence of osteomyelitis, including bone destruction, sclerosis, and irregular cortical thickening, is occasionally seen (see Fig. 8–85).

Myositis Ossificans. Some studies have suggested a higher incidence of infection in patients with ectopic bone.

Persistent Intraarticular Gas. Usually any postoperative gas in the soft tissues is absorbed by about 2 weeks after surgery. Failure of resorption of gas or increasing or developing gas collections indicates infection, communication with the GI tract, or both (Fig. 8–103).

Arthrography

Hip aspiration and arthrography are usually indicated prior to total joint replacement when there is a history of sepsis or previous surgery or when there is continued pain after total hip replacement.[328] Contrast-medium injection permits confirmation of the intraarticular position of the needle tip as well as assessment of local anatomy. Arthrography may demonstrate loosening of prosthetic components or irregular paraarticular cavities virtually diagnostic of infection.

The arthrographic technique used has been described earlier.

Contrast is injected under fluoroscopic monitoring until the joint appears to be full, the patient complains of pain, or there is resistance to injection. A radiograph is then taken, and the needle is withdrawn. Usually less than 15 ml of contrast is sufficient to fill the joint, but considerably more may be necessary. Underfilling may lead to failure to demonstrate abnormal collections of contrast medium or component loosening. This has been confirmed by studies in which injection of contrast agent was accompanied by measurement of intraarticular pressure to ensure that the pressure generated within

473

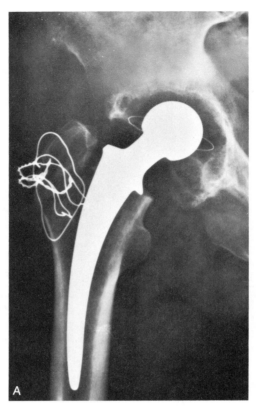

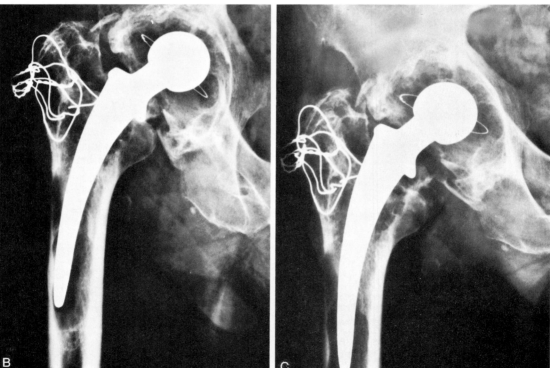

Figure 8–102. Stress Views. *A,* A radiograph 2 weeks postoperatively shows a total hip prosthesis with nonopaque cement around the components. *B* and *C,* Radiographs 7½ years postoperatively show increasing lucency. "Push" *(B)* and "pull" *(C)* films confirm motion of the femoral component, most easily seen by noting the change in the distance between the flange of the prosthesis and the lesser trochanter and the change in position of the tip of the stem within the medullary canal. (From Weissman BNW: *In* Kelley WN, et al. eds.: Textbook of Rheumatology. Philadelphia, WB Saunders, 1981:2032, by permission.)

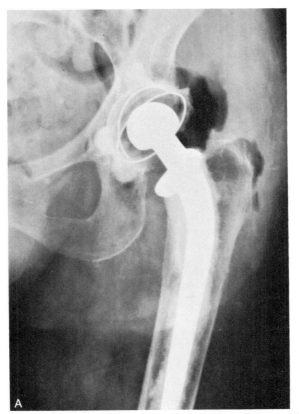

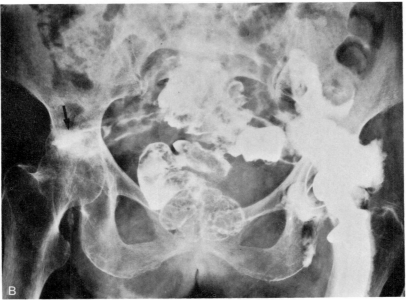

Figure 8–103. Fistula, Due to Diverticulitis, Between the Colon and the Hip. *A,* Several years after a total hip prosthesis, pain began. The AP view shows gas in the hip joint and around the greater trochanter. *B,* Injection of contrast medium into the left hip filled the distal colon and showed extension of contrast material toward the right hip (arrow).

the joint during the arthrogram was as high as occurs under usual stresses, such as walking. A much higher accuracy for the diagnosis of loosening was noted in these cases.[282, 314] Once the needle has been removed, the hip is exercised, and repeat AP and lateral views are taken. AP films with traction applied to the leg may also be done. The patient is then instructed to walk around the room, and AP and lateral radiographs are repeated, with additional views if necessary. Traction films and films after walking have on occasion shown evidence of loosening not demonstrable on standard views.[333, 344]

Anesthetic Injection. Injection of lidocaine at the time of contrast injection has been helpful in separating those patients with pain from loose components or infection from those with extraarticular sources of pain. Burton and co-workers injected a mixture of meglumine diatrizoate diluted with an equal volume of 1 percent lidocaine (5 to 15 ml).[274] Pain relief after lidocaine injection occurred in 95 percent of patients with definite intraarticular abnormalities. Four percent false-positive and 8 percent false-negative cases were noted. The results of lidocaine injection thus were highly accurate in selecting patients who might benefit from reoperation and were more reliable in this respect than were the plain film, arthrogram, or joint fluid culture. Unfortunately, lidocaine may interfere with bacterial cultures, and reaspiration of joint fluid containing lidocaine should not be used for culture.[30]

Subtraction.[267, 298] *Subtraction technique refers to a photographic method used to eliminate densities present on both the preliminary and* the postinjection films so that the injected contrast will be more easily seen. Photographic subtraction is done by making a negative of the film taken prior to contrast medium injection (the subtraction mask) and superimposing this negative on the film obtained after contrast medium injection. This technique is of greatest value in patients with opaque cement around the components of total hip replacements, since the injected contrast and the opaque cement are of similar density (Fig. 8–104). Subtraction technique requires strict patient immobilization, which is often difficult to maintain. In order to minimize the possibility of motion, both preinjection and postinjection films to be used for subtraction are exposed after the needle has been correctly positioned.

A color-subtraction technique is also available (Fig. 8–104).[292] This technique utilizes filters of two opposite primary colors. The films prior to contrast medium injection and following the injection each are placed behind a filter, and a single superimposed image is achieved by means of a beam-splitting mirror. Objects that are identical on both films will appear gray. The

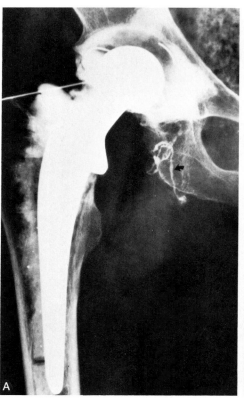
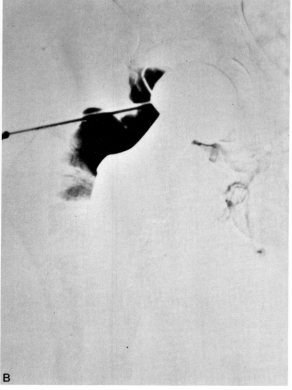

Figure 8–104. Subtraction Technique. *A,* Arthrogram showing lymphatic filling (arrow). Because of the opaque cement around the components, contrast around the cement is difficult to see. *B,* Photographic subtraction (same patient as in *A*) allows differentiation between injected contrast and opaque cement. There is no arthrographic evidence of loosening. (From Weissman BNW: *In* Kelley WN et al., eds.: Textbook of Rheumatology. Philadelphia, WB Saunders, 1981:2033, by permission.)

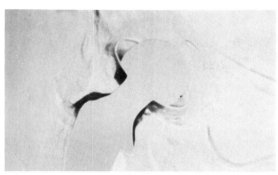

Figure 8–105. Normal Postoperative Hip Arthrogram. Subtraction arthrogram. Contrast medium (black) fills a small pseudocapsule. No contrast material extends along the cement-bone or the metal-cement interface. The entire femoral component should be included on routine examination.

injected contrast will appear in the color of the filter in front of that film. The advantages over photographic subtraction are said to be immediate viewing of the subtracted image and decreased cost. No permanent record is made.

Normal Postoperative Arthrogram. A normal postoperative arthrogram demonstrates filling of a small smooth pseudocapsule that forms within 4 to 5 months postoperatively (Fig. 8–105).[268, 299] Contrast agent parallels the neck of the prosthesis and flares out proximally under the acetabular component and distally along and sometimes under the flanges of the femoral component. In a normal postoperative arthrogram, contrast is not present between the cement and the bone. Aside from the contrast medium just under the femoral flanges, the

medium should not flow between the component and the adjacent cement.

Abnormal Arthrographic Findings. Abnormal arthrographic findings include extension of contrast material along the cement-bone or prosthesis-cement interface, filling of irregular cavities, and lymphatic filling (Table 8–16).[293, 299, 300, 328, 344, 347]

Extension of Contrast Along the Cement-Bone or Metal-Cement Interface. In 1971 Salvati, Freiberger, and Wilson introduced arthrography as a means of detecting complications in patients with pain after total joint replacement.[344] The appearance of contrast material between the acrylic cement and the bone seemed to prove the presence of loosening (Figs. 8–106 and 8–107). Surgical or clinical confirmation of their arthrographic findings in 30 hips (31 arthrograms) revealed only one instance in which a loose femoral component was not demonstrated by arthrography. They concluded that although "a normal arthrogram does not definitely rule out the presence of a complication, a positive arthrogram appears to be diagnostic."

Subsequent studies have compared arthrographic evidence of loosening (contrast material at the cement-bone or metal-cement interface) with evidence of motion of components following manual stress at the time of surgical reexploration. The results are not as optimistic as this first report suggested (Table 8–17). The study by Murray and Rodrigo in 1975 is of particular interest; the conclusion reached was that "arthrographic evidence of loosening may not identify the cause of pain after total hip

Table 8–17. **Correlation of Arthrographic Evidence of Loosening (with or Without Infection) with Clinical or Surgical Findings (Total Hip Replacement)**

	Patients	True Positive Rate	False Positive Rate
Salvati et al., 1971	29 (30 hips) 8 not loose 7 loose 9 loose and infected 2 infected not loose 3 miscellaneous conditions	16/17	0/13
Selby, Brown, and Knickerbocker, 1973	16 surgically proven cases	13/14	1/2
Murray and Rodrigo, 1975	12 with pain and reoperation	7/9	3/3
McLaughlin and Whitehill, 1977	5 with acetabular loosening and re-operation	5/5	
Gelman et al., 1978	9 with painful total hip replacements and surgical evidence of 14 loose components	14/14	1/4
Weighted average		55/59 = 90%	5/22 = 23%

Source: from Weissman BNW: Radiographic evaluation of total joint replacement. *In* Kelley WN et al., eds. Textbook of Rheumatology. Philadelphia, WB Saunders, 1981: 2035, by permission.

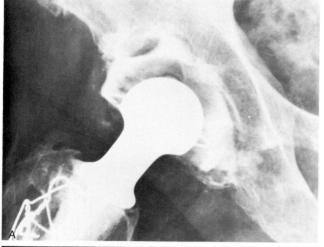

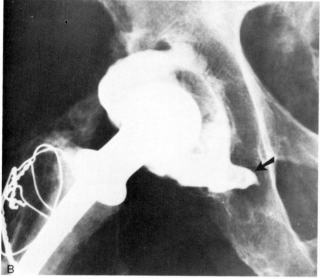

Figure 8–106. Acetabular Loosening. A, The wide cement-bone interface indicates loosening of the acetabular component. B, Contrast agent injected during arthrography fills most of the width of the cement-bone lucency (arrow).

replacement. . . .''[333] These investigators compared the arthrographic findings in 53 asymptomatic total hip prostheses (42 patients) with those in 25 painful total hip prostheses (21 patients). Arthrographic evidence of loosening of the acetabular component was noted in 22.6 percent of asymptomatic hips. No asymptomatic patients demonstrated loosening of the femoral component. Twelve patients with pain underwent reoperation. In 7 patients, loosening demonstrated by arthrography was confirmed at surgery (true positive rate 78 percent).* There were 3 patients in whom loosening of the acetabular component was demonstrated at arthrography but not at surgery and 2 patients

with normal arthrograms but loosening demonstrated at surgery. Thus acetabular loosening may be asymptomatic, and loosening demonstrated on arthrography may not correlate with loosening demonstrated at the time of surgery.

The accuracy of the arthrogram in demonstrating loosening is complicated by ambiguity in the term *loosening*. According to Amstutz and colleagues loosening can be defined (1) mechanically when there is inadequate bonding between materials of different elasticity, (2) radiographically when there is a crack in the methylmethacrylate or development of a lucency at the metal-cement or cement-bone interface, or (3) when gross motion of prosthetic components is demonstrated by applying force to these components at the time of initial surgery or at reoperation.[266]

---

*The authors state that their true positive rate of 58 percent is not calculated in the standard manner.

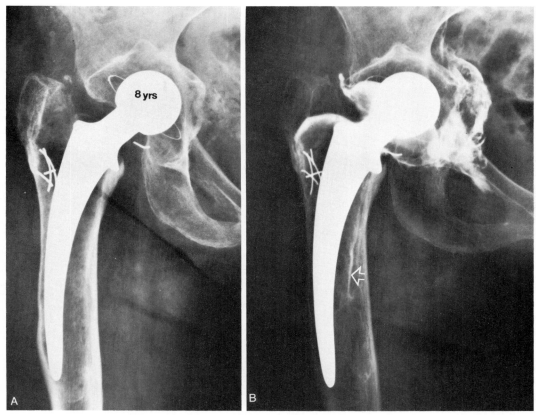

Figure 8–107. Arthrographic Demonstration of Loosening. *A,* Eight years after total hip replacement, settling of the femoral component and an acetabular protrusio deformity have developed. *B,* Injection of contrast agent into the joint shows filling along the femoral (arrow) and acetabular cement-bone interfaces, indicating loosening.

Logic suggests that contrast medium along the cement-bone or metal-cement interface denotes poor bonding between these materials and that in this sense they are loose. The long-term consequence of such an abnormality is still unknown. Pending the outcome of such long-term studies correlating arthrographic findings with clinical outcome, it seems prudent to evaluate carefully each arthrogram for evidence of loosening and to consider the arthrographic findings only in light of the patient's clinical symptoms. Demonstration of contrast material at the cement-bone interface of the femoral component seems more reliable than a similar finding on the acetabular side.

Filling of Irregular Paraarticular Cavities or Fistulous Tracts. These findings are considerably less controversial. The filling of these cavities or fistulae indicates infection (see Fig. 8–85). For example, of the patients reviewed by Dussault and co-workers, who demonstrated filling of such cavities, infection was found in all 5.[293] It should be noted, however, that infection may be present in the absence of abnormal radio-graphic findings (e.g., cavities, fistulae, or loosening).

In patients with draining sinus tracts, contrast agent injected into the tract usually, but not always, demonstrates any communication with the joint. When such a communication is suspected but not shown on the sinogram, arthrography is indicated and will occasionally demonstrate the connection.

Lymphatic Opacification. This condition was seen in 12 patients studied by Dussault and co-workers; 4 had no loosening or infection, 3 had both loosening and infection, and 5 had loosening only.[293] As discussed by Coren, Curtis, and Dalinka,[285] resorption of injected contrast material from normal joints occurs through venous and lymphatic channels. Lymphatic visualization can be noted when the resorption rate is increased, apparently because of increased permeability of the synovial lining and hyperplasia of the lymphatic system. Although it is usually associated with rheumatoid arthritis, these workers suggest that lymphatic visualization is a nonspecific sign of inflammation (Fig. 8–104).

Other Findings. Arthrography following surgery for total hip prosthesis may also demonstrate filling of the trochanteric bursa suggesting trochanteric bursitis (Fig. 8–104), occult fracture of the femoral stem, nonunion of the greater trochanter, and postoperative hematoma preventing reduction of a dislocated femoral component.

Stereophotogrammetry

At the University of California, San Francisco, stereophotogrammetry has been developed to detect and quantify small amounts of motion between prosthetic components and bone. Using a stereo film pair obtained with the extremity on a metal cage (to allow measurement of tube shift and other radiographic parameters) and metal markers implanted in the bone at the time of surgery to identify precise bony locations, computer analysis of the position of prosthetic components relative to bone can be carried out.[278, 316] Such a system is capable of detecting component displacement of 0.8 mm or more at the 95 percent confidence level.[316]

Scintigraphy

Bone scanning has been used in the evaluation of patients with pain following total hip arthroplasty. Campeau, Hall, and Miale performed serial technetium-99m bone scans on patients undergoing total hip replacement and found increased isotopic activity in the acetabular and femoral shaft regions in all patients during the first 3 months.[276] By 6 months the activity returned to normal levels in patients without complication. Patients with increased activity 6 months or more postoperatively all had loosening or infection or both, but often the plain radiographs were normal. No patient with proven complications had a normal scan. Similarly, Feith and associates used strontium-87m scans to evaluate patients with pain following total hip arthroplasty and showed that patients with positive scans generally went on to require surgery, whereas patients with normal scans responded to conservative therapy with gradual diminution in symptoms.[297]

A negative scan virtually excludes the presence of significant loosening or infection.[326, 355] A few false-negative studies, are, however, reported, particularly on the acetabular side.[300, 353, 355]

The distribution of abnormal isotopic activity may help distinguish between infection and aseptic loosening.[359] Focal uptake at the proximal and distal ends of the femoral component is an indication of aseptic loosening (Fig. 8–108). In contrast, diffuse uptake around the femoral

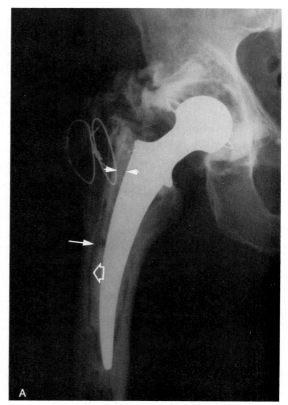

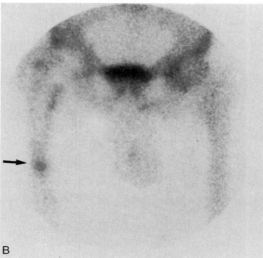

Figure 8–108. Loosening of Acetabular and Femoral Components of a Total Hip Prosthesis. *A,* There are a cement fracture (arrow) and wide cement-bone (open arrow) and metal-cement (arrowheads) lucent zones, indicating loosening of the femoral component. Acetabular loosening, as documented by the presence of an abnormally wide cement-bone lucent zone, is also present. *B,* A bone scan documents loosening of the femoral component, with focal isotope uptake shown proximally and distally (arrow). No evidence of acetabular loosening was apparent, despite the positive radiographic findings. There is some increase in isotope uptake lateral to the femoral neck, owing to the presence of ectopic bone.

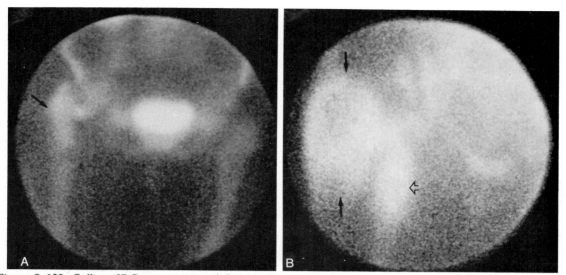

Figure 8–109. Gallium-67 Demonstration of Osteomyelitis and Soft-Tissue Abscess Associated with a Total Hip Prosthesis. The plain films showed evidence of femoral component loosening. *A,* The bone scan shows increased uptake in the proximal femur (arrow). *B,* Gallium-67 scan shows marked incongruent increase in femoral uptake (open arrow) and a circular soft-tissue region of increased uptake typical of an abscess (arrows).

component or diffuse activity around both the femoral and acetabular components may indicate infection. In one series this diffuse uptake pattern about both components correctly iden-

tified all infected prostheses.[353] Therefore, Teranzedeh and associates suggest that evaluation for pain following total joint replacement consist of standard radiographs followed by bone scan-

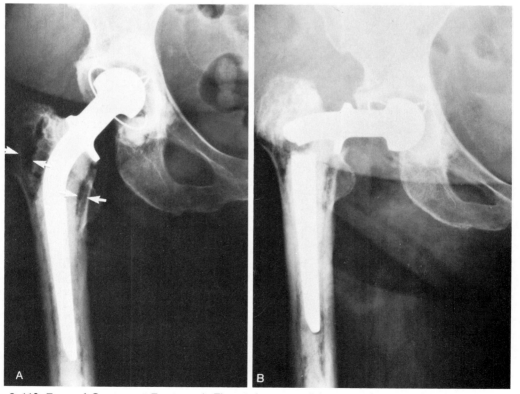

Figure 8–110. Femoral Component Fracture. *A,* There is loosening of the proximal portion of the femoral component, documented by wide cement-bone lucent zones (arrows). The distal portion of the stem does not appear to be loose. *B,* Fracture of the femoral stem occurred.

ning.[353] Joint aspiration and arthrography are then suggested only for patients with diffuse isotopic uptake, which raises the possibility of infection.

Gallium-67 scanning may be of considerable help in differentiating instances of loosening alone from those associated with infection. Gallium-67 scans must be correlated with the technetium-99m bone scan, since the factors that increase the uptake of bone tracer will also increase the uptake of gallium. Infection is highly likely when there is intense uptake or an incongruent distribution of gallium in relation to the technetium bone scan (that is, gallium uptake occurring in areas that are not "hot" on bone scan) (Fig. 8–109). Thus, using both gallium-67 and ^{99m}Tc methylene diphosphonate scans for a study of patients with different types of orthopedic hardware allowed Rosenthall and coworkers to distinguish three groups of patients.[343] In the first group the gallium image was negative, and the technetium bone scan was positive or negative; none of these patients had inflammatory disease. In the second group the gallium scan was positive, but its distribution was similar to the uptake on bone scan. Fifteen of the 16 patients in this category had no inflammatory disease, and the sixteenth had a sterile bursitis. In the third group the gallium scan was positive in an "incongruent" spatial distribution in comparison with the technetium bone scan; all 18 patients had inflammatory disorders, including osteomyelitis, cellulitis, and nonseptic synovitis. Similarly, Reing and associates noted positive gallium citrate Ga 67 scans in 18 of 19 patients subsequently proved at surgery to have infected prostheses.[340] There were no false-positive gallium scans.

Indium-111–labeled leukocytes have been used with some success to identify patients with infection following total hip replacement.[340] In comparison with gallium citrate Ga 67, indium-111–labeled white cells have better imaging characteristics and a higher abscess-to-blood-activity ratio. The test is time consuming, and clinical experience is thus far limited.

Femoral Stem Fractures. Fractures of the femoral component usually are fatigue fractures,

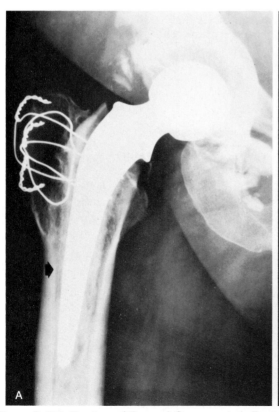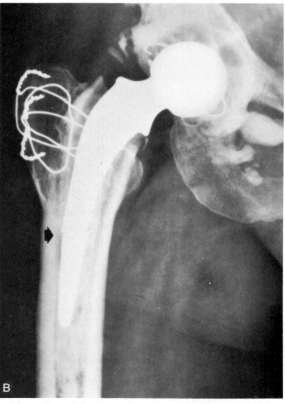

Figure 8–111. Fracture of Femoral Component. *A,* Proximal loosening of the femoral component is documented by a lateral metal-cement lucent zone. No loosening of the tip of the prosthesis is evident. A discontinuity in the femoral stem (arrow) was overlooked. *B,* Follow-up examination 3 months later shows the stem fracture (arrow) to advantage, owing to the increased displacement of the proximal stem. (From Weissman BNW: *In* Kelley WN, et al., eds.: Textbook of Rheumatology. Philadelphia, WB Saunders, 1981:2036, by permission.)

resulting from poor support of the femoral stem. As summarized by Bechtol,[269] poor blood supply to the medial femoral neck results in loosening of the cement-bone bond and medial bone resorption from the proximal femur. The resulting stress placed on the unsupported cement may lead to cement fracture and prosthetic subsidence. Over months or years there is widening of the cement-metal lucency along the lateral aspect of the femoral component. If the tip of the prosthesis is fixed, continued unsupported weight bearing by the femoral compo-

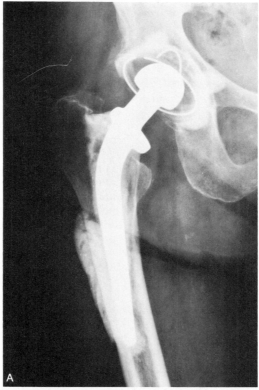

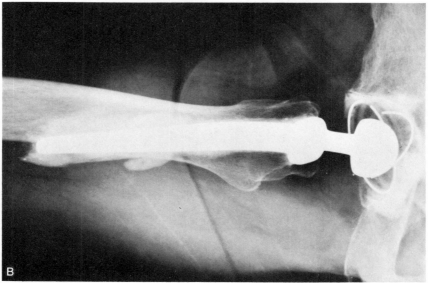

Figure 8–112. Protrusion of the Tip of the Femoral Stem. *A,* The AP view shows cement in the soft tissue adjacent to the femur, indicating femoral fracture. The tip of the femoral component appears close to the lateral femoral cortex. *B,* The frog lateral view shows posterior protrusion of the tip of the femoral component. No clinical sequelae were noted.

nent may eventually result in bending or fracture of the femoral stem (Figs. 8–110 and 8–111).

Several radiographic findings suggest this sequence of events and the need for careful search for radiographically subtle femoral component fracture. Thus, lack of valgus position of the femoral component, resorption of bone along the medial femoral neck, the appearance of a metal-cement lucency laterally along the proximal femoral component, lateral widening of the cement-bone lucency, cement fracture, and early breakage of trochanter wires may precede fracture of the femoral stem. Other factors thought to be associated with increased risk of stem fracture include metallurgical imperfections in the prosthesis and increased patient height or weight or both.[269, 283, 323] However, the actual fracture may be very difficult to demonstrate (Fig. 8–111).

Femoral and Pelvic Fractures. Femoral fractures may occur intraoperatively and are occasionally difficult to recognize on the anteroposterior examination with a mobile x-ray unit. Opaque cement in the soft tissue adjacent to the femoral shaft indicates the presence of a fracture and suggests the need for additional views. Penetration of the femoral cortex by the tip of the prosthesis may also be associated with methylmethacrylate in the soft tissues and may result in apparent foreshortening of the stem of the femoral component on frontal radiographs (Fig. 8–112).

Defects occurring in the inner wall of the acetabulum during preparation of the acetabular bed are identified on postoperative radiographs by the presence of a mass of opaque cement in the pelvic cavity (Fig. 8–113). Usually this extravasation of cement is asymptomatic; however, cases of sciatic nerve entrapment,[277] femoral artery damage[290] or occlusion,[315] defects in the sigmoid colon associated with transient abdominal cramps and bloody diarrhea,[351] bladder fistula,[320] and dyspareunia[295] have been reported. Of particular note are 4 patients, reported by Greenspan and Norman, who developed gross hematuria and dysuria 1 to 2 weeks following total hip replacement.[309] These patients had extravasation of cement into the pelvis, and urographic examination confirmed extrinsic impression on the urinary bladder by the mass of methylmethacrylate. Symptoms were thought to be related to inflammatory changes in the bladder caused by local temperature increases associated with the polymerization of methylmethacrylate. The symptoms disappeared rapidly with conservative therapy.

On postoperative radiographs methylmethacrylate that appeared to be in a draining vein has been seen (Fig. 8–114). No symptoms seemed to be attributable to this finding.[357]

Postoperative fractures have been divided into three categories by McElfresh and Coventry:[325] stress fractures, fractures caused by stress-raisers in the femoral shaft, and fractures due to severe trauma.

Stress fractures occur in patients with severe

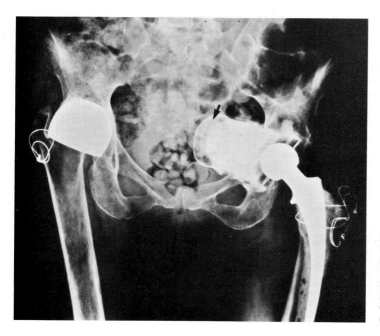

Figure 8–113. Cement Extravasation into the Pelvis. There has been extrusion of cement into the pelvis, pushing medially a femoral-head bone graft (arrow). On the right is a cup arthroplasty. (From Weissman BNW: In Kelley WN, et al., eds.: Textbook of Rheumatology. Philadelphia, WB Saunders, 1981:2037, by permission.)

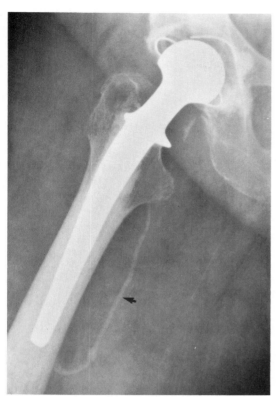

Figure 8–114. Intravenous Methylmethacrylate. A post-operative frog lateral view shows contrast medium extending into the medial soft tissues in the configuration of a draining vein (arrow). No symptoms were attributable to this occurrence. (From Weissman BN, et al.: J Bone Joint Surg (Am) 66:443, 1984, by permission.)

trauma sufficient to fracture a normal limb. Fractures occurring near a femoral component are often treated with closed reduction if adequate alignment and apposition of fracture fragments can be achieved. Since the endosteal blood supply has been compromised during joint replacement surgery, open reduction with stripping of the periosteum may jeopardize the blood supply to the proximal fragment.[325] Methylmethacrylate itself does not appear to interfere with fracture healing.

Paraarticular Ossification. Bone develops within the paraarticular soft tissues in up to 39 percent of patients undergoing total hip replacement.[345] Although in most instances this appears to be of little clinical consequence, Beckenbaugh and Ilstrup have noted lower hip scores in these patients.[270] In a few cases surgical intervention is necessary to remove ectopic bone that significantly interferes with joint motion. The cause of ectopic bone formation is obscure. It is histologically similar to that associated with paraplegia or myositis ossificans progressiva, and trabecular bone eventually develops. Radiological examination shows irregular, poorly defined densities developing 2 to 3 weeks postoperatively, primarily in the region of the abductor muscles

osteopenia, such as those with long-standing rheumatoid arthritis.[346] These fractures appear to be related to the increased activity made possible by joint replacement, and as such they should probably be termed insufficiency fractures, since they are the result of normal stresses applied to abnormal bone. Ipsilateral inferior pubic ramus fracture is one type of stress fracture that may be a source of postoperative hip pain.[341]

The second type of fracture results from *local factors that increase stress* at a particular point. For example, fractures may occur following relatively minor trauma if there is any defect in the femoral cortex, such as may be produced during reaming of the femur in an osteoporotic patient or by prior surgery (e.g., a screw hole). McElfresh and Coventry recommend having methylmethacrylate around the tip of the prosthesis and extending distally at least 2 cm in order to prevent undue stress concentration at the tip of the prosthesis (Fig. 8–115).[325]

The third category of fracture occurs following

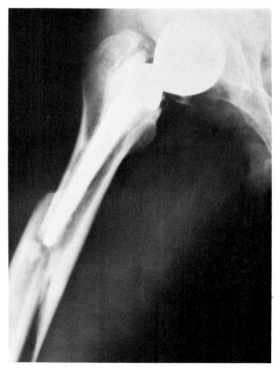

Figure 8–115. Femoral Fracture After Hip Replacement. An oblique fracture through the cement adjacent to the tip of the femoral stem has occurred. (Same patient as in Fig. 8–80.)

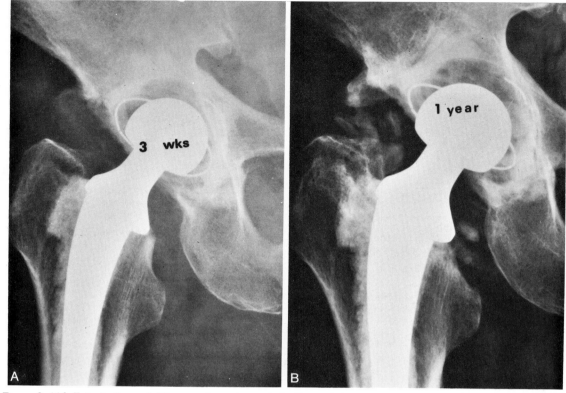

Figure 8–116. Ectopic Bone. *A,* Three weeks postoperatively. Faint calcification is visible laterally. *B,* One year postoperatively. Areas of bone are present in the soft tissues (class 1). No restriction of motion resulted. (From Weissman BNW: *In* Kelley WN, et al., eds.: Textbook of Rheumatology. Philadelphia, WB Saunders, 1981:2038, by permission.)

(Fig. 8–116).[335] Progression to complete bony bridging may occur in about 12 weeks.

Brooker and Bowerman have graded the amount of ectopic bone that is present on radiographs as follows:[273]

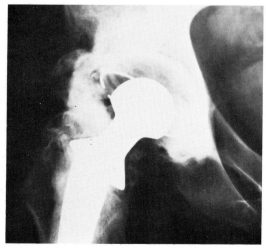

Figure 8–117. Ectopic Bone After Total Hip Replacement. Severe (class 4) ectopic bone is present in the soft tissues around this total hip replacement. Surgical removal of this bone was necessary in order to restore motion.

Class 1—islands of bone within the soft tissues
Class 2—bony projections from the pelvis or proximal femur with 1 cm between bony margins
Class 3—less than 1 cm remaining between opposing bony surfaces
Class 4—apparent bony ankylosis (Fig. 8–117)

Bone scanning has been shown to demonstrate paraarticular ossification prior to its appearance on radiographs.[350] Tanaka and associates performed serial technetium Tc-99m polyphosphate bone scans on quadriplegic and paraplegic patients with paraarticular ossification in an effort to gauge the maturity of the heterotopic bone.[352] Isotopic uptake in the area of heterotopic bone was compared with that in a control area (e.g., spine, sacrum, or ilium), and this ratio was followed with time. In order to decrease the incidence of recurrence, it was suggested that surgical removal of ectopic bone should be done after 2 to 3 months of steady uptake. No assessment of bone maturity could be made from a single examination. Application of these data to patients with total joint replacement has not been reported.

References
Normal Structure and Function
Essential Anatomy
1. Catto M: A histological study of avascular necrosis of the femoral head after transcervical fracture. J Bone Joint Surg (Br) 47:749–776, 1965.
2. Crock HV: The Blood Supply of the Lower Limb Bones in Man. Baltimore, Williams & Wilkins, 1967.
3. Garden RS: The structure and function of the proximal end of the femur. J Bone Joint Surg (Br) 43:576–589, 1961.
4. Hulth A: The vessel anatomy of the upper femur and with special regard to the mechanism of origin of different vascular disorders. Acta Orthop Scand 27:192–209, 1958.
5. Radin EL: Biomechanics of the human hip. Clin Orthop 152:28–34, 1980.
6. Roaas A, Anderson GBJ: Normal range of motion of the hip, knee and ankle joints in male subjects, 30–40 years of age. Acta Orthop Scand 53:205–208, 1982.
7. Rosenthal DI, Scott JA: Biomechanics important to interpret radiographs of the hip. Skeletal Radiol 9:185–188, 1983.
8. Sevitt S, Thompson RG: The distribution and anastomoses of arteries supplying the head and neck of the femur. J Bone Joint Surg (Br) 47:560–573, 1965.
9. Trueta J, Harrison MHM: The normal vascular anatomy of the femoral head in adult man. J Bone Joint Surg (Br) 35:442–461, 1953.
10. Williams PL, Warwick R: Gray's Anatomy, 36th Br ed. Philadelphia, WB Saunders, 1980.

Normal Radiographic Findings
Soft Tissues
11. Brown I: A study of the "capsular" shadow in disorders of the hip in children. J Bone Joint Surg (Br) 57:175–179, 1975.
12. Drey L: A roentgenographic study of transitory synovitis of the hip joint. Radiology 60:588–591, 1953.
13. Fredensborg N, Nilsson BE: The joint space in normal hip radiographs. Radiology 126:325–326, 1978.
14. Guerra J Jr, Armbuster TG, Resnick D, et al.: The adult hip: an anatomic study. Part II. The soft-tissue landmarks. Radiology 128:11–20, 1978.
15. Hefke HW, Turner VC: The obturator sign as the earliest roentgenographic sign in the diagnosis of septic arthritis and tuberculosis of the hip. J Bone Joint Surg 24:857–869, 1942.
16. Pogrund H, Bloom R, Mogle P: The normal width of the adult hip joint: The relationship of age, sex, and obesity. Skeletal Radiol 10:10–12, 1983.
17. Reichmann S: Roentgenologic soft tissue appearances in hip joint disease. Acta Radiol [Diagn] 6:167–176, 1967.
18. Seltzer SE, Finberg HJ, Weissman BN: Arthrosonography—technique, sonographic anatomy and pathology. Invest Radiol 15:19–28, 1980.
19. Weston WJ: Synovial lesions in the adult hip joint in rheumatoid arthritis. Acta Radiol [Diagn]10:326–331, 1970.
20. Wilson DJ, Green DJ, MacLarnon JC: Arthrosonography of the painful hip. Clin Radiol 35:17–19, 1984.
21. Evans WA Jr: The roentgenological demonstration of the true articular space with particular reference to the knee joint and the internal semilunar cartilage. AJR 43:860–864, 1940.
22. Gershon-Cohen J: Internal derangements of the knee joint. The diagnostic scope of soft tissue roentgen examinations and the vacuum technique demonstration of the menisci. AJR 54:338–347, 1945.

Arthrography
23. Jacobs P, Goei The HS, Bijlsma A, et al.: Rheumatoid synovial cyst of the hip. Letter. Arthritis Rheum 26:814–815, 1983.
24. Klein A, Sumner TE, Volberg FM, Orbon RJ: Combined CT-arthrography in recurrent traumatic hip dislocation. AJR 138:963–964, 1982.
25. Lequesne M, Becker J, Bard M, Witvoet J, et al.: Capsular constriction of the hip. Arthrographic and clinical considerations. Skeletal Radiol 6:1–10, 1981.
26. Martel W, Poznanski AK: The value of traction during roentgenography of the hip. Radiology 94:497–503, 1970.
27. McCauley RGK, Wunderlich BK, Zimbler S: Air embolism as a complication of hip arthrography. Skeletal Radiol 6:11–13, 1981.
28. Murphy WA, Siegel MS, Gilula LA: Arthrography in the diagnosis of unexplained chronic hip pain with regional osteopenia. AJR 129:283–287, 1977.
29. Razzano CD, Nelson CL, Wilde AH: Arthrography of the adult hip. Clin Orthop 99:86–94, 1974.
30. Schmidt RM, Rosenkranz HS: Antimicrobial activity of local anesthetics lidocaine and procaine. J Infect Dis 121:597–607, 1970.
31. Staple TW: Arthrographic demonstration of iliopsoas bursa. Radiology 102:515–516, 1972.

Bony Structures
32. Armbuster TG, Guerra J Jr, Resnick D, et al.: The adult hip: An anatomic study. Part 1. The bony landmarks. Radiology 128:1–10, 1978.
33. Griffin JB: The calcar femorale redefined. Clin Orthop 164:211–214, 1982.
34. Harty M: The calcar femorale and the femoral neck. J Bone Joint Surg (Am) 39:625–630, 1957.
35. Johnstone WH, Keats TE, Lee ME: The anatomic basis for the superior acetabular roof notch 'superior acetabular notch'. Skeletal Radiol 8:25–27, 1982.
36. Jowsey J: Metabolic Diseases of Bone. Philadelphia, WB Saunders, 1977: 99–101.
37. Osborne D, Effmann E, Broda K, Harrelson J: The development of the upper end of the femur, with special reference to its internal architecture. Radiology 137:71–76, 1980.
38. Pauwels F: Biomechanics of the Normal and Diseased Hip. Theoretical Foundation Technique and Results of Treatment. An Atlas. New York, Springer-Verlag, 1976: 34–37.
39. Singh M, Nagrath AR, Maini PS: Changes in trabecular pattern of the upper end of the femur as an index of osteoporosis. J Bone Joint Surg (Am) 52:457–467, 1970.
40. Singh M, Riggs BL, Beabout JW, et al.: Femoral trabecular pattern index for evaluation of spinal osteoporosis: a detailed methodologic description. Mayo Clin Proc 48:189–194, 1973.

Anteversion
41. Billing L: Roentgen examination of the proximal femur end in children and adolescents. Acta Radiol [Suppl 110], 1954.
42. Budin E, Chandler E: Measurement of femoral neck anteversion by a direct method. Radiology 69: 209–213, 1957.
43. Chevrot A: Technique radiologique simplifiée dans la mesure de l'angle d'antéversion du fémur et de l'angle cervico-diaphysaire. J Radiol (Frc) 57:545–548, 1976.
44. Dunlap K, Shands AR Jr, Hollister LC Jr, et al.: A new method for determination of torsion of the femur. J Bone Joint Surg (Am) 35:289–311, 1953.

45. Dunn DM: Anteversion of the neck of the femur. A method of measurement. J Bone Joint Surg (Br) 34:181–186, 1952.

46. Edgren W, Laurent LE: A method of measuring the torsion of the femur in congenital dislocation of the hip in children. Acta Radiol 45:371–376, 1956.

47. Hernandez RJ, Tachdjian MO, Noznanski AK: CT determination of femoral torsion. AJR 137:97–101, 1981.

48. Hubbard DD, Staheli LT: The direct radiographic measurement of femoral torsion using axial tomography: technic comparison with an indirect radiographic method. Clin Orthop 86:16–20, 1972.

49. LaGasse DJ, Stahell LT: The measurement of femoral anteversion: A comparison of the fluoroscopic and biplane roentgenographic methods of measurement. Clin Orthop 86:13–15, 1972.

50. Magilligan DJ: Calculation of the angle of anteversion by means of horizontal lateral roentgenography. J Bone Joint Surg (Am) 38:1231–1246, 1956.

51. Ogata K, Goldsand EM: A simple biplanar method of measuring femoral anteversion and neck-shaft angle. J Bone Joint Surg (Am) 61:846–851, 1979.

52. Ozonoff MB: Calculation of Femoral Anteversion. Pediatric Orthopedic Radiology. Philadelphia, WB Saunders, 1979: 481–484.

53. Reynolds TG, Herzer FE: Anteversion of the femoral neck. Clin Orthop 14:80–88, 1959.

54. Rogers SP: A method for determining the angle of torsion of the neck of the femur. J Bone Joint Surg 13:821–824, 1931.

55. Rogers SP: Observations of torsion of the femur. J Bone Joint Surg 16:824–829, 1934.

56. Ruby L, Mital MA, O'Connor J, Patel U: Anteversion of the femoral neck. Comparison of methods of measurement in patients. J Bone Joint Surg (Am) 61:46–51, 1979.

57. Ryder CT, Crane L: Measuring femoral anteversion: the problem and a method. J Bone Joint Surg (Am) 35:321–328, 1953.

58. Stewart SF, Karshner RG: Congenital dislocation of the hip: a method of determining the degree of antetorsion of the femoral neck. AJR 15:258–260, 1926.

59. Vanhoutte JJ, Raeside DE: A generalization of Chevrot's method for determining anteversion and cervicodiaphyseal angles. Radiology 128:251–252, 1978.

60. Weiner DS, Cook AJ, Hoyt WA Jr, et al.: Computed tomography in the measurement of femoral anteversion. Orthopedics 1:299–306, 1978.

Soft Tissue Abnormalities: Cartilage-Space Narrowing in Adults

61. Dwosh IL, Resnick D, Becker MA: Hip involvement in ankylosing spondylitis. Arthritis Rheum 19:683–692, 1976.

62. Martel W, Braunstein EM: The diagnostic value of buttressing of the femoral neck. Arthritis Rheum 21:161–164, 1978.

63. Resnick D: Patterns of migration of the femoral head in osteoarthritis of the hip. Roentgenographic-pathologic correlation and comparison with rheumatoid arthritis. AJR 124:62–74, 1975.

Intracapsular Fractures

64. Albright JP, Weinstein SL: Treatment for fixation complications: femoral neck fractures. Arch Surg 110:30–36, 1975.

65. Arnold WD, Lyden JP, Minkoff J: Treatment of intracapsular fractures of the femoral neck: with special reference to percutaneous Knowles pinning. J Bone Joint Surg (Am) 56:254–262, 1974.

66. Askin SR, Bryan RS: Femoral neck fractures in young adults. Clin Orthop 114:259–264, 1976.

67. Baker GI, Barrick EF: Follow-up notes on articles previously published in the journal: Deyerle treatment for femoral neck fractures. J Bone Joint Surg (Am) 60:269–271, 1978.

68. Banks HH: Factors influencing the result in fractures of the femoral neck. J Bone Joint Surg (Am) 44:931–964, 1962.

69. Banks HH: Nonunion in fractures of the femoral neck. Orthop Clin North Am 5:865–885, 1974.

70. Barnes R, Brown JT, Garden RS, Nicoll EA: Subcapital fractures of the femur: a prospective review. J Bone Joint Surg (Br) 58:2–24, 1976.

71. Barr JS Jr: Experiences with a sliding nail in femoral neck fractures. Clin Orthop 92:63–67, 1973.

72. Barr JS Jr: Diagnosis and treatment of infections following internal fixation of hip fractures. Orthop Clin North Am 5:847–864, 1974.

73. Bentley G: The case for internal fixation of impacted femoral neck fractures. Orthop Clin North Am 5:729–742, 1974.

74. Bingold AC: The science of pinning the neck of the femur. Ann R Coll Surg Engl 59:463–469, 1977.

75. Brodell JD, Leve AR: Disengagement and intrapelvic protrusion of the screw from a sliding screw-plate device. J Bone Joint Surg (Am) 65:697–700, 1983.

76. Casteleyn PP, Melon C, Opdecam P: Treatment of intracapsular femoral neck fractures by femoral prostheses. Acta Orthop Belg 43:693–701, 1977.

77. Chapman MW, Stehr JH, Eberle CF, et al.: Treatment of intracapsular hip fractures by the Deyerle method: a comparative review of one hundred and nineteen cases. J Bone Joint Surg (Am) 57:735–744, 1975.

78. Colbert DS, Chater EH, Wilson AL, et al.: A study of fracture of the neck of the femur in the west of Ireland. 1968–1973. Ir Med J 17:1–12, 1976.

78a. Deyerle WM: Absolute fixation with contact compression in hip fractures (a new fixation device). Clin Orthop 13:279–298, 1959.

79. Dozier JK Jr: Fractures of the femoral neck: a review article. Tex Med 73:50–57, 1977.

80. Duncan TR, Gerlock AJ Jr, Muhletaler CA, et al.: Pseudopathologic hip fracture: anatomic explanation. AJR 135:801–802, 1980.

81. Dykes RG: Gas gangrene after hip nailing. Aust NZ J Surg 47:790–792, 1977.

82. El-Khoury GY, Wehbe MA, Bonfiglio M, et al.: Stress fractures of the femoral neck: a roentgen sign for early diagnosis. Skeletal Radiol 6:271–273, 1981.

83. Fielding JW: Pugh nail fixation of displaced femoral neck fractures: a long term follow-up. Clin Orthop 106:107–116, 1975.

84. Frandsen PA, Jorgensen F: Osteosynthesis of medial fractures of the femoral neck by sliding nail-plate fixation. Acta Orthop Scand 48:57–62, 1977.

85. Garden RS: Selective surgery in medial fractures of the femoral neck: a review. Injury 9:5–7, 1977.

86. Garden RS: Low angle fixation in fractures of the femoral neck. J Bone Joint Surg (Br) 43:647–663, 1961.

87. Garden RS: Stability and union in subcapital fractures of the femur. J Bone Joint Surg (Br) 46:630–647, 1964.

88. Garden RS: Malreduction and avascular necrosis in subcapital fractures of the femur. J Bone Joint Surg (Br) 53:183–197, 1971.

89. Garden RS: Reduction and fixation of subcapital frac-

tures of the femur. Orthop Clin North Am 5:683–712, 1974.

90. Heppenstall RB: Fractures and dislocations of the hip. *In* Heppenstall RB, ed. Fracture Treatment and Healing. Philadelphia, WB Saunders, 1980.

91. Hunter G: Treatment of fractures of the neck of the femur. CMA Journal 117:60–61, 1977.

92. Jacobs B, Wade PA, Match R: Intracapsular fracture of the femoral neck treated by the Pugh nail. J Trauma 5:751–960, 1965.

93. Jarry L: Transarticular nailing for fractures of the femoral neck: a preliminary report. J Bone Joint Surg (Br) 46:674–676, 1964.

94. Jeffery CC: Spontaneous fractures of the femoral neck. Orthop Clin North Am 5:713–727, 1974.

95. Johnson JTH, Crothers O: Nailing versus prosthesis for femoral-neck fractures: A critical review of long-term results in two hundred and thirty-nine consecutive private patients. J Bone Joint Surg (Am) 57:686–692, 1975.

96. Knowles FL: Fracture of the neck of the femur. Wis Med J 35:106–109, 1936.

97. Lowell JD: Fractures of the hip. N Engl J Med 274:1418–1425, 1966.

98. Lowell JD: Fractures of the hip (concluded). N Engl J Med 271:1480–1489, 1966.

99. Massie WK: Functional fixation of femoral neck fractures: telescoping nail technic. Clin Orthop 12:230–255, 1958.

100. Matin P: The appearance of bone scans following fractures, including immediate and long-term studies. J Nucl Med 20:1227–1231, 1979.

101. McElvenny RT: Roentgenographic interpretation of what constitutes adequate reduction of femoral neck fractures. Surg Gynecol Obstet 80:97–106, 1945.

102. McNeill DH: Hip fractures—influence of delay in surgery on mortality. Wis Med J 74:129–130, 1975.

103. Meyers MH, Harvey JP Jr, Moore TM: Delayed treatment of subcapital and transcervical fractures of the neck of the femur with internal fixation and a muscle pedicle bone graft. Orthop Clin North Am 5:743–756, 1974.

104. Meyers MH, Harvey JP Jr, Moore TM: The muscle pedicle bone graft in the treatment of displaced fractures of the femoral neck: indications, operative technique, and results. Orthop Clin North Am 5:779–792, 1974.

105. Meyers MH, Downey NT, Moore TM: Determination of the vascularity of the femoral head with technetium 99m-sulphur colloid: diagnostic and prognostic significance. J Bone Joint Surg (Am) 59:658–664, 1977.

106. Muckle DS: Fractures of the femoral neck. *In* Muckle DS, ed. Femoral Neck Fractures and Hip Joint Injuries. New York, John Wiley, 1977.

107. Naimark A, Lander P: The tumbling bolt. A new sign of deep soft-tissue abscess following Richards fixation. Radiology 129:30, 1978.

108. Nieminen S, Satokari K: Classification of medical fractures of the femoral neck. Acta Orthop Scand 46:775–781, 1975.

109. Pope TL Jr, Keats TE, Stelling CB, et al.: Pseudopathologic fracture of the femoral neck. Skeletal Radiol 7:129–131, 1981.

110. Roback DL: Posttraumatic osteolysis of the femoral neck. AJR 134:1243–1244, 1980.

111. Rosen JF, Wolin DA, Finberg L: Immobilization hypercalcemia after single limb fractures in children and adolescents. Am J Dis Child 132:560–564, 1978.

112. Salvati EA, Artz T, Aglietti P, et al.: Endoprostheses in the treatment of femoral neck fractures. Orthop Clin North Am 5:757–777, 1974.

113. Schultz RJ: The Language of Fractures. Baltimore, Williams & Wilkins, 1972.

114. Shaw JA: Preventing unrecognized pin penetration into hip joint. Orthop Rev 13:142–152, 1984.

115. Sisk TD: Fractures. *In* Edmonson AS, Crenshaw AH, eds. Campbell's Operative Orthopaedics. St. Louis, CV Mosby, 1980.

116. Sunami Y, Nagano K, Hara Y, et al.: A new nail-plate for treatment of fracture of the neck of the femur. Acta Med Okayama 31:383–391, 1977.

117. Takagi LR, Lerch JW: Dystocia and broad ligament hematoma secondary to hip pinning. J Reprod Med 14:80–81, 1975.

118. Tronzo RG: Hip nails for all occasions. Orthop Clin North Am 5:479–491, 1974.

119. Volz RG, Martin MD: Illusory biplane radiographic images. Radiology 122:695–697, 1977.

120. Walters R, Simon SR: Joint destruction, a sequel of unrecognized pin penetration in patients with slipped capital femoral epiphyses. *In* Hip Society, Open Scientific Meeting, 8th. The Hip: Proceedings, St. Louis, CV Mosby, 1980.

121. Weinstein SL: Femoral neck fractures: complications of internal fixation. J Iowa Med Soc 65:17–20, 1975.

122. Zuckerman JD: The internal fixation of intracapsular hip fractures. A review of the first one hundred years. Orthop Rev 11:85–95, 1982.

Extracapsular Fractures

123. Ashby ME, Anderson JC: The use of the Zickel device for a malunited subtrochanteric femur fracture. J Natl Med Assoc 69:623–624, 1977.

124. Baker DM: Fractures of the femoral neck after healed intertrochanteric fractures: a complication of too short a nail plate fixation. Report of three cases. J Trauma 15:73–81, 1975.

125. Beaver RH, Back PH: Zickel nail: a retrospective study of subtrochanteric fractures. South Med J 71:146–149, 1978.

126. Bisla RS, Louis HJ: Intertrochanteric fracture of the hip. Ariz Med 32:401–407, 1975.

127. Boyd HB, Griffin LL: Classification and treatment of trochanteric fractures. Arch Surg 58:853–866, 1949.

128. Clawson DK: Trochanteric fractures treated by the sliding screw plate fixation method. J Trauma 4:737–752, 1964.

129. Cuthbert H, Howat TW: The use of the Kuntscher Y nail in the treatment of intertrochanteric and subtrochanteric fractures of the femur. Injury 8:135–142, 1976.

130. Dimon JH III, Hughston JC: Unstable intertrochanteric fractures of the hip. J Bone Joint Surg (Am) 49:440–450, 1967.

131. Doppelt SH: The sliding compression screw—today's best answer for stabilization of intertrochanteric hip fractures. Orthop Clin North Am 11:507–523, 1980.

132. Ebong WW: False aneurysm of the profunda femoris artery following internal fixation of an intertrochanteric femoral fracture. Injury 9:249–251, 1978.

133. Evans EM: The treatment of trochanteric fractures of the femur. J Bone Joint Surg (Br) 31:190–203, 1949.

134. Fielding JW, Magliato HJ: Subtrochanteric fractures. Surg Gynecol Obstet 122:555–560, 1966.

135. Flynn M: A new method of reduction of fractures of the neck of the femur based on anatomical studies of the hip joint. Injury 5:309–317, 1974.

136. Hanson GW, Tullos HS: Subtrochanteric fractures of

the femur treated with nail-plate devices: a retrospective study. Clin Orthop 131:191–194, 1978.

137. Holland WR, Weiss AB, Daniel WW: Medial displacement osteotomy for unstable intertrochanteric femoral fractures. South Med J 70:576–578, 1977.

138. Hughston JC: Intertrochanteric fractures of the femur (hip). Orthop Clin North Am 5:585–600, 1974.

139. Hunter GA, Mehta A: Subcapital fracture of the hip: a rare complication of intertrochanteric fracture of the femur. Can J Surg 20:165–169, 1977.

140. Hunter GA, Krajbich IJ: The results of medial displacement osteotomy for unstable intertrochanteric fractures of the femur. Clin Orthop 137:140–145, 1978.

141. Hunter GA: The results of operative treatment of trochanteric fractures of the femur. Injury 6:202–205, 1975.

142. Jacobs RR, Armstrong HJ, Whitaker JH, et al.: Treatment of intertrochanteric hip fractures with a compression hip screw and a nail plate. J Trauma 15:599–603, 1976.

143. Jensen JS: A photoelastic study of a model of the proximal femur. A biomechanical study of unstable trochanteric fractures I. Acta Orthop Scand 49:54–59, 1978.

144. Jensen JS: A photoelastic study of the hip nail-plate in unstable trochanteric fractures: A biomechanical study of unstable trochanteric fractures II. Acta Orthop Scand 49:60–64, 1978.

145. Kaufer H, Matthews LS, Sonstegard DA: Fixation mechanics of intertrochanteric fracture. *In* The Hip Society, Open Scientific Meeting, 6th. The Hip: Proceedings, vol 6. St. Louis, CV Mosby, 1978.

146. Kolind-Sorensen V: Comminuted intertrochanteric fracture of· the femoral neck. Acta Orthop Scand 46:651–653, 1975.

147. Laros GS: Current views of hip fracture: a symposium on hip fracture. Arch Surg 110:18–19, 1975.

148. Lowell JD: Trochanteric fractures: clinical implications and management. The Hip Society, Open Scientific Meeting, 6th. The Hip: Proceedings, vol 6. St. Louis, CV Mosby, 1978.

149. Modny MT, Kaiser AJ: A special guide for insertion of multiple pins for fracture of the hip: experience with 200 cases. Clin Orthop 137:144–147, 1978.

150. Morrison D, Mrstik LL, Weingarden TL: Management of unstable intertrochanteric fractures of the hip. J Am Orthop Assoc 77:793, 802, 1978.

151. Muckle DS: Fractures of the femoral neck. *In* Muckle DS, ed. Femoral Neck Fractures and Hip Joint Injuries. New York, John Wiley, 1977.

152. Mulholland RC, Gunn DR; Sliding screw plate fixation of intertrochanteric femoral fractures. J Trauma 12:581–591, 1972.

153. Peltier LF: The diagnosis of fractures of the hip and femur by ausculatatory percussion. Clin Orthop 123:9–11, 1977.

154. Puranen J, Koivisto E: Perforation of the urinary bladder and small intestine caused by a trochanteric plate. Acta Orthop Scand 49:65–67, 1978.

155. Rennie W, Mitchall N: Compression fixation of peritrochanteric fractures and early weight-bearing. Clin Orthop 121:157–162, 1976.

156. Sarmiento A: Intertrochanteric fractures of the femur. 150–degree-angle fixation and early rehabilitation: a preliminary report of 100 cases. J Bone Joint Surg (Am) 45:706–722, 1963.

157. Sarmiento A: Unstable intertrochanteric fractures of the femur. Clin Orthop 92:77–85, 1972.

158. Sarmiento A, Williams EM: The unstable intertrochanteric fracture: treatment with a valgus osteotomy and

159. Schatzker J, Ha'eri GB, Chapman M: Methylmethacrylate as an adjunct in the internal fixation of intertrochanteric fractures of the femur. J Trauma 18:732–735, 1978.

160. Seinsheimer F: Subtrochanteric fractures of the femur. J Bone Joint Surg (Am) 60:300–306, 1978.

161. Shelton ML: Subtrochanteric fractures of the femur. Arch Surg 110:41–48, 1975.

162. Sonstegard DA, Kaufer H, Matthews LS: A biomechanical evaluation of implant, reduction, and prosthesis in the treatment of intertrochanteric hip fractures. Orthop Clin North Am 5:551–570, 1974.

163. Stevens DB: Method of operative treatment for intertrochanteric fracture of the femur. Curr Pract Orthop Surg 7:56–77, 1977.

164. Tronzo RG: Symposium on fractures of the hip. Special considerations in management. Orthop Clin North Am 5:571–583, 1974.

165. Valasco RU, Comfort TH: Analysis of treatment problems in subtrochanteric fractures of the femur. J Trauma 18:513–523, 1978.

166. Wang C-J: False aneurysm of the profundus femoral artery following nail-plate fixation for intertrochanteric fracture of the hip. J Med Soc NJ 72:623–624, 1975.

167. Wolfgang GL: Stress fracture of the femoral neck in a patient with open capital femoral epiphyses: A case report. J Bone Joint Surg (Am) 59:680–681, 1977.

168. Zickel RE: An intramedullary fixation device for the proximal part of the femur: nine years' experience. J Bone Joint Surg 58:866–872, 1976.

169. Zickel RE, Mouradian WH: Intramedullary fixation of pathological fractures and lesions of the subtrochanteric region of the femur. J Bone Joint Surg (Am) 58:1061–1066, 1976.

Ender's Nailing

170. Bohler N, Kuderna H: Ergebnisse der Endernagelung in Osterreich unter spezieller Berucksichtigung der Falle des Lorenz-Bohler-Krankenhauses. Arch Orthop 88:339–346, 1977.

171. Corzatt RD, Bosch AV: Internal fixation by the Ender method. JAMA 240:1366–1367, 1978.

172. Ender HG: Treatment of pertrochanteric and subtrochanteric fractures of the femur with Ender pins. *In* The Hip Society, Open Scientific Meeting, 6th. The Hip: Proceedings, vol 6. St. Louis, CV Mosby, 1978:187–205.

173. Harris LJ: Condylocephalic nailing of proximal femoral fractures. *In* Evarts CM, ed. AAOS Instructional Course Lectures. St. Louis, CV Mosby, 1983.

174. Herrero FC, Birchs JV, Beltran JE: Condylocephalic nail fixation for trochanteric fractures of the femur: surgical technique and complications. Orthop Clin North Am 5:669–678, 1974.

175. Kuderna H, Bohler N, Collon DJ: Treatment of intertrochanteric and subtrochanteric fractures of the hip by the Ender method. J Bone Joint Surg (Am) 58:604–611, 1976.

176. Von Küntscher U: Zur operativen behandlung der pertrochanteren fractur. Zentralbl Chir 91:281–285, 1966.

177. Poigenfurst J, Schnabl P: Multiple intramedullary nailing of pertrochanteric fractures with elastic nails: operative procedure and results. Injury 9:102–113, 1977.

178. Skilbred LA: Internal fixation by the Ender method. Letter. JAMA 241:1106, 1979.

179. Wynn Jones C, Morris J, Hirschowitz D, Hart GM, Shea J, Arden GP: A comparison of the treatment of

trochanteric fractures of the femur by internal fixation with a nail plate and the Ender technique. Injury: 9:35–42, 1977.

Osteonecrosis

180. Arnoldi CC, Lemperg RK: Fracture of the femoral neck. II. Relative importance of primary vascular damage and surgical procedure for the development of necrosis of the femoral head. Clin Orthop 129:217–222, 1977.
181. Aufranc OE, Jones WN, Harris WH: Undisplaced femoral neck fracture. JAMA 189:314–317, 1964.
182. Bauer GCH: Radiopharmaceutical Imaging of Osteonecrosis of the Femoral Head. *In* The Hip Society, Open Scientific Meeting, 7th. Proceedings, vol 7. St. Louis, CV Mosby, 1979.
183. Bayliss AP, Davidson JK: Traumatic osteonecrosis of the femoral head following intracapsular fracture: incidence and earliest radiological features. Clin Radiol 28:407–414, 1977.
184. Bobechko WP, Harris WR: The radiographic density of avascular bone. J Bone Joint Surg (Br) 42:626–632, 1960.
185. Bohr H, Geerfordt J: Autoradiography and histology in a case of idiopathic femoral head necrosis. Clin Orthop 129:209–212, 1977.
186. Catto M: The histological appearances of late segmental collapse of the femoral head after transcervical fracture. J Bone Joint Surg (Br) 47:777–791, 1965.
187. Catto M: A histological study of avascular necrosis of the femoral head after transcervical fracture. J Bone Joint Surg (Br) 47:749–776, 1965.
188. Coleman SS: Aseptic necrosis of bone due to trauma. Orthop Clin North Am 5:819–831, 1974.
189. Conklin JJ, Alderson PO, Zizic TM, et al.: Comparison of bone scan and radiograph sensitivity in the detection of steroid-induced ischemic necrosis of bone. Radiology 147:221–226, 1983.
190. D'Ambrosia RD, Shoji H, Riggins RS, et al.: Scintigraphy in the diagnosis of osteonecrosis. Clin Orthop 130:139–143, 1978.
191. Danigelis J, Fisher R, Ozonoff M, et al.: Tc-99m polyphosphate bone imaging in Legg-Perthes disease. Radiology 115:407–413, 1979.
192. Deutsch SD, Gandsman EJ, Sparagen SC: Quantitative regional blood-flow analysis and its clinical application during routine bone scanning. J Bone Joint Surg (Am) 63:295–305, 1981.
193. Dihlmann W: CT analysis of the upper end of the femur: the asterisk sign and ischemic bone necrosis of the femoral head. Skeletal Radiol 8:251–258, 1982.
194. Edeiken J, Hodes PJ, Libshitz HI, et al.: Bone ischemia. Radiol Clin North Am 5:515–529, 1967.
195. Enneking WF: The choice of surgical procedures in idiopathic aseptic necrosis. *In* The Hip Society, Open Scientific Meeting, 7th. The Hip: Proceedings, vol 7. St. Louis, CV Mosby, 1979.
196. Ficat RP, Arlet J: Ischemia and Necroses of Bone. Baltimore, Williams & Wilkins, 1980.
197. Glimcher MJ, Kenzora JE: The biology of osteonecrosis of the human femoral head and its clinical implications: an abridged communication. Clin Orthop 130:47–50, 1978.
198. Glimcher MJ, Kenzora JE: The biology of osteonecrosis of the human femoral head and its clinical implications. I. Tissue biology. Clin Orthop 138:284–309, 1979.
199. Glimcher MJ, Kenzora JE: The biology of osteonecrosis of the human femoral head and its clinical implications. II. The pathological changes in the femoral head as an organ and in the hip joint. Clin Orthop 139:283–312, 1979.
200. Glimcher MJ, Kenzora JE: The biology of osteonecrosis of the human femoral head and its clinical implications. III. Discussion of the etiology and genesis of the pathological sequelae; comments on treatment. Clin Orthop 140:273–312, 1979.
201. Hulth A: The vessel anatomy of the upper femur end with special regard to the mechanism of origin of different vascular disorders. Acta Orthop Scand 27:192–209, 1958.
202. Hulth A: Necrosis of the head of the femur: a roentgenological microradiographic and histological study. Acta Chir Scand 122:75–84, 1961.
203. Hungerford DS: Bone marrow pressure, venography, and core decompression in ischemic necrosis of the femoral head. *In* The Hip Society, Open Scientific Meeting, 7th. The Hip: Proceedings, vol 7. St. Louis, CV Mosby, 1979.
204. Hungerford DS, Zizk TM: Alcoholism associated ischemic necrosis of the femoral head. Early diagnosis and treatment. Clin Orthop 130:144–153, 1978.
205. Jacobs B: Epidemiology of traumatic and nontraumatic osteonecrosis. Clin Orthop 130:51–67, 1978.
206. Jaffe HL: Ischemic necrosis of bone. Med Radiogr Photogr 45:58–88, 1969.
207. Johnson JTH, Crothers O: Revascularization of the femoral head: a clinical and experimental study. Clin Orthop 114:364–373, 1976.
208. Korvald E, Sundsfjord AJ: Examination of the vascular disturbance of the femoral head following intracapsular fracture of the hip: a preliminary report using a new isotope complex. Acta Orthop Scand 45:572–578, 1974.
209. Martel W, Poznanski AK: The effect of traction on the hip in osteonecrosis: a comment on the "radiolucent crescent line." Radiology 94:505–508, 1970.
210. Martel W, Sitterley BH: Roentgenologic manifestations of osteonecrosis. Radiology 106:509–522, 1969.
211. Meyers MH: The treatment of osteonecrosis of the hip with fresh osteochondral allografts and with the muscle pedical graft technique. Clin Orthop 130:202–209, 1978.
212. Muckle DS, Bentley G, Deane G, Kemp FH: Basic sciences of the hip. *In* Muckle DS, ed. Femoral Neck Fractures and Hip Joint Injuries. New York, John Wiley, 1977.
213. Norman A, Bullough P: The radiolucent crescent line—an early diagnostic sign of avascular necrosis of the femoral head. Bull Hosp Jt Dis 24:99–104, 1963.
214. Outerbridge RE: Perosseous venography in the diagnosis of viability in subcapital fractures of the femur. Clin Orthop 137:132–139, 1978.
215. Phemister DB: Treatment of the necrotic head of the femur in adults. J Bone Joint Surg (Am) 31:55–66, 1949.
216. Rokkanen P, Slatis P: Devitalization of the femoral head after medial fracture of the femoral neck. Acta Orthop Scand 45:564–671, 1974.
217. Sevitt S: Avascular necrosis and revascularisation of the femoral head after intracapsular fractures: a combined arteriographic and histological necropsy study. J Bone Joint Surg (Br) 46B:270–296, 1964.
218. Sevitt S, Thompson RG: The distribution and anastomoses of arteries supplying the head and neck of the femur. J Bone Joint Surg (Br) 27:560–573, 1965.
219. Siegel BA, Donovan RL, Alderson PO, et al.: Skeletal uptake of 99mTc-diphosphonate in relation to local bone blood flow. Radiology 120:121–123, 1976.
220. Theron J: Superselective angiography of the hip:

technique, normal features, and early results in idiopathic necrosis of the femoral head. Radiology 124:649–657, 1977.
221. Trueta J, Harrison MHM: The normal vascular anatomy of the femoral head in adult man. J Bone Joint Surg (Br) 35:442–461, 1953.
222. Williams JL, Cliff MM, Bonakdarpour A: Spontaneous osteonecrosis of the knee. Radiology 107:15–19, 1973.

Osteotomy
223. Adam A, Spence AJ: Intertrochanteric osteotomy for osteoarthritis of the hip: a review of fifty-eight operations. J Bone Joint Surg (Br) 40:219–226, 1958.
224. Bombelli R: Osteoarthritis of the Hip. Pathogenesis and Consequent Therapy. New York, Springer-Verlag, 1976.
225. Bombelli R: Osteoarthritis of the Hip. Classification and Pathogenesis: the Role of Osteotomy As a Consequent Therapy. 2nd ed. New York, Springer-Verlag, 1983.
226. Braunstein EM, Weissman BN, Sosman JL, et al.: Complications of intertrochanteric rotational osteotomy. Skeletal Radiol 10:258–261, 1983.
227. Ferguson AB Jr: High intertrochanteric osteotomy for osteoarthritis of the hip: a procedure to streamline the defective joint. J Bone Joint Surg (Am) 46:1159–1175, 1964.
228. Ford LT: Osteotomies: nomenclature and uses. Radiol Clin North Am 13:79–92, 1975.
229. McMurray TP: Osteo-arthritis of the hip joint. J Bone Joint Surg 21:1–11, 1939.
230. Pauwels F: Biomechanics of the Normal and Diseased Hip. Theoretical Foundation, Technique and Results of Treatment. An Atlas. New York, Springer-Verlag, 1976:146–164.
231. Poss R: Current concepts review. The role of osteotomy in the treatment of osteoarthritis of the hip. J Bone Joint Surg (Am) 66:144–151, 1984.
232. Reigstad A, Gronmark T: Osteoarthritis of the hip treated by intertrochanteric osteotomy. J Bone Joint Surg (Am) 66:1–6, 1984.
233. Sugioka Y: Transtrochanteric anterior rotational osteotomy of the femoral head in the treatment of osteonecrosis affecting the hip: a new osteotomy operation. Clin Orthop 130:191–201, 1978.

Mold Arthroplasty
234. Aufranc OE: Constructive hip surgery with the vitallium mold: A report on 1,000 cases of arthroplasty of the hip over a fifteen-year period. J Bone Joint Surg (Am) 39:237–248, 1957.
235. Clouse ME, Aufranc OE, Weber AL: Roentgenologic and clinical evaluation of vitallium mold arthroplasty of the hip. Surg Gynecol Obstet 127:1042–1050, 1968.
236. Gibson A, Williams TH: Changes in the femoral head underlying a vitallium cup. J Bone Joint Surg (Br) 33:119–121, 1951.
237. Hamblen DL, Harris WH: Myositis ossificans as a complication of hip arthroplasty. J Bone Joint Surg (Br) 53:764, 1971.
238. Harmon PH: Arthroplasty of the hip for osteoarthritis utilizing foreign-body cups of plastic. Surg Gynecol Obstet 12:347–365, 1943.
239. Law WA: Late results in vitallium-mold arthroplasty of the hip. J Bone Joint Surg (Am) 44:1497–1517, 1962.
240. Smith-Petersen MN: Evolution of mold arthroplasty of the hip joint. J Bone Joint Surg (Br) 30:59–75, 1978.

Hemiarthroplasty
241. Anderson LD, Hamsa WR, Waring TL: Femoral-head prostheses. J Bone Joint Surg (Am) 46:1049–1065, 1964.
242. Andersson G, Nielsen JM: Results after arthroplasty of the hip with Moore's prosthesis. Acta Orthop 43:397–410, 1972.
243. Apley AG, Millner WF, Porter DS: A follow-up study of Moore's arthroplasty in the treatment of osteoarthritis of the hip. J Bone Joint Surg (Br) 51:638–647, 1969.
244. Buxton JD, Waugh W: Radiographic bone changes at the hip after insertion of an acrylic prosthesis. J Bone Joint Surg (Br) 36:50–56, 1954.
245. Freedman MT: Radiologic aspects of femoral head replacements and cup mold arthroplasties. Radiol Clin North Am 13:45–56, 1975.
246. Judet J, Judet R: The use of an artificial femoral head for arthroplasty of the hip joint. J Bone Joint Surg (Br) 32:166–173, 1950.
247. Moore AT: The self-locking metal hip prosthesis. J Bone Joint Surg (Am) 39:811–827, 1957.
248. Sarmiento A: Austin Moore prosthesis in the arthritic hip. Clin Orthop 82:14–23, 1972.
249. Thompson FR: Two-and-a-half years experience with a vitallium intramedullary hip prosthesis. J Bone Joint Surg (Am) 36:489–500, 1954.

Bipolar Endoprostheses
250. Anderson PR, Milgram JW: Dislocation and component separation of the Bateman hip endoprosthesis. JAMA 240:2079–2080, 1978.
251. Drinker H, Mall JC: Radiologic aspects of the new universal proximal femoral hip prosthesis. AJR 129:531–533, 1977.
252. Giliberty RP: Low-friction bipolar hip endoprosthesis. Int Surg 62:38–41, 1977.
253. Giliberty RP, Trenkle WA, Licon O: A retrospective study of the bipolar hip endoprosthesis. Orthop Rev 7:27–31, 1978.

Surface Replacement
254. Amstutz HC, Graff-Radford A, Gruen TA, et al.: Tharies surface replacements: a review of the first 100 cases. Clin Orthop 134:87–101, 1978.
255. Bierbaum BE, Sweet R: Complications of resurfacing arthroplasty. Orthop Clin North Am 13:761–765, 1982.
256. Cabanela ME, Campbell DC II, Henderson ED: Total joint arthroplasty. The hip. Mayo Clin Proc 54:559–563, 1979.
257. Capello WN, Wilson N, Wellman H: Bone imaging: a means of evaluating hip surface replacement arthroplasty. In The Hip Society, Open Scientific Meeting, 8th. The Hip: Proceedings, vol 8. St. Louis, CV Mosby, 1980.
258. Capello WN, Ireland PH, Trammell TR, et al.: Conservative total hip arthroplasty. A procedure to conserve bone stock. Part I. Analysis of sixty-six patients. Part II. Analysis of failures. Clin Orthop 134:59–74, 1978.
259. Freeman MAR: Some anatomical and mechanical considerations relevant to the surface replacement of the femoral head. Clin Orthop 134:19–24, 1978.
260. Freeman MAR, Cameron HU, Brown GC: Cemented double cup arthroplasty of the hip: a 5-year experience with the ICLH prosthesis. Clin Orthop 134: 45–52, 1978.
261. Furuya K, Tsuchiya M, Kawachi S: Socket-cup arthroplasty. Clin Orthop 134:41–44, 1978.

262. Hedley AK, Clarke IC, Bloebaum RD, Moreland J, Gruen T, Coster I, Amstutz HC: Viability and cement fixation of the femoral head in canine hip surface replacement. *In* The Hip Society, Open Scientific Meeting, 7th. The Hip: Proceedings, vol 7. St. Louis, CV Mosby, 1979.

263. Steinberg ME: Symposium on Surface Replacement Arthroplasty of the Hip. Orthop Clin North Am 13:661–666, 1982.

264. Trentani C, Vaccarino F: The Paltrinieri-Trentani hip joint resurface arthroplasty. Clin Orthop 134:36–40, 1978.

265. Wagner H: Surface replacement arthroplasty of the hip. Clin Orthop 134:104–130, 1978.

Total Hip Replacement

266. Amstutz HC, Markolf KL, McNeice GM, et al.: Loosening of total hip components: cause and prevention. *In* The Hip Society, Open Scientific Meeting, 4th. The Hip: Proceedings, vol 4. St. Louis, CV Mosby, 1976.

267. Anderson LS, Staple TW: Arthrography of total hip replacement using subtraction technique. Radiology 109:470–472, 1973.

268. Beabout JW: Radiology of total hip arthroplasty. Radiol Clin North Am 13:3–19, 1975.

269. Bechtol CO: Failure of femoral implant components in total hip replacement operations. Orthop Rev 4:23–29, 1975.

270. Beckenbaugh RD, Ilstrup DM: Total hip arthroplasty. A review of three hundred and thirty-three cases with long follow-up. J Bone Joint Surg (Am) 60:306–313, 1978.

271. Bergstrom B, Lindberg L, Persson BM, et al.: Complications after total hip arthroplasty according to Charnley in a Swedish series of cases. Clin Orthop 95:91–95, 1973.

272. Bone Ingrowth and Uncemented THPs. *In* Royal Society of Medicine. Symposium on Cementless Fixation of Implants. 1981.

273. Brooker AF, Bowerman JW, Robinson RA, et al.: Ectopic ossification following total hip replacement: incidence and a method of classification. J Bone Joint Surg (Am) 55:1629, 1973.

274. Burton DS, Propst-Proctor SL, Schurman DJ: Anesthetic hip arthrography in the diagnosis of postoperative hip pathology. Contemp Orthop 7:17–25, 1983.

275. Campbell RE, Marvel JP Jr: Concomitant dislocation and intraarticular foreign body: a rare complication of the Charnley total hip arthroplasty. AJR 126: 1059–1062, 1976.

276. Campeau RJ, Hall MF, Miale A Jr: Detection of total hip arthroplasty complications with Tc-99m pyrophosphate. J Nucl Med 17:526, 1976.

277. Casagrande PA, Danaby PR: Delayed sciatic-nerve entrapment following the use of self-curing acrylic. J Bone Joint Surg (Am) 53:167–169, 1971.

278. Chafetz N, Baumrind S, Murray WR, et al.: Femoral prosthesis subsidence in asymptomatic patients. A stereophotogrammetric assessment. Invest Radiol 19:235–241, 1984.

279. Chandler HP, Reneck T, Wixson RL, et al.: Total hip replacement in patients younger than thirty years. J Bone Joint Surg (Am) 63:1426–1434, 1981.

280. Charnley J, Cupic Z: The nine and ten year results of the low-friction arthroplasty of the hip. Clin Orthop 95:9–25, 1973.

281. Charnley J, Halley DK: Rate of wear in total hip replacement. Clin Orthop 112:170–171, 1975.

282. Clarke IC, Black K, Rennie C, et al.: Can wear in total hip arthroplasties be assessed from radiographs? Clin Orthop 121:126–142, 1976.

283. Collis DK: Femoral stem failure in total hip replacement. J Bone Joint Surg (Am) 59:1033–1041, 1977.

284. Cone RO, Yaru N, Resnick D, et al.: Intracapsular pressure monitoring during arthrographic evaluation of painful hip prosthesis. AJR 141:885–889, 1983.

285. Coren GS, Curtis J, Dalinka M: Lymphatic visualization during hip arthrography. Radiology 115:621–623, 1975.

286. Daffner RH, Carden TS Jr, Gehweiler JA: Complications of unrecognized dislocation of Charnley-Muller hip prosthesis. Importance of early roentgen diagnosis. Radiology 108:323–324, 1973.

287. DeLee JG, Charnley J: Radiological demarcation of cemented sockets in total hip replacement. Clin Orthop 121:20–32, 1976.

288. DeSmet AA, Kramer D, Martel W: The metal-cement interface in total hip prostheses. AJR 129:279–282, 1977.

289. Dolinskas C, Campbell RE, Rothman RH: The painful Charnley total hip replacement. AJR 121:61–68, 1974.

290. Dorr LD, Conaty JP, Kohl R, Harvey JP: False aneurysm of the femoral artery following total hip surgery. J Bone Joint Surg (Am) 56:1059–1062, 1974.

291. Drinker H, Mall JC: Radiologic aspects of the new universal proximal femoral hip prosthesis. AJR 129:531–533, 1977.

292. Drinker H, Turner RH, McKenzie JD, et al.: Color subtraction arthrography in the diagnosis of component loosening in hip arthroplasty. Orthopedics 1:224–229, 1978.

293. Dussault RG, Goldman AB, Ghelman G: Radiologic diagnosis of loosening and infection in hip prostheses. J Can Assoc Radiol 28:119–123, 1977.

294. Eftekhar N: Low-friction arthroplasty: indications, contraindications and complications. JAMA 218:705–710, 1971.

295. Evanski PM, Waugh TR, Orofino CF: Total hip replacement with the Charnley prosthesis. Clin Orthop 95:69–72, 1973.

296. Fackler CD, Poss R: Dislocation in total hip arthroplasties. Clin Orthop 151:169–178, 1980.

297. Feith R, Slooff TJ, Kazem I, et al.: Strontium 87mSR bone scanning for the evaluation of total hip replacement. J Bone Joint Surg (Br) 58:79–83, 1976.

298. Firooznia H, Baruch H, Seliger G, et al.: The value of subtraction in hip arthrography after total hip replacement. Bull Hosp Joint Dis 35:36–41, 1974.

299. Gelman MI: Arthrography in total hip prosthesis complications. AJR 126:743–750, 1976.

300. Gelman MI, Coleman RE, Stevens PM, et al.: Radiography, radionuclide imaging, and arthrography in the evaluation of total hip and knee replacement. Radiology 128:677–682, 1978.

301. Ghelman B: Radiographic localization of the acetabular component of a hip prosthesis. Radiology 130:540–542, 1979.

302. Giliberty RP: Low friction bipolar hip endoprosthesis. Int Surg 62:38–41, 1977.

303. Gilula LA, Staple TW: Miniature atlas of total hip prostheses. Radiol Clin North Am 13:21–44, 1975.

304. Georgen TG, Resnick D: Evaluation of acetabular anteversion following total hip arthroplasty: necessity of proper centering. Br J Radiol 48:259–260, 1975.

305. Goldring SR, Schiller AL, Roelke M, et al.: The synovial-like membrane at the bone-cement interface in loose total hip replacements and its proposed role

in bone lysis. J Bone Joint Surg (Am) 65:575–584, 1983.

306. Goodman L, McGee JW: Eccentric femoral heads in total hip prosthesis. Radiology 111:235, 1974.

307. Gore DR, Murray MP, Gardner GM, et al.: Roentgenographic measurements after Muller total hip replacement. J Bone Joint Surg (Am) 59:948–953, 1977.

308. Green DL: Complications of total hip replacement. South Med J 69:1559–1564, 1976.

309. Greenspan A, Norman A: Gross hematuria: a complication of intrapelvic cement intrusion in total hip replacement. AJR 130:327–329, 1978.

309a. Griffiths HJ, Lovelock JE, Evarts CM, et al.: The radiology of total hip replacement. Skeletal Radiol 12:1–11, 1984.

310. Gruen TA, McNeice GM, Amstutz HC: "Modes of failure" of cemented stem-type femoral components. A radiographic analysis of loosening. Clin Orthop 141:17–27, 1979.

311. Harris WH: Total joint replacement. N Engl J Med 297:650–651, 1977.

312. Harris WH, Jones WH: The use of wire mesh in total hip replacement surgery. Clin Orthop 106:117–121, 1975.

313. Harris WH, McCarthy JC Jr, O'Neill DA: Femoral component loosening using contemporary techniques of femoral cement fixation. J Bone Joint Surg (Am) 64:1063–1067, 1982.

314. Hendrix RW, Wixson RL, Rana NA, et al.: Arthrography after total hip arthroplasty: a modified technique used in the diagnosis of pain. Radiology 148:647–652, 1983.

315. Hirsch SA, Robertson H, Gorniowsky M: Arterial occlusion secondary to methylmethacrylate use. Arch Surg 111:204, 1976.

316. Hunter JC, Baumrind S, Genant HK, et al.: The detection of loosening in total hip arthroplasty: description of a stereophotogrammetric computer assisted method. Invest Radiol 14:323–329, 1979.

317. Jackson DM: Total hip prosthesis: real and apparent dislocation. Clin Radiol 26:63–65, 1975.

318. Lane EJ, Proto AV, Phillips TW: Mach bands and density perception. Radiology 121:9–17, 1976.

319. Ling RSM: Prevention of loosening of total hip components. In The Hip Society, Open Scientific Meeting, 8th. Riley LH Jr, ed. The Hip: Proceedings, vol 8. St. Louis, CV Mosby, 1980:292–307.

320. Lowell JD, Davies JAK, Bennett AH: Bladder fistula following total hip replacement using self-curing acrylic. Clin Orthop 111:131–133, 1975.

321. Magilligan DJ: Calculation of the angle of anteversion by means of horizontal lateral roentgenography. J Bone Joint Surg (Am) 38:1231–1246, 1956.

322. Markolf KL: In vitro and technical considerations in femoral component insertion. In The Hip Society, Open Scientific Meeting, 8th. Riley LH Jr, ed. The Hip: Proceedings, vol 8. St. Louis, CV Mosby, 1980:121–141.

323. Martens M, Aernoudt E, de Meester P, et al.: Factors in the mechanical failure of the femoral component in total hip prosthesis: report of six fatigue fractures of the femoral stem and results of experimental loading tests. Acta Orthop Scand 45:693–710, 1974.

324. Matisonn A, Weber FA: Radiological assessment of the Charnley total hip arthroplasty. S Afr Med J 49:1299–1302, 1975.

325. McElfresh EC, Coventry MB: Femoral and pelvic fractures after total hip arthroplasty. J Bone Joint Surg (Am) 56:483–492, 1974.

326. McInerney DP, Hyde ID: Technetium 99Tcm pyro-phosphate scanning in the assessment of the painful hip prosthesis. Clin Radiol 29:513–517, 1978.

327. McLaren RH: Prosthetic hip angulation. Radiology 107:705–706, 1973.

328. McLaughlin RE, Whitehill R: Evaluation of the painful hip by aspiration and arthrography. Surg Gynecol Obstet 144:381–386, 1977.

329. Moreland JR, Gruen TA, Mai L, et al.: Aseptic loosening of total hip replacement: incidence and significance. In The Hip Society, Open Scientific Meeting, 8th. Riley LH Jr, ed. The Hip: Proceedings, vol 8. St. Louis, CV Mosby, 1980:281–291.

330. Mountford PJ, Hall FM, Coakley AJ, et al.: Assessment of the painful hip prosthesis with 111 In-labelled leucocyte scans. Letter. Br J Radiol 55:378, 1982.

331. Mullins MF, Sutton RN, Lodwick GS: Complications of total hip replacement. A roentgen evaluation. AJR 121:55–60, 1974.

332. Murray WR: Total joint prostheses: complications with emphasis on hips. In Symposium on Osteoarthritis. St. Louis, CV Mosby, 1974:103–122.

333. Murray WR, Rodrigo JJ: Arthrography for the assessment of pain after total hip replacement. J Bone Joint Surg (Am) 57:1060–1065, 1975.

334. Nicholson OR: Total hip replacement. An evaluation of the results and technics 1967–1972. Clin Orthop 95:217–223, 1973.

335. Nollen AJG, Slooff TJJH: Para-articular ossifications after total hip replacement. Acta Orthop Scand 44:230–241, 1973.

336. Pepper HW, Noonan CD: Radiographic evaluation of total hip arthroplasty. Radiology 108:23–29, 1973.

337. Pettersson H, Gentz C-F, Lindberg HO, et al.: Radiologic evaluation of the position of the acetabular component of the total hip prosthesis. Acta Radiol [Diagn] 23:259–263, 1982.

338. Radin EL, Paul IL, Rose RM, et al.: Wear and loosening of total joint replacements. Acta Orthop Belg 40:831–835, 1974.

339. Reckling FW, Dillon WL: The bone-cement interface temperature during total joint replacement. J Bone Joint Surg (Am) 59:80–82, 1977.

340. Reing CM, Richin PF, Kenmore PI: Differential bone-scanning in the evaluation of a painful total joint replacement. J Bone Joint Surg 61:933, 1979.

341. Resnick D, Guerra J Jr: Stress fractures of the inferior pubic ramus following hip surgery. Radiology 137:335–338, 1980.

342. Riley LH Jr, Hughes JL: Total replacement of the hip joint. Surg Annu 5:157–167, 1973.

343. Rosenthall L, Lisbona R, Hernandez M, et al.: 99m Tc-PP and 67-Ga imaging following insertion of orthopedic devices. Radiology 133:717–721, 1979.

344. Salvati EA, Freiberger RH, Wilson PD Jr: Arthrography for complications of total hip replacement. A review of thirty-one arthrograms. J Bone Joint Surg (Am) 53:701–709, 1971.

345. Salvati EA, Im VC, Aglietti P, et al.: Radiology of total hip replacements. Clin Orthop 121:75–82, 1976.

346. Schneider R, Kaye JD: Insufficiency and stress fractures of the long bones occurring in patients with rheumatoid arthritis. Radiology 116:595–599, 1975.

347. Selby Brown C, Knickerbocker WJ: Radiologic studies in the investigation of the causes of total hip replacement failures. J Can Assoc Radiol 24:245–253, 1973.

348. Stauffer RN: Ten-year follow-up study of total hip replacement: with particular reference to roentgenographic loosening of the components. J Bone Joint Surg (Am) 64:983–990, 1982.

349. Sutherland CJ, Wilde AH, Borden LS, et al.: A ten-

year follow-up of one hundred consecutive Muller curved-stem total hip-replacement arthroplasties. J Bone Joint Surg (Am) 64:970–982, 1982.

350. Suzuki Y, Hisada K, Takeda M: Demonstration of myositis ossificans by 99mTc pyrophosphate bone scanning. Radiology 111:663–664, 1974.

351. Switzer PJ, Cooperberg PL, Knickerbocker WJ: Defects in the sigmoid colon caused by placement of a left hip prosthesis. J Can Assoc Radiol 25:151–153, 1974.

352. Tanaka T, Rossier AB, Hussey RW, et al.: Quantitative assessment of para-osteo-arthropathy and its maturation on serial radionuclide bone images. Radiology 123:217–221, 1977.

353. Tehranzadeh J, Schneider R, Freiberger RH: Radiological evaluation of painful total hip replacement. Radiology 141:355–362, 1981.

354. Weber FA, Charnley J: A radiological study of fractures of acrylic cement in relation to the stem of a femoral head prosthesis. J Bone Joint Surg (Br) 57:297–301, 1975.

355. Weiss PE, Mall JC, Hoffer PB, et al.: 99m Tc-methylene diphosphonate bone imaging in the evaluation of total hip prostheses. Radiology 133:727–729, 1979.

356. Weissman BN: The radiology of total joint replacement. In Kelley WN, Harris ED, Ruddy S, et al., eds. Textbook of Rheumatology. Philadelphia, WB Saunders, 1981.

357. Weissman BN, Sosman JL, Braunstein EM, et al.: Intravenous methylmethacrylate after total hip replacement. J Bone Joint Surg (Am) 66:443–450, 1984.

358. Willert HG, Ludwig J, Semlitsch M: Reaction of bone to methacrylate after hip arthroplasty. J Bone Joint Surg (Am) 56:1368–1382, 1974.

359. Williams F, McCall IW, Park WM, et al.: Gallium-67 scanning in the painful total hip replacement. Clin Radiol 32:431–439, 1981.

360. Williamson BRJ, McLaughlin RE, Wang G-J, et al.: Radionuclide bone imaging as a means of differentiating loosening and infection in patients with a painful total hip prosthesis. Radiology 133:723–725, 1979.

Chapter 9

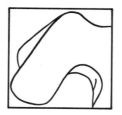

The
KNEE

NORMAL STRUCTURE AND FUNCTION

Essential Anatomy

Femorotibial Articulation

The knee joint is composed of femorotibial and patellofemoral articulations that allow flexion-extension motion and rotation. The pattern of flexion and extension differs from that of a true hinge joint in that, because of the spiral contours of the femoral condyles, the axis of motion is not fixed but shifts upward and forward in extension and downward and backward in flexion. Also, rotation occurs between the tibia and femur, with the tibia rotating laterally during the last 30 degrees of knee extension. With flexion the tibia internally rotates on the femur, and the menisci slide posteriorly on the tibial plateau. The medial meniscus is firmly fixed to the joint capsule; therefore, it moves less than the more loosely attached lateral meniscus.[106]

Bony Anatomy

The distal femur consists of a supracondylar portion extending from the metaphyseal-dia-

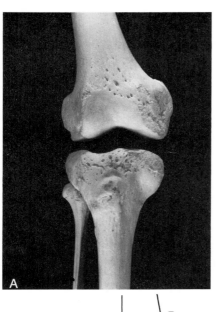

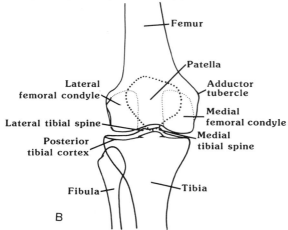

Femur

Patella

Lateral
femoral condyle

Adductor
tubercle

Medial
femoral condyle

Lateral tibial spine

Medial
tibial spine

Posterior
tibial cortex

Fibula

Tibia

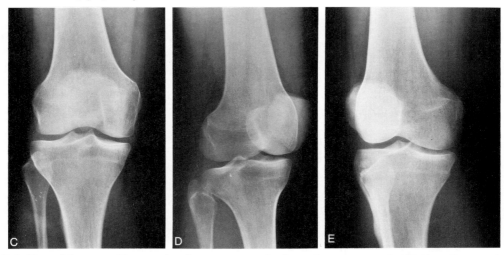

Figure 9–1. Normal Anatomy. Photographic, diagrammatic, and radiographic anatomy in the AP *(A to C);* internal oblique *(D);* external oblique *(E);* tunnel *(F,G);* and lateral *(H to L)* views (arrow = Blumensaat's line; asterisk = groove for popliteus).

Illustration continued on opposite page

498

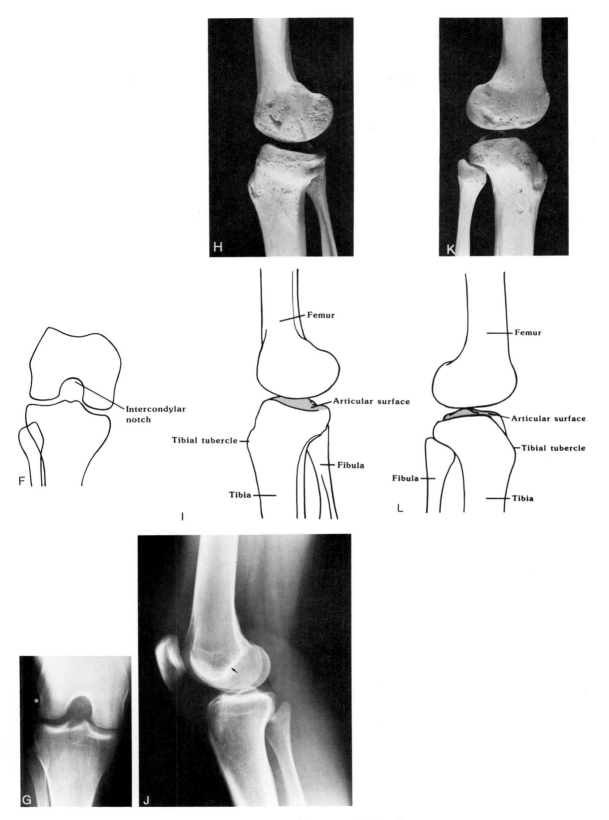

Figure 9–1. Normal Anatomy *Continued.*

physeal junction to the femoral condyles (Fig. 9–1). The medially located adducter tubercle is proximal to the medial epicondyle and is the site of insertion of the adductor magnus (Fig. 9–2). The curved femoral condyles are of slightly different shapes, with the articular surface of the medial condyle longer than that of the lateral condyle (Fig. 9–3).[7] The trochlea is the portion of femur located anteriorly between the condyles, for articulation with the patella. Articular cartilage covers the femoral condyles and the trochlea and is normally thicker over the medial than over the lateral condyle.[6]

The proximal tibia consists of medial and lateral condyles and a central nonarticular intercondylar eminence to which the cruciate ligaments and menisci attach. The medial (anterior) and the lateral (posterior) tibial spines are part of the nonarticular area. The cruciate ligaments attach to the adjacent bone, rather than to the tibial spines per se, and are covered by synovial reflections (Fig. 9–4). Articular cartilage covers the upper surfaces of the tibia and extends upward, along the outer margins of the tibial spines. The lateral tibial articular surface is almost circular in configuration and is smaller than the more oval medial surface (Fig. 9–4). The muscle attachments on the tibia are shown in Figure 9–5.

Soft-Tissue Anatomy
The quadriceps tendon consists of four components—the rectus femoris, the vastus medialis, the vastus lateralis, and the vastus intermedius tendons that insert on the superior border of the patella (Fig. 9–6). The quadriceps tendon continues over the anterior aspect of the patella to join the patellar tendon.

The anterior cruciate ligament extends from the lateral femoral condyle to the tibia anterior to the medial tibial tubercle. The posterior cruciate ligament originates from the medial femoral condyle and inserts on the posterior tibia (Fig. 9–4). It is central in location and is the fundamental stabilizer of the knee in flexion, in extension, and in rotation.

The menisci are crescent-shaped fibrocartilaginous structures that lie on the articular surface of the tibia (Fig. 9–7). The *medial meniscus* is C-shaped but wider posteriorly than anteriorly. The anterior end is attached to the tibia in front of the anterior cruciate ligament; the posterior end attaches behind the insertion of the lateral meniscus and in front of the posterior cruciate ligament.[4] The outer margin of the medial meniscus blends with the joint capsule.

The *lateral meniscus* is more circular in configuration. It is attached anteriorly to the tibia, behind and lateral to the anterior cruciate ligament with which it blends. Posteriorly, it is attached to the tibia, anterior to the insertion of the medial meniscus. The peripheral attachment of the lateral meniscus to the capsule is interrupted posteriorly by the tendon and sheath of the popliteus muscle.

The menisci are covered by reflections of the synovial membrane that lines the joint capsule.[4] Cross sections of the menisci show their typical triangular shape, which corresponds to the triangular appearance of the meniscus viewed tangentially at arthrography. Only the peripheral margins have a vascular supply.

Several functions are attributed to the menisci, including those of increasing joint stability, promoting joint lubrication, bearing weight and distributing weight-bearing forces, and preventing capsular and synovial impingement during motion.[85, 179]

There are two major types of supporting structures in the knee, the static and the dynamic stabilizers.[9] The static stabilizers consist of the ligaments and are subdivided into two layers, capsular and noncapsular (Figs. 9–1 and 9–8). The dynamic stabilizers consist of the muscles and their tendons and aponeuroses.

The Patellofemoral Joint
The patella is a sesamoid bone in the quadriceps tendon. It functions as a spacer, increasing the distance of the extensor apparatus from the axis of a flexion-extension motion and thereby increasing the force of extension by 30 to 50 percent.[3] Considerable compressive force, which can reach 3.5 times body weight during stair descent, is generated at the patellofemoral joint.[125] It is therefore not surprising that the patellar cartilage is the thickest in the body and that damage to the cartilage is frequent.

The patellar articular surface is subdivided into medial and lateral facets by a bony prominence, the median ridge, which is covered by cartilage 5.4 to 6.4 mm thick.[21] The medial facet is further subdivided into a smaller medial (odd) facet and a medial facet proper by a cartilaginous prominence (Fig. 9–9). The odd facet may not be apparent on tangential patellar views but can be seen on arthrography.[3]

Usually, the lateral patellar facet is larger than the medial, although variations in size and shape led Wiberg to describe three patellar configurations (Fig. 9–10).[21]

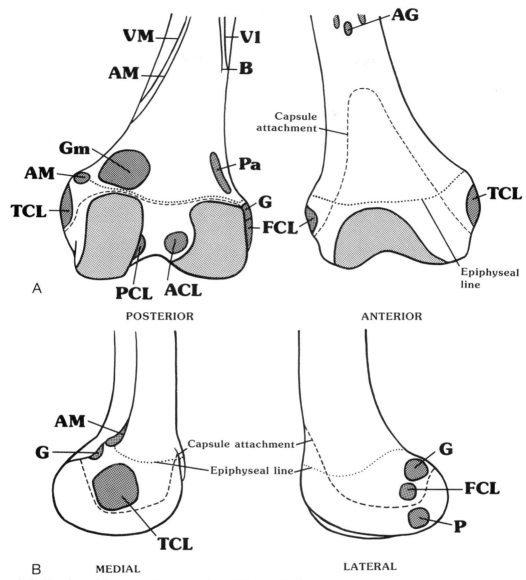

Figure 9–2. Muscle and Ligament Insertions, Distal Femur. *A,* Posterior and anterior; *B,* medial and lateral. ACL = anterior cruciate ligament; AG = articular muscle; AM = adductor magnus; B = biceps, short head; FCL = fibular collateral ligament; G = gastrocnemius; Gm = gastrocnemius medial head; P = popliteus; Pa = plantaris; PCL = posterior cruciate ligament; TCL = tibial collateral ligament; VI = vastus intermedius; VM = vastus medialis.

Type I—Medial and lateral facets of equal size

Type II—A smaller medial facet

Type III—A small medial facet with a steeply sloped contour

The patellar trabeculae are arranged in a parallel fashion, perpendicular to the coronal plane of the patella and, therefore, oblique to the subchondral cortex (Fig. 9–11).[3] The subchondral bone is normally thicker along the lateral facet.

The femoral side of the patellofemoral joint (the trochlea) has a large lateral articular surface that projects farther anteriorly than the medial surface. The cartilage covering is thicker laterally (about 2 to 3 mm) than medially, but the femoral cartilage overall is thinner than the patellar articular cartilage.[3]

The proximal three fourths of the posterior surface of the patella articulates with the femur, but only a small portion of the articular surface is in contact with the femur at any particular degree of flexion. With the knee in maximum

Text continued on page 508

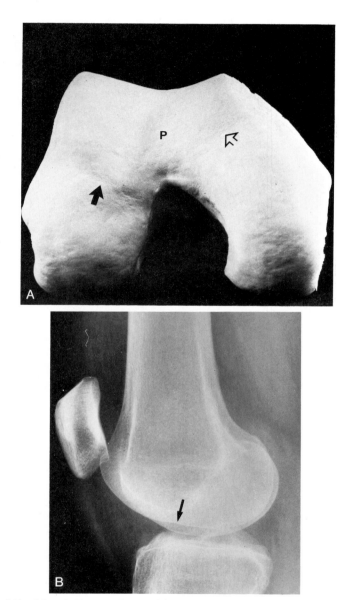

Figure 9–3. The Femoral Condyles. *A,* Tangential view of the articular surface of the distal femur shows the condylopatellar sulcus (groove) that separates the patellar (P) and tibial articular surfaces. The groove is located between the anterior and middle thirds of the medial condyle (open arrow) and between the anterior and posterior halves of the lateral condyle (solid arrow). *B,* The lateral femoral condyle projects farther anteriorly. The lateral condylopatellar sulcus (arrow) is seen between the anterior and posterior halves of the femoral condyle.

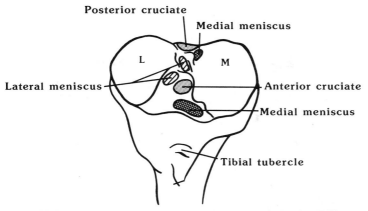

Figure 9–4. The Cruciate and Meniscal Attachments and the Upper Surface of the Tibia. The sites of cruciate attachment on the tibia are shown. The configuration of the lateral tibial articular surface is almost circular, whereas the medial surface is nearly oval. L = lateral articular surface, M = medial.

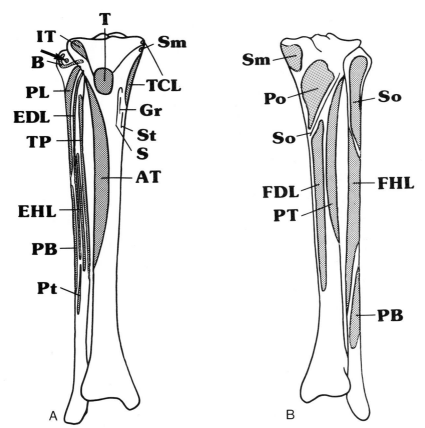

Figure 9–5. Muscle Insertions, Tibia. *A,* Anterior view; *B,* posterior view. AT = anterior tibial; B = biceps femoris; EDL = extensor digitorum longus; EHL = extensor hallucis longus; FDL = flexor digitorum longus; FHL = flexor hallucis longus; Gr = gracilis; IT = iliotibial tract; PB = peroneus brevis; Po = popliteus; PL = peroneus longus; Pt = peroneus tertius; PT = posterior tibial; So = soleus; Sm = Semimembranosus; St = Semitendinosus; T = patellar tendon; TCL = tibial collateral ligament; → = fibular collateral ligament.

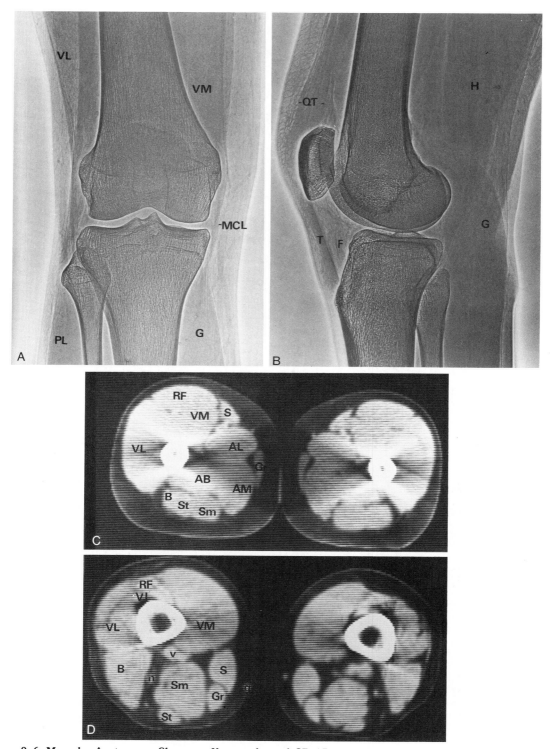

Figure 9–6. Muscular Anatomy as Shown on Xerography and CT. AP xerogram *(A)*; lateral xerogram *(B)*. CT images through the upper femur *(C)*; lower third of femur *(D)*.

Illustration continued on opposite page

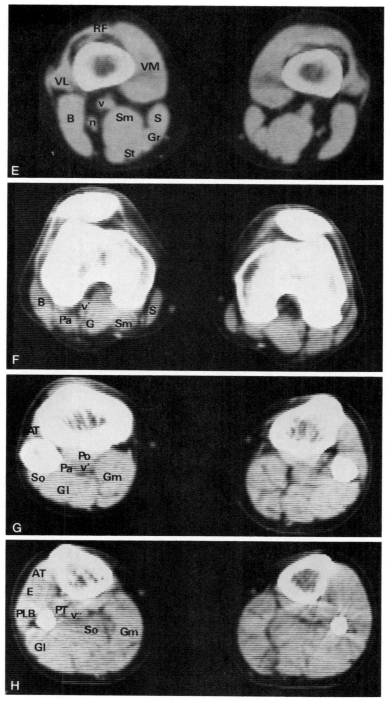

Figure 9–6. Muscular Anatomy as Shown on Xerography and CT *Continued.* Distal femur *(E);* knee (femoral condyles) *(F);* proximal tibia *(G);* more distal tibia *(H).* AT = Tibialis anterior; AB = adductor brevis; AL = adductor longus; AM = adductor magnus; B = biceps femoris; E = extensor digitorum longus; F = infrapatellar fat pad; g = greater saphenous vein; Gr = gracilis; G = gastrocnemius (Gm = medial, Gl = lateral head); H = hamstrings (biceps femoris, semimembranosus, semitendinosus); MCL = medial collateral ligament; n = nerves (tibial and common peroneal); Po = popliteus; Pa = plantaris; PL, PLB =peroneus longus; peroneus longus and brevis; PT = posterior tibial; QT = quadriceps tendon; RF = rectus femoris; S = sartorius; Sm = semimembranosus; So = soleus; St = semitendinosus; T = patellar tendon; v = deep femoral vein and artery; v' = popliteal artery and vein; v" = peroneal and posterior tibial arteries and veins; VI = vastus intermedius; VL = vastus lateralis; VM = vastus medialis.

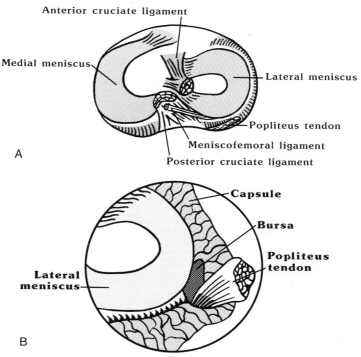

A

B

Figure 9–7. The Menisci. The medial meniscus is attached to the joint capsule throughout its periphery, whereas the attachment of the lateral meniscus is interrupted posteriorly by the popliteus tendon and sheath. The medial meniscus is C-shaped and wider posteriorly than anteriorly. The lateral meniscus has a more circular shape. *A,* Menisci from above. *B,* Detailed view of relationship of the lateral meniscus and the popliteus tendon.

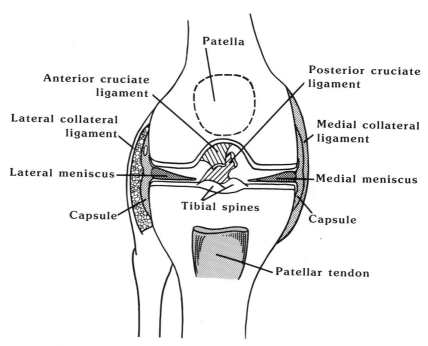

Figure 9–8. Ligamentous Anatomy. The medial collateral ligament is intimately related to the joint capsule. The lateral collateral ligament is separated from the joint capsule by fat and also by the lateral inferior genicular vessels and nerve (not shown). The cruciate ligaments are covered by synovial reflections and therefore are extraarticular.

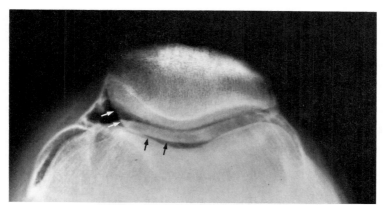

Figure 9–9. The Patellar Facets. The patella has medial and lateral facets, separated by a median ridge. The medial facet is further subdivided by the contour of the articular cartilage into odd (white arrows) and medial (black arrows) facets.

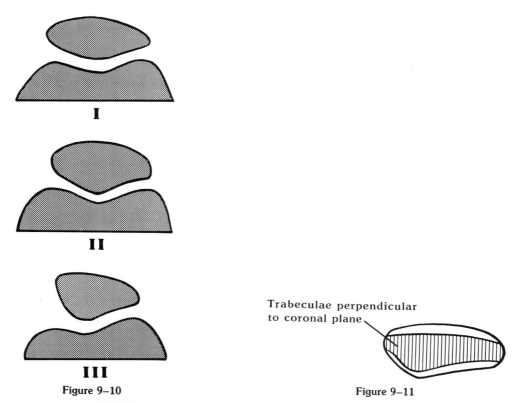

Figure 9–10

Figure 9–11

Figure 9–10. The Wiberg Classification of Patellar Shapes. Type I, in which the medial and lateral facets are equal in size; type II, in which the medial facet is smaller than the lateral; type III, in which the medial facet is small and vertical.

Figure 9–11. Patellar Trabeculae. The patellar trabeculae are perpendicular to the coronal plane of the patella. The subchondral cortex is thicker along the lateral facet. (After Ficat RP, Hungerford DS: Disorders o the Patello-Femoral Joint. Baltimore, Williams & Wilkins, 1977.)

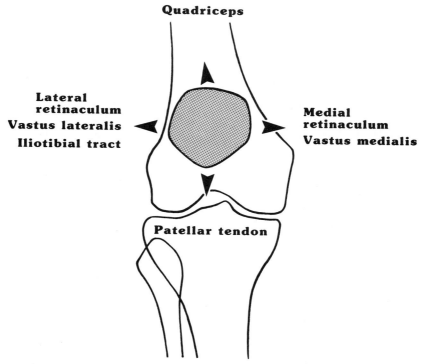

Figure 9–12. Forces Acting on the Patella. (Redrawn from Ficat RP, Hungerford DS: Disorders of the Patello-Femoral Joint. Baltimore, Williams & Wilkins, 1977.)

extension the patella does not articulate with the femur at all but rests against the prefemoral fat pad. As the knee is flexed to 90 degrees, different areas of the patella come into contact with the femur.[3, 21, 118] The odd facet does not make contact with the femur until marked flexion

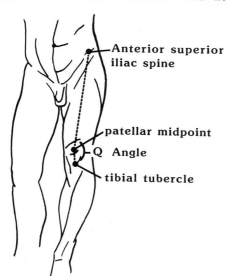

Figure 9–13. The Q Angle. This angle is measured clinically from the anterior superior iliac spine to the center of the patella and from the center of the patella to the tibial tubercle. The Q angle is normally 15 to 20 degrees.

(greater than 110 degrees) is achieved, at which time the patella rotates on its long axis, allowing the odd facet to contact the medial femoral condyle.[125] Thus the odd facet is not usually a contact area, and this relative disuse is suggested as the cause of nonprogressive surface degeneration (fibrillation) of the articular cartilage in this region.[118]

The soft-tissue attachments to the patella that influence its position are summarized in Figure 9–12, adapted from Ficat and Hungerford.[3] In extension the valgus angle of the knee theoretically produces an increased lateral pull on the patella. This tendency is related to the orientation of the quadriceps and the patellar tendons when the knee is in extension, the angle between these two tendons being described *clinically* as the Q angle (Fig. 9–13). The tendency for the patella to dislocate laterally is counteracted by the medial ligaments, the shapes of the patellar and trochlear articular surfaces, and the pull of the vastus medialis muscle.[3] The Q angle and the tendency for lateral dislocation decrease as the knee is flexed.

Normal Radiographic Appearances

The standard radiographic series for evaluation of the knee usually consists of lateral, anteroposterior supine, and tunnel views (see Fig. 9–1). The examination is supplemented by oblique, standing, or tangential patellar views, depending upon the clinical circumstances.

Anteroposterior View

On the supine AP view most of the femorotibial cartilage space is not shown in profile, because although the radiograph is taken with the x-ray beam perpendicular to the knee, the tibial articular surface actually tilts downward posteriorly (Fig. 9–14). A more accurate demonstration of the cartilage space can therefore be obtained by tilting the x-ray tube caudally about 5 degrees. Lines drawn along the articular surfaces of the tibia and femur are parallel.

The thin subchondral bony plate of the tibia is visible and is of particular interest, since its appearance and that of the underlying cancellous bone reflect the incident stress. Normally, stress is evenly distributed on both tibial plateaus, and the subchondral bone is therefore of equal thickness medially and laterally. Moderately increased stress in a compartment results in increased bone under the subchondral cortex (subchondral sclerosis) and in increased thickness of the underlying trabeculae. Marked increase in stress results in eventual bone resorption. Complete cartilage loss from both the femoral and the tibial surfaces results in subchondral sclerosis on both sides of the joint, which is the radiographic correlate of eburnation noted at surgery (see Fig. 9–57).

Some normal appearances may be confusing. For example, the lateral tibial margin may be irregular, erroneously suggesting periostitis; therefore, the marginal irregularity is termed pseudoperiostitis. The lateral femoral indentation for the popliteus tendon may mimic erosion.

Standing Anteroposterior View

Evaluation of knee alignment and of the true width of the cartilage space are obviously important in clinical decision making and operative planning. Standing views have been used in an attempt to more accurately define these features. Standing radiographs may be done with the patient standing only on the leg to be radiographed (stork view) or with weight evenly distributed on both legs. Especially in the latter circumstance, spurious findings may result from bracing one leg against the other or favoring one leg. Even the stork views, however, may occasionally provide erroneous information and also may be difficult for infirm patients or patients with severe joint damage. Despite these limitations, the technique has strong advocates.

The Mechanical Axis. Maquet notes that standing views of the entire leg, not only the knee, are necessary for assessing overall alignment.[134] Such standing views of a normal leg demonstrate that the centers of the femoral head, knee, and ankle form a straight line, the mechanical axis (Fig. 9–15). This axis is angled slightly lateral to the line of the body weight.[2] The tibia is in line with the mechanical axis of

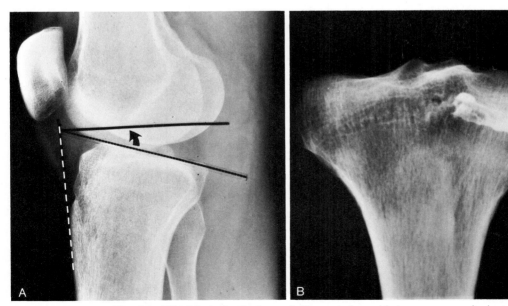

Figure 9–14. Posterior Tilt of the Tibial Articular Surfaces. *A,* The angle (arrow) between a perpendicular to the anterior tibia and the tibial articular surface is shown. *B,* An AP view of a tibia shows the posterior, medial cortical rim (marked with barium) to be projected below the anterior cortex.

the leg. The transverse plane of the knee (defined by a line through the distal femoral subchondral bone) should be perpendicular to the mechanical axis and also to the tibia.

Varus-Valgus Angulation. The shape of the femoral shaft is such that the axis of the shaft is angled 5 to 7 degrees lateral to the mechanical axis. But rather than viewing the relationship in this way, the femur is seen as being straight, and the tibia as being angled. Thus when lines drawn along the femoral and tibial shafts intersect at an angle of 5 to 7 degrees (Fig. 9–15), this juncture is termed 5 to 7 degrees of valgus angulation of the tibia. However, despite this designation, the ends of the tibia (at the knee and ankle) are parallel to each other and the ground.

Subluxation. Lines along the axes of the femur and tibia normally intersect at the knee. If they intersect proximal to the joint line, lateral subluxation of the tibia is said to be present.[2] Vainionpaa and co-workers quantify the amount of subluxation by measuring the distance be-

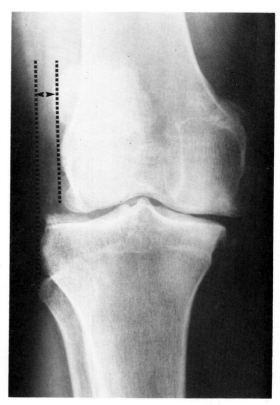

Figure 9–16. Femorotibial Subluxation in Osteoarthritis. The degree of medial femoral subluxation is indicated by the separation between parallel lines drawn along the most lateral margins of the femur and tibia. A more accurate measurement would have been obtained with the leg less externally rotated and with weight-bearing. In this patient complete medial cartilage loss is documented by the presence of subchondral sclerosis on each side of the medial cartilage space.

tween parallel lines drawn along the most lateral margins of the femur and tibia (Fig. 9–16).[140]

Articular Cartilage and Soft Tissues. On standing views the cartilage space is of uniform thickness and measures between 5 and 11 mm in height.[131]

Tunnel View

Tunnel views of the knee are taken with the knee flexed and the x-ray tube angled so that the intercondylar notch is well seen, unobscured by the patella or tibia. The posterior articular surfaces of the femoral condyles are brought into profile.

Lateral View

A wealth of information is available from the lateral view.

Bony Structures. On examination of the distal femur a dense white line (Blumensaat's line) representing the surface of the intercondylar notch that is tangential to the x-ray beam is

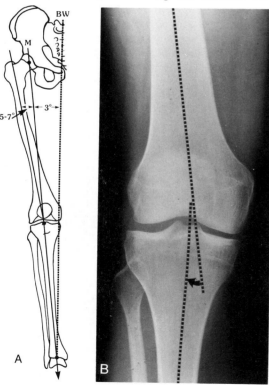

Figure 9–15. The Mechanical Axis. *A*, Normally, a line drawn from the center of the femoral head to the center of the tibial plafond intersects the center of the knee. This straight line is termed the mechanical axis (M). Note the 5 to 7 degrees of normal valgus. BW = body weight. *B*, Normal mild valgus (arrow) is present. (*A*, Redrawn from Maquet PG. *In* Freeman MA, ed. Arthritis of the Knee: Clinical Features and Surgical Management. Heidelberg, Springer-Verlag, 1980.)

seen. This line and the lines denoting the limits of anterior intercondylar surface and the site of the old epiphyseal plate define a triangular region on the lateral film that is normally relatively radiolucent.[13] Increased density of this area may provide a subtle clue to the presence of bony abnormalities (particularly tumors) that may otherwise be difficult to detect.

The superimposed femoral condyles can usually be differentiated, since the lateral femoral condyle is usually flatter than the medial condyle and has a groove (condylopatellar sulcus) located in approximately the middle of its curve that separates the articular surface for the patella from that for the tibia (see Fig. 9–4).[13] A similar but more anterior groove is present on the medial aspect of the medial femoral condyle, between its anterior and middle thirds. These grooves may be confused with abnormal conditions, such as osteochondritis dissecans.[7]

The position of the femoral condyles in relation to the long axis of the femur can be deduced by noting the angle formed by a line drawn down the anterior aspect of the femoral cortex and Blumensaat's (intercondylar) line (Fig.

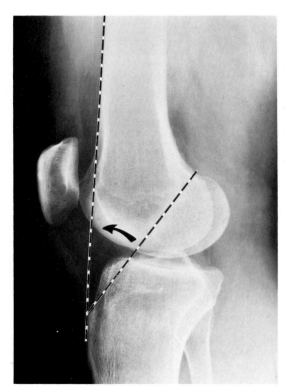

Figure 9–17. Determining the Position of the Femoral Condyles. The position can be assessed by noting the angle formed between lines drawn along the anterior femoral cortex and Blumensaat's intercondylar line. Normally, this angle is 34 ± 0.5 degrees.

9–17). This angle ranges from 26 to 44 degrees and normally averages 34 ± 0.5 degrees.[15] This method helps quantify any deformity resulting from a supracondylar fracture of the femur.

On the lateral view the medial tibial spine is the highest bony projection. The anterior cruciate ligament inserts along the ascending slope of bone that rises to the medial tibial spine (Figs. 9–18 and 9–19).[5] The articular surface of the tibia slopes posteriorly downward at an angle (the tibial plateau angle) that can be measured on the lateral view. This angle may be helpful in the evaluation of tibial plateau fractures. The medial and lateral tibial plateaus can be differentiated, since the lateral side continues posteriorly to form a smooth convex arch, whereas the medial plateau extends abruptly downward.[11] Also, the medial tibial condyle projects farther posteriorly and has a more squared shape than the lateral condyle. A small bony spur (Parson's knob) is sometimes seen just anterior to the medial tibial spine; it indicates the site of insertion of the anterior horn of the medial meniscus.[5]

On the true lateral view of the tibia a dense line, the top part of which is the posteromedial aspect of the lateral tibial condyle, is noted (Fig. 9–18). It continues inferiorly and anteriorly toward the tibial articular surface of the tibiofibular joint.[20] Normally, this dense line is projected over the midportion of the fibular head. The tibiofibular joint itself may be oriented in a horizontal or oblique fashion,[19] and it is often best seen on 45- to 60-degree internal oblique views.[5] In 10 percent of adults a communication exists between this joint and the knee joint.

The Patella. Lateral views are helpful for assessing the vertical location of the patella. Abnormally high patellar position (patella alta) has been noted to be associated with recurrent subluxation, chondromalacia, Sinding-Larsen-Johansson syndrome, and cerebral palsy.[3] The opposite abnormality (patella baja) is less frequent. It may be seen in achondroplasia, polio, and juvenile rheumatoid arthritis and also as a complication of tibial tubercle transposition or trauma.[3]

Commonly used measures of patellar position include:

Blumensaat's line. A lateral view taken with the knee in 30 degrees of flexion is said to demonstrate normal patellar position if the lower pole of the patella is at the level of a line extended anteriorly from the intercondylar notch (Blumensaat's line). However, this measure has been found to be inaccurate.[10, 12]

Method of Insall and Salvati.[10] The length of the patellar tendon (LT, measured from the

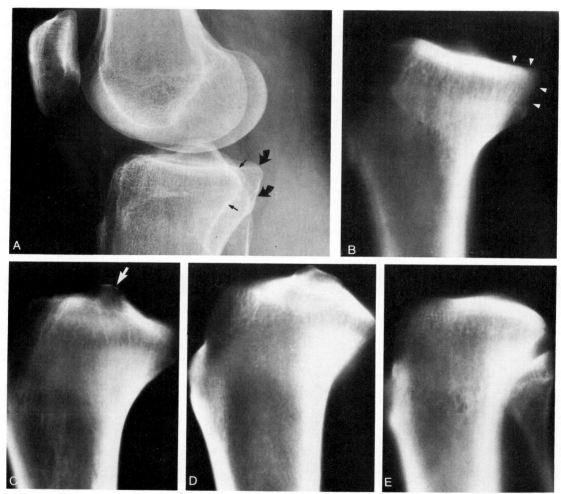

Figure 9–18. Tibial Anatomy. *A,* Normal tibia. The continuation of the lateral (posterior) tibial spine into the cortex of the tibiofibular joint (arrows) is seen. The medial tibial plateau (curved arrows) is squared in contour. *B,* Tomography of tibial specimen. The medial tibial plateau is in focus. It ends in a squared contour (arrowheads). *C,* The medial (anterior) tibial spine (arrow). *D,* The lateral (posterior) tibial spine continues in a straight line obliquely downward. *E,* The lateral tibial plateau is higher than the medial plateau and is posteriorly more rounded.

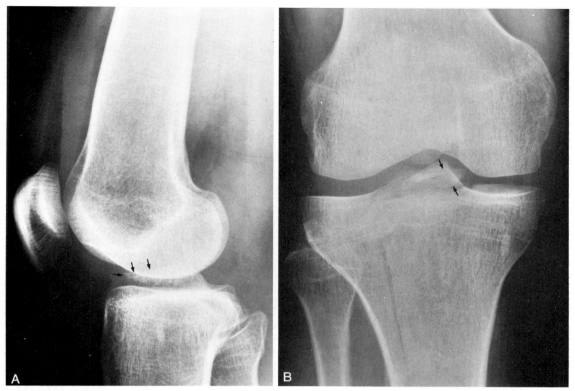

Figure 9–19. Anterior Cruciate Avulsion. *A,* The lateral view shows a joint effusion and a flat-fluid level. There is an elevated bony fragment (arrows) anterior to the tibial spines. *B,* AP view. The bony fragment (arrows) is superimposed on the tibial spines. A split fracture of the lateral tibial plateau is also present.

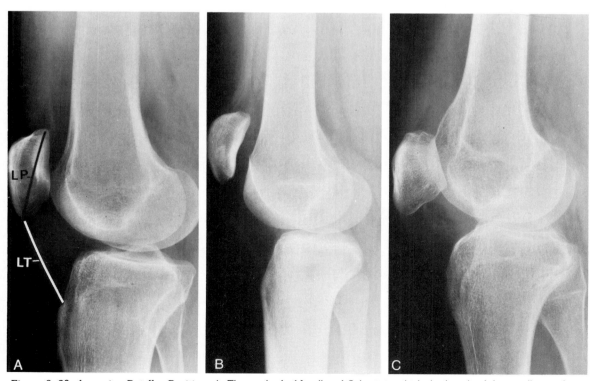

Figure 9–20. Assessing Patellar Position. *A,* The method of Insall and Salvati, in which the length of the patellar tendon (LT) is compared with the diagonal length of the patella (LP), is shown. *B,* Patella alta. The ratio is higher than 1.3:1. *C,* Patella baja. The patella is in an abnormally low position in this patient with juvenile rheumatoid athritis. Note the abnormally square patellar shape.

513

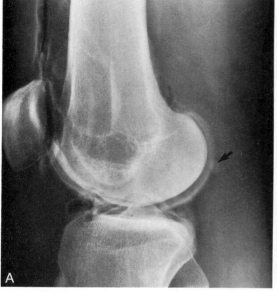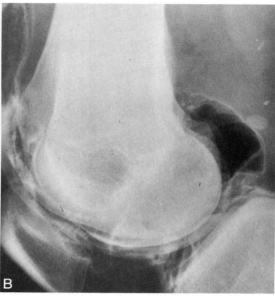

Figure 9–21. Fabellar Relationships to the Joint Capsule. *A,* A cross-table lateral view after double-contrast arthrography shows the fabella (arrow) closely related to the femoral condyles. *B,* With the knee flexed the joint capsule distends posteriorly, and the fabella is positioned farther from the lateral femoral condyle.

lower pole of the patella to the notch of the tibial tubercle) is compared with the diagonal length of the patella (LP; Fig. 9–20). Usually, these measurements are equal. An LT:LP ratio of more than 1.3:1 is abnormally high.[10] The lateral views for this assessment are taken in mild flexion.

The Fabella. A small sesamoid bone, the fabella (little bean), is noted in up to 18 percent of the population; it is bilateral slightly more than 70 percent of the time. It is located in the posterior joint capsule at the insertion of the lateral head of the gastrocnemius muscle. This location makes it susceptible to displacement by effusion and to changes due to arthritis, particularly osteoarthritis (Fig. 9–21). Enlargement of

the fabella has been noted in acromegaly (a sign analogous to the sesamoid sign in the hands). Occasionally, fractures of the fabella occur (Fig. 9–22).[178]

Tangential Patellar Views

Tangential patellar views are usually necessary for evaluation of the patellofemoral joint. Methods for obtaining these views are anything but standard. Ficat and Hungerford recommend a series of tangential patellar views with the knees in 30, 60, and 90 degrees of flexion.[3] The 30-degree position allows the detection of subluxation that may be reduced on views obtained with increased flexion. The 60-degree film shows the central contact area best. The patient is

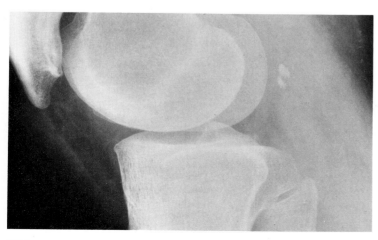

Figure 9–22. Fabellar Fracture. The fabellar fragments are slightly separated.

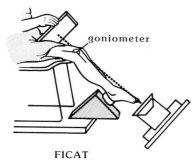

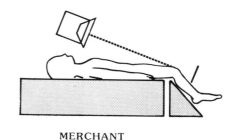

FICAT

MERCHANT

Figure 9–23. Methods of Obtaining Patellofemoral Views. *A,* Ficat method. *B,* Merchant method. A film holder is necessary.

seated on a platform or chair placed on the x-ray table; his or her legs, flexed to the desired angle, rest on a platform or cushion (Fig. 9–23). The x-ray beam is directed from the feet, angled about 10 degrees toward the tibia; the cassette is held on the thighs, perpendicular to the beam, by the patient. The feet and toes are plantar flexed. The knees and feet are pressed together to control rotation. The quadriceps must be relaxed, since muscular contraction may reduce a patellar subluxation.[17] While this examination may be optimal, it is necessary only in selected cases. However, in order to provide a consistently good examination, the method must be practiced frequently. It is not applicable to many infirm or arthritic patients.

Merchant and co-workers suggest obtaining films with the patient supine, the knees flexed over the end of the table and resting on a support (Fig. 9–23).[17] The beam is directed toward the feet, and the film is held on the shins in a specially constructed holder. This technique is less reliable with lesser degrees of knee flexion (e.g., 30 degrees), and special equipment is required.

A number of normal measurements and relationships can be studied on tangential patellar views, but the most frequently used are the following:

Position of the Patellar Apex. The patella is centered when its apex is directly above the depth of the trochlear sulcus.

Sulcus Angle. The sulcus angle is formed by the highest points of the medial and lateral femoral condyles and the lowest point of the intercondylar sulcus (Fig. 9–24). Shallow sulcus angles (greater measurements) are related to recurrent patellar dislocation. The normal value is 138 plus or minus 6 degrees.[3, 17]

Congruence Angle.[17] The congruence angle helps to define the position of the patella within the femoral sulcus (trochlea). The sulcus angle is drawn and bisected to establish a reference line. A line is then drawn from the posterior

point of the patella to the apex of the sulcus angle. The angle between the reference line and the patellar line is the congruence angle (Fig. 9–24). Medial patellar deviation is considered

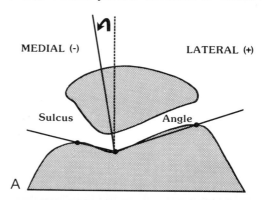

MEDIAL (-) LATERAL (+)

Sulcus   Angle

A

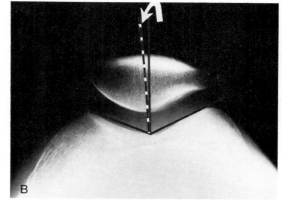

B

Figure 9–24. Sulcus Angle and Congruence Angle. *A,* The sulcus angle is formed by connecting the highest points of the medial and lateral femoral condyles and the lowest point of the intercondylar sulcus. The congruence angle (arrow) is measured between a line bisecting the sulcus angle and a line (dashed) from the posterior point of the patella to the apex of the sulcus angle. Lateral deviation of the patella by more than 16 degrees (angle > 16 degrees) is abnormal. *B,* An example in which the lowest point on the patella is difficult to find. The approximate angle between the reference line (black) and a line (dashed) through the patellar apex is within the normal range. (*A,* Redrawn from Merchant AC, et al.: J Bone Joint Surg (Am) 56:1391, 1974.)

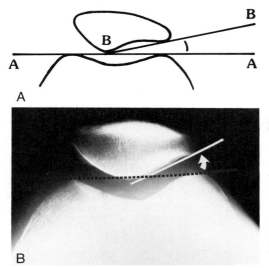

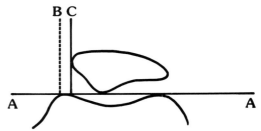

Figure 9–27. Lateral Patellar Displacement. A line is drawn through the highest points of the medial and lateral femoral condyles (AA). A perpendicular to that line, at the medial edge of the medial femoral condyle (B), normally lies 1 mm or less medial to the patella (line C). (After Laurin CA, Dussault R, Levesque HP: Clin Orthop 144:16, 1979.)

Figure 9–25. The Lateral Patellofemoral Angle. A, Two lines, one connecting the apices of the femoral condyles (AA) and another along the lateral patellar facet (BB), are drawn. The angle of intersection of these lines (arrow) usually opens laterally, or, rarely, the lines are parallel. B, Example. (After Laurin CA, Dussault R, Levesque HP: Clin Orthop 144:16, 1979.)

negative (−), and lateral deviation positive (+). A congruence angle greater than + 16 degrees is abnormal.

The next three observations are applicable only to films obtained in 20 degrees of flexion.

Lateral Patellofemoral Angle (Fig. 9–25).[14]

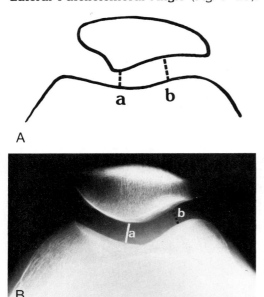

Figure 9–26. The Lateral Patellofemoral Index. A, This index is the ratio between the narrowest medial patellofemoral distance measured at the lateral edge of the medial facet (a) and the narrowest lateral patellofemoral distance (b). The ratio is normally 1 or less. B, Example. (After Laurin CA et al: Clin Orthop 144:16, 1979.)

Two lines, one joining the apices of the femoral condyles and one joining the limits of the lateral patellar facet, are drawn. Normally, the angle of intersection of these lines is open laterally, but the lines may rarely be parallel. In patients with patellar subluxation the lines are parallel or open medially.

Patellofemoral Index (Fig. 9–26).[14] [14a] The patellofemoral index is the quotient obtained by dividing the narrowest medial patellofemoral distance measured at the lateral edge of the medial facet by the narrowest lateral patellofemoral distance. This index is normally less than or equal to 1.0. A patellofemoral index of more than 1.0 is noted in patients with chondromalacia patellae.

Laurin Method of Measuring Lateral Patellar Displacement (Fig. 9–27).[14] A line is drawn at the medial edge of the medial femoral condyle, perpendicular to a line through the highest points of the medial and lateral femoral facets. In normal situations the medial edge of the patella is medial to the line or, at most, 1 mm lateral to it. Lateral patellar position is noted in about one third of cases of chondromalacia, in one half of patients with subluxing patellae, and in patients with lateral patellofemoral cartilage loss (Fig. 9–27).

Normal Soft Tissues

The lateral view is exceptionally good for evaluating the soft tissues around the knee, particularly when high-kv films are obtained. The quadriceps and patellar tendons are easily identified anteriorly, and the hamstring muscles and tendons and the heads of the gastrocnemius muscle are seen posteriorly.[28] Normal muscular anatomy is shown on xerography and on computed tomography in Figure 9–6.

On the lateral radiograph, between the femur and the quadriceps femoris tendon, a thin soft-tissue density is normally seen extending superiorly from behind the patella to the inferior

In the infrapatellar area a thin rim of soft-tissue density may be seen between the anterior portion of the femoral condyles and the infrapatellar fat pad. This rim represents the combined densities of the articular cartilage, the joint capsule, and any fluid within the joint. In adults this density measures less than 5 mm.[25]

Posteriorly, thin layers of extrasynovial fat parallel the curve of the femoral condyles and continue inferiorly around the popliteus tendon. The union of these fat lines forms the shape of a figure 3.[29] In the midline the posterior capsule may be visible because of fat anterior and posterior to it (Fig. 9–28). This posterior capsule line is seen behind the 3-shaped lucency on the lateral view.[29]

Arthrography

Indications. The situations in which arthrography is used are much influenced by the preferences of the referring physician and the skill and experience of the arthrographer. Arthrography provides a low-risk means of assessing the menisci as well as most other intraarticular structures. Even when surgical intervention is planned, arthrography may provide additional information about areas difficult to see on arthrotomy or arthroscopy, and it may provide information about unsuspected areas of abnormality.

Contraindications. Contraindications include prior severe reactions to contrast agent and uncontrolled bleeding disorders.

Technique. Several recent textbooks have been written about arthrography and are recommended to the interested reader.[86, 93, 112, 116] What follows are some highlights of arthrographic technique and interpretation and a discussion of the relevance of the athrographic finding of a meniscal or cruciate tear.

The technique used at the Brigham and Women's Hospital is a modification of the fluoroscopic technique developed by Butt and McIntyre in 1969.[90] The modifications primarily involve the use of intraarticular epinephrine to retard contrast absorption and of fluoroscopy to ensure correct needle placement. Each of these steps has been found helpful in ensuring high-quality examinations in a teaching institution.

Preliminary AP, lateral, and tangential patellar views of the knee are obtained if they have not been done recently.

The procedure is discussed with the patient, and a brief history and physical examination are performed. The patient is then placed supine on the x-ray table with the knee slightly flexed over an angle sponge, and the knee is washed with iodinated soap solution and draped with sterile

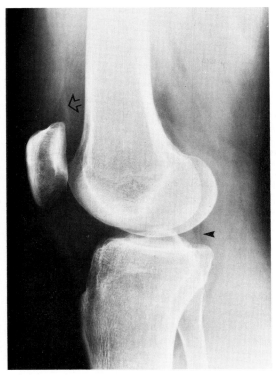

Figure 9–28. Normal Joint Capsule. The nondistended suprapatellar pouch is seen as a thin threadlike density (arrow) continuing from behind and extending proximal to the patella. The posterior joint capsule in the midline is made visible anteriorly and posteriorly (arrowhead) by the adjacent fat.

aspect of the quadriceps tendon (Fig. 9–28). This density represents the cephalad extension of the joint (the suprapatellar pouch). It is normally thin (measuring 1 or 2 mm) and is optimally seen on films in full or near-full extension.[29] These films can be taken with the patient lying on the side of the knee to be radiographed. A 5-degree cephalad tube angulation is said to be helpful, since without it the lateral femoral condyle is projected above the longer medial condyle and may obscure the base of the suprapatellar pouch.[25]

Another method for lateral radiography is to obtain cross-table lateral films with the patient supine and the knee in maximum extension. A bolster is placed under the knee to elevate it so that all of the posterior soft tissues can be included on the radiograph and any effusion present will be pushed from the dependent posterior recesses into the suprapatellar pouch. This view has the advantages of allowing a fat-fluid level to be shown, if present, and of being a more comfortable position for an injured patient to assume. We recommend it for routine use.

towels. While the solution dries on the skin, the following materials are assembled:

1. Three ml of contrast material (Reno-M-60) mixed with 0.1 to 0.3 ml of 1:1000 epinephrine is drawn up into a 5 ml syringe and then attached to connector tubing. The connector tubing reminds the examiner that this is the syringe with contrast medium, not lidocaine (Xylocaine).

2. Four ml (2 ampules) of 1 percent lidocaine are drawn into a syringe and attached to a short 25-gauge needle. The needle serves to remind

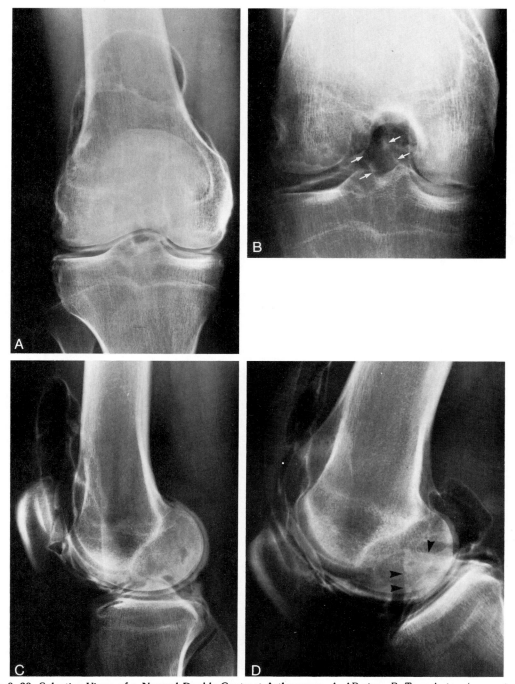

Figure 9–29. Selective Views of a Normal Double-Contrast Arthrogram. *A,* AP view. *B,* Tunnel view (arrows indicate the synovial reflections along the anterior cruciate ligament). *C,* Cross-table lateral view. *D,* Spot film of cruciate ligaments. The single arrowhead is on the posterior cruciate, the double arrowhead is on the anterior cruciate reflection.

Illustration continued on opposite page

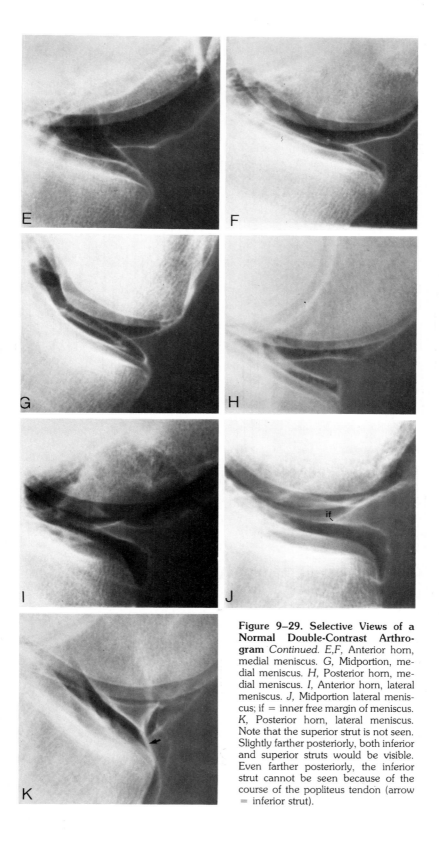

Figure 9–29. Selective Views of a Normal Double-Contrast Arthrogram *Continued. E,F,* Anterior horn, medial meniscus. *G,* Midportion, medial meniscus. *H,* Posterior horn, medial meniscus. *I,* Anterior horn, lateral meniscus. *J,* Midportion lateral meniscus; if = inner free margin of meniscus. *K,* Posterior horn, lateral meniscus. Note that the superior strut is not seen. Slightly farther posteriorly, both inferior and superior struts would be visible. Even farther posteriorly, the inferior strut cannot be seen because of the course of the popliteus tendon (arrow = inferior strut).

the examiner that this is the syringe containing Xylocaine.

With particularly anxious individuals it may be wise to prepare the syringes outside the examining room before the procedure begins so that the syringes, needles, and so on are not seen by the patient.

We usually use a lateral approach. Lidocaine is introduced into the skin and the subcutaneous tissues at a point just behind and proximal to the midpoint of the patella. Then, while the patella is pushed laterally, a 20-gauge needle is advanced toward the patella and cephalad, into the joint. If any fluid is present, it is aspirated as thoroughly as possible and sent for culture only if it is unusual in appearance or if there has been recent joint aspiration. Additional studies, such as examination for crystals, are done if clinically indicated. If no fluid is obtained, a small amount of lidocaine is injected. When the needle is intraarticular in location, almost no resistance to injection will be felt. We also routinely confirm intraarticular needle position by injecting contrast material under fluoroscopic control. If the needle is properly positioned, the contrast material immediately flows away from the needle tip. All the contrast material, followed by approximately 40 ml of room air, is then injected until the joint feels full. The patient is notified that the knee will suddenly become full when the air is introduced but that this will not be painful. There appears to be no advantage to massively distending the knee joint. The needle is then removed; the knee is exercised briefly in the supine position; and the patient is then repositioned prone with the knee in a brace, for spot filming. By use of distraction and varus or valgus stress against the brace, the knee is turned so that about 12 tangential views of each meniscus are obtained (Fig. 9–29). Spot films are then checked, and any questionable areas are reexamined. The knee is then flexed in order to fill a small popliteal cyst if one is present and to identify the cruciate reflections. Spot films in the lateral projection with the knee slightly flexed, AP, and tunnel views, are obtained. A 30 degree tangential patellar view is taken with the patient supine.

Following the procedure the patient is instructed not to engage in strenuous athletics for 12 to 24 hours, although there is no documented evidence that such activity is harmful. The patient is told that the swelling will decrease gradually but that some swelling may persist for about a week. If the swelling increases or fever develops, he or she is to call the doctor who did the examination.

This technique has worked for us and is modified appropriately for particular clinical situations. As newer contrast agents are introduced and experience is gained, our technique will probably change. In fact, even now some controversy exists as to the optimal method for examination. For example, the following points are debated:

1. Which gas should be used and how much? Estimates of the amount of gas needed for double-contrast arthrography vary. Butt and McIntyre use 20 to 30 ml of room air and 60 to 80 ml of carbon dioxide. This combination has been suggested so that joint distension can initially be obtained for filming, and rapid absorption of the carbon dioxide will then allow the patient to go home without much distension. Enough air does remain, however, for repeat spot filming to be done if necessary. Mink and Dickerson note that pain is more common and severe if carbon dioxide is used and relate this increased discomfort to a decrease in intraarticular pH.[104] Goldberg, Hall, and Wyshak have noted that 20 percent of patients studied (with 50 ml of either CO_2 or air and 1.6 ml of contrast agent) had increased pain during the 24 hours following the examination. Several authors have been able to obtain consistently good quality studies with about 40 ml of air,[93] but patients who were studied with CO_2 experienced slightly greater immediate pain.[97] Aspiration of the joint after arthrography has no apparent beneficial effect.

2. Are single or double-contrast studies better? In particular situations, such as for the identification of loose bodies or the demonstration of synovial abnormalities, single-contrast studies, using either dilute positive or negative contrast material, have been suggested.[93] Tegtmeyer and associates have noted equal and excellent accuracy in the diagnosis of meniscal tears when either double- or single-contrast examinations are performed.[110] One study suggests following a double-contrast examination with supine positive-contrast films, since in several patients tears were demonstrated on these latter films that were not seen on the initial double-contrast series.[107]

3. Should epinephrine be added? In 1974 Hall reported improvement in the clarity of intraarticular structures when 0.35 ml of 1:1000 epinephrine was added to the injected contrast material.[98] This improvement has been confirmed and has been shown to be the result of a decrease in both the absorption of contrast material from the joint and the dilution of contrast from the inflow of fluid into the joint.[109]

Multiple other modifications—including the use of bandages to compress the suprapatellar pouch, air drawn through a sterile gauze, and so on—all have proponents, but their value is unproven. The optimal examination for each clinical situation and each institution must be individually assessed.

Accuracy

Meniscal Tears. In general, the literature supports the idea that arthrography is a highly accurate procedure for the diagnosis of meniscal tears.[89, 94, 103, 111] Butt and McIntyre noted that in 142 verified cases there were 1 false-positive and 8 false-negative studies.[90] The accuracy of single- and double-contrast arthrographic techniques was assessed by Tegtmeyer and colleagues in 722 surgically excised menisci.[110] When the double-contrast method was used, a 95 percent overall accuracy in the diagnosis of medial meniscal tears, a 90 percent accuracy in the diagnosis of lateral meniscal tears, and a 93 percent accuracy in combined tears were noted. The accuracy was slightly better with single-contrast examinations. Many other studies have confirmed that the sensitivity of arthrography (the proportion of actually torn menisci identified on arthrography as torn) is high, averaging 94 percent, and the specificity (the proportion of normal menisci called normal on arthrography) averages almost 97 percent.[89]

In contrast, however, other studies have shown less satisfactory clinical-radiological correlations.[96] Particular difficulties seem to arise in the correlation between the description of a tear on arthrography and the diagnosis established at the time of surgery. The exact description of the type of tear may not be as important, however, as the identification and localization of a tear. Unfortunately, in one series even the site of abnormality described on arthrography did not always correlate with the site of the lesion found at surgery.[96] Braunstein and associates have noted that a normal arthrogram in a clinically equivocal case provides reassuring evidence that surgery is not necessary.[87]

It is clearly difficult to establish the accuracy of arthrography in general. Rather, each examiner must find the technique that he or she is most comfortable with and document its accuracy. As experience accrues, this evaluation will be a necessary and, it is hoped, a rewarding endeavor.

Other Lesions. Lesions other than meniscal tears are more difficult to demonstrate. Loose bodies, for example, are often difficult to identify and were detected in only 18 percent of patients with them in one series.[89] Similarly, areas of cartilage damage are often missed, since not all

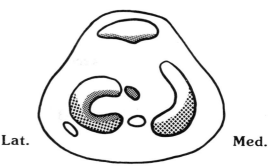

Figure 9–30. Areas of Difficulty on Arthrography and Arthroscopy. The lightly stippled areas indicate regions in which abnormalities are demonstrated with difficulty on arthrography. The crosshatched areas are those difficult to evaluate on arthroscopy. (Redrawn from Levinsohn EM, Baker BE: AJR 134:107, 1980.)

the cartilage surfaces are viewed tangentially. When a focal lesion is demonstrated, however, it can usually be documented at surgery or arthroscopy. Failure to demonstrate such a lesion on arthrography does not exclude its presence.

Arthrography Versus Arthroscopy. The place of arthrography is undergoing reevaluation in light of the increased use and availability of arthroscopy. Although differences of opinion exist, several studies suggest that these examinations are complementary rather than competitive. Ireland and co-workers determined the combined accuracy of these procedures to be 98 percent, whereas the accuracy of arthrography alone was 86 percent, and arthroscopy alone, 84 percent.[100]

Thijn found arthrography to be superior to arthroscopy (from an anterolateral approach) in the diagnosis of medial meniscal tears (94 percent versus 81 percent positive correlations).[111] Arthrography was less efficacious than arthroscopy in diagnosing lateral meniscal lesions (90 percent versus 94.5 percent), chondromalacia patellae (55 versus 99.5 percent), and cruciate ligament tears (69 versus 97 percent).

Levinsohn and Baker (also using an anterolateral approach) noted that arthroscopy was more accurate for diagnosing tears of the central edge and the anterior horns of the menisci and for anterior cruciate tears, whereas arthrography was more accurate for midbody and peripheral meniscal tears (Fig. 9–30).[103]

ABNORMAL CONDITIONS

Soft Tissue Abnormalities

Effusion

Small synovial effusions can be detected first in the suprapatellar pouch.[22] The anterior and pos-

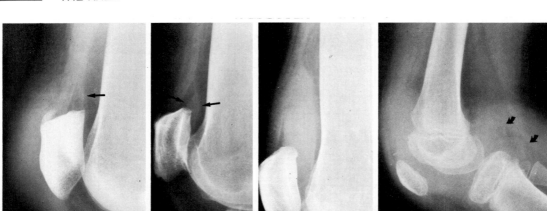

Figure 9–31. Abnormal Soft Tissues. *A,* Prepatellar bursitis. Following a fall there is marked swelling of the prepatellar soft tissues. No intraarticular fluid is seen; the suprapatellar pouch (arrow) remains thin. *B,* Mild swelling. A coned view of the suprapatellar area in a patient with rheumatoid arthritis shows a mildly widened suprapatellar pouch (arrows). *C,* Marked effusion. There is marked widening of the suprapatellar pouch and increased density around the femoral condyles (arrow) and the tibia. *D,* A child with marked effusion; the knee held in flexion shows distension of the posterior capsule producing a 3-configuration (arrows). Marked anterior swelling is also seen.

terior walls of the suprapatellar pouch are separated by the fluid, and on the lateral view the normally threadlike shadow of the suprapatellar pouch is widened (Fig. 9–31). Hall correlated various radiographic findings with the results of fluid aspiration prior to arthrography.[25] When the width of the base of the suprapatellar pouch was 10 mm or more, 10 ml or more of fluid was aspirated in almost all cases. Measurements of 5 to 10 mm were noted in 20 of 21 patients with 1 to 9 ml of aspirated fluid. When the base of the suprapatellar pouch measured less than 5 mm, joint effusion could be excluded with an accuracy of 90 percent. Other abnormalities, such as synovial membrane thickening, may explain some of the cases in which the suprapatellar pouch appears wide but no fluid can be aspirated. Even greater accuracy is expected if the affected knee can be compared with a normal opposite side.

All other signs of knee effusion are less sensitive than widening of the suprapatellar pouch (Table 9–1). However, one sign that may be useful clinically is the increased soft-tissue density (>5 mm) around the anterior portions of the femoral condyles in patients with large (>20 ml) effusions. This finding may allow the diagnosis of effusion when the suprapatellar area is not adequately seen. Soft-tissue density localized to the infrapatellar area (without distension of

the suprapatellar pouch) suggests a localized mass, such as pigmented villonodular synovitis, rather than joint effusion.

Widening of the joint space, bowing of the quadriceps tendon, anterior displacement of the patella, and bulging of the posterior capsule are evidence of relatively large effusions. Another sign of effusion is posterior displacement of the

Table 9–1. Findings Suggesting Knee Effusion

Lateral View
  Thick suprapatellar pouch (as compared with other side, or ≥ 5 mm)*
  Blurring of posterior aspect of quadriceps tendon
  Increased soft tissue around anterior femoral condyles (≥ 5 mm)*
  Wide joint space
  Bowing of quadriceps tendon
  Anterior displacement of patella
  Bulging of posterior fat lines
  Displacement of fabella
Frontal View
  Visible fat around suprapatellar bursa
  Widened cartilage space
Tangential Patellar View (Prone)
  Filling in of medial patellofemoral fatty space*
  Bulging of medial soft tissues (> 3 mm difference from other side)*
  Tilting of patella
  Separation of patella and femur

*Features seen with small effusions if comparison films are available.

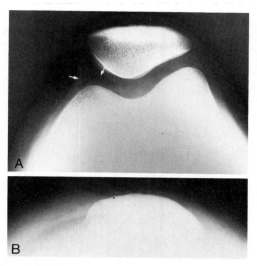

Figure 9–32. Tangential Patellar View for Joint Effusion. *A*, The normal tangential patellar view has fat medially visible (arrows). *B*, In this patient with effusion the fat is displaced by soft-tissue density.

fabella.[24] The fabella normally moves posteriorly as the knee is flexed; therefore, a correction factor has been devised to accommodate the degree of knee flexion (Fig. 9–21).[24] Given the same degree of flexion, or using the correction factor, the fabellar positions as measured from the center of the fabella to the closest edge of the lateral femoral condyle should be bilaterally symmetrical, and an increase of more than 1.2 mm on one side suggests effusion on that side.

Frontal radiographs have also been used to detect joint effusion. Harris and Hecht noted that displaced fat around a distended suprapatellar pouch could be identified on the AP view as curvilinear lucent lines medial or lateral to the distal femur.[26] We have found this sign to be of little clinical utility.

Joint effusion may also be detected on tangential patellar views obtained with the patient in the prone position.[23] Increased soft-tissue density in the normally fatty area between the medial aspects of the patella and the femur has been noted in patients with effusion (Fig. 9–32). Differences of more than 3 mm in the thickness of the soft tissue adjacent to the medial femoral condyle also suggest effusion. With large fluid collections lateral tilting of the patella and separation of the patella and the femur are noted.

Lipohemarthrosis

Intraarticular fractures may result in the liberation into the joint of marrow fat that can be identified by joint aspiration or radiography.

Cross-table lateral films will permit demonstration of a fat-fluid level in the suprapatellar pouch, and this view should routinely be obtained in patients with knee injuries. Occasionally, confusion arises because of the juxtaposition of the normal anterior fat and the suprapatellar pouch. Differentiation can usually be made by noting that a true fat-fluid level often continues under the patella, whereas a normal fat pad ends at the superior pole of the patella.

If cross-table lateral views are not available, fat within the joint can sometimes be diagnosed by seeing the wall of the suprapatellar pouch defined by fat on either side.[33] This view is analogous to the visibility of the wall of a bowel loop when both intraluminal and extraluminal gas are present.

The fracture itself may be difficult to identify and may seem small in comparison with the large amount of fat observed (Figs. 9–19 and 9–33). When a lipohemarthrosis or an acute effusion associated with pain is present and standard and oblique views are normal, pluridirectional tomography is the most efficacious way of demonstrating an underlying fracture.[30]

Popliteal Cysts

Popliteal cysts have been classified as primary or secondary. Primary cysts are unassociated with intraarticular abnormalities; they are most often seen in children, and they may be bilateral. Cysts in adults are usually secondary to intraarticular abnormalities in which joint effusion occurs.

Childress emphasized the association of popliteal cysts with tears of the posterior medial meniscus and noted that the cysts usually resolve after treatment of the underlying meniscal abnormality.[38] Cysts have also been noted in association with systemic lupus erythematosus,[60] gout, osteoarthritis, psoriatic arthritis, Reiter's syndrome, Sjögren's syndrome,[48] tuberculosis, brucellosis, and pigmented villonodular synovitis,[36] but they are most frequently seen in patients with rheumatoid arthritis. In fact, popliteal cysts have been found on arthrography in up to 63 percent of patients with rheumatoid arthritis.[57, 60]

The cysts are usually located posteromedially, deep to the medial head of the gastrocnemius muscle,[5] but they may occasionally extend into the lateral or anterior medial calf, or they may reach posteriorly into the thigh.[51, 52, 58] Cysts may also originate from the apex of the suprapatellar pouch and expand proximally into the anterior soft tissues of the thigh.[56]

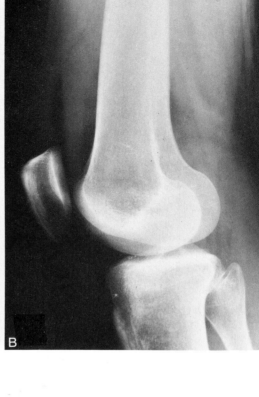

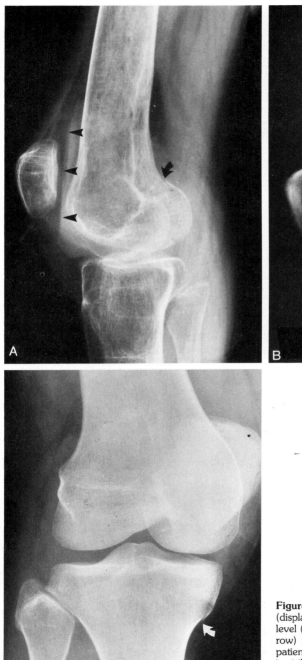

Figure 9–33. Fat-Fluid Levels. *A,* A cross-table lateral (displayed as a routine lateral) view shows a fat-fluid level (arrowheads). A nondisplaced femoral fracture (arrow) is seen. *B,* A cross-table lateral view of another patient also shows a fat-fluid level although no fracture is visible. *C,* An oblique view was necessary to demonstrate the tibial fracture (arrow).

Anatomical and Pathophysiological Considerations. Most popliteal cysts are thought to represent distended gastrocnemio-semimembranosus bursae that usually communicate with the joint through a posterior defect in the joint capsule. Such a communication has actually been noted in 17 of 30 cadaver dissections.[59]

This channel tends to close when the knee is extended and to open when the knee is flexed. A valvular mechanism allows fluid to pass from the knee joint to the cyst but may prevent transmission of fluid in the opposite direction, thus limiting the elevation of intraarticular pressure.[46]

Histological studies show that some cysts do have a synovial lining, but the majority are lined with fibrous tissue, and some have an inflammatory component.[36, 43] The walls of the inflammatory cyst are thick, and the inner surface is sometimes shaggy and irregular, with fibrin and amorphous material adhering to the lining.

Symptoms. Most popliteal cysts are asymptomatic. For example, Zizic and associates noted synovial cysts on arthrography in 19 of 30 hospitalized patients with rheumatoid arthritis, but only 3 patients had associated signs or symptoms.[60] Rupture of a popliteal cyst may be associated with acute symptoms mimicking thrombophlebitis.[35, 39a, 41, 43, 44, 47, 55] Some of these cases result from an inflammatory response that occurs in patients with rheumatoid arthritis when the joint fluid ruptures into the calf. On the other hand, Dixon and Grant used human plasma to distend the knee joints of five normal volunteers, and although joint rupture occurred in two instances, no symptoms were produced.[39a] This finding supports the concept that the symptoms depend not only upon the dissection of fluid into the calf but also upon the type of fluid, e.g., rheumatoid synovial fluid in contrast to plasma. Venous thrombosis is probably not the source of symptoms, since almost all surgically explored cases have shown no evidence of thrombosis. Hemorrhage into the cyst, inflammation or synovitis of the cyst wall, and rheumatoid nodules in the cyst wall have been suggested as possible sources of acute calf pain. A large nondissecting cyst extending into the calf may also produce relatively acute pain,[53] although the onset of pain in these patients is more gradual and less severe than that accompanying cyst rupture.[42]

Arthrography. In most patients a communication between the knee joint and the cyst is present, and knee arthrography is therefore usually diagnostic (Fig. 9–34). Ten to 20 or more ml of positive contrast medium is injected into the suprapatellar pouch until it is distended. The knee is flexed and extended; the cyst is often noted to fill only on flexion. If there is doubt as to whether the entire cyst is filled, the patient is asked to exercise the leg and to walk, and repeat films are obtained. Usually at least a portion of the cyst will fill, although its entire length may not always be delineated. Hench and co-workers noted that during the phase of subsiding inflammation communication to the knee joint may be obliterated.[44] In these patients or in instances in which the entire cyst does not appear to be filled, direct cyst puncture may be done.

In a patient with rheumatoid arthritis and acute calf pain and swelling, demonstration of a cyst, with or without extravasation, is taken as confirmatory evidence that the symptoms are related to the cyst. Venography is not usually performed. Recently, however, a patient with both deep venous thrombosis and a large dissecting popliteal cyst was reported.[54]

Ultrasonography. Most studies have shown ultrasound to be a fairly accurate method for confirming the presence of a popliteal cyst (Table 9–2). Advantages over athrography include the noninvasive nature of ultrasonography (which allows it to be repeated during treatment); the ability to detect cysts that do not communicate with the knee joint; and the potential for differentiating a cyst from other masses, including solid tumors and popliteal artery aneurysms (Fig. 9–35). On the other hand, cysts of less than 1 cm in internal diameter and cysts that have ruptured and decompressed may not be demonstrable on ultrasound examination. In addition, it may be difficult to differentiate debris within a cyst from a solid mass. Hermann and colleagues examined 100 consecutive patients with knee trauma and found 27 cases in which the arthrogram demonstrated a cyst, but the ultrasound study did not (Table 9–2).[45] None of these patients had a palpable mass or symptoms referable to the popliteal area. In contrast, all the cysts detected on ultrasound examination were associated with either pain or a mass. The applicability of these data to patients with rheumatoid arthritis is untested. Arthrography is still suggested in rheumatoid patients when a popliteal cyst is clinically likely, but there is a negative ultrasound examination. CT may also be used to document the presence of a cyst.[55a]

Table 9–2. Correlation Between Arthrography and Ultrasonography in the Diagnosis of Popliteal Cysts

	% Cases with Cysts Diagnosed by			
	Arthrogram	+	+	−	−
Study	*Ultrasound*	+	−	+	−
Meire et al., 1974 (24 cases)[50]		79	4	4	13
Carpenter et al., 1976 (34 cases)[37]		47	6	6	41
Gompels and Darlington 1979 (49 cases)[40]		29	17	10	44
Hermann et al., 1981 (100 cases)[45]		15	27	0	58

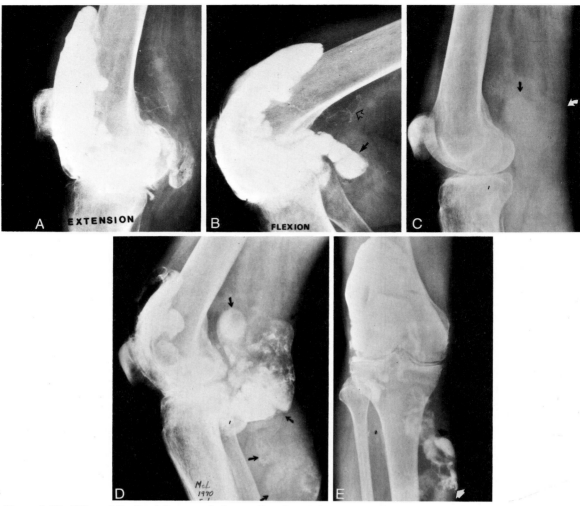

Figure 9–34. Filling of Popliteal Cysts on Arthrography. *Case 1:* In extension *(A)* the cyst is minimally filled, whereas in flexion *(B)* it is well filled (arrow). The changes of rheumatoid arthritis, including irregular enlargement of the joint capsule, filling defects, and lymphatic filling (open arrow) are present. *Case 2: C,* The preliminary lateral view shows the upper margins of a soft-tissue mass (arrow) posteriorly. *D,* The arthrogram confirms a large popliteal cyst (arrows). *Case 3: E,* The typical medial location of the cyst (arrows) is shown on this AP view.

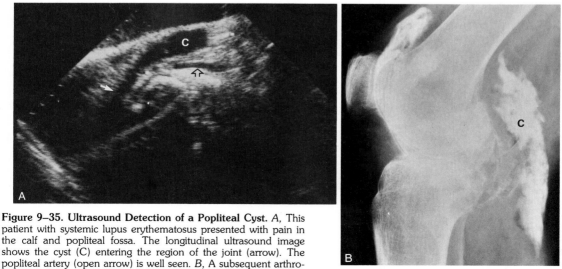

Figure 9–35. Ultrasound Detection of a Popliteal Cyst. *A,* This patient with systemic lupus erythematosus presented with pain in the calf and popliteal fossa. The longitudinal ultrasound image shows the cyst (C) entering the region of the joint (arrow). The popliteal artery (open arrow) is well seen. *B,* A subsequent arthrogram confirms the cyst (C) and documents its irregular contour (suggesting dissection into adjacent soft tissue) as well as multiple filling defects.

Synovial Plicae

Synovial septa that divide the joint into three compartments are present during embryological development of the knee joint: a superior femoropatellar and two inferior femorotibial compartments.[65] Portions of these septa may persist into adulthood and are then called synovial plicae.

The three plicae—suprapatellar, mediopatellar, and infrapatellar (ligamentum mucosum)—are shown in Figure 9–36. Plicae have been seen in up to 60 percent of examined knees.[67]

Symptoms may be associated with an unusually large, thick medial patellar plica. Patel notes an increased incidence of chondromalacia of the medial facet of the patella and the medial femoral condyle in these cases, but the relationship between the presence of this plica and the chondromalacia is unclear. The medial plica may actually impinge on these areas as the knee is flexed, interfere with the normal quadriceps mechanism, or be the focus of localized synovitis.[66, 67] On physical examination tenderness is noted medial to the patella, and a snapping sensation can be elicited with knee motion. The

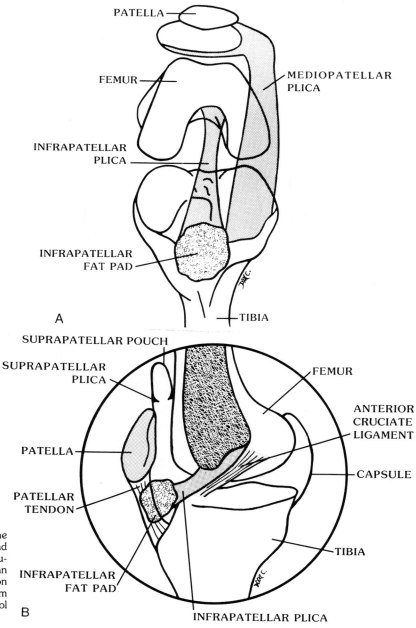

Fig. 9–36. Synovial Plicae. The mediopatellar, suprapetellar, and infrapatellar (ligamentum mucosum) plicae are shown on an exploded, tunnel view (A) and on a sagittal view (B). (Redrawn from Apple JS et al. Skeletal Radiol 7:251, 1982.)

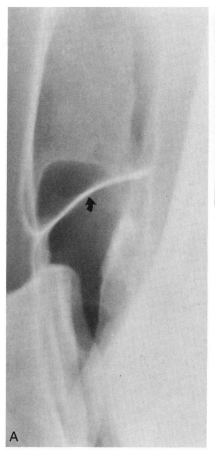

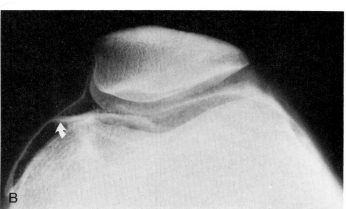

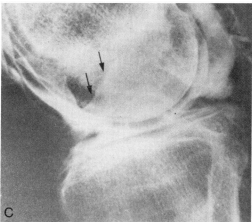

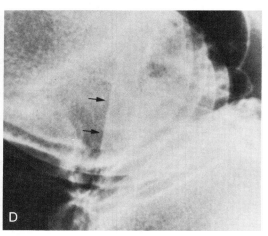

Figure 9–37. Synovial Plicae Demonstrated on Arthrography. *A,* A lateral view of the suprapatellar pouch shows a transverse septum, the suprapatellar plica (arrow). The presence of contrast and air above and below the plica confirms its being incomplete (fenestrated). *B,* The medial patella plica (arrow) is shown on this tangential view of the patellofemoral joint. *C,* The infrapatellar plica (arrows) extends from the anterior fat pad to the area of origin of the anterior cruciate. *D,* A normal anterior cruciate (arrows) is shown for comparison with *C.* (*C* and *D* are from Brody GA, Pavlov H, Warren RF, et al.: AJR 140:767, 1983, by permission.)

medial patellar plica can be identified on tangential patellar views or on computed tomography obtained after double-contrast arthrography (Fig. 9–37).[62] The relationship between the presence of a plica and the presence of symptoms has not been determined. Medial patellar plicae have been divided at arthroscopy or at arthrotomy with improvement in symptoms.[66, 67]

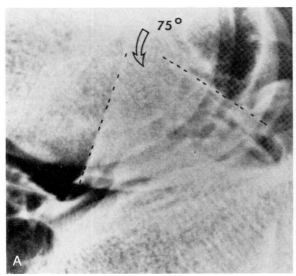
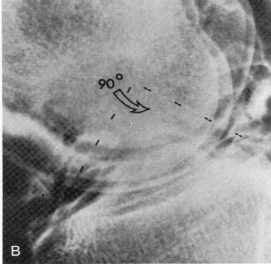

Figure 9–38. The Infrapatellar Plica, the Posterior and the Anterior Cruciate Ligaments. As demonstrated by Brody and associates, the angle between the anterior and the posterior cruciates is < 90 degrees *(A)*, whereas the angle between the infrapatellar plica and the posterior cruciate is > 90 degrees *(B)*. (From Brody GA, Pavlov H, Warren, RF et al: AJR 140:767, 1983, by permission.)

It is important to recognize the infrapatellar plica on arthrography because its course parallels that of the anterior cruciate ligament, and the plica may be confused with the ligament.[64] Brody and co-workers noted that the angle between the normal anterior and posterior cruciate ligaments is less than 90 degrees, whereas the angle between the inferior plica and the posterior cruciate is greater than 90 degrees (Fig. 9–38).[63] When the inferior patellar plica was seen at arthrography, an anterior cruciate tear was uniformly present. Therefore, the radiological distinction between the inferior patellar plica and the anterior cruciate is more than a mere academic exercise. The suprapatellar plica is usually an incidental finding on arthrography.

Ruptures of the Extensor Mechanism

Quadriceps Tendon Rupture. Rupture of the quadriceps tendon results from sudden violent contraction of the quadriceps during an attempt to stop a fall or from acute and marked flexion of the knee from a force applied to the foot or toes.[80] A number of conditions have been noted to predispose to tendon rupture, including obesity, gout,[74] systemic lupus erythematosus,[74, 79, 83] rheumatoid arthritis,[76] hyperparathyroidism,[77] renal failure,[78, 84] and diabetes mellitus.[68] Often, the patients are elderly, and degenerative changes of the tendon that predispose to rupture are present.

Tears may be partial or complete. The central anterior portion of the tendon tears first, and if the force continues, the tear extends medially and laterally. The area 1.3 to 2 cm above the patella is usually involved.

Diagnosis may be difficult on clinical examination. The characteristic finding is an inability to extend the knee actively. Bleeding into the area may obscure an otherwise palpable defect in the tendon, and only after swelling subsides may the defect become apparent.[81] Bilateral rupture may also occur.

Radiological Findings. This is a difficult radiographic diagnosis. Abnormalities are confined to the lateral view (Table 9–3). Hemarthrosis and blurring of the normally sharply defined margins of the quadriceps tendon caused by adjacent hemorrhage are noted.[84] The finding of a suprapatellar soft-tissue mass with calcification within it provides an important diagnostic clue (Figs. 9–39 and 9–40). The mass represents the retracted portion of the tendon; the calcification may be a consequence of prior degenerative change in the tendon or of newly avulsed fragments from the patella. Although the patellar position should be low, this is not

Table 9–3. **Radiographic Signs of Quadriceps Rupture**

Hemarthrosis
Blurring of margins of quadriceps tendon
Suprapatellar soft-tissue mass with calcification
Low patellar position

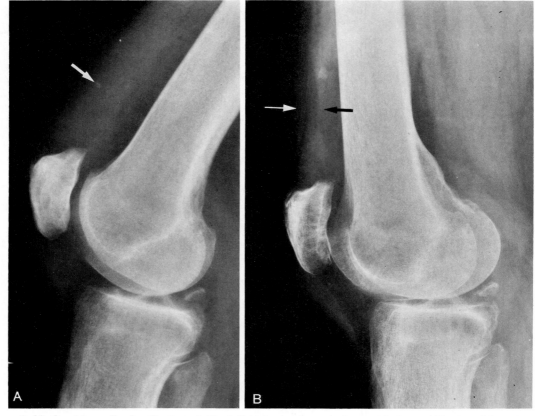

Figure 9–39. Quadriceps Tendon Rupture. *A,* The initial lateral radiograph shows widening and blurring of the soft tissues in the area of the quadriceps tendon. A small calcification (arrow) is noted. There is mild fullness in the suprapatellar pouch. A loose body is present in the joint posteriorly. *B,* One year later, the swelling has subsided, leaving an abnormally thin quadriceps tendon shadow (arrows). Muscle retraction has resulted in the more proximal location of the calcification.

always apparent on radiographs obtained in the supine position. Laxity of the patellar tendon may be demonstrable.

Injection of contrast material into the suprapatellar pouch can confirm the diagnosis (Fig. 9–40). In full-thickness tears the contrast medium will leak into the soft tissues anterior to the patella and then downward, sometimes filling the prepatellar and infrapatellar bursae.[70, 82]

Patellar Tendon Rupture. As in patients with quadriceps tendon rupture, rupture of the patellar tendon produces a deficit in active knee extension. Patients with patellar tendon rupture are often younger than those with quadriceps rupture.[81] Swelling around the patellar tendon with obliteration of its normally sharp adjacent fat lines and an abnormally high patellar position

are characteristic radiographic features (Fig. 9–41; Table 9–4).

Meniscal Tears

Classification. Meniscal tears more commonly involve the less mobile medial meniscus and are more common posteriorly than anteriorly. However, lateral tears are noted in up to one third of patients,[89] and combined medial and lateral tears occur in between 3 and 9 percent of patients.[89, 90] In a small number of patients tears of an asymptomatic meniscus are found.

There are many classifications of meniscal tears. The Groh classification has been advocated by Ricklin and associates.[106] In this classification tears are grouped according to etiology:

1. *Spontaneous detachment* (primary degeneration) occurs in menisci that are abnormal as a result of aging or of abnormal stress over long periods. The orientation is usually horizontal, hence the designation "horizontal cleavage lesions."[175]

2. *Fresh traumatic tears* occur in younger

Table 9–4. **Radiographic Signs of Patellar Tendon Rupture**

Blurring of margins of patellar tendon
High patellar position

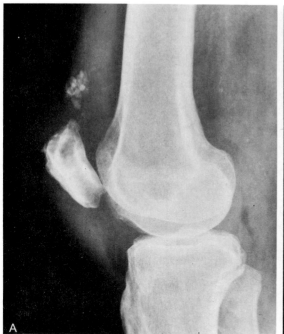
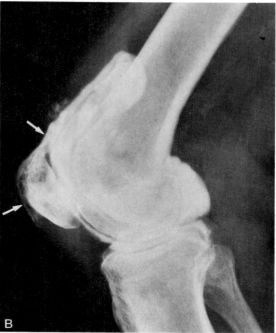

Figure 9–40. Quadriceps Tendon Rupture. *A,* The lateral view shows calcification in the area of the quadriceps tendon. There is soft-tissue swelling anterior and inferior to the patella, and there is a joint effusion. The upper pole of the patella is abnormally tilted anteriorly. *B,* Injection of positive contrast medium into the suprapatellar pouch was accompanied by anterior leakage of the contrast medium (arrows), thus confirming the presence of a defect in the quadriceps tendon.

individuals and may be associated with joint locking. They are longitudinal, bucket-handle, or peripheral tears.

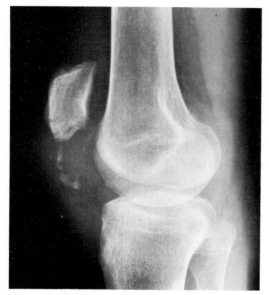

Figure 9–41. Patellar Tendon Rupture. This patient has chronic renal disease. Weeks after a fall, the lateral radiograph shows an abnormally high patellar position and ossification in the area of the patellar tendon. A previously noted joint effusion has subsided. There is a nondisplaced fracture of the inferior pole of the patella.

3. *Late changes after a traumatic tear* may result from enlargement of a tear or from degeneration of an already torn meniscus.

4. *Late changes after ligamentous damage* usually involve the posterior horn of the meniscus, medially in patients with anteromedial instability, and laterally in patients with anterolateral laxity.

Tears may also be classified by their morphology (Figs. 9–42 and 9–43):[94]

1. *Vertical tears.* These include two types: (a) *Concentric tears* parallel the contour of the meniscus. The bucket-handle tear is a vertical tear in the substance of the meniscus, rather than at its periphery. The radiological appearance depends on the degree of displacement of the inner fragment. With minimal displacement of the inner fragment both the inner and the outer fragments are seen. When the inner fragment is displaced into the intercondylar notch, it may be obscured, and only the deformity of the outer fragment suggests the diagnosis. (b) *Radial tears* are vertical tears that are roughly perpendicular to the circumference of the meniscus. Accumulated contrast medium makes the involved inner portion of the meniscus appear abnormally dense.

2. *Horizontal tears* occur parallel to the tibial articular surface. A line of increased density

531

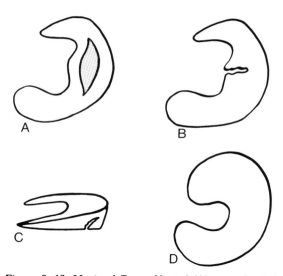

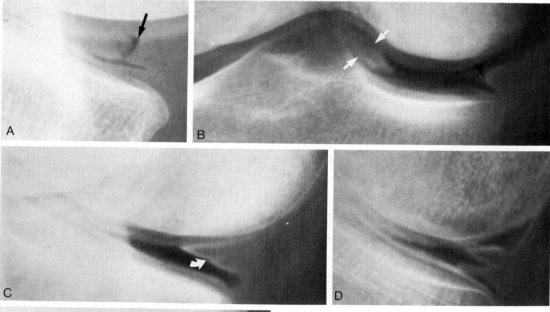

Figure 9–42. Meniscal Tears. Vertical *(A),* vertical radial *(B),* and oblique *(C)* tears are shown. The abnormal contour of a discoid meniscus is shown in *D.* (Redrawn from Freiberger RH, Killoran PJ, and Cardona G: AJR 97:736, 1966.)

extending into the meniscus from its inner superior or inferior surface will be noted.

3. *Tears in a discoid meniscus* are evident from the abnormal discoid shape of the meniscus. The lateral side is usually involved, although rare cases involving the medial meniscus are reported.

Freiberger, Killoran, and Cardona noted that most tears are complex combinations of these types.[94] They therefore make no attempt to classify the tears except as to location. However, there is probably some merit in trying to classify lesions, and there is a definite need to localize them. For example, degenerative tears are often horizontal in configuration (horizontal cleavage lesions) and are quite frequent in older populations. Smillie suggests removal of all these menisci to avoid subsequent osteoarthritis, but this practice is not universal.[99, 169, 175] Also, arthroscopic surgery may be appropriate in some instances, such as the removal of the inner fragment of a bucket-handle tear when the

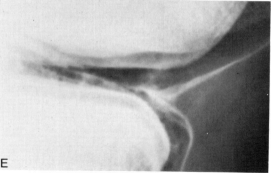

Figure 9–43. Examples of Meniscal Tears and Post-surgical Deformity. *A,* Complex vertical tear (arrow), base of posterior medial meniscus. *B,* Vertical tear, bucket-handle type. The displaced inner fragment (arrows) is seen, and the inner margin of the peripheral fragment is blunted (arrowhead). *C,* Oblique tear, inferior surface medial meniscus (arrow). This type may be difficult to confirm on arthroscopy. *D,* Horizontal tear. The tear divides the meniscus into upper and lower fragments. *E,* After medial meniscectomy, the anterior horn appears thinner than usual, consistent with the appearance of a regenerated meniscus.

remainder of the meniscus is normal. Preoperative arthrography is helpful in deciding on this approach.

Menisectomy

Indications. The criteria for menisectomy are changing. On the one hand, the functional role of the meniscus is increasingly appreciated, and the high incidence of postmenisectomy osteoarthritis and functional limitation is noted.[85, 108] On the other hand, failure to remove a damaged meniscus may also result in the development of osteoarthritis.

The type of tear—deduced by clinical, arthroscopic, and arthrographic examinations—is taken into consideration. In young patients, healing of tears in the well-vascularized peripheral zone may occur.[99, 105] Alternatives to menisectomy are being tried—for example, surgical repair of the medial meniscus has been done at the time of repair of a torn medial collateral ligament.[105] Portions of a damaged meniscus may be removed during arthroscopy.

Complications and Radiographic Follow-up. Immediate local complications of menisectomy include damage to adjacent nerves and vessels or to articular cartilage, incomplete removal of the meniscus, hemarthrosis, and

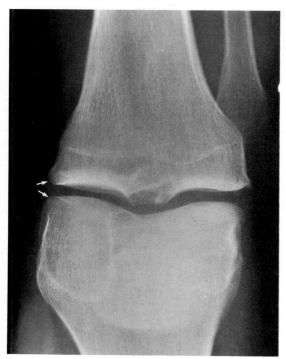

Figure 9–44. Postmenisectomy Changes. Years after medial menisectomy, there is mild squaring of the bony margins (arrows). Osteophytes and subchondral sclerosis have developed laterally. There is mild lateral cartilage-space narrowing.

infection.[85] Later, osteoarthritis may develop. Fairbank evaluated the preoperative and postoperative radiographs of 107 menisectomy patients and noted the development of a hypertrophic ridge of bone from the margin of the femoral condyle of the involved compartment, flattening of the femoral articular surface, and narrowing of the joint space on the side of operation (Fig. 9–44).[92] There was mild sharpening of the articular margin of the tibia. Long-term studies have shown these changes, indicative of osteoarthritis, to be the rule rather than the exception.

Menisectomy may be either complete or partial. Complete menisectomy is done through the peripheral attachment of the meniscus to facilitate regeneration of a fibrocartilaginous meniscus.[85] The regenerated meniscus is thinner and narrower than the normal one.[99] In partial menisectomy, only the torn portion is removed, preserving the more normal peripheral portion to provide some continued meniscal function. It is anticipated that partial menisectomy will avoid or ameliorate the deleterious changes ascribed to complete menisectomy.

Alignment Abnormalities

Chondromalacia Patellae

The term *chondromalacia* is used extensively but is seldom defined. It has been used to describe all stages and types of degenerative disease of the patellar cartilage but is often misapplied to a painful condition in young adults. The term should be reserved to describe pathological findings of soft cartilage on the patellae, as the name implies. This pathological finding may or may not be associated with the clinical syndrome of anterior knee pain.

Pathology. Goodfellow, Hungerford, and Woods noted two apparently separate pathological processes involving the patella.[119] The first, termed age-dependent surface degeneration, occurs in habitual noncontact areas, such as the odd facet of the patella. Fibrillaton of the cartilage begins at the surface, with gradual thinning of the cartilage. It is suggested that such surface degeneration, limited to the odd facet, is not a cause of patellofemoral pain. However, a similar lesion in areas of contact may result in osteoarthritis in later middle age.

The second lesion, basal degeneration, begins, as the name implies, in the deep layers of cartilage; the cartilaginous surface is involved late. The ridge separating the odd facet from the medial facet and the ridge between the medial and lateral facets are the areas predominantly

upside down ?.

involved. Goodfellow and colleagues suggest that this lesion may produce symptoms in young patients. This condition would therefore seem to correspond to the clinical term *chondromalacia.*

Etiology. In view of the absence of a uniform definition for *chondromalacia,* it is not surprising that a number of mechanisms have been suggested to cause the condition. Both overuse (including aging) and habitual disuse have been suggested as causes. Insall, Falvo, and Wise suggest that trauma is a major initiating factor, since all patients in their series had a history of meniscal tears, abnormal patellar alignment, or direct injury to the patella.[122] Laurin and coworkers explain the origin of the disorder as a structural or a functional imbalance or both that leads to poor patellar tracking or to patellofemoral malalignment, resulting in decreased pressure on the medial aspect of the patellofemoral joint and increased pressure laterally.[14] Medial hypopressure leads to malnutrition of the medial side of the patellofemoral joint, to release of degradative enzymes, to chemical synovitis, and to effusion. Eventually, damage to the lateral patellofemoral cartilage occurs as a result of the combined effects of chondrolytic enzyme release and excessive mechanical compression of the lateral side of the joint.[14]

Symptoms and Signs. The symptoms of chondromalacia may mimic those of medial meniscal tears. Typically, adolescents and young adults, females predominating, are affected.[119] Pain in the area of the patella occurs and may be exacerbated by loading the joint in flexion, typically when going up or down stairs.[119, 125] Prolonged sitting with the knee in flexion produces pain (the "theatre sign"). Older patients with patellofemoral pain usually have osteoarthritis with typical radiological and clinical features.

Several alignment abnormalities are noted in association with chondromalacia, including an

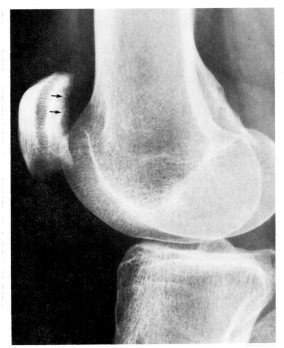

Figure 9–45. Chondromalacia. There is loss of subchondral bone from the patella (arrows).

abnormal Q angle and an abnormally high patella (patella alta). **Q** *angle* refers to the angle formed by the quadriceps and the patellar tendons. It is measured clinically from the anterior superior iliac spine to the center of the patella and from this point to the tibial tubercle (see Fig. 9–13). Normally, this angle measures 15 to 20 degrees,[122, 125] and measurements of greater than 20 degrees are considered abnormal. An increased angle represents an increased tendency for the patella to deviate laterally and an increase in lateral pressure on the patella with flexion.

Radiographic Findings

Alignment Abnormalities. A number of alignment abnormalities are noted on radio-

Table 9–5. Patellar Position As Shown on Tangential Films in 20 Degrees of Flexion

% in Various Conditions	Patellofemoral Index		Patellar Tilt			Patellar Displacement	
			Lateral Patellofemoral Angle			Medial to or Touching Reference Line	Lateral to Reference Line
	≤1.0	> 1.0	Open Laterally	Parallel	Open Medially		
% of Normal controls	100	0	97	3	0	100	0
% of Subluxing patellae	0	100	0	60	40	47	53
% of Chondromalacia patellae	3	97	90	10	0	70	30

Source: Laurin CA, Dussault R, Levesque HP: Clin Orthop 144:16, 1979; personal communication, Carroll A. Laurin, M.D., 1985.

graphic examination of patients with chondromalacia. These including the following:

Patella alta: This state is most easily evaluated on lateral views by dividing the length of the patellar tendon by the diagonal length of the patella. Ratios of more than 1.3:1 are abnormally high.[10, 12] (See section on normal radiographic appearances and Figure 9–20.)

Lateral tilt or lateral patellar subluxation: These states have been evaluated by Laurin and associates on tangential views in 20 degrees of flexion (see the section Normal Radiographic Appearances). Ninety-seven percent of patients with chondromalacia have patellofemoral indices of more than 1.6, indicating some tilt of the patella (usually not as much as seen in patients with subluxing patellae and therefore not enough to produce an abnormal lateral patellofemoral angle; Table 9–5).

Lateral patellar displacement: Lateral patellar displacement is noted in some patients with chondromalacia as well as in some with subluxing patellae (Table 9–5).

Structural Changes. Early lesions are confined to the cartilage, and no bony changes are seen. Small cyst-like areas in the patella, however, may suggest this diagnosis. Later findings are those of osteoarthritis, with cartilage narrowing, sclerosis, bone loss, and hypertrophic lipping (Fig. 9–45). Bone loss is sometimes suggested on the lateral film, with the changes in the femur (femoral gouging) even more apparent than those in the patella (Fig. 9–46; Table 9–6).

Table 9–6. Radiographic Findings of Chondromalacia

Plain Films
± Patella alta
± Patellar subluxation
Patellar tilt (patellofemoral index > 1.0)
Cystic changes in patella
Thickening of bony trabeculae
Focal or diffuse osteoporosis
Osteoarthritis
Arthrography
Focal or diffuse increase in cartilage thickness
Irregular or cracked cartilage surface
Contrast within cartilage
Decreased cartilage thickness

Arthrography. The proper role for arthrography in the evaluation of chondromalacia is debated.[114, 116] Ficat and associates advocate single-contrast arthrography with tangential patellofemoral views at 30, 45, 60, and 90 degrees of flexion for evaluation of patellar cartilage.[118] Horns performed double-contrast arthrography with multiple lateral and oblique spot-films of the patella and a tangenital patellar view; in patients with chondromalacia, localized nodular elevations of the cartilage surface or more diffuse increase in its thickness, irregularity of or distinct cracks in the surface, and contrast material within the confines of the cartilage were noted.[120] Eventually, the thickness of articular cartilage is decreased (Fig. 9–47). Such changes were found in arthrographic studies of 24 patients; they were confirmed by palpation at the time of surgery in 87.5 percent of the patients.[120]

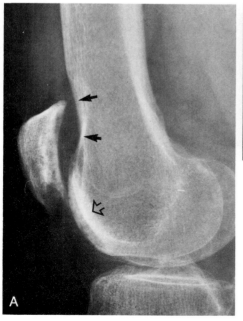

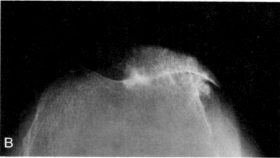

Figure 9–46. Patellofemoral Osteoarthritis. *A,* The lateral view shows marked erosion of the anterior femur (arrows). The patella is thinned, and there is subchondral sclerosis and lucency of the patella and the femur (open arrow). *B,* The tangential patellar view confirms complete patellofemoral cartilage loss and also shows lateral patellar subluxation and osteophytes.

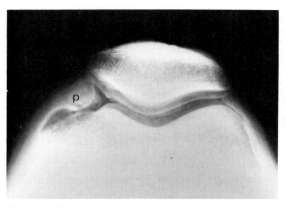

Figure 9–47. Chondromalacia. Tangential patellar view after arthrography shows thinning and slight roughening of the patellar cartilage, especially medially. The mediopatellar plica (p) is noted to be markedly thickened.

Boven and colleagues performed computed tomography after double-contrast arthrography and found this combination to improve the accuracy of assessing chondromalacia.[113] Cartilage irregularity was better demonstrated by CT than by arthrography alone and permitted diagnosis of probable or definite chondromalacia in 17 of 18 patients later shown to have the disease. Knee arthrography is helpful in detecting associated meniscal tears; the presence of both a meniscal lesion and chondromalacia is not uncommon.[116]

Treatment. Conservative measures, consisting of resting the knee, avoiding excessive flexion under load, and exercising the muscles to strengthen them, are the first line of treatment. If these measures fail, a number of surgical procedures have been advocated.

Realignment procedures include proximal soft-tissue surgery (such as tightening of a lax medial capsule or releasing tight lateral structures) and moving part or all of the insertion of the patellar tendon to a more medial location to decrease the Q angle. The Hauser,[126] the Elmslie-Trillat, and the Maquet procedures are examples of these distal procedures.[123, 135] (See Treatment under Recurrent Patellar Subluxation and Dislocation, later in this section.)

Localized defects in the patellar cartilage may be treated by excising the full thickness of involved cartilage; holes are drilled in the subchondral bone, allowing reparative granulation tissue to grow through them and replace damaged cartilage with fibrocartilage.[124, 125] In cases in which surgical procedure has failed or in which damage is more severe, patellectomy has been recommended. Patellectomy, however, is often followed by persistent weakness and by quadriceps atrophy.[124]

Arthroscopy has been used for the diagnosis and sometimes for the treatment of chondromalacia.[114] In addition to evaluation of the articular cartilage, patellofemoral anatomy, patellar tracking, and patellar mobility can be assessed. Shaving rough edges of cartilage and releasing tight lateral capsules have been done through the arthroscope.

Excessive Lateral Pressure Syndrome[3]

Excessive lateral pressure syndrome (ELPS) is characterized clinically by the presence of pain and radiologically by a tilting of the patella laterally on the tangential patellar view without lateral subluxation. The excessive lateral pull on the patella may be thought as resulting from a tight lateral retinaculum. Increased stress on the lateral facet results in lateral patellofemoral cartilage-space narrowing, subchondral sclerosis of the lateral facet, and reorientation of the lateral trabeculae (Table 9–7). Increased tension on the lateral ligaments produces lateral patellar osteophytes and calcification in the lateral retinaculum. The lateral patellar tilt is documented by an abnormal patellofemoral index.[14] Treatment choices are the same as for recurrent patellar subluxation and dislocation.

Recurrent Patellar Subluxation and Dislocation

A number of associated soft-tissue and bony abnormalities have been noted to be associated with recurrent patellar subluxation or dislocation, including a shallow femoral articular surface, a flatter than normal patella (often a Wiberg type III), patella alta, and traumatic injury to the medial soft tissues (Fig. 9–48).[3] At the time of subluxation or dislocation fragments of bone, cartilage, or both may be knocked off the patella, or the pull from the medial soft tissues may avulse a small medial patellar fragment. These fragments provide radiological confirmation of prior dislocation (Fig. 9–48). Posttraumatic cal-

Table 9–7. **Findings on Tangential Patellar Views in Excessive Lateral Pressure Syndrome (ELPS)**

Normal
Lateral patellofemoral cartilage-space narrowing
Subchondral sclerosis, lateral patella
Osteoporosis of medial patella
Subchondral cysts
Reorientation of lateral trabeculae
Lateral osteophytes and calcification
Lateral margin fractures

Source: Ficat RP, Hungerford DS: Disorders of the Patello-Femoral Joint. Baltimore, Willimas & Wilkins, 1977.

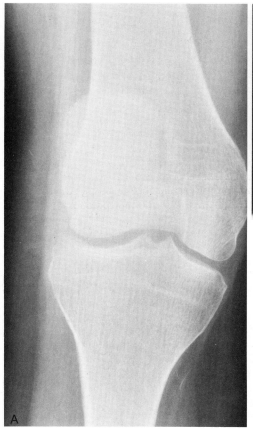

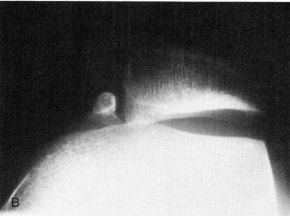

Figure 9–48. Abnormal Patellofemoral Joint and Absent Fibula. *A,* The AP view shows absence of the fibula, a smaller than normal medial tibial articular surface, and a relatively long medial femoral condyle. *B,* The tangential patellar view shows flat patellar and femoral articular surfaces. The medial bony fragment is evidence of a prior dislocation.

cification may also be noted in the medial soft tissues.

Patellar malposition may be difficult to detect radiologically. In most cases, the patella is displaced laterally (Figs. 9–49 and 9–50). Views in minimal flexion (20 or 30 degrees) with the quadriceps relaxed may be necessary to confirm subluxation, since increased flexion or muscle tightening may result in patellar recentering. Subluxation can be documented by noting (1) the lateral edge of the patella displaced lateral to the femoral condyle or lateral deviation of the

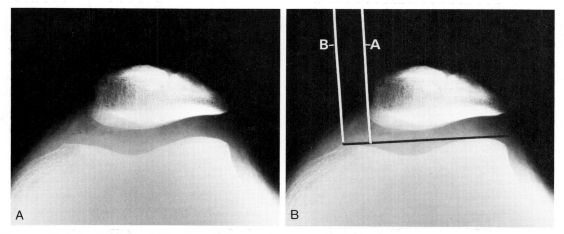

Figure 9–49. Lateral Patellar Subluxation. *A,* The patella seems to be displaced laterally, and the articular surfaces are flat. *B,* The degree of subluxation may be measured as the distance between lines A and B. (See Fig. 9–27.)

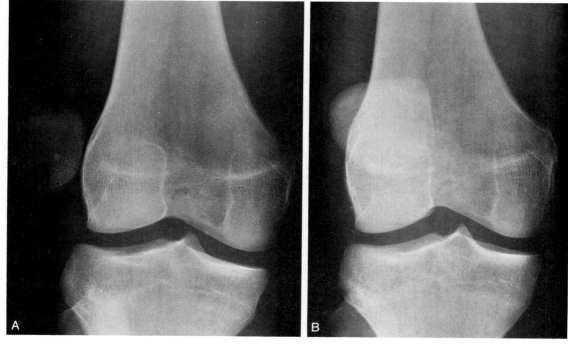

Figure 9–50. Patellar Dislocation. *A,* The patella is dislocated laterally. *B,* AP view after reduction.

medial aspect of patella from a line drawn through the medial femoral condyle (Fig. 9–49);[14] (2) widening of the medial joint space; (3) displacement of the apex of the patella lateral to the deepest point of the femoral groove; (4) a congruence angle of more than 16 degrees; and (5) a lateral patellofemoral angle that is

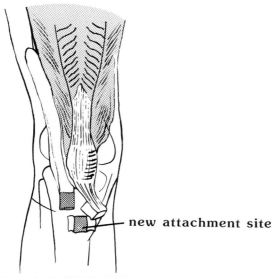

— new attachment site

Figure 9–51. The Hauser Procedure. The distal end of the patellar tendon and the attached bone are shifted medially and distally. The soft tissues are divided laterally. (After Hauser E: Surg Gynecol Obstet 66:199, 1938.)

open medially (40 percent) or is parallel (60 percent) on 20-degree flexion views.[17, 124]

Treatment. Initial treatment consists of conservative measures, including modification of activity, salicylates, and exercise. Several surgical procedures can be used in situations in which conservative programs fail. Surgical treatments include lateral retinacular release, proximal or distal realignment, tibial tubercle elevation, and patellectomy.

The Hauser Procedure (Figs. 9–51 and 9–52). In this procedure the patellar tendon and ½ inch of bone at its distal attachment are shifted medially and distally and fixed into a corresponding depression created in the tibia.[126] The original site of the patellar tendon insertion is filled with bone removed from the new site of attachment. According to Murray, however, this repositioning of the tibial tubercle actually places the tubercle more posteriorly, which increases the forces across the patellofemoral joint and the wear on the articular surface.[123]

Maquet Advancement of the Tibial Tuberosity (Figs. 9–53 and 9–54).[123, 134, 135] Anterior displacement of the tibial attachment of the patellar tendon increases the lever arm through which the tendon works and therefore increases the efficiency of the extensor mechanism. It also increases the angle at which the forces generated act on the patella. For both of these reasons a

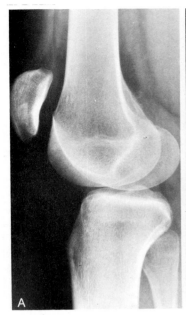 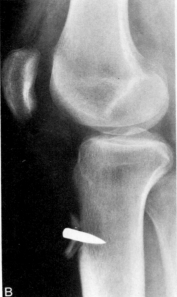 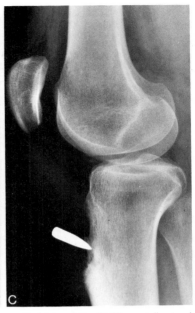

Figure 9–52. Hauser Procedure. *A,* A lateral view in extension shows an abnormally high patella. *B,* The patellar tendon and adjacent bone have been transplanted distally (and medially). The patellar position is improved. *C,* Weeks later, after an automobile accident, the staple has pulled loose from the tibia, and the patella has shifted proximally.

reduction in the compressive forces across the patellofemoral joint results. The anterior displacement may be combined with medial displacement of the tibial tubercle to relocate a subluxed patella.

Tibial tubercle elevation is accomplished by separating the tibial crest from the underlying bone and inserting iliac grafts, the largest piece of which is placed as far proximally as possible beneath the tibial tubercle. Relative forward position of the tibial tubercle can also be achieved during a tibial osteotomy.

Elmslie-Trillat Procedure. The tibial tubercle is detached proximally and then rotated medially (Fig. 9–55).

Arthritis

Osteoarthritis
The knee is the most frequent site of osteoarthritis (OA, osteoarthrosis, or degenerative joint disease), the pathogenesis of which depends heavily on alterations in normal biomechanics.[2] In the normal knee force applied across the joint falls on the center of the knee. The equal distribution of stress onto the medial and lateral compartments is reflected by the uniform thickness of the subchondral bone of both tibial plateaus.

Development of varus or valgus alignment abnormalities leads to increased stress on one side of the joint and to eventual degenerative changes.[129] For example, displacement of force toward the medial side of the knee joint (possibly caused by varus deformity or medial meniscal loss) leads to increased stress on the medial side of the joint. At first, this results in bone apposition (subchondral sclerosis) and then to cartilage-space narrowing. This narrowing further increases the varus deformity and shifts stress onto the medial compartment. Eventually, increased stress leads to bone resorption (predominantly from the tibia in varus deformity), creating even greater distortion. Lateral ligamentous laxity and medial subluxation of the femur on the tibia eventually occur.[129, 134, 135]

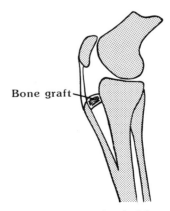

Figure 9–53. Maquet Tibial Tubercle Advancement. The tibial tubercle is elevated and bone graft inserted between the tubercle and the underlying tibia.

Bone graft

539

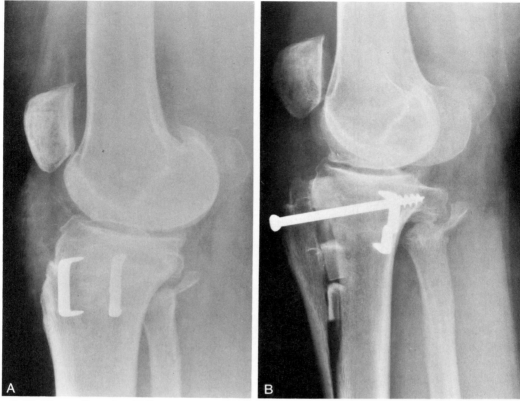

Figure 9–54. Maquet Procedure Following High-Tibial Osteotomy. *A,* Lateral view after high-tibial osteotomy; patellofe-moral pain was disabling. *B,* The tibial tubercle has been elevated and bone graft placed beneath it. A cancellous screw maintains the position of the fragments.

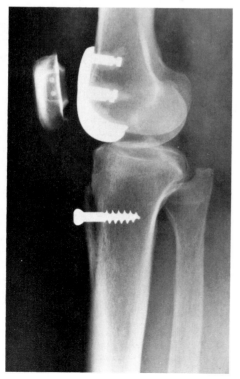

Figure 9–55. Elmslie-Trillat Procedure. A cancellous screw holds the medially shifted tibial tubercle in place. A patellofemoral prosthesis for severe patellofemoral osteoarthritis has been inserted.

Table 9–8. **Sequence of Radiographic Findings in Osteoarthritis of the Medial Compartment**

1. Subchondral sclerosis of tibial condyle (due to tibial articular cartilage loss)
2. Sclerosis of femoral condyle (due to femoral articular cartilage loss)
3. Bone loss from femoral and tibial articular surfaces
4. Subluxation

Source: Ahlback S: Acta Radiol [Diagn] (Suppl) 277:7, 1968.

Table 9–9. **Findings Confirming Cartilage Narrowing on Standing Views**

Cartilage space < 3 mm
Cartilage space (≤ one-half width that of opposite normal knee
Cartilage space narrower on standing than on supine examination

Source: Ahlback S: Acta Radiol [Diagn] (Suppl) 277:7, 1968.

Radiological Changes. Radiographs reflect the preceding biomechanical alterations.

Subchondral Sclerosis. This term refers to the development of increased density under the articular cortex. When seen in a tibial plateau, subchondral sclerosis is an early indicator of abnormal stress on that compartment. Ahlback correlated this radiographic finding with loss of tibial articular cartilage (Table 9–8; Fig. 9–56).[127]

Cartilage-Space Narrowing. Cartilage-space narrowing in OA most often involves the medial and patellofemoral compartments.[139] Cartilage loss is documented by cartilage-space narrowing that is sometimes more accurately demonstrated on weight-bearing than on supine views (Fig.

9–57). According to Ahlback, cartilage-space narrowing is present when the cartilage space measures less than 3 mm, or half or less than the same area of the contralateral normal knee, or when there is cartilage-space narrowing on weight-bearing as compared with nonweight-bearing views (Table 9–9).[127] Standing views, particularly those obtained of both legs simultaneously, may, however, show a spuriously normal cartilage space, even when severe cartilage loss is present. Usually, the presence of sclerosis on both the femoral and tibial sides of the joint or flattening of the articular surfaces provides evidence that severe cartilage loss is actually present (Figs. 9–56 and 9–57). Standing

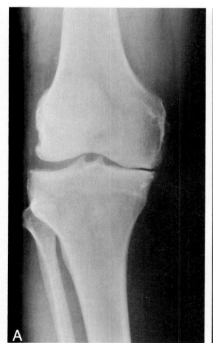
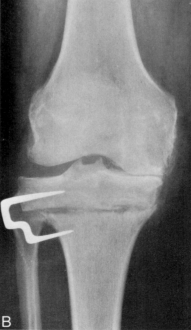
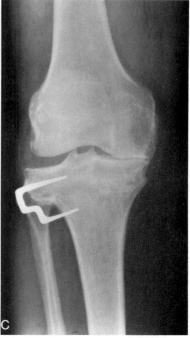

Figure 9–56. Osteotomy for Osteoarthritis. *A,* A standing view shows severe medial cartilage-space narrowing, with flattening of articular surfaces and subchondral sclerosis. There is varus deformity. *B,* Six weeks after high-tibial osteotomy: Correction is insufficient with only neutral alignment achieved. *C,* Further healing is seen at 10 months. There has been collapse at the osteotomy site, producing varus deformity. Despite apparent continued medial bony apposition, symptoms were improved.

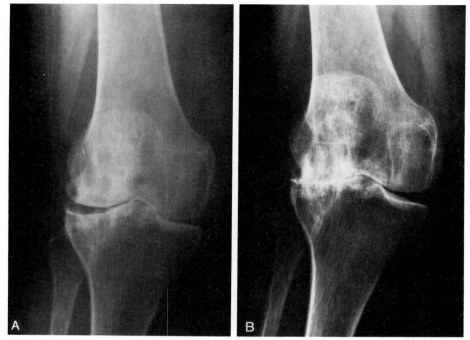

Figure 9–57. Osteoarthritis. *A,* The supine view shows valgus alignment. Sclerosis and subchondral lucencies are seen laterally, and there is more than the usual concavity of the lateral tibial plateau, all findings indicating severe lateral compartment cartilage loss (without the necessity of obtaining a standing view). *B,* The standing view confirms complete lateral cartilage loss.

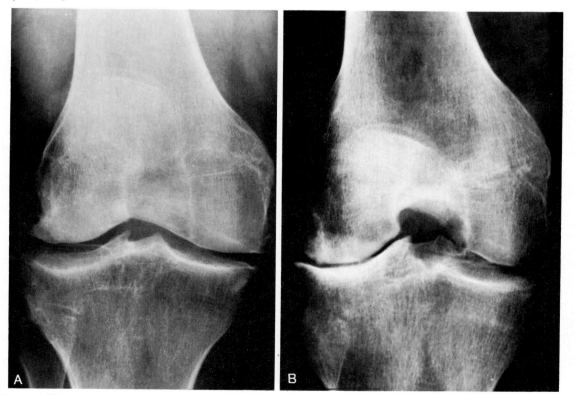

Figure 9–58. Osteoarthritis Best Demonstrated on the Tunnel View. *A,* The AP supine radiograph shows osteophytes from the joint margins. There is mild medial compartment cartilage-space narrowing. *B,* The tunnel view documents severe posterior lateral cartilage loss.

views with the knees slightly flexed (standing tunnel views) or routine tunnel views may show posterior cartilage-space narrowing not seen on standard AP or on weight-bearing films (Fig. 9–58).[136, 138]

Subchondral Cysts. In the knee, subchondral cysts occurring in patients with OA are smaller than those associated with rheumatoid arthritis. In fact, the presence of a large subchondral cyst in the knee should suggest the possibility of an alternative or underlying diagnosis, such as RA or calcium pyrophosphate dihydrate deposition disease (see Fig. 9–69). The cysts are found in the subchondral bone, surrounded by a zone of sclerosis and often apparently pointing toward the joint. Hypotheses regarding their development include (1) intrusion of synovial fluid into the bone through a defect in articular cartilage; and (2) bone degeneration from accumulated microfractures of overloaded trabeculae.[130] The latter theory is the more plausible one. The absence of filling of these cysts during arthrography suggests that any communication to the joint space that may have been present has been obliterated.

Effusion. Joint effusion is not a prominent feature of OA. Large effusions should suggest additional considerations, particularly rheumatoid arthritis and infection.

Osteophytes. Early cartilage damage in OA stimulates the development and ingrowth of blood vessels into the subchondral bone and cartilage. This stage is followed by subchondral bone formation, including the production of osteophytes, which are localized projections of cortical and cancellous bone continuous with adjacent normal bone and covered by hyaline cartilage.

Osteotomy for Osteoarthritis

The clinical goal of osteotomy is to relieve pain and correct deformity in patients with OA that is predominantly unicompartmental. On mechanical grounds the goal of osteotomy is to realign the leg to reduce and to redistribute stresses over the largest possible articular surface. Overcorrection of the deformity is usually required in order to shift the stresses of weight-bearing onto the more normal compartment. Failure to change the distribution of stress is associated with inevitable progression of damage.

When varus deformity is present, tibial osteotomy is usually done, whereas when valgus deformity is present, femoral osteotomy is preferred. Successful results are accompanied by a decrease in symptoms and by radiological evidence of healing. Follow-up arthrographic and histological studies in these cases have shown the development of a fibrocartilaginous joint surface on areas of previously denuded bone.[136]

Some of the available osteotomy techniques are reviewed in the following section. Postoperative fixation may be accomplished by internal fixation (e.g., blade-plate or staples) or by external compression.

Coventry High-Tibial Osteotomy. Coventry advocates high-tibial osteotomy in the cancellous bone proximal to the patellar tendon insertion.[129] The benefits of using this site are said to be (1) the site is near the site of deformity (the knee), (2) cancellous bone heals rapidly, (3) staples are all that is necessary for fixation, (4) postoperative immobilization is short, (5) there is almost no incidence of nonunion or delayed union, (6) weight-bearing and quadriceps contraction aid in compressing the osteotomy site, and (7) the collateral ligaments can be tightened.

In OA with varus deformity the surgical procedure is done through a lateral approach. A wedge of bone that is wider laterally is removed (Fig. 9–59). The upper arm of the wedge is parallel to the knee joint and 2 cm below it. The site of the lower limit of the wedge is determined

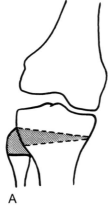
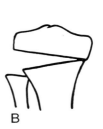
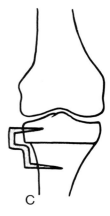

Figure 9–59. Coventry High-Tibial Osteotomy. *A* and *B,* A wedge of bone proximal to the patellar tendon insertion is removed from the tibia. *C,* The tibial fragments are then brought together, increasing the valgus angulation of the leg.

A   B   C

from preoperative radiographs. After the wedge is removed the medial tibia is perforated in a few places so that the medial cortex can be fractured. The leg is then realigned by valgus force and the bone margins held in apposition by 1 or 2 staples.

The amount of bone to be removed is determined from preoperative standing radiographs as follows (Fig. 9–60):

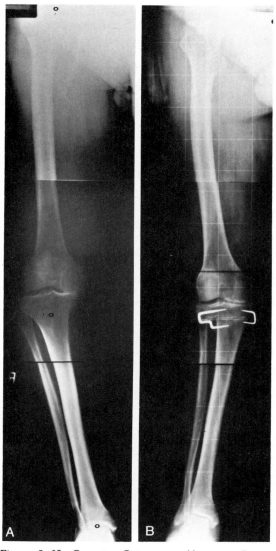

Figure 9–60. Coventry Osteotomy: Alignment Determined from Standing Views of the Entire Leg. *A,* The preoperative deformity is determined by drawing lines from the center of the femoral head (o) to the proximal tibia in the region of planned osteotomy (o) to the center of the tibial plafond (o) and noting the angle of intersection. This degree of varus angulation plus the normal valgus plus a 4-degree overcorrection defines the desired degree of correction. *B,* After osteotomy, overall valgus alignment is present.

1. The degree of deformity of the knee is defined by drawing lines from the centers of the femoral and the tibial shafts to a chosen point at the knee, such as the center of the intercondylar notch.

2. The degree of deformity is compared with the uninvolved side or to the standard normal situation, in which about 7 degrees of valgus is present. The number of degrees of correction necessary to change the abnormal leg to the normal degree of valgus is calculated (e.g., if there is 5 degrees of varus deformity, then 12 degrees of correction would be necessary to achieve 7 degrees of valgus alignment).

3. Overcorrection of 4 degrees is added to this figure, so that the apex of the wedge of resected bone is 12 degrees plus 4 degrees, or 16 degrees. Thus the angle of the wedge to be resected is a combination of the degree of varus deformity, the degree of valgus to be achieved, and a 4-degree overcorrection factor. This method is applicable to varus or valgus osteotomies and to high-tibial or low-femoral osteotomies. At surgery the size of the wedge can be determined by inserting Kirschner wires, obtaining radiographs or views on an image-intensifier, and measuring the angle formed until the measured angle equals the desired angle.

Radiologically detectable complications include medial or lateral shifts in the position of the fragments, loss of correction, nonunion or delayed union, and fracture into the joint (Figs. 9–56 and 9–61).

Maquet (Barrel Vault) Osteotomy. This technique may be used in patients with medial compartment osteoarthritis, even when severe deformity is present (Fig. 9–62). Maquet advocated weight-bearing films of the entire extremity (rather than the knee alone) for preoperative evaluation.[134, 135] Lines are drawn, one from the center of the femoral head to the middle of the tibia at the level of the osteotomy and one from this tibial site to the center of the talus (or tibial plafond). The angle formed by the intersection of these lines should be zero, and any deviation reflects the angular deformity (α) present (see Mechanical Axis, in Normal Radiographic Apperances).[134] The correction needed is calculated by adding 3 to 5 degrees to this angle and rotating a tracing of the knee until the desired correction is obtained. At surgery, Steinmann pins are introduced through the upper third of the tibial shaft and under the tibial plateau, forming an angle of α plus 3 to 5 degrees. The distal fragment is rotated (and brought forward) until the two pins are parallel on AP radiographs. Compression clamps are placed over the pins.

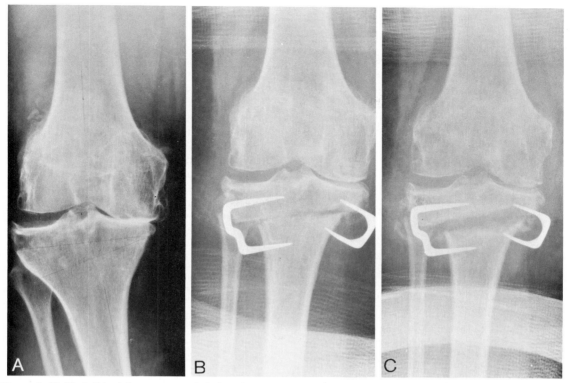

Figure 9–61. High-Tibial Osteotomy with Delayed Union. *A,* This standing view shows severe osteoarthritis involving the medial compartment, with a varus deformity of 10 degrees. *B,* After a high-tibial valgus osteotomy, the overall alignment is 7 degrees of valgus. *C,* A follow-up film at about 4 months shows marked bone resorption at the osteotomy site; fluoroscopy confirmed motion there. Healing occurred after further immobilization.

The anterior position of the distal fragment is thought to reduce compression forces on the femorotibial and patellofemoral joints.

Tibial osteotomy may also be done at a level below the tibial tubercle.[141] Osteotomy of the fibula is usually performed to facilitate tibial realignment.

It is of interest that the calculated degree of

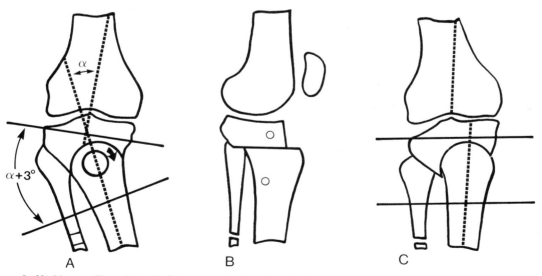

Figure 9–62. Maquet (Barrel Vault) Osteotomy. *A,* Two lines (dashed) are drawn, one from the center of the femoral head to the planned site of osteotomy and one from this point to the ankle. These lines should coincide, and any deviation (angle α) reflects the angular deformity that is present. Pins are placed through the tibia proximal and distal to the osteotomy site. The distal fragment is displaced forward *(B)* and rotated *(C)* until the pins are parallel. (Redrawn from Maquet PGJ: Treatment of Osteoarthritis of the Knee by Osteotomy. *In* Weil VH, ed. Progress in Orthopedic Surgery, Vol 4. Joint Preserving Procedures of the Lower Extremities. Heidelberg, Springer-Verlag, 1980.)

angular deformity of the knee may differ considerably, depending on whether the angle is determined from the centers of the femoral head, the tibia, and the ankle or from the axes of the femoral and the tibial shafts as seen on the standard upright view of the knee.

Distal Femoral Osteotomy. Distal femoral osteotomies may be used for correction of a number of alignment abnormalities, including varus or valgus deformities, rotational deformities, flexion contractures, and genu recurvatum.[135] Osteoarthritis with valgus deformity is more often treated with distal femoral than with proximal tibial osteotomy.

As for tibial osteotomy, the angular deformity may be calculated from the standing view of the leg by constructing lines from the center of the femoral head to the level of the planned osteotomy site proximal to the femoral condyles and then to the center of the ankle. Tracings are used to plan the surgical procedure.

At surgery two Steinmann pins are inserted in parallel through the femoral condyles (with the distal one near the joint) and another set of pins is inserted through the femoral shaft. The angle between these sets of pins corresponds to the measured deformity. The osteotomy is done in the supracondylar part of the femur, and the fragments are then rotated so that the proximal fragment sinks into the distal fragment and the four pins are parallel. Compression clamps or a blade-plate hold the fragments in position.[141] Depending on the deformity to be corrected, several others types of supracondylar osteotomy (e.g., opening wedge) can be performed.

Rheumatoid Arthritis

Soft-tissue swelling is the most frequent finding in knees of patients with RA. In a review of early cases of RA with abnormal radiographs, 80 percent showed soft-tissue swelling as the only abnormality.[143] Marginal erosion occurs less frequently in the knee than in the smaller joints. Uniform cartilage-space narrowing involving medial, lateral, and patellofemoral compartments is typical (Fig. 9–63).

Pigmented Villonodular Synovitis

This entity was first described by Simon in 1865 as xanthoma of the synovial lining.[145] In 1941 Jaffe, Lichtenstein, and Sutro reviewed the subject and renamed the condition pigmented villonodular synovitis (PVNS).[147] PVNS is a benign proliferative disorder that may produce either *diffuse* abnormalities with hyperplasia of all synovial villi or *localized* and nodular involvement. Microscopically, both forms contain giant cells,

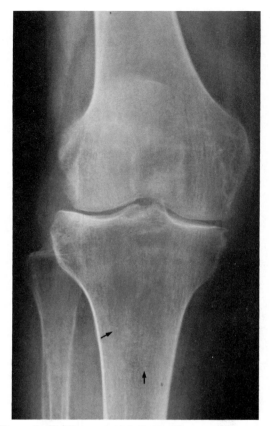

Figure 9–63. Rheumatoid Arthritis. There is uniform medial and lateral compartment cartilage narrowing. A small medial tibial erosion is present (with some secondary osteophyte formation). A central tibial lucency (arrows) suggests a large cyst.

foam cells, proliferative synovial villi, histiocytes, collagen, and areas of hyaline degeneration. Although the cause is still unclear, possible etiologies include trauma, hemorrhage, or a disturbance of lipid metabolism with a low-grade inflammatory response.

Young adults are most often affected, the clinical presentation varying according to site and type of the disease. In the diffuse form monarticular involvement of the knee or, occasionally, the hip, the ankle, the wrist, or the shoulder is noted. Symptoms include chronic swelling and stiffness. The localized form may be intra- or extraarticular. The extraarticular form is most common in the hand, producing nodular tenosynovitis. The intraarticular form of localized disease is most often found in the knee; it may present as a palpable mass, or it may simulate internal derangement.

Plain film radiographic diagnosis of intraarticular disease may be very difficult, since calcification is extremely rare. Classic radiographic findings include (1) monarticular involvement;

Table 9–10. Radiographic Features of Diffuse PVNS

Type of Evaluation	Features
Plain Films	Monarticular
	Soft-tissue swelling around joint, especially if lobulated
	No calcification of the soft-tissue mass
	Normal bony mineralization
	Normal cartilage spaces
CT	High attenuation number
Arthrography	Large joint capsule
	Filling defects

(2) soft-tissue swelling around a joint, particularly if this swelling is lobulated or nodular in character; (3) lack of calcification within the soft-tissue masses; (4) normal bony mineralization;

and (5) preservation of cartilage spaces (Table 9–10; Fig. 9–64). Bone erosion caused by extrinsic pressure from the soft-tissue masses and cyst-like lesions caused by expansion of the process into the relatively soft cancellous bone may occur. These occurrences are less common in the knee than they are in other joints (such as the fingers) because of the larger capacity of the synovial recesses of the knee. When present, the bone lesions appear as sharply circumscribed erosions and single or multiple lucent lesions with thin sclerotic margins.[144]

The introduction of double-contrast arthrography of the knee has improved the preoperative diagnosis of PVNS.[146, 151] Characteristically, joint aspiration discloses a brown-tinged joint effusion. In the diffuse form of PVNS the arthrographic findings of enlargement of the joint

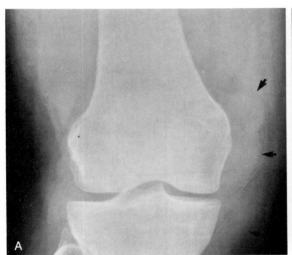

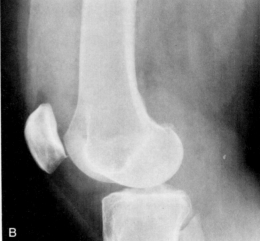

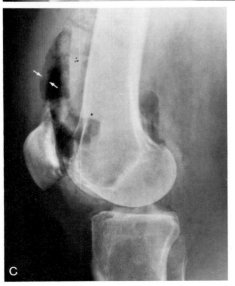

Figure 9–64. Pigmented Villonodular Synovitis. AP *(A)* and lateral *(B)* views show lobulated soft-tissue swelling (arrows). *C,* A lateral view from the double-contrast arthrogram shows intraarticular filling defects and thickening of the synovial lining (arrows).

547

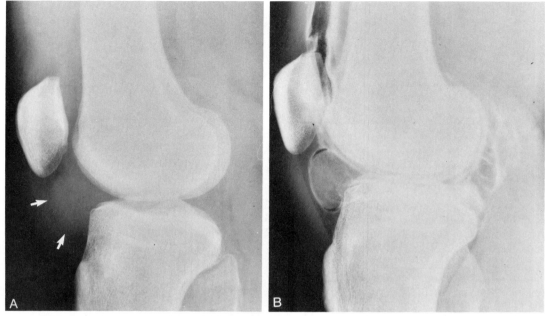

Figure 9–65. Localized Pigmented Villonodular Synovitis. *A,* The lateral radiograph shows a lobulated soft-tissue mass (arrows) in the infrapatellar region, continuous with the intraarticular soft tissues. There is mild fullness in the suprapatellar pouch. *B,* The arthrogram better defines the intraarticular nature of the mass, which proved to be focal pigmented villonodular synovitis.

cavity and multiple filling defects are typical (Fig. 9–64). Other causes of filling defects—such as synovial chondromatosis, synovial hemangioma, lipoma arborescens, and rheumatoid arthritis—may, however, produce similar filling defects.

Goergen and co-workers studied two patients with localized PVNS of the knee and noted in each a single mass located anteriorly, adjacent to the fat pad (Fig. 9–65).[146] Differential diagnostic considerations based on the arthrogram alone include enlargement of the fat pad caused by recurrent trauma and inflammation, displacement of the fat pad by a torn fragment of medial meniscus, adjacent loose bodies, and tumors—such as fibromas, hemangiomas, and intraarticular ganglia.

The increase in iron content in PVNS results in high absorption numbers on computed tomography,[149] a feature that can be helpful in differential diagnosis and in evaluating recurrence of the disease.

Synovial Chondromatosis

Synovial chondromatosis, or osteochondromatosis, is a rare, characteristically monarticular disease in which there is synovial metaplasia characterized by the formation of numerous cartilaginous nodules that may calcify or ossify. In the older literature many other names were

used for this condition, including synovial chondromata, diffuse enchondroma of the joint capsule, and chondromatosis of the joint capsule.

The knee is the most commonly affected joint, but reports of hip, shoulder, elbow,[153] ankle,[154] and even metacarpophalangeal joint involvement can be found. Tendon sheaths may also be involved. Milgram examined 20 cases and proposed three separate phases of this condition:[158] (1) active intrasynovial disease without loose bodies; (2) transitional lesions with osteochondral nodules in the synovial membrane and loose bodies; and (3) numerous free loose bodies (calcified or not) with quiescent intrasynovial disease.

In the past controversy raged as to whether this entity was premalignant or not. Although there have been cases of reported malignant degeneration,[159] doubt now exists as to whether the histologically identified chondrosarcoma actually originated within clearly defined areas of synovial chondromatosis or not.

Different theories exist as to the initial stimulus for metaplasia. These include the preexistence of primitive embryonic rests, infection (disputed by Jeffreys, who obtained numerous negative cultures of surgical specimens),[155] and some type of either noted or occult trauma. The last is now the most widely accepted theory.

The disorder is not familial and is most com-

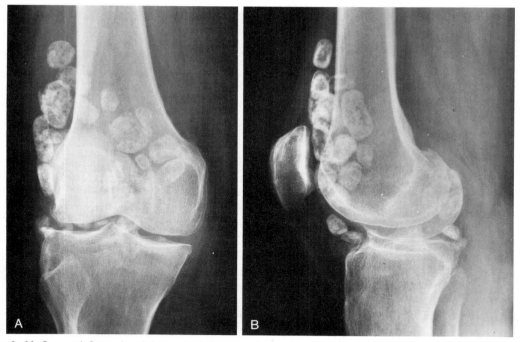

Figure 9–66. Synovial Osteochondromatosis. AP *(A)* and lateral *(B)* views show multiple calcified and ossified densities. There is hypertrophic lipping (osteophytes) but only minimal cartilage space-narrowing.

mon in adults aged 20 to 50. Occurrence in males outnumbers that in females by at least 2:1. Symptoms are nonspecific and include a history of pain, swelling, decreased motion, and sometimes locking of or clicking in the involved joint.

Diagnosis can be made on plain radiographs if the loose bodies are calcified. The classic picture is that of numerous calcified bodies of different sizes and shapes that conform to the expected location of the joint capsule (Fig. 9–66). When calcification is not seen on plain films, arthrography may be useful in demonstrating numerous small, sharply defined filling defects, either free-floating or attached to the synovial lining.[161]

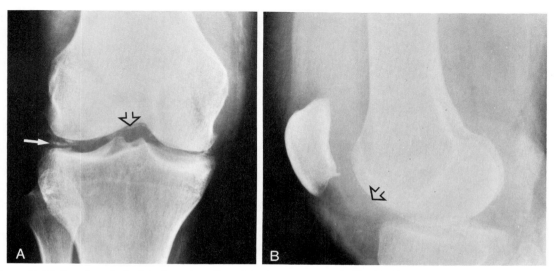

Figure 9–67. Pseudogout. Acute pain and swelling of the knee were noted. The AP *(A)* and lateral *(B)* radiographs show articular (open arrows) and meniscal (closed arrow) calcification and a large joint effusion.

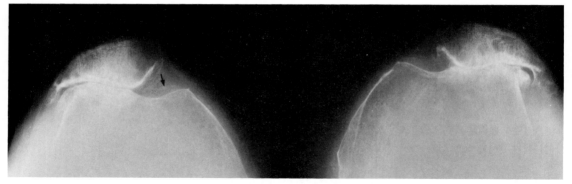

Figure 9–68. Patellofemoral Osteoarthritis and CPPD. The tangential patellar view shows faint chondrocalcinosis (arrow), lateral patellar subluxation, severe cartilage-space narrowing, sclerosis, and lateral osteophytes. The medial- and lateral-compartment cartilage spaces were normal.

The significance of this entity lies mainly in the loss of function, the discomfort, and the secondary degenerative changes that may occur. Treatment is surgical, with removal of loose bodies usually accompanied by either partial or complete synovectomy.

Calcium Pyrophosphate Dihydrate Deposition Disease

Calcification of hyaline cartilage or fibrocartilage or both (chondrocalcinosis) may be caused by the presence of calcium pyrophosphate, ortho-phosphate, or hydroxyapatite.[164] The deposits associated with calcium pyrophosphate di-hydrate (CPPD) deposition disease are typically bilateral and symmetrical. Diagnosis is established by a characteristic x-ray diffraction pattern of joint crystals obtained at aspiration or biopsy, or it is established by the presence of polyartic-ular chondrocalcinosis on radiographs and the identification of the characteristic crystals that have absent or weakly positive birefringence on compensated polarized light microscopy.[163] Symptoms that mimic other disorders, including rheumatoid arthritis ("pseudorheumatoid"), gout ("pseudogout"), or neuropathic ("pseu-doneuropathic") arthropathy, may occur (Fig. 9–67).

Two types of radiographic findings, calcification and arthropathy, may be present. Calcification includes chondrocalcinosis and sometimes synovial and periarticular deposits (often bilateral). The arthropathy resembles osteoarthritis but may be distinguished from it in some cases by disproportionately severe patellofemoral damage and by the presence of subchondral cysts that are larger and more numerous than in typical osteoarthritis (Figs. 9–68 and 9–69). Clinically and radiographically, the knee is the most frequent area of involvement.

Osteochondritis Dissecans

This entity is recognized by its typical radiographic appearance. Young men are most often affected, and the condition may be bilateral.[165] In about 85 percent of cases the intercondylar aspect of the medial femoral condyle is involved. Other areas in which the condition has been seen include the lateral femoral condyle, the femoral head, the capitellum and radial head,

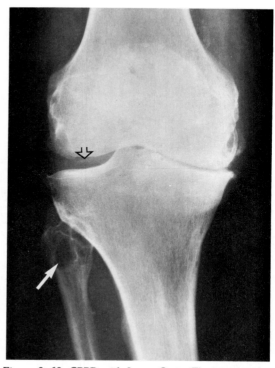

Figure 9–69. CPPD with Large Cysts. There is complete medial cartilage loss. Chondrocalcinosis is noted laterally (open arrow), and there are marginal osteophytes. Large cysts are present in the proximal fibula (arrow). The appearances were bilaterally similar.

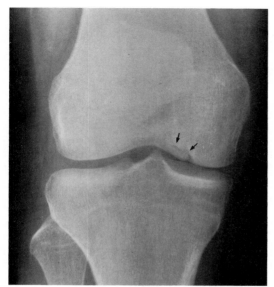

Figure 9–70. Osteochondritis Dissecans. A small bony fragment with an adjacent lucent zone is noted in the lateral aspect of the medial femoral condyle. A sclerotic reaction is present (arrows).

the talus, the posterior surface of the patella, the first metatarsal head, and the phalanges.[165]

Radiographic findings are diagnostic and consist of a localized area of lucency in the subchondral region, often demarcated from the

adjacent normal cancellous bone by a rim of sclerosis and lying deep to a dense, sharply marginated fragment (Fig. 9–70). The proximal lucent zone is composed of fibrocartilage,[166] and the dense fragment is avascular bone or calcified cartilage. The subchondral cortex and the overlying cartilage may become partially or completely detached, leaving an irregular depression in the articular surface.

Spontaneous Osteonecrosis

Spontaneous osteonecrosis (osteochondritis dissecans of the elderly) is characterized by radiographic evidence of a lesion identical to that of osteochondritis dissecans but occurring in the weight-bearing area of the medial femoral condyle in patients over the age of 60.[175] Women are more frequently affected. The history is noteworthy in that the onset of pain is sudden and severe, and often the patient can recall the exact day and circumstance of its onset. A history of prior minor injury can sometimes be obtained. Pain occurs both with activity and at rest.

Diagnosis is usually established by the clinical history and confirmatory bone scan or radiographic findings (Table 9–11). Intense isotopic uptake in the medial femoral condyle (or, occasionally, the medial tibial condyle) is charac-

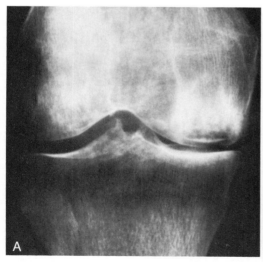

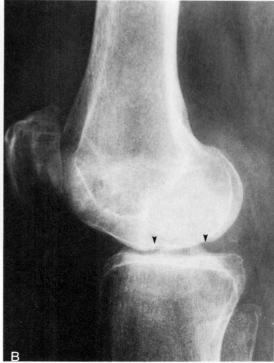

Figure 9–71. Spontaneous Osteonecrosis. *A,* The AP view shows a cortical fragment with adjacent lucency and sclerosis in the medial femoral condyle. The weight-bearing area is involved. *B,* The lateral view confirms involvement of the weight-bearing area of the medial femoral condyle with flattening of its contour (arrowheads). The smooth cortex of the lateral condyle is partially superimposed.

Table 9–11. **Radiographic and Scintigraphic Findings in Spontaneous Osteonecrosis***

Time Elapsed	Findings
Days after symptoms begin	Intense isotopic uptake on all phases of scan
Months	Subchondral radiolucency
	Flattening of subchondral cortex
Months to years	Osteoarthritis

*The medial femoral condyle is most commonly involved.

teristically present on bone scan within days after the onset of symptoms.[167, 170] These acute cases show increased uptake in all phases of the three-phase radionuclide study (angiogram, blood pool, and delayed.)[168] The intensity and the focal distribution of uptake allow the diagnosis to be established and the disorder to be differentiated from potentially confusing clinical conditions such as osteoarthritis and meniscal tears.

Radiographic diagnosis may be delayed, since up to 8 months may elapse before typical radiological features are present. According to Norman and Baker, the earliest changes are either a radiolucent area in the subchondral bone or a flattening of the weight-bearing aspect of the medial femoral condyle.[173] Eventually, the characteristic large lucent zone surrounded by a reparative zone of sclerosis is noted (Figs. 9–71 and 9–72). A sequestrum of dead subchondral cortex (and attached nonopaque cartilage) may be noted within the lucency, or the subchondral cortex may be flattened. Periosteal new bone has been seen proximal to the area of involvement.[173]

Norman and Baker noted meniscal tears on arthrography in 78 percent of patients with spontaneous osteonecrosis, and the edge of the meniscal fragment was noted to correspond to the area of bone abnormality.[173] They postulated a causal relationship between the meniscal tear and the development of spontaneous osteonecrosis.[169] Controversy exists, however.[167, 169]

Secondary osteoarthritis occurs earlier and is more severe in patients with larger lesions. Therefore, osteotomy or osteotomy plus arthrotomy to remove a separate articular fragment has been suggested for lesions larger than 5 cm² on AP and lateral views. Muheim and Baker suggest conservative management if the lesion measures less than 3.5 cm², with removal of any sequestrum that develops.[171]

Fractures and Dislocations

Patellar Fractures

Fractures of the patella may result from direct or indirect trauma.[179] Direct injuries are usually

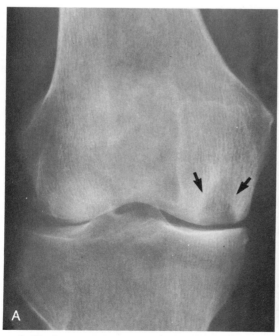
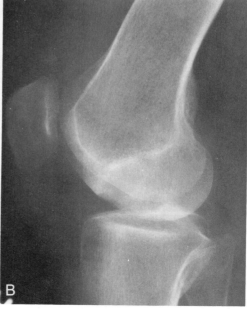

Figure 9–72. Spontaneous Osteonecrosis. A lucency with adjacent sclerosis (arrows) is present in the medial femoral condyle. The medial cartilage space is narrowed. *A*, AP view; *B*, lateral view.

Figure 9–73. Patellar Fractures. Patellar fractures are classified according to their configuration.

  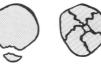

Undisplaced   Transverse   Lower or Upper Pole   Comminuted   Vertical

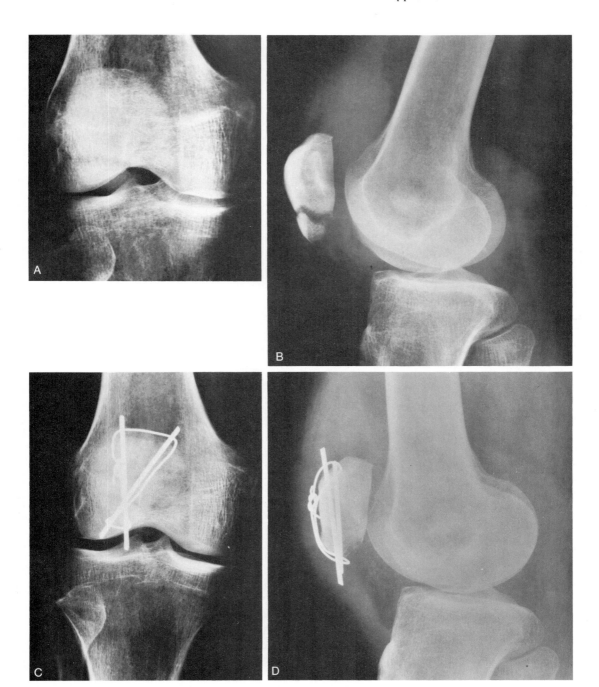

Figure 9–74. Patellar Fracture. AP *(A)* and lateral *(B)* views show a displaced fracture through the inferior pole of the patella. The articular surface is intact. There is a large joint effusion. AP *(C)* and lateral *(D)* views after tension banding with almost anatomical reduction.

nondisplaced because the medial and lateral soft tissues (retinacula) are intact, and this limits the degree to which the fragments can be separated. Indirect injuries occur when sudden active muscular contraction—for example, during an attempt to break a fall—pulls the patella apart. Since the adjacent retinacula are torn in these injuries, displacement of fracture fragments is possible. Combined injuries may occur.

Classification. Patellar fractures are classified by their configuration (Fig. 9–73). Indirect forces typically produce transverse fractures, but direct injury results in nondisplaced, stellate, or comminuted fractures. Transverse and oblique fractures are most frequent (50 to 80 percent), stellate and comminuted fractures next (30 to 35 percent), and vertical fractures least frequent (12 to 27 percent).

Clinical and Radiographic Findings. Clinical examination demonstrates local tenderness and swelling. The fracture defect may be palpable. Routine lateral radiographs usually confirm the diagnosis and demonstrate any displacement of fracture fragments or incongruity of the posterior articular surface (Fig. 9–74). The frontal view is often difficult to evaluate because of the superimposed femur, but oblique and tangential patellar views may be of considerably more help.

Treatment. Nonoperative treatment may be used for patients with nondisplaced fractures in which the articular surface is fairly smooth and the extensor mechanism (as tested by the patient's ability to actively and fully extend the knee) is not disrupted. Two to 3 mm of separation and a 2- to 3-mm step-off in the articular surface may be acceptable.[176, 179] In other cases, including those with osteochondral fracture fragments displaced into the joint, surgical intervention is necessary. Numerous methods have been developed for maintaining the fracture fragments in position, including use of a circumferential wire loop (cerclage) or of wires passed through longitudinal or transverse drill holes in the patella.[179] Screws have also been used for fixation. With AO tension-band wiring, a figure-of-eight wire is threaded through the patellar and quadriceps tendons and onto the anterior aspect of the patella (Fig. 9–74). This method produces a posterior gap between the fracture fragments that closes postoperatively with quadriceps con-

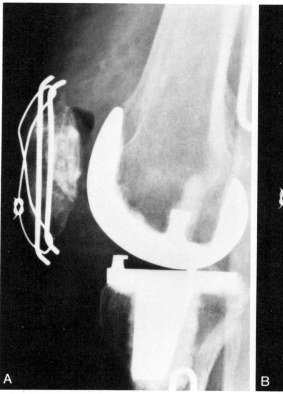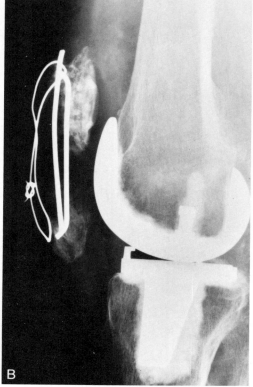

Figure 9–75. Patellar Fracture, Tension Banding, and Loss of Fixation. *A,* Tension banding after patellar fracture in a patient with a total-knee prosthesis, including a patellar component, has produced complete reduction of fracture fragments. *B,* The fragments have separated, and the tension-band system is disrupted.

traction.[182] This technique is applicable to transverse fractures (Chap. 1, Figs. 1–31 and 1–32).

It is possible to excise a small fragment or fragments of the patella and salvage one large fragment to be used in the repair of the extensor mechanism. Patellectomy is occasionally used when other treatments fail or when fractures are very severely comminuted.

Complications. Postoperative complications include the separation or the change in position of fracture fragments, refracture, and fracture through a fibrous union (Fig. 9–75). Osteonecrosis generally involves the proximal pole of the patella and is usually asymptomatic. It is first seen radiographically 1 to 2 months after injury as an increase in density of the proximal patellar fragment. This resolves by about 6 months, and healing of the fracture occurs. Osteonecrosis has

been noted in 25 percent of transverse patellar fractures.[183]

Tibial Plateau Fractures

These fractures have been referred to as bumper or fender fractures and, indeed, about half are caused by automobiles striking pedestrians.[179] Almost 75 percent of these injuries involve the lateral tibial condyle alone, with the remaining cases involving isolated injury of the medial plateau or both plateaus.

In most cases injury results from the prominent anterior portion of the lateral femoral condyle being driven into the lateral tibial plateau.[190, 195] The configuration of the subsequent fracture depends on the magnitude and direction of the applied force, the site of impact, and the resistance of the bone.[195] Experimental work has shown that a pure abduction force (valgus)

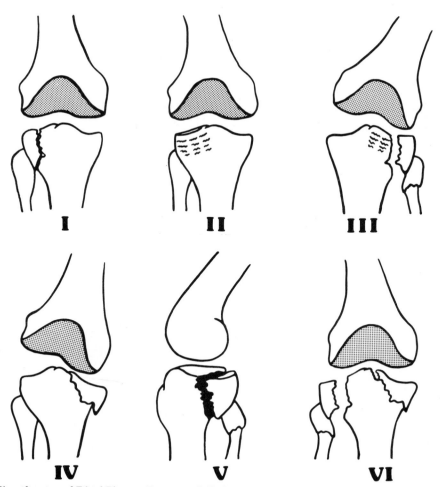

Figure 9–76. Classification of Tibial Plateau Fractures. *I.* Undisplaced. *II.* Local depression (central depression). *III.* Local depression (split depression). *IV.* Total depression. *V.* Split. *VI.* Comminuted. (Redrawn from Hohl M: J Bone Joint Surg (Am) 49:1455, 1967.)

applied to the knee results in a split fracture of the lateral tibial condyle, but a pure compression force produces compression of the lateral tibial plateau.[190] The site of a compression injury depends on the degree of knee flexion at the time of impact, with greater degrees of flexion leading to more posterior lesions. Severe fractures of both condyles occur when great compression force is applied. Dissection of specimens with compression fractures or mixed fractures has shown considerably more disruption of the articular surface than was appreciable on standard specimen radiographs.[190]

Classification. The most widely used classification is that proposed by Hohl.[188] Fractures are first grouped as undisplaced (less than 3 mm of displacement and minimal impaction) or displaced. Displaced fractures are subdivided into four types: local depression, total depression, split, and comminuted, as shown in Figure 9–76. If there is to be appropriate classification and treatment, the necessity for identifying depression of the tibial plateau on preoperative radiographs is apparent.

Radiological Examination (Figs. 9–77 to 9–79). There are difficulties in the identification and delineation of tibial plateau fractures. A tibial plateau fracture can usually be identified from AP and lateral radiographs. Cross-table lateral views (rather than standard vertical-beam films) of the knee are recommended as routine for patients with a history of knee trauma, since this technique makes possible the identification of a fat-fluid level, the presence of which provides strong evidence of an intraarticular fracture (Fig. 9–79). If the fracture itself is not seen, oblique views and tomography are indicated.

Once a fracture is identified, its characterization is necessary for treatment planning. Multiple studies have shown, however, that the presence and degree of depression or displacement of fracture fragments is not accurately determined on standard films.[186, 187, 190, 192, 196] In order to define the amount of depression of fracture fragments more accurately, tilting of the x-ray tube along the plane of the tibial plateau (about 14 degrees caudad) has been suggested.[192]

Tomography. Tomography has been shown to be the most accurate method for evaluating tibial plateau fractures (Figs. 9–77 and 9–78). Tomography should be done in both the frontal and the lateral projections at about 0.5 cm intervals.[196] Although bandages and splints should be removed, we have obtained adequate studies through plaster using complex motion tomography.

In addition to accurately describing the location and type of fractures, several other findings should be noted, including (1) identification of small, comminuted fracture fragments that may be loose in the joint or attached to ligaments; (2) description of the location of depressed

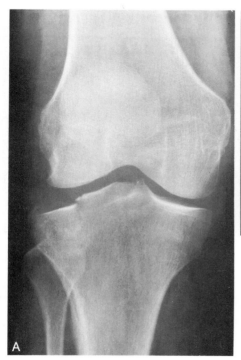

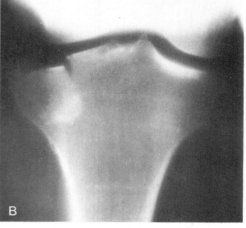

Figure 9–77. Tibial Plateau Fracture. *A,* A portion of the lateral tibial articular surface is depressed. *B,* Tomography confirms a depression of only a few millimeters in the tibial articular surface. Nonoperative treatment was used with a good clinical result.

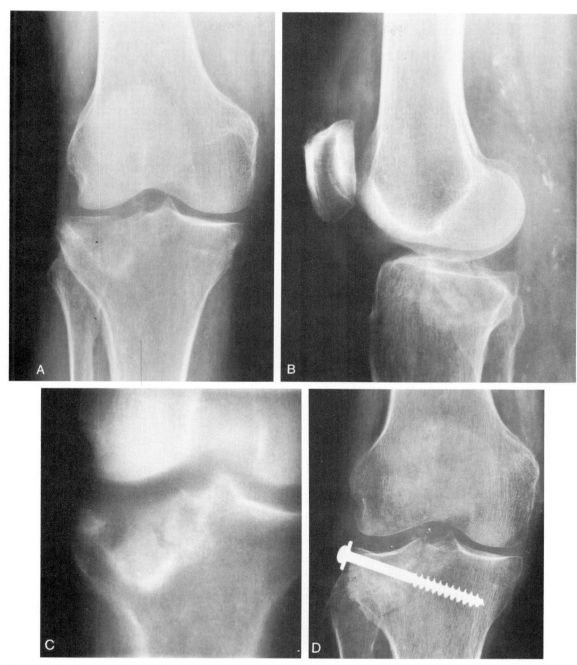

Figure 9–78. Tomography for Evaluation of a Tibial Plateau Fracture, Type II, Central Depression. *A*, The AP view shows mild valgus with apparent narrowing of the lateral cartilage space. A zone of lucency and adjacent sclerosis involving the lateral tibial plateau is noted. *B*, The lateral view shows a joint effusion with a probable flat-fluid level in the suprapatellar pouch. Multiple fracture fragments involving the posterior and midportions of the tibia are suggested. *C*, Tomography in the anteroposterior projection confirms marked depression and fragmentation of the subchondral cortex and the cancellous bone. *D*, AP radiograph after elevation of one large fragment and bone grafting. The clinical result was good.

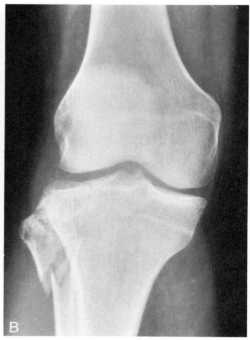

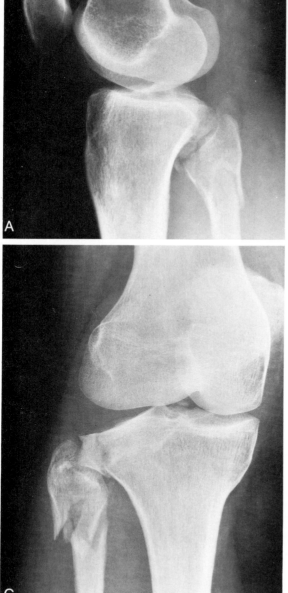

Figure 9–79. Tibial Plateau Fracture, Type III, Split Depression. *A,* A fat-fluid level is present in the suprapatellar pouch. There is a proximal fibular fracture and irregularity of the posterior tibia. *B,* The AP view suggests a slight depression of the lateral subchondral cortex and a vertical fracture line. *C,* An internal oblique view better demonstrates a split fracture of the posterolateral tibia. There is faint sclerosis of the cancellous bone, suggesting some compression as well.

fragments; (3) definition of the integrity of the anterior tibial cortex, which is helpful in planning a surgical approach; (4) identification of comminution about the tibial spines and, therefore, avulsion of the cruciate ligaments; and (5) identification of chip fractures at the sites of collateral ligament insertions.[186]

Stress Views. Ligamentous rupture may occur in association with tibial plateau fractures, especially the split-depression type; this finding is one indication that surgical correction is necessary.[189, 195] Rasmussen noted that in a series of 260 tibial plateau fractures 5.4 percent of patients had rupture of the anterior cruciate ligament, 3.8 percent had rupture of the medial collateral ligament, and 0.4 percent had posterior cruciate or lateral collateral ligament tears.[195]

Stress views are usually obtained under spinal or general anesthesia. Widening of the medial joint space indicates a medial collateral ligamentous tear. The production of valgus deformity alone does not reliably indicate a ligamentous injury, since such a deformity may be the result of the sinking of the femur into the deformed tibial plateau.[190] Development of calcification near the origin of the medial collateral ligament (Pellegrini-Stieda calcification) is evidence of prior ligamentous injury.[195]

Post-treatment results correlate poorly with the final anatomical position of the tibial plateau as demonstrated radiographically. Overall, a larger number of adequate clinical results than might be expected from evaluation of the anatomical result are noted.[185] These outcomes are partially explained by the laying down of fibrocartilage or the thickening of an overlying meniscus, both of which have been shown on autopsy specimens to fill in the bony defects and to improve articular congruity.[185] The development of secondary osteoarthritis, angular deformity, and instability better correlate with the clinical outcome.

Treatment. Treatment varies according to the extent of bone and soft-tissue injury. Nondisplaced fractures may be treated without surgery if the ligamentous structures can be shown to be intact on clinical and radiological examination.[179] For evaluation, stress radiographs, taken after induction of spinal or general anesthesia, may be necessary. Follow-up radiographs are necessary to exclude changes in the position of fracture fragments.[179]

The treatment of fractures with 5 to 10 mm of depression is somewhat controversial. Hohl notes that depression of the lateral articular surface by 5 to 10 mm usually results in valgus instability. Comparable results have, however, been found in operated and nonoperated cases.[191] Larson suggests open reduction in patients with more than 8 mm of articular depression or in young patients with less articular depression but more than 5 degrees of increased valgus with the leg extended.[179] In general, local depression of a plateau by 10 mm or more is considered an indication for surgery to elevate or remove depressed fragments.[188]

When the entire tibial plateau is depressed, comminution of the articular surface is not usually present, and nonoperative methods or internal fixation may be used. Careful radiological follow-up is necessary to exclude displacement of the fracture fragments.

Hohl suggests internal fixation of split fractures when the fragment is displaced by 5 mm or more or when it is depressed below the articular surface.[188] Comminuted fractures may be treated by operative or nonoperative means (especially traction).

Characteristics of a good result after a tibial plateau fracture are a knee that is strong and stable and has nearly full motion and normal or almost normal alignment.[179] Several factors associated with a poor result after tibial plateau fracture include instability from residual depression of the articular surface or ligamentous laxity, loss of articular cartilage, osteoarthritis, and failure to begin early motion. Late pain may be due to the development of osteoarthritis or to ligamentous strain on the convex side of the deformity. A higher incidence of osteoarthritis has been noted following bicondylar fractures and in patients with residual angular deformity or instability. No correlation has been found between the development of osteoarthritis and residual depression of the articular surface.[195]

Tibial Shaft Fractures

The tibia is the most frequently fractured long bone.[198] Fractures occur as a result of direct trauma (e.g., in automobile accidents) or indirect injury (e.g., falling or turning with the foot fixed in position). With greater force the fibula, too, is fractured.

Classification

Ellis: Fractures are classified according to the degree of displacement, of angulation, and of comminution and according to the presence of an open wound as follows:[197, 198]

Minor severity	No (0 to 50 percent)* displacement
	No angulation
	Minor comminution
	Minor open wound

*Numbers in parentheses are modifications by Leach.

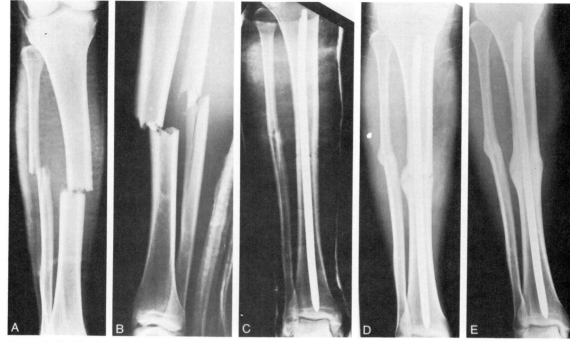

Figure 9–80. Tibial Shaft Fracture with Acute Compartment Syndrome. Initial AP *(A)* and lateral *(B)* radiographs show a midtibial fracture with half a shafts width posterior displacement and one fourth a shafts width lateral displacement of the distal fragment. A fibular fracture is present. Decreased sensation was noted, and the patient underwent fasciotomy of all four compartments, open reduction, and intramedullary rodding of the tibial fracture. *C,* At 18 days after injury the position of the fracture fragments is almost anatomical. *D,* At 4 months healing has progressed. *E,* Further healing is evident at 1 year.

Moderate severity	Total (50 to 100 percent)* displacement
	Minor comminution
	Open wound
Major severity	Complete displacement
	Major comminution or major open wound

Weissman: This classification is based on the degree of displacement and angular deformity present:[199]

Minimal displacement	Less than one fifth of a shafts width displacement
	Ten-degree or less angulation
Mild	One to two fifths of a shafts width displacement
	Between 10 and 30 degrees angulation
Marked	More than 50 percent horizontal displacement
Severe	Total horizontal displacement

Radiographic Examination. Usually, AP and lateral views that include both the knee and the ankle are sufficient for evaluation. As with other long-bone fractures, the location of the fracture and its degree of comminution, displacement,

and angular deformity are assessed. The degree of rotation is difficult to define radiologically, although marked changes in the diameters of the adjacent fracture margins suggest rotational malalignment.

Treatment. Closed reduction with casting is the usual treatment in mild or moderate cases. When residual angular deformity is present, cutting an appropriate wedge from the cast may correct the deformity. Moderate to severe injuries may be treated with pins that are placed above and below the fracture site and incorporated into the plaster cast (Fig. 1–42, Chap. 1).

Open reduction with compression plating or intramedullary rodding more or less depends on surgical preference (Fig. 9–80). Segmental fractures more often require the use of these methods.

Acceptable Reduction.[198] General guidelines for acceptable reduction include the absence of rotational deformity and no more than 5 degrees of angular deformity in either the AP or the medial-lateral plane. Shortening of 5 to 7.5 mm is apparently acceptable, but no distraction is tolerable, since this lengthens the time to healing. The degree of displacement is less critical, and fractures will heal with even one shafts width displacement (Fig. 9–81).

---

*Numbers in parentheses are modifications by Leach.

Prognosis and Healing. Fractures with little or no displacement, no comminution, and no open wound have the most favorable prognosis. An intact fibula generally indicates a less severe injury and a better prognosis.

Leach notes the approximate time for healing of an uncomplicated fracture to be 10 to 13 weeks, of a displaced fracture, 13 to 16 weeks, and of an open or comminuted fracture, 16 to 26 weeks.[198]

Complications. Complications include delayed union, nonunion, malunion, infection, vascular injury, and compartment syndrome.

Delayed Union. This complication is a fairly frequent occurrence, particularly in comminuted or displaced fractures. Leach defines delayed union as the absence of bony union by 20 weeks, but he notes that other authors use a longer time interval (e.g., 26 weeks) before making that diagnosis.[198] No radiographic evidence of nonunion should be present.

Nonunion. This designation indicates that healing has stopped. As in other areas, both clinical features (e.g., pain on weight-bearing and local tenderness) and radiographic features are used to make the diagnosis. Radiographic findings are designated atrophic (with no evidence of callus formation) or hypertrophic (with sclerosis and smoothing of the bone ends). Infection may be a complicating factor.

Malunion. Malunion, a deformity that interferes with function or is cosmetically unacceptable, is uncommon (Fig. 9–81).

Compartment Syndrome. The term *compartment syndrome* refers to a condition in which high pressure develops in a closed fascial space (muscular compartment), resulting in reduction of capillary perfusion to levels below that necessary for tissue viability. The causes of compartment syndrome are categorized as those that decrease compartment size (e.g., constrictive dressings, casts, and burns) and those that increase compartment contents (e.g., postischemic swelling, prolonged immobilization, fractures, and osteotomies).[204] Fractures are the most common cause, particularly tibial fractures and especially those with little displacement or comminution (see Fig. 9–80). Compartment

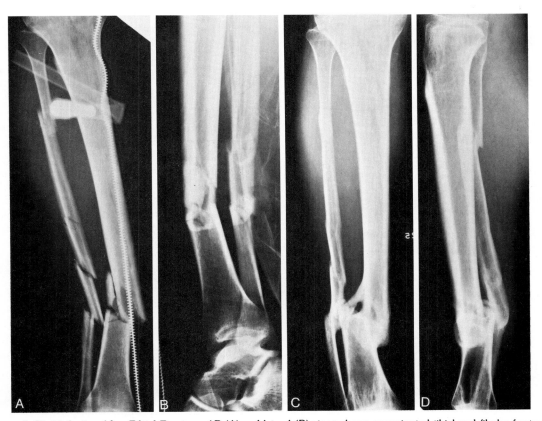

Figure 9–81. Malunion After Tibial Fracture. AP *(A)* and lateral *(B)* views shows comminuted tibial and fibular fractures. This was an open wound, treated with debridement and open reduction. Additional closed reduction was done in an attempt to correct angular deformity. AP *(C)* and lateral *(D)* views 3 years later show residual angular deformity (15 degrees varus and 15 degrees posterior bow) and displacement. The patient remains moderately symptomatic.

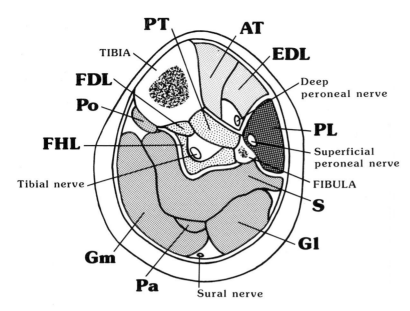

Figure 9–82. The Compartments of the Leg. Cross-section of right leg viewed from above. Deep posterior compartment (light stipples), anterior compartment (medium light), superficial posterior compartment (medium dark), lateral compartment (dark stipples). AT = anterior tibial; EDL = extensor digitorum longus; FDL = flexor digitorum longus; FHL = flexor hallucis longus; Gl = gastrocnemius lateral head; Gm = gastrocnemius medial head; Pa = plantaris; PL = peroneus longus; Po = popliteus; PT = posterior tibial; S = soleus. (After Williams P, Warwick R: Gray's Anatomy, 36th Br. ed. Edinburgh, Churchill Livingstone, 1980.)

syndrome also occurs in the forearm following humeral fracture (Volkmann's contracture), and in the hand, arm, shoulder, thigh, and buttock.[204]

There is a nerve within each of the four compartments of the leg, and neurological damage is an important clue to diagnosis. Contents of the leg compartments are as follows (Fig. 9–82):

Anterior Compartment	Deep peroneal nerve
	Anterior tibial muscle
	Extensor digitorum longus muscle
	Extensor hallucis longus muscle
	Peroneus tertius muscle
	Anterior tibial artery
Lateral Compartment	Superficial peroneal nerve
	Peroneus brevis muscle
	Peroneus longus muscle
Superficial Posterior Compartment	Sural nerve
	Soleus muscle
	Plantaris muscle
	Gastrocnemius muscle
	Posterior tibial nerve
	Posterior tibial muscle
	Popliteus muscle
Deep Posterior Compartment	Flexor hallucis longus
	Flexor digitorum longus
	Posterior tibial artery
	Peroneal artery

Compartment syndrome is a difficult clinical diagnosis. Characteristic features include pain out of proportion to the injury, a sensory deficit, and palpable pulses. The compartment may feel swollen. With an anterior compartment syndrome, paresthesias are noted over the dorsum of the foot, and pain occurs on flexing the great toe (thus stretching the extensor muscles). Deep posterior compartment syndrome is characterized by leg pain, weak toe flexion, painful passive toe extension, and plantar numbness.[203, 204] Elevated compartment pressures (above 30 mm Hg) establish the diagnosis. Treatment consists of fasciotomy.

Imaging techniques may help confirm the diagnosis. Ultrasound examination has shown disorganized muscle patterns, with both solid and cystic areas.[195] Computed tomography localizes the areas of necrosis, which appear as areas of low attenuation (20 to 30 Hounsfield units) with little or no enhancement following intravenous administration of contrast material.[208] Rydholm and associates noted muscle enlargement in a patient with compartment syndrome involving the tensor fasciae latae.[206] Years after a compartment syndrome has occurred, dense calcification may remain in the area (Fig. 9–83).[207]

Proximal Tibiofibular Dislocations

Four types of traumatic dislocation of the tibiofibular joint may be distinguished, depending on the final position of the fibula.[19, 20]

Anterolateral dislocation is the most common type and is often the result of a violent twisting injury. On the AP radiograph the fibular head is laterally displaced and therefore may not overlap the lateral aspect of the tibia. The lateral view will show the fibular head to be anterior to the

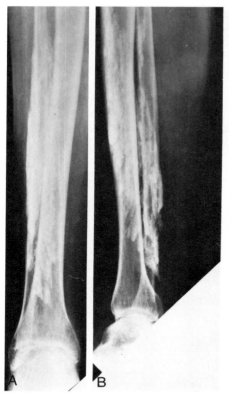

Figure 9–83. Calcification after Compartment Syndrome. This patient suffered a femoral fracture and neurovascular disruption of the right knee. She underwent vascular repair but did not recover neurological function of the common peroneal nerve and continued to have leg pain. AP *(A)* and lateral *(B)* radiographs years later showed a large area of calcification in the lateral aspect of the leg. Vascular clips are seen. At surgery the muscles of the anterior compartment were extensively calcified.

sloping cortical line that marks the posterior aspect of the lateral tibial condyle. (Normally this line points to the midportion of the fibular head.) This dislocation may be reduced by closed means, but secondary osteoarthritis may occur.

Posteromedial dislocations may be due to direct trauma, such as the lateral aspect of the knee striking a gate post (hence the term *horseback rider's knee*). On the AP radiograph the fibular head is superimposed on the tibia, and on the lateral view the fibula is behind the dense line of the posterior medial aspect of the lateral tibial condyle. Open reduction is often necessary.

Superior dislocation of the entire fibula may occur in association with tibial shaft fractures.

Subluxation, defined by Ogden as excessive symptomatic anteroposterior motion without frank dislocation, may occur in younger individuals and often heals spontaneously.[19]

Total-Knee Replacement

Three categories of prostheses may be distinguished by the degree of stability that they provide (Fig. 9–84).[237] In the first group stability is provided entirely by the prosthesis. The hinge prostheses (e.g., Guepar, Walldius, Shiers) and the spherocentric knee fall into this category. Such prostheses have the highest incidence of loosening. The second group of prostheses provides some stability (partial constraint to motion) by virtue of the fit of the prosthetic surfaces to each other. The geometric, the UCI, and the Freeman-Swanson prostheses are in this group (Fig. 9–85). The third group provides minimal or no constraint (stability) to knee motion. This group includes the PCA, kinematic, and Insall-Burstein prostheses. The incidence of loosening should be least in this group, but the possibility of instability should be greatest (Fig. 9–86).

Hinge Prostheses

These prostheses resurface the joint and provide stability. Radiographic examination should show the hinge parallel to the ground on weight-bearing views. It is usual to find sclerosis of the weight-bearing bone adjacent to the tibial and femoral articular surfaces. When cement is not used, the components often settle into the femur, the tibia, or both, and this may produce gradually increasing deformity. Detectable loosening of uncemented prostheses is frequent, and it is routine to see a 2- to 3-mm lucent zone around the stems of uncemented Walldius prostheses followed 5 years or longer.[252] If opaque cement is used around the components, a wide or widening lucency at the cement-bone interface suggests loosening (with or without infection) that may be confirmed on occasion by stress films or athrography (Figs. 9–87 and 9–88). Complications include infection, fracture of bone or prosthesis, metal synovitis, and tendon rupture (Fig. 9–89). Rupture of the quadriceps or the patellar tendons is suggested by a localized soft-tissue mass with obliteration of adjacent fat lines and appropriate change in patellar position (Fig. 9–90). Calcification within the tendon is occasionally seen.

Nonconstrained and Partially Constrained Prostheses

Normal Appearances

Newer Prostheses. The newer metal-to-plastic total-knee prostheses (e.g., the Kinematic, Brigham, PCA, Insall-Burstein) share several radiographic features (Figs. 9–91 to 9–93).

Text continued on page 574

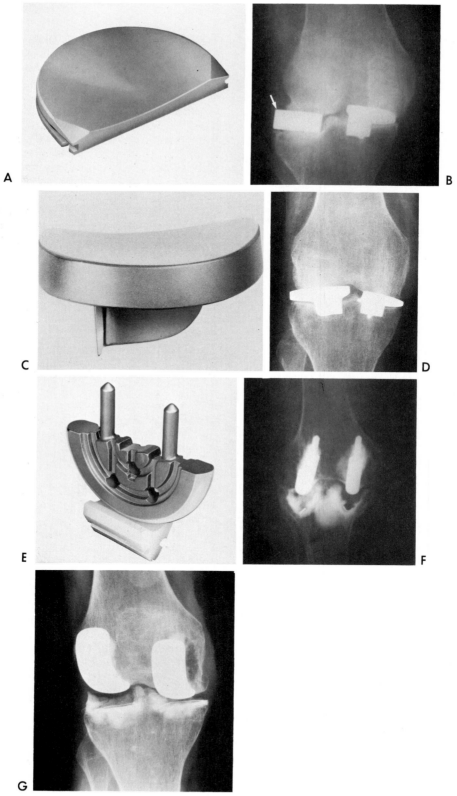

Figure 9–84. Various Total Knee Prostheses, Nonconstrained.
A,B: McIntosh (Howmedica);
C,D: McKeever (Howmedica);
E,F: Polycentric (Howmedica);
G: Marmor (Richards).

Illustration continued on opposite page

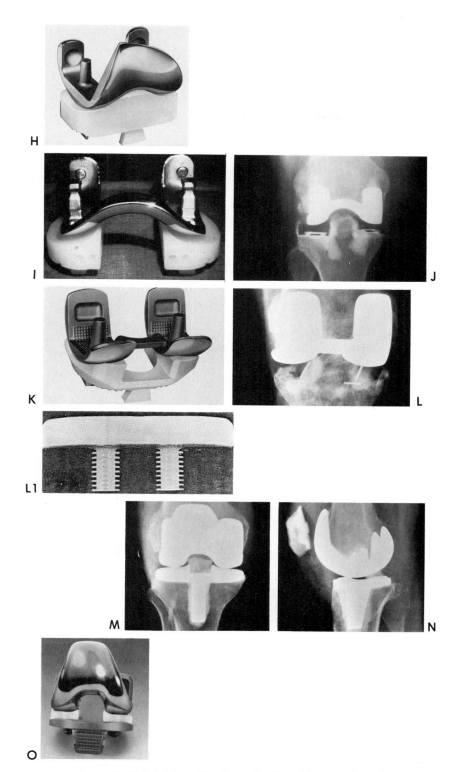

Figure 9–84. Total Knee Prostheses *Continued* **Semiconstrained.**
   H: Anametric (Howmedica);
   I,J: Duocondylar (Johnson & Johnson);
   K,L: Geomedic (Howmedica);
   L1: ICLH tibial component;*
   M,N: Kinematic (Howmedica);
   O: Kinematic II (anteriorly joined) (Howmedica).   *Illustration continued on following page*

*(From Freeman MA, Bloha JD, Bradley GW, et al.: Orthop Clin North Am 13:141, 1982.)

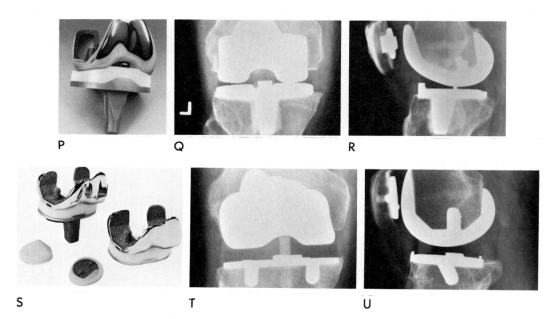

Figure 9–84. Total Knee Prostheses, Semiconstrained *Continued.*
P,Q,R: Kinematic II, total condylar (Howmedica);
S,T,U: PCA (Howmedica).

Illustration continued on opposite page.

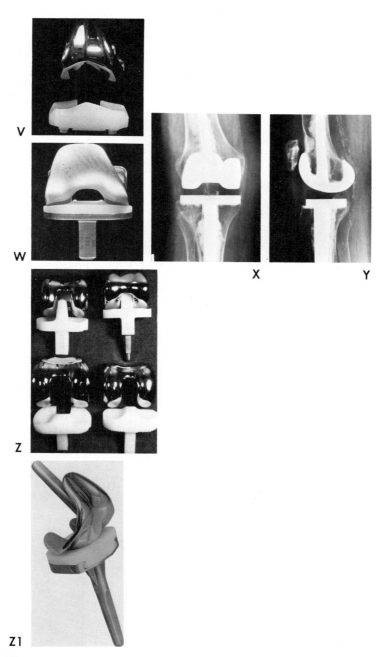

Figure 9–84. Total Knee Prostheses, Semiconstrained *Continued.*

   V: Richards;

W,X,Y: Robert Breck Brigham (Johnson & Johnson);

    Z: Total condylar (Johnson & Johnson—*Upper left,* Total condylar III; *Upper right,* Stabilocondylar; *Lower left,* Duopatellar; *Lower right,* Total condylar);

   Z1: Variable Axis (Howmedica).

Illustration continued on following page.

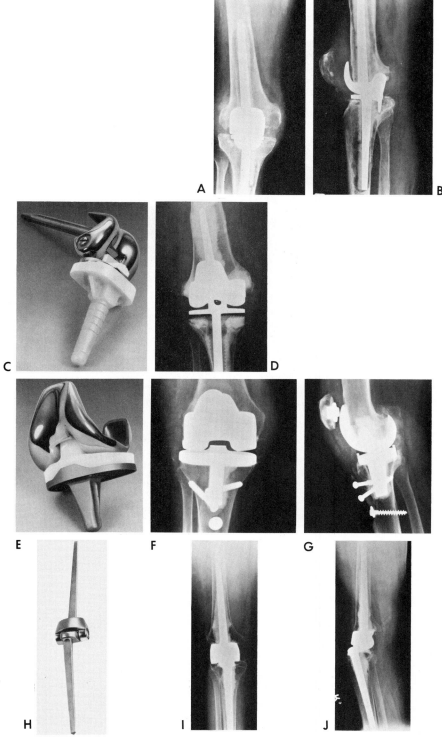

Figure 9–84. Total Knee Prostheses *Continued* **Constrained.**
    A,B: Guepar (Howmedica);
    C,D: Kinematic rotating hinge (Howmedica);
  E,F,G: Kinematic stabilizer (Howmedica);
    H,I,J: Shiers (Howmedica);

Illustration continued on opposite page.

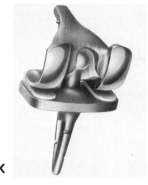

K

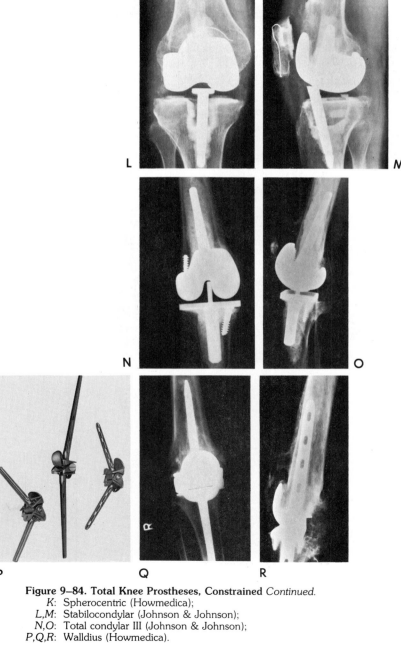

Figure 9–84. **Total Knee Prostheses, Constrained** *Continued.*
    K: Spherocentric (Howmedica);
    L,M: Stabilocondylar (Johnson & Johnson);
    N,O: Total condylar III (Johnson & Johnson);
    P,Q,R: Walldius (Howmedica).

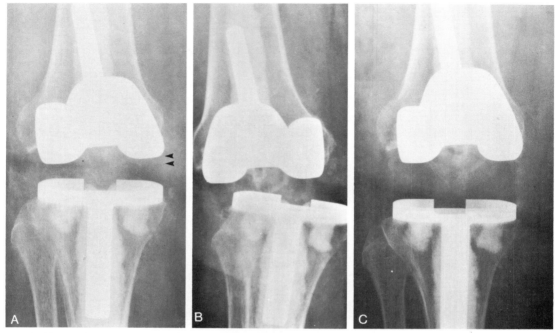

Figure 9–85. Instability Following Semiconstrained Total-Knee Prosthesis. *A*, The first postoperative film shows more than usual soft-tissue density between the medial femoral component and the tibial component (arrowheads). *B*, Ligamentous laxity was confirmed clinically and led to lateral femoral subluxation. *C*, A thicker nonopaque tibial component was inserted, and stability was achieved.

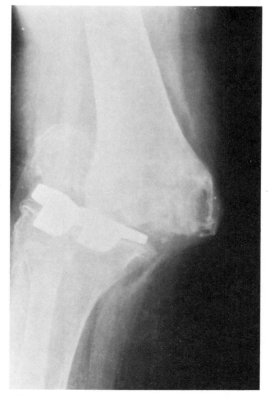

Figure 9–86. Instability After McKeever Arthroplasty. This patient had severe rheumatoid arthritis with ligamentous damage. After McKeever prostheses were inserted, medial femoral subluxation occurred.

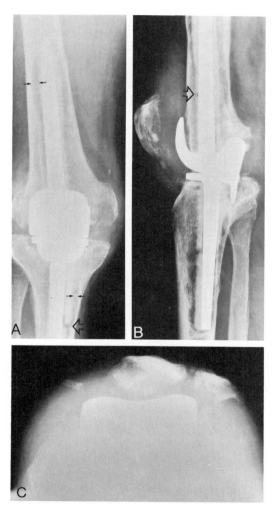

Figure 9–87. Loose Hinge Prosthesis (Guepar). *A,* AP radiograph. Opaque cement has been used for fixation. Wide cement-bone lucencies (arrows) and a cement fracture (open arrow) are present. *B,* Lateral radiograph. In addition to wide cement-bone lucencies and a femoral cement fracture (open arrow), a large effusion and patellar erosion are seen. *C,* The tangential patellar view shows patellar erosion and fragmentation.

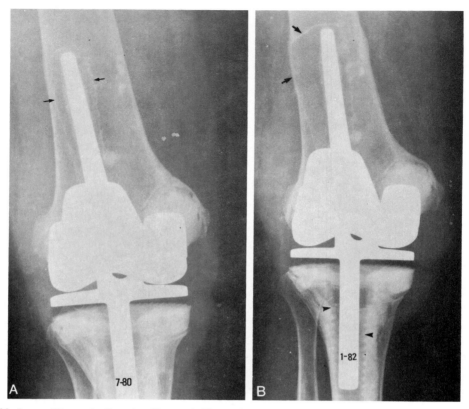

Figure 9–88. Loose Kinematic Rotating Hinge. *A,* The wide cement-bone lucency (arrows) around the femoral stem documents loosening. The lucent zone under the metal of the tibial component is a nonopaque polyethylene sleeve. *B,* One and a half years later the lucent zone around the femoral stem has progressed (arrows). A 2-mm lucency is noted proximally along the tibial-component cement. The nonopaque polyethylene sleeve (arrowheads) is better seen silhouetted by the metal femoral stem and the opaque cement.

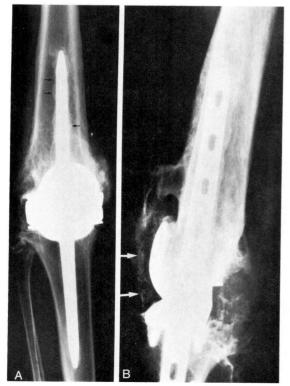

Figure 9–89. Metal Synovitis. *A,* The AP view shows a Walldius prosthesis in place. No cement was used, but increased density (due to metal debris) is seen around the femoral stem (arrows). *B,* In addition to the increased density present about the femoral stem, there is density in the soft tissue, also caused by metal-particle deposition (arrows). (Courtesy of Dr. Arthur Newberg, New England Baptist Hospital, Boston, Mass.)

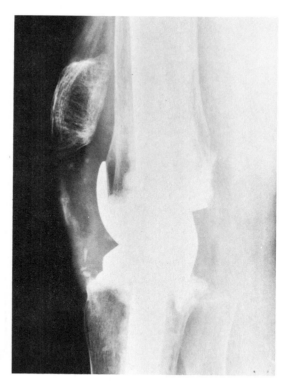

Figure 9–90. Patellar Tendon Rupture After Hinge Arthroplasty. The patella is in an abnormally high position, and there is calcification of the patellar tendon. Slight soft-tissue swelling is present near the patellar tendon insertion on the tibia.

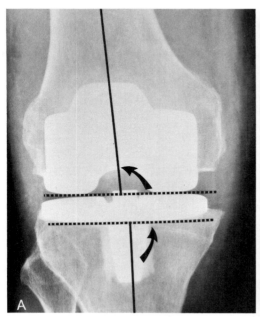

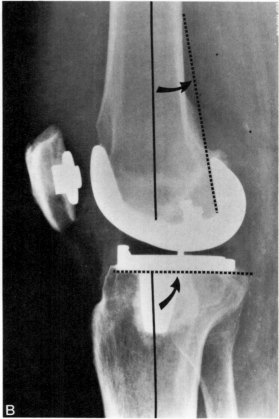

Figure 9–91. A Method of Measuring Component Position. Lines (dashed) are drawn along the prosthesis and the femoral and tibial axes (black). *A,* AP view. As the angles (arrows) increase, the components are in increased valgus alignment. *B,* Lateral view. In this case, the alignment of components is excellent. Ideally, however, the components should completely cover the resected end of the tibia.

573

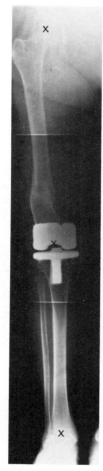

Figure 9–92. Standing View of Entire Leg After Total-Knee Replacement. A femoral fracture was followed by osteoarthritis. After total knee replacement the centers of the femoral head, knee, and ankle (x) are aligned.

Standing frontal radiographs show the overall knee alignment to be in about 7 degrees of valgus because of a valgus orientation of the femoral component. The tibial component(s) should be parallel to the ground on both the anteroposterior and the lateral views. The positions of both components should remain unchanged on serial examinations. Tangential patellar views should be routinely obtained and should show a good fit of the patella or the patellar prosthesis into the femoral groove.

Unicompartment Replacement. At the Brigham and Women's Hospital a unicondylar prosthesis, consisting of a cam-shaped metallic femoral component and a high-density polyethylene tibial component, is used in selected elderly patients with osteoarthritis confined to a single compartment (Fig. 9–94). On the anteroposterior view the femoral component is positioned in the center of the involved femoral condyle. On the lateral view this component covers the posterior part of the condyle and extends anteriorly far enough to cover the weight-bearing surface in extension. On the anteroposterior view the tibial component should be directly under its femoral counterpart and perpendicular to the long axis of the tibia. On the lateral view the tibial component should also be perpendicular to the long axis of the tibia or its posterior aspect should be directed distally as much as 10 degrees to permit the femur to slide posteriorly on the tibia in flexion.

Complications of Total-Knee Replacement

Loosening. Loosening of prosthetic components causes the largest number of total-knee replacement failures.[237] The tibial components are most often involved, usually at the cement-bone interface. As seen in patients with total hip replacement, thin lucencies may develop at the cement-bone interface in asymptomatic individuals. However, a wide (2 mm or more) or widening lucency, collapse of the underlying trabecular bone, fragmentation of underlying cement, change in the position of a component, and change in the degree of knee angulation on weight-bearing views are radiographic features suggestive of loosening (Figs. 9–95 to 9–97). Occasionally, loosening at the metal-cement interface of the femoral component may be seen. Tilting of the tibial component on immediate postoperative radiographs has been noted to be more frequent in patients who go on to develop loosening.[216]

Arthrography may be useful in documenting loosening or infection.[217] Single-contrast arthrography is preferred. A sample of joint fluid is aspirated for culture. Contrast material is then injected until the suprapatellar pouch is full (at least 15 ml is usually necessary). After the needle is removed the knee is flexed and extended several times and films are taken in AP, oblique, and lateral projections. Additional films may be taken after exercise. If subtraction is to be done, the initial film is taken after proper needle placement is confirmed, and the second anteroposterior film is taken immediately after contrast material injection, before the patient has moved. As in hip arthrography, contrast agent filling the cement-bone lucency indicates an abnormal bond at this interface (Fig. 9–96).

Bone scintigraphy can also demonstrate loosening or infection and is particularly useful in evaluating the femoral component (Fig. 9–98).[227] However, increased isotopic activity

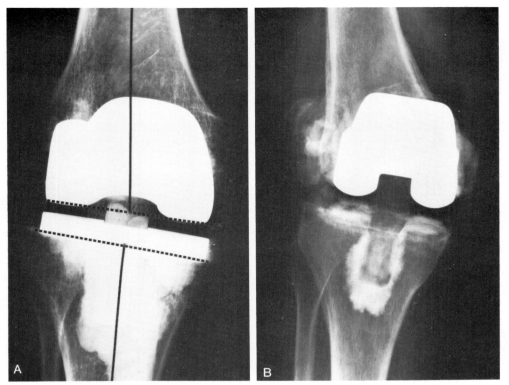

Figure 9–93. Component Malposition. *A,* The femoral component is in valgus, and the tibial component in varus. Surgery was performed again. *B,* Another patient has severe femoral component valgus with patellar dislocation.

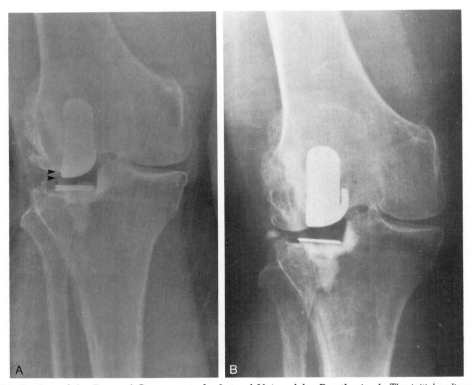

Figure 9–94. Settling of the Femoral Component of a Lateral Unicondylar Prosthesis. *A,* The initial radiograph shows overall valgus alignment. The margins of the bone and the profile of the femoral component in this view are indicated by arrowheads. *B,* Increased valgus resulting from the impaction of the femoral component into the femur is noted. This is best appreciated by noting the change in distance from the femoral component to the femoral cortex (see arrowheads in *A*) on the two examinations. Laterally, a cement fragment is noted.

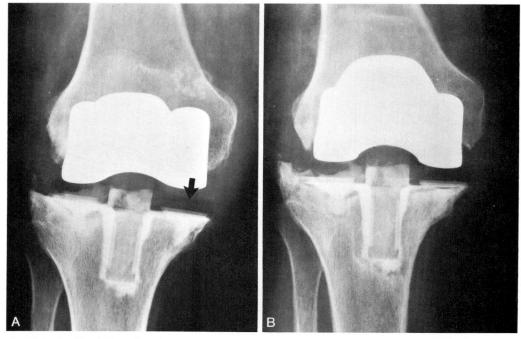

Figure 9–95. Loose Total-Knee Prosthesis. *A,* The initial view after surgery shows a greater than usual soft-tissue gap (arrow), medially, between the femoral and the tibial components, suggesting ligamentous laxity. *B,* One and a half years later there is loosening of the tibial component, with wide cement-bone lucencies and sinking of the tibial component into the lateral tibial plateau.

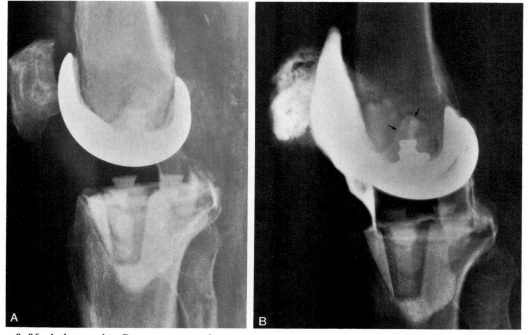

Figure 9–96. Arthrographic Documentation of a Loose Total-Knee Prosthesis. *A,* Lateral view shows slightly wide cement-bone lucent zones around the tibial and the femoral components. *B,* The arthrogram shows contrast-medium filling some of these lucencies (arrows).

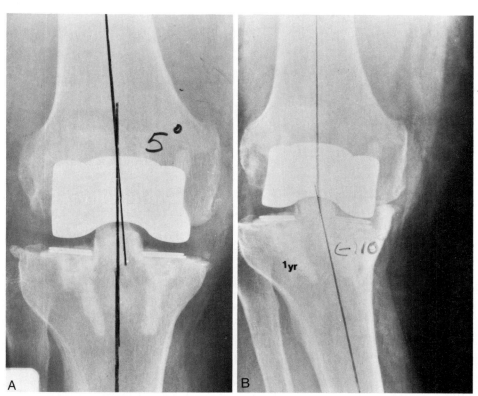

Figure 9–97. Change in Knee Alignment As a Result of Component Loosening. *A,* The postoperative radiograph shows no evidence of loosening. Overall knee alignment is 5 degrees of valgus. *B,* The 1 year follow-up radiograph shows a change to varus alignment caused by the sinking of the medial tibial component.

THE KNEE

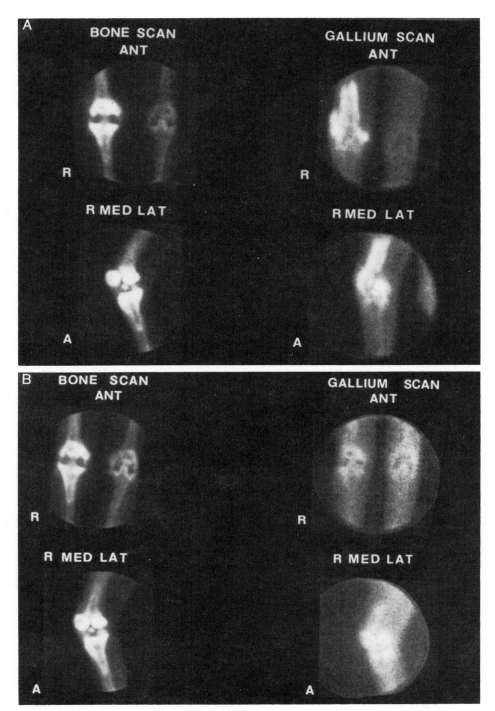

Figure 9–98. Scintigraphic Findings of an Infected Total-Knee Prosthesis. *A,* At the time of acute infection there is increased isotopic uptake of bone agent around the prosthetic components. There is incongruent uptake of gallium in the femoral shaft. *B,* One month later, after treatment, the bone scan remains abnormal, but increased uptake on the gallium scan has subsided. (Courtesy of Barbara J. McNeil, M.D., Brigham and Women's Hospital, Boston, Mass.)

over the femoral component on the anterior scan may be the result of patellar damage, and, therefore, lateral scans should always be done for localization. One review of a small number of patients with painful total-knee prostheses indicated an accuracy of 100 percent for both knee arthrography and scanning,[219] although other studies are much less optimistic.[227]

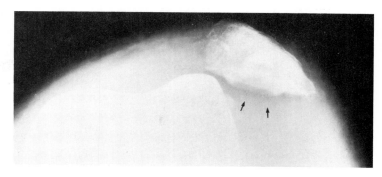

Figure 9–99. Patellar Dislocation After Total-Knee Replacement. The patella is dislocated laterally. Arrows indicate the prosthetic patellar-articular surface.

Infection. Deep infection is the second most frequent cause for failure of a total-knee replacement and may be immediate or delayed. Radiographic findings consist of prosthetic loosening and soft-tissue swelling.

Patellar Complications. Complications noted postoperatively at the patellofemoral joint include subluxation or dislocation of the patella, progressive damage to the articular surface of the patella, and catching of the patella on an overhanging shelf of the femoral condyle or on an anteriorly positioned femoral component.[222] Patellar resurfacing may be complicated by patellar fracture (0.2 to 5 percent of cases) or by loosening of the prosthesis (Figs. 9–99 to 9–102).[215] Mechanical factors, such as making the patella too thin or the anchoring hole too

large, and vascular compromise of the patella, predispose to postoperative fracture (Fig. 9–103).[215]

Fracture. Fractures related to osteoporotic bone, to trauma, or to the presence of factors increasing stress may occur in patients with total-knee replacement. A subtle change in the position of one of the components may be a clue to this diagnosis.

Uncemented Prostheses

With porous-coated prostheses it is hoped that bony ingrowth will fix the components to bone. Excellent apposition at the bone-prosthetic interface and immobilization at that interface appear to be required for successful bony ingrowth. Fibrous tissue, rather than bony ingrowth, may

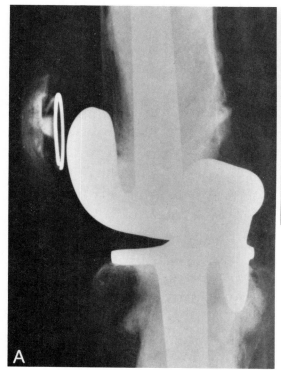

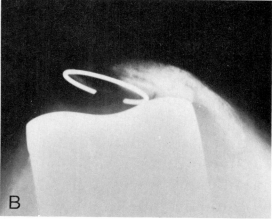

Figure 9–100. Loose (Separated) Patellar Component, Total-Knee Prosthesis (Guepar). A, The lateral view shows a wide separation between the metal marker wire and the cement. B, The tangential patellar view shows medial displacement of the patellar component, apparently caused by fracture through the cement-bone and the prosthesis-cement interfaces.

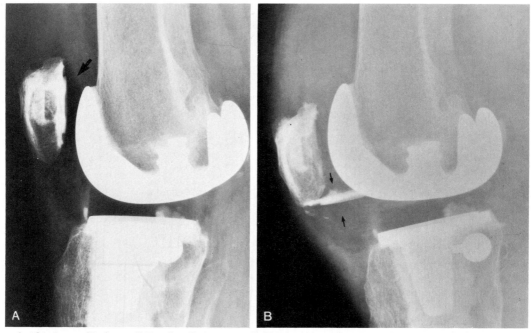

Figure 9–101. Loose (Dislocated) Patellar Component. *A,* The initial lateral view shows no abnormality. The nonopaque surface of the patellar component is seen (arrow). *B,* Follow-up examination shows the patellar prosthesis and some cement to be dislocated inferiorly (arrows). An effusion is present.

be seen, particularly if there is motion of the prosthesis.

The porous-coated anatomical total-knee prosthesis (PCA) developed by Hungerford and co-workers has porous-coated fixation surfaces with a double layer of chrome-cobalt beads.[226] The components are press-fitted, but eventual stability depends on the ingrowth of bone into the prosthetic surfaces.[226] The presence of insufficient, sclerotic, or poorly vascularized bone

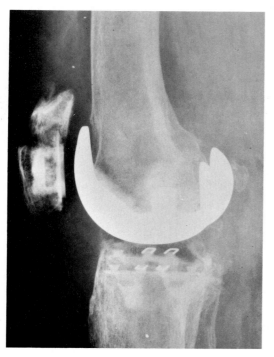

Figure 9–102. Patellar Fracture After Total-Knee Prosthesis. A fracture has occurred at the cement-bone interface of the patellar component.

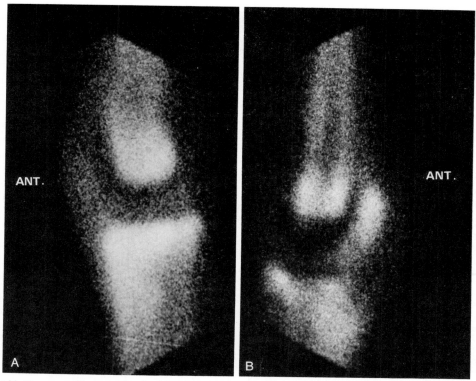

Figure 9–103. Decreased Isotopic Uptake After Total-Knee Prosthesis with Lateral Patellar Release. There is a decrease in isotopic uptake in the patella on the operated *(A)*, as compared with the other (previously operated) *(B)*, side (ANT. = Anterior).

may hinder bony ingrowth; such conditions are therefore contraindications to the use of this prosthesis. Radiographs should show intimate contact between the bone and the prosthesis, with a well-defined trabecular pattern that apparently testifies to the transmission of stress from the prosthesis to the bone. Currently, this prosthesis is approved for use with cement (where its irregular surface increases cement contact), and its use without cement is limited to certain centers of clinical investigation.

Another type of prosthesis, in which stability is related to the interdigitation of the prosthesis and the adjacent bone (termed immediate osseointegration), has been developed. The tibial component of the ICLH prosthesis has two high-density polyethylene pegs from which a series of flanges project (see Fig. 9–84).[218] These projections flex as the peg is forced into a drill hole. Thereafter, the flanges either remain in this position against the bone or relax to fill any adjacent gap. The effect is said to be analogous to that of the barb of a fish hook. Radiographic evaluation of these prostheses is limited, since the component itself is radiolucent; consequently, an adjacent radiolucent zone will not be appreciated. Changes in the angle of the prosthesis may be evaluated. Within the limits

of these considerations Freeman and colleagues noted no evidence of loosening or sinking of these prostheses.[218] A zone of increased density was noted near the interface around the fixation pegs or under the tibial plateau in about 40 percent of knees, and adjacent lucency was noted in 3 percent.

References
Normal Structure and Function
1. Chiu LC, Schapiro RL: Atlas of Computed Body Tomography. Normal and Abnormal Anatomy. Baltimore, University Park Press, 1980.
2. Freeman MAR: The surgical anatomy and pathology of the arthritic knee. *In* Freeman MAR, ed. Arthritis of the Knee. Clinical Features and Surgical Management. New York, Springer-Verlag, 1980: 31–56.
3. Ficat RP, Hungerford DS: Disorders of the Patello-Femoral Joint. Baltimore, Williams & Wilkins, 1977.
4. Williams PL, Warwick R, eds. Gray's Anatomy, 36th Br ed. Philadelphia, WB Saunders, 1980.
5. Guerra J, Newell J, Danzig L, Resnick D, Broderick T, Georgen TG, Niwayama G: The knee: anatomic-radiographic-pathologic correlation. Part I: The bony landmarks. Chicago, RSNA Exhibit, 1978.
6. Hall FM, Wyshak G: Thickness of articular cartilage in the normal knee. J Bone Joint Surg (Am) 62:408–413, 1980.
7. Harrison RB, Wood MB, Keats TE: The grooves of the distal articular surface of the femur—a normal variant. AJR 126:751–754, 1976.

8. Houston CS, Swischuk LE: Occasional notes. Varus and valgus—no wonder they are confused. N Engl J Med 302:471–472, 1980.

9. Hughston JC, Andrews JR, Cross MJ, Moschi A: Classification of knee ligament instabilities. Part I. The medial compartment and cruciate ligaments. J Bone Joint Surg (Am) 58:159–179, 1976.

10. Insall J, Salvati E: Patella position in the normal knee joint. Radiology 101:101–104, 1971.

11. Jacobsen K: Radiologic technique for measuring instability in the knee joint. Acta Radiol [Diagn] 18:113–125, 1977.

12. Jacobsen K, Bertheussen K: The vertical location of the patella. Fundamental views on the concept patella alta, using a normal sample. Acta Orthop Scand 45:436–445, 1974.

13. Kohler A: Borderlands of the Normal and Early Pathologic in Skeletal Roentgenology. New York, Grune & Stratton, 1956.

14. Laurin CA, Dussault R, Levesque HP: The tangential x-ray investigation of the patello-femoral joint: x-ray technique, diagnostic criteria and their interpretation. Clin Orthop 144:16–26, 1979.

14a. Laurin CA: Personal Communication, 1985.

15. Lindahl O, Movin A: Roentgenologic angulation measurement in supracondylar fractures of the femur. Acta Radiol [Diagn] 10:108–112, 1970.

16. Martinez S, Korobkin M, Fondren FB, Hedlund LW, Goldner JL: Computed tomography of the normal patellofemoral joint. Invest Radiol 18:249–253, 1982.

17. Merchant AC, Mercer RI, Jacobsen RH, Cool CR: Roentgenographic analysis of patellofemoral congruence. J Bone Joint Surg (Am) 56:1391–1396, 1974.

18. Newberg AH, Seligson D: The patello-femoral joint: 30°, 60° and 90° views. Radiology 137:57–61, 1980.

19. Ogden JA: Subluxation and dislocation of the proximal tibio-fibular joint. J Bone Joint Surg (Am) 56:145–154, 1974.

20. Resnick D, Newell JD, Guerra J Jr, Danzig LA, Niwayama G, Goergen TG: Proximal tibiofibular joint: Anatomic-pathologic-radiologic correlation. AJR 131:133–138, 1978.

21. Wiberg G: Roentgenographic and anatomic studies on the femoropatellar joint. With special reference to chondromalacia patellae. Acta Orthop Scand 12:319–411, 1941.

Joint Effusion

22. Bachman AL: Roentgen diagnosis of knee-joint effusion. Radiology 46:462–469, 1946.

23. Engelstad BL, Friedman EM, Murphy WA: Diagnosis of joint effusion on lateral and axial projections of the knee. Invest Radiol 16:188–192, 1981.

24. Friedman AC, Naidich TP: The fabella sign: fabella displacement in synovial effusion and popliteal fossa masses. Normal and abnormal fabello-femoral or fabello-tibial distances. Radiology 127:113–121, 1978.

25. Hall FM: Radiographic diagnosis and accuracy in knee joint effusions. Radiology 115:49–54, 1975.

26. Harris RD, Hecht HL: Suprapatellar effusions. A new diagnostic sign. Radiology 97:1–4, 1970.

27. Lewis RW: Roentgenographic study of soft tissue pathology in and about the knee joint. AJR 65:200–220, 1951.

28. Weston WJ, Palmer DG: Soft Tissues of the Extremities. A Radiologic Study of Rheumatic Disease. New York, Springer-Verlag, 1978.

29. Weston WJ: The extrasynovial and capsular fat pads on the posterior aspect of the knee joint. Skeletal Radiol 2:87–93, 1977.

Lipohemarthrosis

30. Apple JS, Martinez S, Allen NB, Caldwell DS, Rice JR: Occult fractures of the knee: tomographic evaluation. Radiology 148:303–387, 1983.

31. Holmgren BS: Flussiges Fett im Kniegelenk nach Trauma. Acta Radiol 23:131–137, 1942.

32. Peirce CB, Eaglesham DC: Traumatic lipo-hemarthrosis of the knee. Radiology 39:655–662, 1942.

33. Sacks BA, Rosenthal DI, Hall FM: Capsular visualization in lipohemarthrosis of the knee. Radiology 122:31–32, 1977.

34. Saxton HM: Lipohaemarthrosis. Br J Radiol 35:122–127, 1962.

Popliteal Cysts

35. Bowerman JW, Muhletaler C: Arthrography of rheumatoid synovial cysts of the knee and wrist. J Can Assoc Radiol 24:24–32, 1973.

36. Burleson RJ, Bickel WH, Dahlin DC: Popliteal cyst: a clinicopathologic survey. J Bone Joint Surg (Am) 38:1265–1274, 1956.

37. Carpenter JR, Hattery RR, Hunder GG, et al.: Ultrasound evaluation of the popliteal space. Comparison with arthrography and physical examination. Mayo Clin Proc 51:498–503, 1976.

38. Childress HM: Popliteal cysts associated with undiagnosed posterior lesions of the medial meniscus: the significance of age in diagnosis and treatment. J Bone Joint Surg (Am) 52:1487–1492, 1970.

39. Cooperberg PL, Tsang IT, Truelove L, Knickerbocker WJ: Gray scale ultrasound in the evaluation of rheumatoid arthritis of the knee. Radiology 126:759–763, 1978.

39a. Dixon A St.J, Grant C: Acute synovial rupture in rheumatoid arthritis: clinical and experimental observations. Lancet 1:742–745, 1964.

40. Gompels BM, Darlington LG: Evaluation of popliteal cysts and painful calves with ultrasonography: comparison with arthrography. Ann Rheum Dis 41:355–359, 1982.

41. Good AE: Rheumatoid arthritis, Baker's cyst and thrombophlebitis. Arthritis Rheum 7:56–64, 1964.

42. Hall AP, Scott JT: Synovial cysts and rupture of the knee joint in rheumatoid arthritis. An arthrographic study. Ann Rheum Dis 25:32–40, 1966.

43. Harvey JP Jr, Corcos J: Large cysts in lower leg originating in the knee occurring in patients with rheumatoid arthritis. Arthritis Rheum 3:218–228, 1960.

44. Hench PK, Reid RT, Reames PM: Dissecting popliteal cyst simulating thrombophlebitis. Ann Intern Med 64:1259–1264, 1966.

45. Hermann G, Yeh H-C, Lehr-Janus C, et al.: Diagnosis of popliteal cyst: double contrast arthrography and sonography. AJR 137:369–372, 1981.

46. Jayson MI, Dixon A: Valvular mechanisms in juxtaarticular cysts. Ann Rheum Dis 29:415–420, 1970.

47. Kilcoyne RF, Imray TJ, Stewart ET: Ruptured Baker's cyst simulating acute thrombophlebitis. JAMA 240:1517–1518, 1978.

48. Lapayowker MS, Cliff MM, Tourtellotte CD: Arthrography in the diagnosis of calf pain. Radiology 95:319–323, 1970.

49. Lawson TL, Mittler S: Ultrasonic evaluation of extremity soft-tissue lesions with arthrographic correlation. J Can Assoc Radiol 29:58–61, 1978.

50. Meire GB, Lindsay DJ, Swinson DR, et al.: Comparison of ultrasound and positive contrast arthrosonography in the diagnosis of popliteal and calf swellings. Ann Rheum Dis 33:221–224, 1974.

51. Meurman KOA, Luppi A, Turunen MJ: A giant retrofemoral Baker's cyst. Br J Radiol 51:919–920, 1978.

52. Palmer DG: Antero-medial synovial cysts at the knee joint in rheumatoid disease. Australas Radiol 16:79–83, 1972.

53. Perri JA, Rodnan GP, Mankin HJ: Giant synovial cysts of the calf in patients with rheumatoid arthritis. J Bone Joint Surg (Am) 50:709–719, 1968.

54. Prescott SM, Pearl SE, Tikoff G: 'Pseudo-pseudo-thrombophlebitis': ruptured popliteal cyst with deep venous thrombosis. Letter. N Engl J Med 299:1192–1193, 1978.

55. Schwimmer M, Edelstein G, Heiken JP, et al.: Synovial cysts of the knee: CT evaluation. Radiology 154:175–177, 1985.

56. Seidl G, Scherak O, Hofner W: Antefemoral dissecting cysts in rheumatoid arthritis. Radiology 133:343–347 1979.

57. Taylor AR: Arthrography of the knee in rheumatoid arthritis. Br J Radiol 42:493–497, 1969.

58. Taylor AR, Ansell BW: Arthrography of the knee before and after synovectomy for rheumatoid arthritis. J Bone Joint Surg (Br) 54:110–115, 1972.

59. Wilson PD, Eyre-Brook AL, Francis JD: A clinical and anatomical study of the semimembranosus bursa in relation to popliteal cyst. J Bone Joint Surg 20:963–984, 1938.

60. Zizic TM, Whelton JC, Bowerman JW, Stevens MB: Arthrographic diagnosis of synovial pathology. Arthritis Rheum 17:326, 1974.

Plicae

61. Apple JS, Martinez S, Hardaker WT, Daffner RH, Gehweiler JA: Synovial plicae of the knee. Skeletal Radiol 7:251–254, 1982.

62. Boven F, DeBoeck M, Potvliege R: Synovial plicae of the knee on computed tomography. Radiology 147:805–809, 1983.

63. Brody GA, Pavlov H, Warren RF, Ghelman B: Plica synovialis infrapatellaris: arthrographic sign of anterior cruciate ligament disruption. AJR 140:767–769, 1983.

64. Dalinka MK, Garofola J: The infrapatellar synovial fold: a cause for confusion in the evaluation of the anterior cruciate ligament. AJR 127:589–591, 1976.

65. Deutsch AL, Resnick D, Dalinka MK, Gilula L, Danzig L, Guerra J Jr, Dunn FH: Synovial plicae of the knee. Radiology 141:627–634, 1981.

66. Patel D: Arthroscopy of the plicae—synovial folds and their significance. Am J Sports Med 6:217–225, 1978.

67. Reid GD, Glasgow M, Gordon DA, Weight TA: Pathological plicae of the knee mistaken for arthritis. J Rheumatol 7:573–576, 1980.

Quadriceps and Patellar Tendon Rupture

68. Brotherton BJ, Ball J: Bilateral simultaneous rupture of the quadriceps tendons. Br J Surg 62:918–920, 1975.

69. Duncan AM: Arthrography in rupture of the suprapatellar bursa with pseudocyst formation. AJR 121:89–93, 1974.

70. Jelaso DV, Morris GA: Rupture of the quadriceps tendon: diagnosis by arthrography. Radiology 116:621–622, 1975.

71. Kricun R, Kricun ME, Arangio GA, Salzman GS, Berman AT: Patellar tendon rupture with underlying systemic disease. AJR 135:803–807, 1980.

72. McLaughlin HL, Francis KC: Operative repair of injuries to the quadriceps extensor mechanism. Am J Surg 91:651–653, 1956.

73. MacDonald JA: Bilateral subcutaneous rupture of the quadriceps tendon: report of a case with delayed repair. Can J Surg 9:74–76, 1966.

74. Morgan J, McCarty DJ: Tendon ruptures in patients with systemic lupus erythematosus treated with corticosteroids. Arthritis Rheum 17:1033–1036, 1974.

75. Newberg A, Wales L: Radiographic diagnosis of quadriceps tendon rupture. Radiology 125:367–371, 1977.

76. Peiro A, Ferrandis R, Garcia L, Alcazar E: Simultaneous and spontaneous bilateral rupture of the patellar tendon in rheumatoid arthritis. A case report. Acta Orthop Scand 46:700–703, 1975.

77. Preston ET: Avulsion of both quadriceps tendons in hyperparathyroidism. JAMA 221:406–407, 1972.

78. Preston FS, Adicoff A: Hyperparathyroidism with avulsion of three major tendons. Report of a case. N Engl J Med 266:968–971, 1962.

79. Rascher JJ, Marcolin L, James P: Bilateral, sequential rupture of the patellar tendon in systemic lupus erythematosus. A case report. J Bone Joint Surg (Am) 56:821–822, 1974.

80. Scuderi C: Ruptures of the quadriceps tendon. Study of twenty tendon ruptures. Am J Surg 95:626–634, 1958.

81. Siwek CW, Rao JP: Ruptures of the extensor mechanism of the knee joint. J Bone Joint Surg (Am) 63:932–937, 1981.

82. Smason JB: Post-traumatic fistula connecting prepatella bursa with knee joint. Report of a case. J Bone Joint Surg (Am) 54:1553–1554, 1972.

82a. Turner DA, Prodromos CC, Petasnick JP, et al.: Acute injury of the ligaments of the knee: magnetic resonance evaluation. Radiology 154:717, 1985.

83. Twining RH, Marcus WY, Garey JL: Tendon rupture in systemic lupus erythematosus. JAMA 189:377–378, 1964.

84. Wilson JN: Bilateral rupture of the rectus femoris tendons in chronic nephritis. Br Med J 1:1402–1403, 1957.

Meniscal Tears and Arthrography

85. Allen WC: Medial meniscus injuries: Mechanism, diagnosis and treatment. In Funk, FJ, ed.: AAOS Symposium on the Athlete's Knee. 1982: 131–140.

86. Arndt RD, Horns JW, Gold RH: Clinical Arthrography. Baltimore, Williams & Wilkins, 1981.

87. Braunstein EM, Matthews LS, Kaplan RJ, Martel W: Clinical utility of knee arthrography. J Can Assoc Radiol 34:125–127, 1983.

88. Braunstein EM: Anterior cruciate ligament injuries: a comparison of arthrographic and physical diagnosis. AJR 138:423–425, 1982.

89. Brown DW, Allman FL Jr, Eaton SB: Knee arthrography: a comparison of radiographic and surgical findings in 295 cases. Am J Sports Med 6:165–172, 1978.

90. Butt WP, McIntyre JL: Double-contrast arthrography of the knee. Radiology 92:487–499, 1969.

91. Dalinka MK, Brennan RE: The technique, evaluation and significance of knee arthrography. Weekly Radiol Sci Update 3:1–5, 1976.

92. Fairbank TJ: Knee joint changes after meniscectomy. J Bone Joint Surg (Br) 30:664–670, 1948.

93. Freiberger RH, Kaye JJ: Arthrography. New York, Appleton-Century-Crofts, 1979.

94. Freiberger RH, Killoran PJ, Cardona G: Arthrography of the knee by double contrast method. AJR 97:736–747, 1966.

95. Furuya M, Harrison-Stubbs MO, Freiberger RH: Arthrography of the knee: analysis of 2101 arthrograms

and 623 surgical findings. Rev Hosp Spec Surg 2:11–21, 1972.

96. Gillies H, Seligson D: Precision in the diagnosis of meniscal lesions: a comparison of clinical evaluation, arthrography, and arthroscopy. J Bone Joint Surg (Am) 61:343–346, 1979.

97. Goldberg RP, Hall FM, Wyshak G: Pain in knee arthrography: comparison of air vs CO2 and reaspiration vs. no reaspiration. AJR 136:377–379, 1981.

98. Hall FM: Epinephrine-enhanced knee arthrography. Radiology 111:215–217, 1974.

99. Hohl M, Larson RL: Fractures and dislocations of the knee. In Rockwood CA Jr, Green DP, eds. Fractures. Philadelphia, JB Lippincott, 1975.

100. Ireland J, Trickey EL, Stoker DJ: Arthroscopy and arthrography of the knee: a critical review. J Bone Joint Surg (Br) 62:3–6, 1980.

101. Korn MW, Spitzer RM, Olsson HE: Arthrographic, clinical and surgical analysis of 100 problem knees. Am J Sports Med 5:63–66, 1977.

102. Larson RL: Dislocations and ligamentous injuries of the knee. In Rockwood CA Jr, Green DP, eds. Fractures. Philadelphia, JB Lippincott, 1975: 1182–1184.

103. Levinsohn EM, Baker BE: Prearthrotomy diagnostic evaluation of the knee. Review of 100 cases diagnosed by arthrography and arthroscopy. AJR 134:107–111, 1980.

104. Mink JH, Dickerson R: Air or CO_2 for knee arthrography? AJR 134:991–993, 1980.

105. Price CT, Allen WC: Ligament repair in the knee with preservation of the meniscus. J Bone Joint Surg (Am) 60:61–65, 1978.

106. Ricklin P, Ruttimann A, DelBuono MS: Meniscus Lesions. Practical Problems of Clinical Diagnosis, Arthrography and Therapy. New York, Grune & Stratton, 1971.

107. Salazar JE, Sebes JI, Scott RL: The supine view in double-contrast knee arthrography. AJR 141:585–586, 1983.

108. Sim FH: Complications and late results of meniscectomy. In Funk FJ, ed.: AAOS Symposium on the Athlete's Knee. 1982: 141–152.

109. Spataro RF, Katzberg RW, Burgener FA, Fischer HW: Epinephrine enhanced knee arthrography. Invest Radiol 13:286–290, 1978.

110. Tegtmeyer CJ, McCue FC 3d, Higgins SM, Ball DW: Arthrography of the knee: a comparative study of the accuracy of single and double contrast techniques. Radiology 132:37–41, 1979.

111. Thijn CJP: The accuracy of double-contrast arthrography and arthroscopy of the knee joint. Skeletal Radiol 8:187–192, 1982.

112. Thijn CJP: Arthrography of the Knee Joint. New York, Springer-Verlag, 1979.

Chondromalacia

113. Boven F, Bellemans M-A, Geurts J, DeBoeck H, Potviliege R: The value of computed tomography scanning in chondromalacia patellae. Skeletal Radiol 8:183–185, 1982.

114. Cassells SW: The arthroscope in the diagnosis of disorders of the patellofemoral joint. Clin Orthop 144:45–50, 1979.

115. Cave EF, Rowe CR: The patella: its importance in derangement of the knee. J Bone Joint Surg (Am) 32:542–553, 1950.

116. Dalinka MK: Arthrography. New York, Springer-Verlag, 1980.

117. Ficat RP, Philippe J, Hungerford DS: Chondromalacia patellae: a system of classification. Clin Orthop 144:55–62, 1979.

118. Goodfellow J, Hungerford DS, Zindel M: Patellofemoral joint mechanics and pathology: 1. Functional anatomy of the patello-femoral joint. J Bone Joint Surg (Br) 58:287–290, 1976.

119. Goodfellow J, Hungerford DS, Woods C: Patellofemoral joint mechanics and pathology: 2. Chondromalacia patellae. J Bone Joint Surg (Br) 58:291–299, 1976.

120. Horns JW: The diagnosis of chondromalacia by double contrast arthrography of the knee. J Bone Joint Surg (Am) 59:119–120, 1977.

121. Insall J, Bullough PG, Burstein AH: Proximal "tube" realignment of the patella for chondromalacia patellae. Clin Orthop 144:63–69, 1979.

122. Insall J, Falvo KA, Wise DW: Chondromalacia patellae: a prospective study. J Bone Joint Surg (Am) 58:1–8, 1976.

123. Murray JWG: The Maquet principle. Its application in severe chondromalacia patellae, patellofemoral and global knee osteoarthritis. Orthop Rev 5:29–36, 1976.

124. Outerbridge RE, Dunlop JA: The problem of chondromalacia patellae. Clin Orthop 110:177–196, 1975.

125. Sledge CB: Chondromalacia patellae. Harvard Orthopedic Radiology Course Syllabus, March 1978: 20–24.

Patellar Subluxation and Dislocation

126. Hauser E: Total tendon transplant for slipping patella. A new operation for recurrent dislocation of the patella. Surg Gynecol Obstet 66:199–214, 1938.

Osteoarthritis and Osteotomy

127. Ahlback S: Osteoarthritis of the knee. A radiographic investigation. Acta Radiol [Diagn] (Suppl)277:7–72, 1968.

128. Brueckmann FR, Kettelkamp DB: Proximal tibial osteotomy. Orthop Clin 13:3–16, 1982.

129. Coventry BM: Osteotomy about the knee for degenerative and rheumatoid arthritis: indications, operative technique and results. J Bone Joint Surg (Am) 55:23–48, 1973.

130. Landells JW: The bone cysts of osteoarthritis. J Bone Joint Surg (Br) 35:643–649, 1953.

131. Leach RE, Gregg T, Siber FJ: Weight-bearing radiography in osteoarthritis of the knee. Radiology 97:265–268, 1970.

132. Mankin HJ: The reaction of articular cartilage to injury and osteoarthritis. Part I. N Engl J Med 291:1285–1292, 1974.

133. Mankin HJ: The reaction of articular cartilage to injury and osteoarthritis. Part II. N Engl J Med 291:1335–1340, 1974.

134. Maquet PGJ: Osteotomy. In Freeman MAR, ed. Arthritis of the Knee. Clinical Features and Surgical Management. New York, Springer-Verlag, 1980: 143–183.

135. Maquet PGJ: Treatment of osteoarthritis of the knee by osteotomy. In Weil VH, ed. Progress in Orthopedic Surgery, vol. 4, Joint Preserving Procedures of the Lower Extremities. New York, Springer-Verlag, 1980: 57–73.

136. Marklund T, Myrnerts R: Radiographic determination of cartilage height in the knee joint. Acta Orthop Scand 45:752–755, 1974.

137. Resnick D, Niwayama G, Goergen TG, et al.: Clinical, radiographic and pathologic abnormalities in calcium pyrophosphate dihydrate deposition disease (CPPD): pseudogout. Radiology 122:1–15, 1977.

138. Resnick D, Vint V: The "tunnel" view in assessment of cartilage loss in osteoarthritis of the knee. Radiology 137:547–548, 1980.

139. Thomas RH, Resnick D, Alazraki NP, Daniel D, Greenfield R: Compartmental evaluation of osteoarthritis of the knee. A comparative study of available diagnostic modalities. Radiology 116:585–594, 1975.

140. Vainionpaa S, Laike E, Kirves P, Tiusanen P: Tibial osteotomy for osteoarthritis of the knee. A five to ten-year follow-up study. J Bone Joint Surg (Am) 63:938–946, 1981.

141. Wagner H: Principles of corrective osteotomies in osteoarthritis of the knee. *In* Weil VH, ed. Progress in Orthopedic Surgery, vol. 4, Joint Preserving Procedures of the Lower Extremities. New York, Springer-Verlag, 1980: 75–102.

Rheumatoid Arthritis

142. Weissman BNW, Sosman JL: The radiology of rheumatoid arthritis. Clin Orthop 6:653–674, 1975.

143. Sosman JL: Radiological aspects of the knee in rheumatoid arthritis. International Congress Series, no. 61. Excerpta Medica Fndtn 167–170, 1963.

PVNS

144. Breimer CW, Freiberger RH: Bone lesions associated with villonodular synovitis. AJR 79:618–629, 1958.

145. Docken WP: Pigmented villonodular synovitis: a review with illustrative case reports. Semin Arthritis Rheum 9:1–22, 1979.

146. Georgen JG, Resnick D, Niwayama G: Localized nodular synovitis of the knee. A report of two cases with abnormal arthrograms. AJR 126:647–650, 1976.

147. Jaffe HL, Lichtenstein L, Sutro CJ: Pigmented villonodular synovitis, bursitis and tenosynovitis. Arch Pathol 31:731–765, 1941.

148. Lewis RW: Roentgenographic study of soft tissue pathology in and about the knee joint. AJR 65:200–220, 1951.

149. Rosenthal DI, Aronow S, Murray WT: Iron content of pigmented villonodular synovitis detected by computed tomography. Radiology 133:409–411, 1979.

150. Simon G: Xanthoma of joints. Arch Clin Chir 6:573, 1965.

151. Wolfe RD, Giuliano V: Double-contrast arthrography in the diagnosis of pigmented villonodular synovitis of the knee. AJR 110:793–799, 1970.

Synovial Osteochondromatosis

152. Dalinka MK, Lally JF, Koniver G, Cores GS: The radiology of osseous and articular infection. CRC Crit Rev Clin Radiol Nucl Med 7:1–64, 1975.

153. Giustra PE, Furman RS, Roberts L, Killoran PJ: Synovial osteochondromatosis involving the elbow. AJR 127:347–348, 1976.

154. Holm CL: Primary synovial chondromatosis of the ankle. J Bone Joint Surg (Am) 58:878–880, 1976.

155. Jeffreys TE: Synovial chondromatosis. J Bone Joint Surg (Br) 49:530–534, 1967.

156. Jones HT: Loose body formation in synovial osteochondromatosis with special reference to the etiology and pathology. J Bone Joint Surg 6:407–458, 1924.

157. Lichtenstein L: Tumors of the synovial joints, bursae, and tendon sheaths. Cancer 8:816–830, 1955.

158. Milgram JW: Synovial osteochondromatosis. A histopathological study of thirty cases. J Bone Joint Surg (Am) 59:792–801, 1977.

159. Nixon JE, Frank GR, Chambers G: Synovial osteochondromatosis. With report of four cases, one showing malignant change. US Armed Forces Med J 11:1434–1445, 1960.

160. Paul LW, Juhl JH: The Essentials of Roentgen Interpretation. New York, Harper & Row, 1972.

161. Prager RF, Mall JC: Arthrographic diagnosis of synovial chondromatosis. AJR 127:344–346, 1976.

CPPD

162. Martel W, McCarter DK, Solsky MA, Good AE, Hart WR, Braunstein EM, Brady TM: Further observations on the arthropathy of calcium pyrophosphate crystal deposition disease. Radiology 141:1–15, 1981.

163. McCarty DJ Jr, ed. Proceedings of the Conference on Pseudogout and Pyrophosphate Metabolism. Arthritis Rheum [Suppl] 19:275–502, 1976.

164. Resnick D, Niwayama G, Goergen TG, et al.: Clinical, radiographic and pathologic abnormalities in calcium pyrophosphate dihydrate deposition disease (CPPD): pseudogout. Radiology 122:1–15, 1977.

Osteochondritis Dissecans

165. Lavner G: Osteochondritis dissecans. An analysis of forty-two cases and a review of the literature. AJR 57:56–70, 1947.

166. Milgram JW: Radiological and pathological manifestations of osteochondritis dissecans of the distal femur. A study of 50 cases. Radiology 126:305–311, 1978.

Spontaneous Osteonecrosis

167. Ahlback S, Bauer GCH, Bohne WH: Spontaneous osteonecrosis of the knee. Arthritis Rheum 11:710–733, 1968.

168. Greyson ND, Lotem MN, Gross AE, Houpt JB: Radionuclide evaluation of spontaneous femoral osteonecrosis. Radiology 142:729–735, 1982.

169. Hall FM: Osteonecrosis of the knee and medial meniscal tears. Letter to the editor. Radiology 133:828, 1979.

170. Houpt JB, Alpert B, Lotem M, Freyson ND, Pritzker KPH, Langer F, Gross AE: Spontaneous osteonecrosis of the medial tibial plateau. J Rheumatol 9:81–90, 1982.

171. Muheim G, Gohne WH: Prognosis in spontaneous osteonecrosis of the knee. Investigation by radionuclide scintimetry and radiography. J Bone Joint Surg (Br) 52:605–612, 1970.

172. Norman A, Baker ND: Osteonecrosis of the knee and medial meniscus tears. Reply to letter to the editor. Radiology 133:828–829, 1979.

173. Norman A, Baker ND: Spontaneous osteonecrosis of the knee and medial meniscal tears. Radiology 129:653–656, 1978.

174. Rozing PM, Insall J, Bohne WH: Spontaneous osteonecrosis of the knee. J Bone Joint Surg (Am) 62:2–7, 1980.

175. Smillie IS: Loose bodies: osteochondritis dissecans and conditions of like radiologic appearance. *In* Smillie IS, ed. Diseases of the Knee Joint. New York, Churchill Livingstone, 1980: 387–402.

Patellar and Fabellar Fractures

176. Bostrom A: Fracture of the patella. A study of 422 patellar fractures. Acta Orthop Scand [Suppl] 143:1–80, 1972.

177. Brooke R: The treatment of fractured patella by excision. A study of morphology and function. Br J Surg 24:733–747, 1937.

178. Dashefsky JH: Fracture of the fabella. A case report. J Bone Joint Surg (Am) 59:698, 1977.

179. Hohl M, Larson RL: Fractures and dislocations of the knee. *In* Rockwood CA Jr, Green DP, eds. Fractures. Philadelphia, JB Lippincott, 1975.

180. Jacobsen K: Radiologic technique for measuring instability in the knee joint. Acta Radiol [Diagn]
18:113–125, 1977.
181. Lotke PA, Ecker ML: Transverse fractures of the
patella. Clin Orthop 158:186–190, 1981.
182. Muller ME, Allgower M, Schneider R, Willenegger H:
Manual of Internal Fixation. New York, Springer-
Verlag, 1979.
183. Scapinelli R: Blood supply of the human patella. Its
relation to ischemic necrosis after fracture. J Bone
Joint Surg (Am) 49:563–570, 1967.
184. Sorensen KH: The late prognosis after fracture of the
patella. Acta Orthop Scand 34:198–212, 1964.

Tibial Plateau Fractures

185. Dovey H, Heerfordt J: Tibial condyle fractures. A
follow-up of 200 cases. Acta Chir Scand
137:521–531, 1971.
186. Elstrom J, Pankovich AM, Sassoon H, Rodriguez J:
Use of tomography in the assessment of fractures of
the tibial plateau. J Bone Joint Surg (Am) 58:551–555,
1976.
187. Fagerberg S: Tomographic analysis of depressed fractures within the knee joint, and of injuries to the
cruciate ligaments. Orthop Scand 27:219–227, 1958.
188. Hohl M: Tibial condylar fractures. J Bone Joint Surg
(Am) 49:1455–1467, 1967.
189. Hohl M, Luck JV: Fractures of the tibial condyle. A
clinical and experimental study. J Bone Joint Surg
(Am) 38:1001–1018, 1956.
190. Kennedy JC, Bailey WH: Experimental tibial-plateau
fractures. Studies of the mechanism and a classification. J Bone Joint Surg (Am) 50:1522–1534, 1968.
191. Lucht U, Pilgaard S: Fractures of the tibial condyles.
Acta Orthop Scand 42:366–376, 1971.
192. Moore TM, Harvey JP Jr: Roentgenographic measurement of tibial-plateau depression due to fracture. J
Bone Joint Surg (Am) 56:155–160, 1974.
193. Newberg AH, Greenstein R: Radiographic evaluation
of tibial plateau fractures. Radiology 126:319–323,
1978.
194. Palmer I: Fractures of the upper end of the tibia. J
Bone Joint Surg (Br) 33:160–166, 1951.
195. Rasmussen PS: Tibial condylar fractures. Impairment
of knee joint stability as an indication for surgical
treatment. J Bone Joint Surg (Am) 55:1331–1350,
1973.
196. Schioler G: Tibial condylar fractures with a particular
view to the value of tomography. Acta Orthop Scand
42:462, 1971.

Tibial Shaft Fractures

197. Ellis H: The speed of healing after fracture of the tibial
shaft. J Bone Joint Surg (Br) 40:42–46, 1958.
198. Leach RE: Fractures of the tibia. In Rockwood CA Jr,
Green DP, eds. Fractures. Philadelphia, JB Lippincott,
1975: 1285–1359.
199. Weissman SL, Herold HZ, Engelberg M: Fractures of
the middle two-thirds of the tibial shaft. Results of
treatment without internal fixation in 140 consecutive
cases. J Bone Joint Surg (Am) 48:257–267, 1966.

Compartment Syndrome

200. Auerbach DN, Bowen AD III: Sonography of leg in
posterior compartment syndrome. AJR 136:407–408,
1981.
201. Gelberman RH, Garfin SR, Hergenroeder PT, Mubarak SJ, Menon J: Compartment syndromes of the
forearm: diagnosis and treatment. Clin Orthop
161:252–261, 1981.
202. Hargens AR, Schmidt DA, Evans KI, Gonsalves MR,
Cologne JB, Garfin SR, Mubarak SJ, Hagan PL,
Akeson WH: Quantitation of skeletal-muscle necrosis
in a model compartment syndrome. J Bone Joint Surg
(Am) 63:631–636, 1981.
203. Hayden JW: Compartment syndromes. Early recognition and treatment. Postgrad Med 74:191–202,
1983.
204. Mubarak SJ, Hargens AR: Acute compartment syndromes. Surg Clin North Am 63:539–565, 1983.
205. Pearl AJ: Anterior compartment syndrome: a case
report. Am J Sports Med 9:119–120, 1981.
206. Rydholm U, Brun A, Ekelund L, Rydholm A: Chronic
compartmental syndrome in the tensor fasciae latae
muscle. Clin Orthop 177:169–171, 1983.
207. Viau MR, Pedersen HE, Salciccioli GG, Manoli A II:
Ectopic calcification as a late sequela of compartment
syndrome. Report of two cases. Clin Orthop
176:178–180, 1983.
208. Vukanovic S. Hauser H, Wettstein P: CT localization
of myonecrosis for surgical decompression. AJR
135:1298–1299, 1980.

Total Knee Replacement

209. Aglietti P, et al.: A new patella prosthesis design and
application. Clin Orthop 107:175–187, 1975.
210. Andriacchi TP, et al.: The influence of total knee
replacement design on walking and stair climbing. J
Bone Joint Surg (Am) 64:1328–1335, 1982.
211. Bargar WL, et al.: Results with the constrained total
knee prosthesis in treating severely disabled patients
and patients with failed total knee replacements. J
Bone Joint Surg (Am) 62:504–512, 1980.
212. Bartel DL, et al.: Performance of the tibial component
in total knee replacement. J Bone Joint Surg (Am)
64:1026–1033, 1982.
213. Brause BD: Infected total knee replacement. Orthop
Clin North Am 13:245–249, 1982.
214. Brodersen MP, et al.: Arthrodesis of the knee following
failed total knee arthroplasty. J Bone Joint Surg (Am)
61:181–185, 1979.
215. Chand K: The knee joint in rheumatoid arthritis. IV.
Treatment by nonhinged total knee prosthetic replacement. Int Surg 60:11–18, 1975.
216. Clayton ML, Thirupathi R: Patellar complications after
total condylar arthroplasty. Clin Orthop 170:152–155,
1982.
217. Ducheyne P, et al.: Failure of total knee arthroplasty
due to loosening and deformation of the tibial component. J Bone Joint Surg (Am) 60:384–391, 1978.
218. Freeman MA, Blaha JD, Bradley GW, Insler HP:
Cementless fixation of ICLH tibial component. Orthop
Clin North Am 13:141–154, 1982.
219. Gelman MI, Coleman RE, Stevens PM, Davey BW:
Radiography, radionuclide imaging, and arthrography
in the evaluation of total hip and knee replacement.
Radiology 128:677–682, 1978.
220. Gelman MI, Dunn HK: Radiology of knee joint replacement. AJR 127:447–455, 1976.
221. Gilula LA, Staple TW: Radiology of recently developed
total knee prostheses. Radiol Clin North Am 13:57–66,
1975.
222. Goergen TG, Resnick D: Radiology of total knee
replacement. J Can Assoc Radiol 27:178–185, 1976.
223. Harris WH: Total joint replacement. N Engl J Med
297:650–651, 1977.
224. Hendrix RW, Anderson TM: Arthrographic and radiologic evaluation of prosthetic joints. Radiol Clin North
Am 19:349–364, 1981.

225. Hui FC, Fitzgerald RH: Hinged total knee arthroplasty. J Bone Joint Surg (Am) 62:513–519, 1980.
226. Hungerford DS, Kenna RV, Krackow KA: The porous-coated anatomic total knee. Orthop Clin North Am 13:103–122, 1982.
227. Hunter JC, Hattner RS, Murray WR, Genant HK: Loosening of the total knee arthroplasty: detection by radionuclide bone scanning. AJR 135:131–136, 1980.
228. Insall J: Reconstructive surgery and rehabilitation of the knee. In Kelley WN, Harris ED, Ruddy S, Sledge CB, eds. Textbook of Rheumatology. Philadelphia, WB Saunders, 1981.
229. Insall JN, et al.: The posterior stabilized condylar prosthesis: a modification of the total condylar design. Two- to four-year clinical experience. J Bone Joint Surg (Am) 64:1317–1323, 1982.
230. Insall JN, et al.: A comparison of four models of total knee replacement prostheses. J Bone Joint Surg (Am) 58:754–765, 1976.
231. Kagan A II: Mechanical causes of loosening in knee joint replacement. J Biomech 10:387–391, 1977.
232. Kaufer H, Matthews LS: Spherocentric arthroplasty of the knee. J Bone Joint Surg (Am) 63:545–559, 1981.
233. Lotke PA, Ecker ML: Influence of positioning of prosthesis in total knee replacement. J Bone Joint Surg (Am) 59:77–79, 1977.
234. Mensch JS, Amstutz HC: Knee morphology as a guide to knee replacement. Clin Orthop 112:231–241, 1975.
235. McKenna R, et al.: Thromboembolic disease in patients undergoing total knee replacement. J Bone Joint Surg (Am) 58:929–932, 1976.
236. Murray DG: Editorial. In defence of becoming unhinged. J Bone Joint Surg (Am) 62:495–496, 1979.
237. Peterson L, et al.: Total joint arthroplasty: The knee. Mayo Clin Proc 54:564–569, 1979.
238. Potter TA, et al.: Arthroplasty of the knee in rheumatoid arthritis and osteoarthritis. A follow-up study after implantation of the McKeever and MacIntosh prostheses. J Bone Joint Surg (Am) 54:1–24, 1972.
239. Radin EL: Biomechanics of the knee joint. Its implication in the design of replacements. Orthop Clin North Am 4:539–546, 1973.
240. Radin EL, et al.: Changes in the bone-cement interface after total hip replacement. An in vivo animal study. J Bone Joint Surg (Am) 64:1188–1200, 1982.
241. Reckling FW, et al.: A longitudinal study of the radiolucent line at the bone cement interface following total joint-replacement procedures. J Bone Joint Surg (Am) 59:355–358, 1977.
242. Reing CM, et al.: Differential bone scanning in the evaluation of a painful total joint replacement. J Bone Joint Surg (Am) 61:933–936, 1979.
243. Rosenthall L, et al.: 99mTc-PP and 67Ga imaging following insertion of orthopedic devices. Radiology 133:717–721, 1979.
244. Thomas WH: Total knee replacement with hinged prostheses. Orthop Clin 6:823–829, 1975.
245. Schneider R, et al.: Radiologic evaluation of knee arthroplasty. Orthop Clin North Am 13:225–244, 1982.
246. Scott RD: Duopatellar total knee replacement: the Brigham experience. Orthop Clin North Am 13:89–102, 1982.
247. Scott RD, Turoff N, Ewald FC: Stress fracture of the patella following duopatellar total knee arthroplasty with patellar resurfacing. Clin Orthop 170:147–151, 1982.
248. Scott WN: Foreword, Symposium on total knee arthroplasty. Orthop Clin North Am 13:1–2, 1982.
249. Sledge CB, Walker PS: Total knee replacement in rheumatoid arthritis. In Insall JN, ed. Surgery of the Knee. New York, Churchill Livingstone, 1984.
250. Weissman BNW: Radiographic evaluation of total joint replacement. In Kelley WN, Harris ED, Ruddy S, Sledge CB, eds. Textbook of Rheumatology. Philadelphia, WB Saunders, 1981.
251. Williamson BRJ, et al.: Radionuclide bone imaging as a means of differentiating loosening and infection in patients with a painful total hip prosthesis. Radiology 133:723–725, 1979.
252. Wilson FC: Total replacement of the knee in rheumatoid arthritis. A prospective study of the results of treatment with the Walldius prosthesis. J Bone Joint Surg (Am) 54:1429–1443, 1972.

Chapter 10

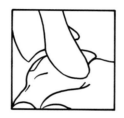

The
ANKLE

NORMAL STRUCTURE AND FUNCTION

Essential Anatomy

Bony Structures

The configuration of the ankle joint is like that of a mortise and tenon, in which a shaped piece of wood (tenon) fits into a slot (mortise) in another piece of wood. Thus the talus (tenon) is embraced by the distal tibia and the medial and the lateral malleolli (mortise; Fig. 10–1).

The inferior articular surface of the tibia is called the tibial plafond (ceiling), and it is medially continuous with the medial malleolus. The talus has three superior articular facets: the trochlea, for articulation with the tibia, and the medial and lateral facets, for articulation with the malleolli. The articular surfaces of the tibia and the talus are wider anteriorly than posteriorly, and longer laterally than medially (Fig. 10–2).

The lateral malleolus is posterior to the medial malleolus and projects about 1 cm distal to it. The coronal plane of the ankle is oriented at 15 to 20 degrees of external rotation with relation to the knee, which explains the necessity for rotating the ankle internally to obtain a true AP (mortise) view of the tibiotalar joint with both malleolli at the same level. A medial facet in the lateral malleolus allows articulation with the talus, and a posterior sulcus is present for the peroneus brevis and the peroneus longus tendons (Figs. 10–3 and 10–4). The medial malleolus has a posterior sulcus for the tibialis posterior and the flexor digitorum longus tendons.

Soft Tissues

Joint Capsule and Articular Cartilage. The ankle joint capsule attaches to the margins of the articular surfaces of the tibia and fibula (Fig. 10–4). The capsule is thin anteriorly and posteriorly, and these portions are most easily displaced by intraarticular fluid. A small synovial recess extends upward between the tibia and fibula.[2] Hyaline cartilage covers the articular surfaces of the talus, tibia, and fibula and extends along the most distal portion of the tibiofibular syndesmosis.

Ligamentous Anatomy. Medial support for the ankle is provided by the strong triangular *deltoid ligament* (also called the medial collateral ligament; Fig. 10–5). This consists of superficial and deep fibers that originate from the medial

Text continued on page 594

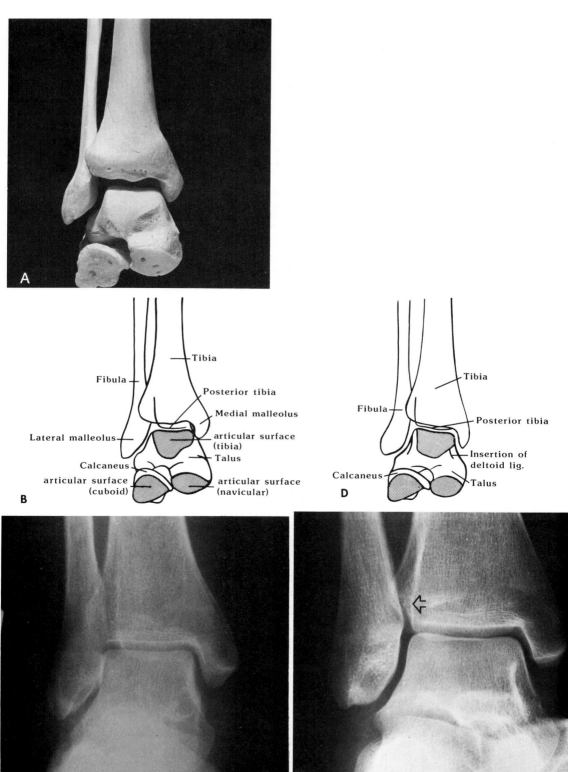

Figure 10–1. Normal Ankle. Photographic, diagrammatic, and radiological anatomy of the ankle in the AP *(A–C)*, internal oblique (mortise) *(D,E)*, and lateral *(F–H)* projections. Note the equal width of the cartilage spaces and the alignment of the lateral talus with the posterior cortex (arrow) on the mortise view.

Illustration continued on opposite page

590

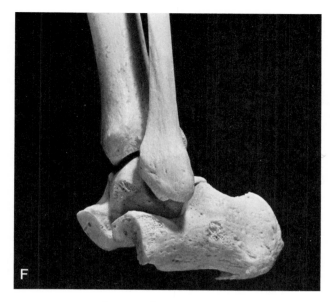

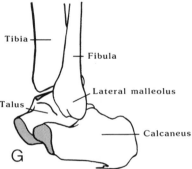

Tibia

Fibula

Lateral malleolus

Talus

Calcaneus

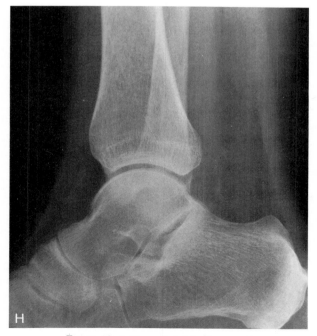

Figure 10–1. Normal Ankle *Continued.*

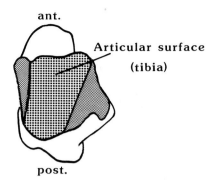

ant.

Articular surface
(tibia)

post.

Figure 10–2. The Normal Talus. The anterior trochlear surface of the talus is wider than the posterior surface.

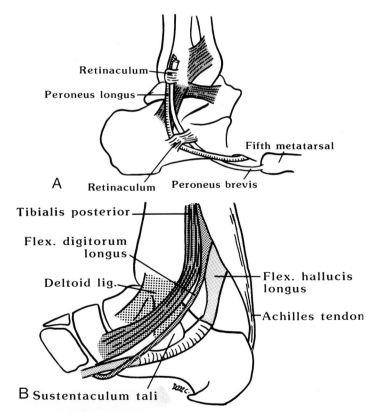

Retinaculum

Peroneus longus

Fifth metatarsal

A   Retinaculum   Peroneus brevis

Tibialis posterior

Flex. digitorum
longus

Deltoid lig.

Flex. hallucis
longus

Achilles tendon

B Sustentaculum tali

Figure 10–3. Tendons. *A,* Lateral view. The tendons of the peroneus brevis and the peroneus longus muscles are shown. These muscles evert the foot. They lie in a common synovial sheath behind the lateral malleolus. The peroneus longus crosses the lateral aspect of the cuboid and the sole and attaches to the lateral sides of the bases of the first metatarsal and the medial cuneiform. The peroneus brevis tendon passes around the lateral malleolus, anterior to the peroneus longus, and inserts on the base of the fifth metatarsal. *B,* Medial view. The posterior tibial tendon, in a separate sheath, passes around the medial melleolus, anterior to the tendon of the flexor digitorum longus. It functions to invert the foot. The tendon of the flexor hallucis longus passes under the sustentaculum tali.

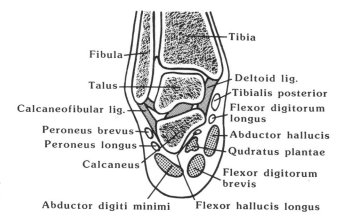

Figure 10–4. Joint Capsule and Related Structures. The tibiotalar joint capsule and adjacent structures are shown.

Labels in Figure 10–4:
Tibia
Fibula
Talus
Deltoid lig.
Calcaneofibular lig.
Tibialis posterior
Flexor digitorum longus
Peroneus brevus
Peroneus longus
Abductor hallucis
Qudratus plantae
Calcaneus
Flexor digitorum brevis
Abductor digiti minimi
Flexor hallucis longus

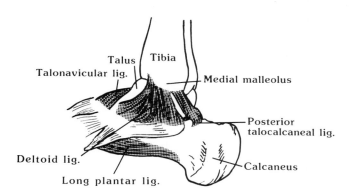

Labels in Figure 10–5:
Talus
Tibia
Talonavicular lig.
Medial malleolus
Posterior talocalcaneal lig.
Deltoid lig.
Calcaneus
Long plantar lig.

Figure 10–5. The Deltoid Ligament.

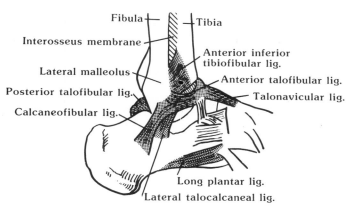

Labels in Figure 10–6:
Fibula
Tibia
Interosseus membrane
Anterior inferior tibiofibular lig.
Lateral malleolus
Anterior talofibular lig.
Posterior talofibular lig.
Talonavicular lig.
Calcaneofibular lig.
Long plantar lig.
Lateral talocalcaneal lig.

Figure 10–6. The Lateral Collateral Ligament. The anterior talofibular, posterior talofibular, and calcaneofibular portions of the lateral collateral ligament are shown.

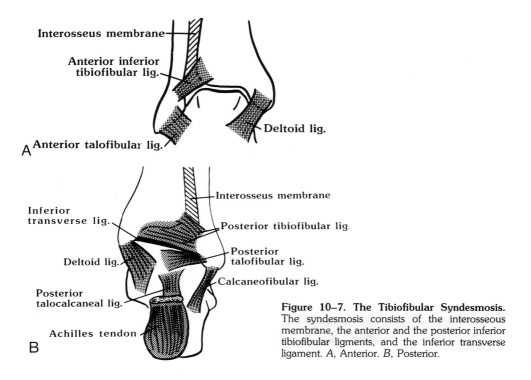

Figure 10–7. The Tibiofibular Syndesmosis. The syndesmosis consists of the interosseous membrane, the anterior and the posterior inferior tibiofibular ligaments, and the inferior transverse ligament. *A*, Anterior. *B*, Posterior.

malleolus. The superficial fibers divide into anterior, middle, and posterior groups, which insert on the navicular, the sustentaculum tali, and the talus. The deep fibers insert on the talus at a site marked by a small concavity in the bone. The deltoid ligament lies beneath the tendons of the tibialis posterior and flexor digitorum longus muscles.

Lateral support is provided by three separate ligaments: *anterior talofibular, posterior talofibular, and calcaneofibular* (Fig. 10–6). The calcaneofibular ligament is under the tendons of the peroneus longus and the peroneus brevis and may blend with their sheaths. It is of primary importance in stabilizing the subtalar joint and it also provides some ankle joint stability.[19, 25]

The tibia and fibula are bound together by four ligaments and the interosseous membrane, which together form the tibiofibular syndesmosis (Fig. 10–7). The *anterior and the posterior inferior ligaments* extend anteriorly and posteriorly between the adjacent margins of the tibia and the fibula. The posterior ligament is the stronger of the two. The *inferior transverse ligament* passes across the posterior portion of the joint, from the lateral malleolus to the posterior margin of the tibial articular surface just below the posterior inferior tibiofibular ligament. It extends below the bony margin of the tibia and forms part of the tibial articular surface. The *interosseous ligament* is the distal part of the interosseous membrane and is the major bond between the tibia and the fibula.

Function

The ankle joint allows flexion-extension motion, which is measured using the foot at a right angle to the tibia as the reference point. From this position 20 degrees of dorsiflexion and about 50 degrees of plantar flexion are normally present (Fig. 10–8).[3] Inversion and eversion of the foot occurs at the tarsal joints, especially at the subtalar articulation.

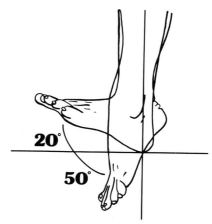

Figure 10–8. Ankle Motion. The tibiotalar joint allows 20 degrees of dorsiflexion and about 50 degrees of plantar flexion.

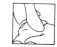

The stability of the ankle results from its ligamentous and bony architecture. Forces of gravity and muscular contraction tend to produce posterior displacement of the talus on the tibia (see Fig. 10–24). This displacement is resisted by the shape of the articular surfaces of the talus and the tibia (which are wider anteriorly than posteriorly) and by the long posterior lip of the tibia. The greater anterior width of the articular surface of the talus also means that more room is required between the malleoli in dorsiflexion than in plantar flexion. This is provided by slight motion of the fibula and stretching of the syndesmosis.[2] Ligamentous restraint to posterior talar subluxation is provided by the medial and the lateral collateral ligaments.[1]

Normal Radiographic Appearances

Standard radiographic examination includes anteroposterior (AP), lateral, and mortise views, the last taken with the foot internally rotated 15 to 20 degrees to bring the more posteriorly located lateral malleolus to the same level as the medial malleolus (Fig. 10–1). On the AP view the long axis of the tibia is continuous with the vertical axis of the talus. The fibula overlies the lateral margin of the tibia, and the subchondral cortices of the tibia and the talus are parallel. In the mortise view the talus should be equidistant from the medial malleolus, the lateral malleolus, and the tibial plafond. The lateral margin of the talus should be aligned with the dense line representing the posterior portion of the lateral tibia. On the lateral view the articular cartilage space should be of uniform width. Virtually no soft tissue density should be seen anterior to the tibiotalar joint.

Arthrography

Technique. Ankle arthrograms are technically rather easy to do; interpretation, however, may be more of a problem. There are several techniques for joint puncture, but the key to success is fluoroscopic monitoring in the lateral projection.[9] The following technique works for us: The ankle is examined, and the course of the dorsalis pedis artery noted. The area is washed with a povidone-iodine (Betadine) solution and draped with sterile towels. Fluoroscopy is then done in the frontal projection, and the sterile tip of a hemostat is placed just below the superomedial aspect of the ankle joint space to mark the site to be infiltrated with 1 percent lidocaine (Xylocaine). Infiltration medial to the extensor hallucis

longus tendon will prevent inadvertent injury to the anterior tibial nerve that is located on the lateral aspect of this tendon.[14] The leg is then turned into the lateral position, and the needle used for joint puncture (usually a 25-gauge, 1½-inch needle) is inserted through the anesthetized area and directed slightly laterally and superiorly until its tip lies between the talus and the tibia. Aspiration of joint fluid is attempted but is usually nonproductive. Any fluid that is aspirated is not saved unless specific clinical indications, such as possible sepsis or pseudogout, are present. The intraarticular needle position is confirmed by noting that injected contrast medium flows immediately away from the needle tip. Six to 8 ml of contrast agent is then injected, the type of agent used depending upon the clinical setting. For example, single positive-contrast examination is used most often for the demonstration of ligament tears. Double-contrast study may be preferable for evaluation of the articular cartilage. In the latter case tomography is often done, and 0.1 to 0.2 ml of a 1:1000 solution of epinephrine may be added to prolong the period during which optimal films can be obtained. Single-contrast examination with air alone is occasionally used when the study is undertaken for the demonstration of intraarticular loose bodies or when the patient has had a prior serious adverse reaction to contrast agent.

After contrast medium injection the needle is removed; the ankle is briefly exercised; and a standard overhead anteroposterior view, internal and external oblique views, and a lateral view with the foot in neutral position are obtained. If the study is undertaken for evaluation of ligamentous damage, varus and valgus stress views and views during an anterior drawer test are obtained,[13] and if the first series of films is negative, the exercise period and filming are repeated. Studies done for assessment of the articular cartilage or for the presence of loose bodies are usually followed by tomography after the initial series of films. Speigel and Staples recommend rest and elevation for several hours after the procedure.[13]

The Normal Arthrogram. The normal ankle arthrogram shows contrast agent over the articular surfaces and filling of anterior and posterior

Table 10–1. **Filling of Adjacent Structures on Ankle Arthrography**

Flexor hallucis longus and flexor digitorum longus	20%
Subtalar joint	10%

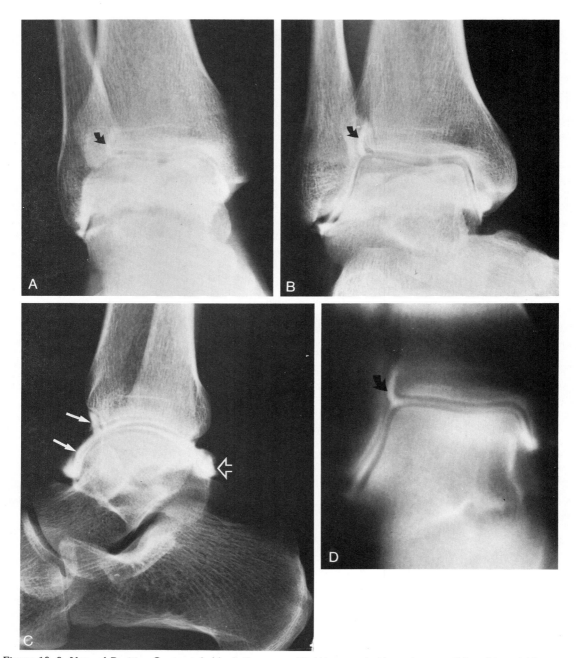

Figure 10–9. Normal Positive Contrast Ankle Arthrogram. AP *(A)*, internal oblique (mortise; *B,*) and lateral *(C)* views and a tomogram *(D)* in the internal oblique projection show contrast agent coating the articular surfaces and filling normally present anterior (white arrow), posterior (open arrow), and syndesmotic (black arrows) recesses. There is no extension of contrast medium into the soft tissue medially or laterally.

recesses of variable size (Fig. 10–9). A syndesmotic recess, extending between the distal tibia and the fibula, is seen on frontal views. It averages 1 to 2.5 cm in length and is smooth in outline.

Contrast medium should be seen only within the confines of the joint capsule. In 20 percent

of apparently normal individuals, however, filling of the tendon sheaths of the flexor hallucis longus, the flexor digitorum longus, or both occurs (Table 10–1).[7, 11] These tendons are located posteromedially, beneath the sustentaculum tali on the lateral view (Fig. 10–10). No tendon sheath filling should normally be present

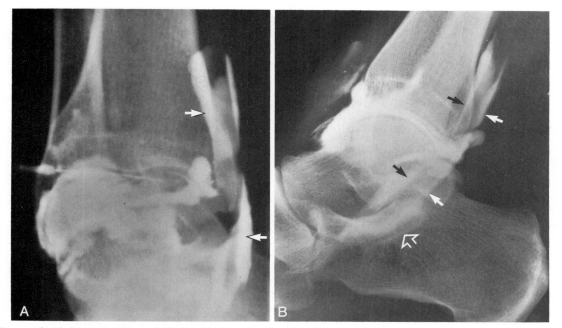

Figure 10–10. Normal Filling of Medial Tendon Sheaths. The sheath of the flexor digitorum longus tendon is filled (arrows). The flexor hallucis longus passes under the sustentaculum tali (open arrow) and is not filled in this case. *A,* AP view. *B,* Lateral view.

on the lateral side of the ankle. In 10 percent of normal subjects contrast material fills the posterior talocalcaneal (subtalar) joint (see Fig. 11–3).

ABNORMAL CONDITIONS

Soft Tissue Abnormalities

Joint Effusion

The lateral view with the foot in neutral position is the most sensitive projection for detecting joint effusion (Fig. 10–11). In the absence of joint distension, only fat should be seen immediately both anterior to and posterior to the ankle on the lateral radiograph.[16, 17] Joint distension due to any cause (e.g., hemarthrosis, rheumatoid arthritis) produces a soft tissue density anteriorly that displaces the pretalar fat pad and extends along the neck of the talus. The presence of this density allows as little as 5 ml of fluid to be detected.[16] The fact that effusion is easier to detect anteriorly than posteriorly is related to the observation that the anterior limit (anterior ligament) of the ankle joint is very thin.[18] Distension of the posterior recess of the ankle joint does occur, however; it is recognizable by the "figure three" configuration it assumes because of bulging of the synovial membrane above and below the indentation of the posterior syndesmotic ligaments.[18]

Saunders and Weston noted the value of AP and oblique projections in detecting soft tissue abnormalities. Normally, the deep fascia between the medial malleolus and the talus is concave. In the presence of effusion or a localized mass the soft tissues in the area assume a convex contour, and the adjacent fat plane is displaced medially.[15]

Ligamentous Injuries

Definitions. Sprains are partial ligament tears. They must be distinguished from complete ligamentous disruption, since untreated complete tears may be followed by degenerative changes in the ankle joint. Displacement of the talus in the ankle mortise without apparent fracture or the presence of instability indicates complete ligament rupture.[23] When clinical evidence of a moderately severe injury is present but no fracture or talar displacement is seen on standard radiographs, stress views may demonstrate instability and confirm ligamentous rupture.

As emphasized by Neer, the bones and ligaments of the ankle mortise form a ring (Fig. 10–12).[27] When displacement of the talus occurs within the mortise, disruption (ligament tear or fracture) of at least two structures must be present. A ligament tear must therefore be present when the talus is displaced and only one fracture is present. The medial deltoid ligament is strong, and its rupture is much less frequent than is avulsion of the medial malleolus.[19]

Of the three divisions of the lateral collateral ligament the anterior talofibular ligament is

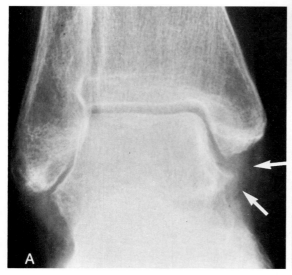
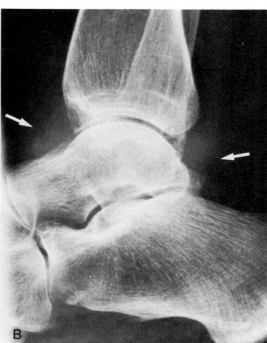

Figure 10–11. Ankle Joint Effusion. The AP view *(A)* shows bulging of the medial soft tissues (arrow). The lateral view *(B)* shows anterior and posterior capsular distension (arrows).

weakest and most often torn. Surgical exploration of severe ligamentous injuries has in fact shown that rupture of the anterior talofibular ligament is the most frequently encountered injury and that the combination of torn anterior talofibular and calcaneofibular ligaments is the second most frequent lesion.[22] Tears of the anterior talofibular ligament are difficult to exclude on physical examination, and there may be no talar tilt on routine radiographs. Inversion

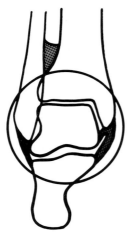

Figure 10–12. Ring Configuration of the Ankle. The bones and ligaments of the ankle form a ring. (After Neer CS: Conn Med 17:580, 1953. Copyright 1985, Conn Med, by permission.)

stress films can, however, confirm the diagnosis. Tears of the anterior joint capsule accompany anterior talofibular ligament tears and explain the positive arthrographic findings in early cases.[19]

Isolated tears of the calcaneofibular ligament are uncommon. Combined tears of the calcaneofibular and talofibular ligaments are more frequent and are most often responsible for tilting of the talus on standard radiographs.

The posterior talofibular ligament almost never tears, since avulsion fracture occurs before ligamentous rupture.[19]

Radiographic Findings

Standard Views. The only abnormality on standard radiographs of patients with ligamentous injuries may be soft tissue swelling. A small flake of detached bone provides specific evidence of avulsion fracture at the site of ligamentous insertion (see Fig. 10–20).[28]

Inversion Stress

Stress Views (Table 10–2). Inversion of the hindfoot is used to test the integrity of the lateral collateral ligament (Fig. 10–13). Complete tear of the anterior talofibular ligament results in abnormal talar tilt on inversion stress films, and this is said to be accentuated if the calcaneofibular ligament is also torn (Fig. 10–14).[25] Sauser and co-workers were unable, however, to differentiate tears of the anterior talofibular liga-

Table 10–2. **Plain Film Findings in Ligament Tears**

Ligament Involved	Routine Views	Varus Stress	Valgus Stress	Anterior Drawer	Ext. Rotation
Lateral					
Anterior talofibular	± Talar tilt			+	
Calcaneofibular	Normal	Normal*			
Combined anterior talofibular and calcaneofibular	Talar tilt	↑ +			
Medial					
Deltoid	> 4-mm joint space medially		+		
Syndesmosis	> 5.5-mm tibiofibular space				+
	Fibular fracture ≥ 3 cm above joint line				
	Avulsion fracture of anterior or posterior tibial tubercles				

*Subtalar tilt may be present.

ment alone from combined talofibular and calcaneofibular tears by evaluating inversion stress views.[12] Section of the calcaneofibular ligament alone produces no talar tilt but does result in subtalar tilt demonstrable on specially angled views.[25] The degree of talar tilt is assessed by noting the angle of insertion of lines drawn along the articular surfaces of the talus and tibia.[25, 29] Difficulty in interpretation results from the ob-

servation that the talus may tilt with inversion stress even in uninjured patients. Laurin and associates found this tilt to average 7 degrees, but values up to 27 degrees were noted.[25] Using a stress apparatus to study patients with acute injury, Sauser and colleagues found a talar tilt of 10 degrees or more to be associated with lateral ligament injury in 99 percent of cases (Table 10–3).[12] The degree of tilt is increased

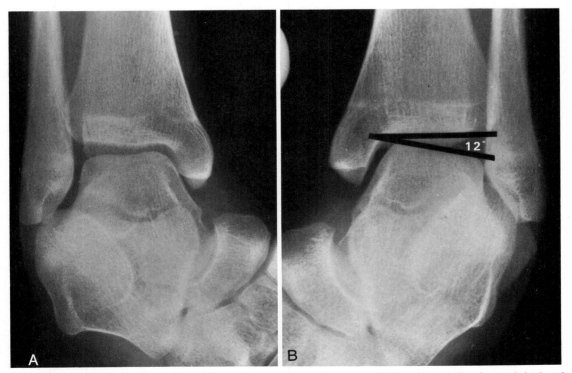

Figure 10–13. Normal Inversion Stress Views. Inversion stress views on each side show similar degrees of talar tilt. Although the measured angle is higher than average, the symmetrical appearance attests to the fact that this is a normal examination.

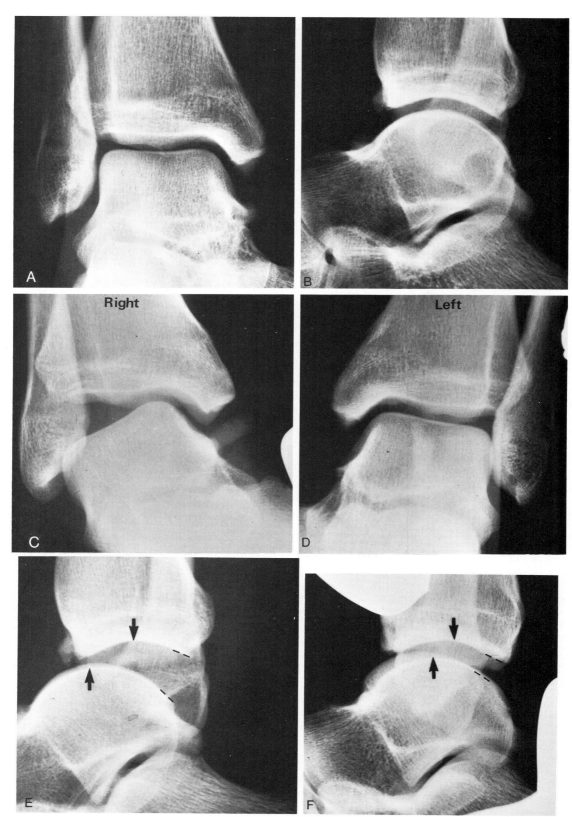

Figure 10–14. *See legend on opposite page.*

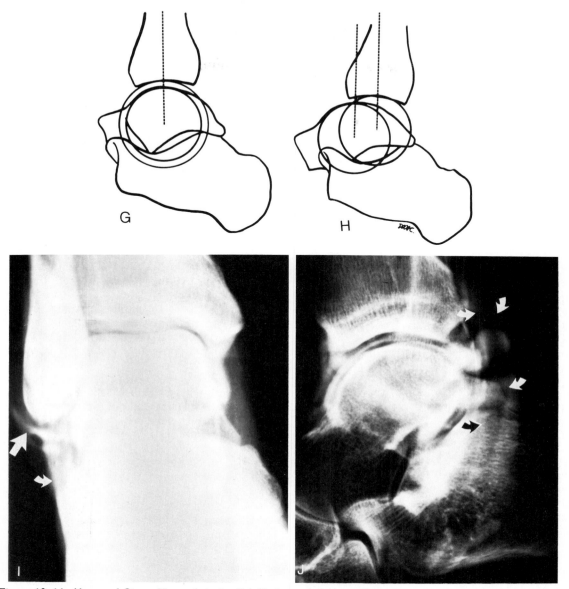

Figure 10–14. Abnormal Stress Views: Anterior Talofibular and Calcaneofibular Ligament Tears. AP *(A)* and lateral *(B)* views of the right ankle show hypertrophic lipping from the anterior tibia and talus. The syndesmosis is slightly wide. Comparison varus stress views of the right *(C)* and left *(D)* ankles show abnormal talar tilt on the right, particularly when compared with the normal left side. This is diagnostic of an anterior talofibular ligament tear on the right, with or without a calcaneofibular ligament tear. The anterior drawer test is abnormal on the right *(E)* as compared with the left *(F)*. Comparison can be made by noting the anterior shift of the midtalus in relation to the midtibia (arrows) on each side, the loss of parallelism of the subchondral cortices on the right, or the marked widening of the posterior joint space (lines) on the abnormal as compared with the normal side. This is consistent with an anterior talofibular ligament tear on the right. Diagrams *(G,H)* of anterior shift. G is normal, H abnormal. The AP *(I)* and lateral *(J)* arthrogram views show filling around the lateral malleolus (arrow), indicating an anterior talofibular ligament tear, and filling of the peroneal tendon sheaths (curved arrows), indicating a calcaneofibular ligament tear. (G and H redrawn from Lindstrand A, Martensson W: Acta Radiol Diagn 18:529, 1977.)

when the foot is held in plantar flexion, since the posterior articular surface of the talus is relatively narrow. Comparison views of both ankles are of particular value, since the degree of talar tilt, although not necessarily identical, is usually within 10 degrees of the other side.[25]

Laurin and colleagues also noted that "normal" talar tilt on inversion stress is accompanied by external rotation of the leg (identified by superimposition of the lateral malleolus on the tibia and talus), even when the films are made with the patella directed upward. In contrast, post-

Table 10–3. **Probability of Acute Lateral Ligament Tear (Based on Talar Tilt on Inversion Stress)**

Measured Angle ≥ (degrees)	Probability of Talofibular or Combined Talofibular/ Calcaneofibular Tear (percent)
0	61
5	76
9	97
10	99

Source: Sauser DD, Nelson RC, Lavine MH, et al: Radiology 148:653, 1983.

traumatic talar tilt is not accompanied by external rotation of the leg. Thus any talar tilt that is markedly asymmetrical is suspect and is even more so if external rotation of the involved leg does not accompany the tilt.

Anterior Drawer Test. Lindstrand and Mortensson suggest that a diagnosis of acute rupture of the anterior talofibular ligament can be made by stress views that attempt to displace the talus anteriorly, the radiological equivalent of the anterior drawer maneuver.[26] In a normal ankle the articular surfaces of the tibia and talus remain parallel on these stress lateral radiographs, but in abnormal cases this parallelism is lost (Fig. 10–14). The degree of anterior displacement of the talus is greater if the calcaneofibular ligament as well as the talofibular ligament is torn. Sauser

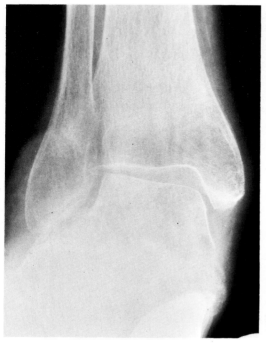

Figure 10–15. Deltoid Ligament Insufficiency. Valgus stress view shows abnormal talar tilt, diagnostic of an abnormal deltoid ligament.

and co-workers noted no statistically significant difference, however, between anterior drawer tests in patients with intact and those with acutely torn lateral ligaments.[12] The presence of muscle spasm may be responsible for a falsely normal test, and anesthesia or the application of weights to the leg may increase the sensitivity of the method.

Eversion Stress. Complete tear of the deltoid ligament is virtually always associated with fracture of the fibula, damage to the tibiofibular syndesmosis, or both.[1] The mortise view is diagnostic of deltoid ligament damage if the distance from the medial malleolus to the talus is greater than 4 mm.[1] Eversion stress tests the deltoid ligament. Partial tears (of the anterior fibers) may produce a 10 degree talar tilt, while a complete tear is associated with a 35 to 45 degree tilt (Fig. 10–15).

Tibiofibular Syndesmosis. The syndesmotic ligaments include the anterior and the posterior inferior tibiofibular ligaments and the interosseous ligament.[1] Complete diastasis involves all of these structures, while partial diastasis involves the anterior inferior tibiofibular ligament, with or without damage to the interosseous ligament.[28]

Standard films that show separation between the medial fibular cortex and the posterior edge of the peroneal groove of more than 5.5 mm suggest diastasis.[1] Pettrone and co-workers noted that tibiofibular overlap of less than 10 mm on the AP view and less than 1 mm on the mortise view suggests widening of the syndesmosis (Fig. 10–16).[47] The level of a fibular fracture also indicates whether or not the anterior inferior tibiofibular ligament is torn. The fibers of this ligament insert on the fibula 2 to 3 cm proximal to the level of the ankle joint. Therefore, fracture of the fibula at or proximal to 3 cm above the joint line indicates that a tear of the anterior inferior tibiofibular ligament has occurred. Fracture of the fibula distal to the ligamentous insertion usually indicates that the ligaments of the syndesmosis are intact.[44] External rotation stress films can be used to test the syndesmosis.

Arthrographic Demonstration of Ligamentous Injury (Table 10–4). Injected contrast material normally remains within the confines of the joint capsule or extends into the medially located tendons of the flexor hallucis longus, the flexor digitorum longus, or both. Extravasation in any other location is abnormal and confirms ligamentous rupture (Fig. 10–17). The location of the extravasated contrast agent is a reliable indicator of the ligament(s) involved.[10, 11] Dem-

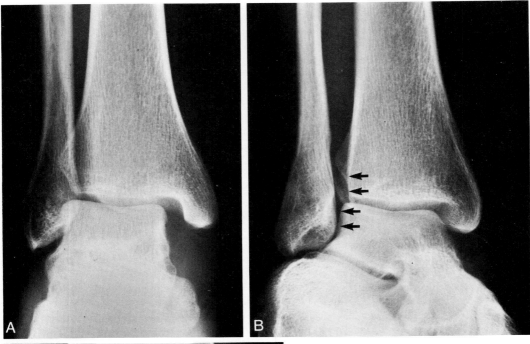

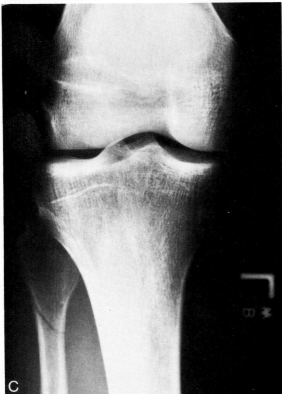

Figure 10–16. Maisonneuve Fracture. *A,* The AP view shows lateral subluxation of the talus, indicated by the wide medial cartilage space. *B,* The internal oblique view confirms lateral talar shift by loss of alignment of the lateral margins of the talus and the posterior tibial (arrows) as well as medial cartilage-space widening. The tibiofibular distance is wide, indicating disruption of the syndesmosis. *C,* An AP view of the proximal fibula confirms a fracture.

Table 10–4. **Ankle Arthrography for Detection of Ligamentous Rupture**

Location	Area of Extravasation	Significance
Lateral	Around tip of lateral malleolus	Tear of anterior talofibular ligament
	Filling of peroneal tendon sheaths	Acute or chronic calcaneofibular ligament tear
Medial	Filling of sheaths of flexor digitorum longus, flexor hallucis longus, or both	Normal
	Around medial malleolus	Deltoid ligament tear (look for other injuries)
Syndesmosis	Extravasation upward from syndesmotic recess	Anterior tibiofibular ligament tear

onstration of ligamentous tears requires that arthrography be done as soon as possible after injury, since false-negative results may occur on delayed studies owing to sealing of the capsular defect. Views taken after exercise or with applied stress may be necessary to demonstrate contrast extravasation.

Patterns of Extravasation (Table 10–4; Fig. 10–17)

Lateral Ligaments. The *anterior talofibular* ligament is the most frequent site of ligamentous disruption in the ankle.[9] Rupture of this ligament is associated with contrast extravasation anterior to, lateral to, and around the tip of the lateral malleolus (Fig. 10–14). The contrast may overlie the area of the syndesmosis on the AP view, but on the lateral view the region of the anterior tibiofibular ligament (see following) will not be opaque.

Calcaneofibular ligament tears are identified by the presence of contrast material in the peroneal tendon sheaths. Acute rupture of the calcaneofibular ligament essentially is always accompanied by rupture of the anterior talofibular ligament. If there is no arthrographic evidence of a talofibular ligament tear and if the arthrogram is done within 48 hours of injury, then presumably the calcaneofibular ligament tear represents an old injury.[9]

Isolated tears of the *posterior talofibular* ligament apparently do not occur. When a posterior talofibular ligament tear occurs in conjunction with rupture of the anterior talofibular and calcaneofibular ligaments, the arthrographic findings are those associated with tears of the two latter ligaments. There will, however, be gross lateral instability present when all three ligaments are torn.[11]

Medial Ligaments. *Deltoid* ligament tears are usually associated with other bone or soft tissue injuries. The tear is usually incomplete, most often involving only the anterior portion of the ligament. Injected contrast material extravasates around the medial malleolus in relation to the location of the tear.

The Syndesmosis. Anterior inferior tibiofibular ligament tears are associated with contrast extravasation upward from the syndesmotic recess. These are not isolated injuries.

Despite the elucidation of these patterns of extravasation, the place of arthrography in the assessment of acute ankle injuries remains controversial. Ala-Ketola and associates describe arthrography as indispensable because it allows accurate classification of ankle injuries into the Lauge-Hansen scheme, which may then be used to select a treatment plan.[4] In contrast with their 300 ankle arthrograms in 6 months, however, we perform virtually no ankle arthrograms in patients with acute injury. Most of our examinations are performed for evaluation of chronic pain following trauma, possible loose bodies, or articular cartilage abnormalities.

Ankle Fractures

The three bones and the associated ligaments of the ankle mortise make up a ring (Fig. 10–12).[44] A single break in the ring without displacement represents a *stable* injury; more than one break in the ring is an *unstable* situation. When a *displaced* malleolar fracture is evident on radiographs, another injury (bony or ligamentous) must be present, and the ring is therefore *unstable*. Talar shift in the AP or the lateral direction is evidence that at least two breaks in the ring are present.

Given a particular initiating force, injury to the ankle mortise follows an orderly sequence. This sequence allows the trained observer to suggest the mechanism of fracture and to identify sites of expected ligamentous injury. The mechanism of fracture production is of some clinical importance, since manipulative reduction is performed

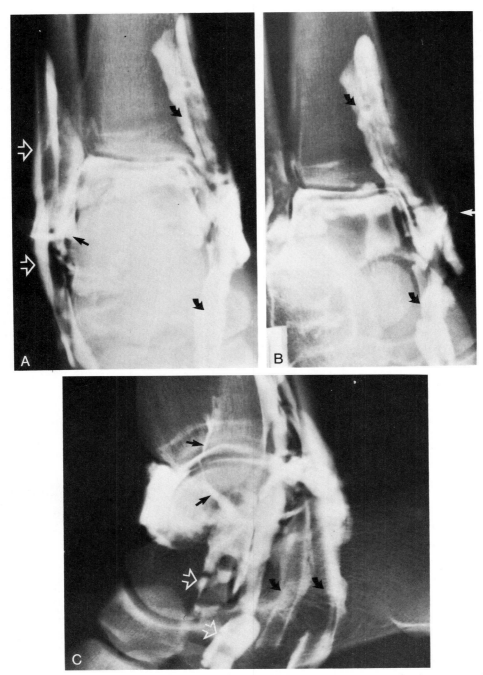

Figure 10–17. Arthrographic Demonstration of Deltoid, Anterior Talofibular, and Calcaneofibular Ligament Tears. AP *(A)*, oblique *(B)*, and lateral *(C)* views demonstrate a tear of the deltoid ligament, with contrast agent extravasation around the medial malleolus (white arrow). A tear of the anterior talofibular ligament has allowed contrast medium to extravasate anterior to, lateral to, and around the tip of the lateral malleolus (black arrows). Filling of the peroneal tendon sheaths (open arrows) indicate a calcaneofibular ligament tear. Normal filling of the flexor hallucis and the flexor digitorum longus tendon sheaths (curved arrows) is noted, and since they pass under the sustentaculum tali, they are projected lower in position than the lateral tendons.

by applying forces opposite to those responsible for creating the injury.[51]

Avulsion fractures are generally transverse, whereas fractures produced by the impact of the talus on a malleolus are oblique.[43, 51] The remaining analysis of the mechanism of a particular fracture is unfortunately complicated by a morass of poorly defined terms. Therefore, a

605

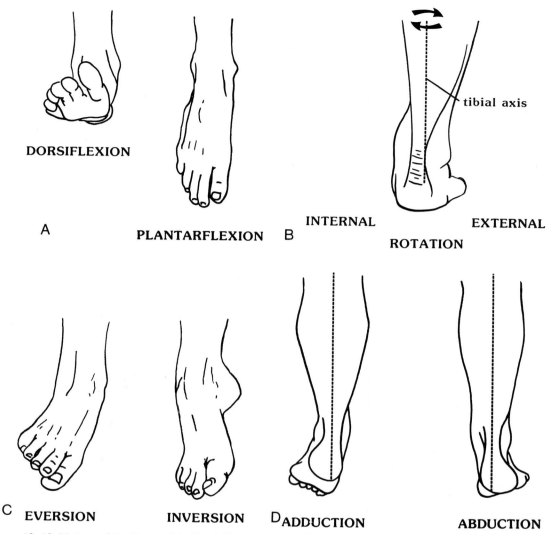

DORSIFLEXION

A   **PLANTARFLEXION**

B

INTERNAL   **EXTERNAL**

ROTATION

tibial axis

C   **EVERSION**   **INVERSION**   D **ADDUCTION**   **ABDUCTION**

Figure 10–18. Motions of the Foot and Ankle. *A, Plantar flexion* and *dorsiflexion* refer to movement of the foot downward or upward. *Supination* and *pronation* refer to rotation of the foot internally or externally around the longitudinal axis of the foot. *B, Internal* and *external* rotation of the foot refer to motion around the vertical axis of the tibia. *C, Eversion* directs the sole laterally, whereas *inversion* refers to rotation of the foot until the sole is directed medially. *D, Adduction* and *abduction* describe motion of the forefoot toward or away from the midline.

review of applied terminology, illustrated in Figure 10–18, precedes a discussion of ankle fractures. Movements of the foot and the ankle are considered as one, although they usually represent the combined motion of several joints. *Dorsiflexion* and *plantar flexion* refer to motion of the foot upward (dorsiflexion) or downward (plantar flexion). Most motion in this plane occurs at the ankle itself. *Supination* and *pronation* refer to rotation of the foot internally (supination) or externally (pronation) around the longitudinal axis of the foot. Actually, supination of the foot includes inward rotation, adduction of the hind foot, and inversion of the forefoot.[43] *External* and *internal rotation* of the foot refer to move-

ment around the vertical axis of the tibia.[41] *Inversion* describes rotating the foot inward until the sole faces medially. Since the sole of the foot tends to rotate upward, supination of the sole accompanies inversion. *Abduction* and *adduction* are terms usually applied to describe motion of the forefoot away from or toward the midline (around the long axis of the talus).[41]

Classification

Ashhurst and Bromer classified fractures according to the postulated mechanism of injury and noted that about 60 percent were due to external rotation forces, 20 percent to abduction forces, and 13 percent to adduction forces.[32] In

1950 Lauge-Hansen performed a series of experiments on amputated extremities in which the foot was placed in a particular position, and various stresses were then applied.[43] From this study evolved a commonly used classification that designates major kinds of injury with two words, the first representing the position of the foot, the second the direction of the applied force. Within each major group stages of injury were designated. Radiographic evaluation often allows the injury to be categorized and the severity of the injury (the stage) to be documented.

Lauge-Hansen Classification of Ankle Fractures[43]

Supination-Adduction *(Supination-Inversion;* Fig. 10–19)*

Stage 1—detachment of collateral ligaments from the tip of the lateral malleolus (most often) or horizontal transverse fracture of the lateral malleolus.

Stage 2—fracture at the base of the medial malleolus.

Supination-Eversion *(Supination–External Rotation; Supination–Lateral Rotation; Figs. 10–20 and 10–21)*

Stage 1—anterior inferior tibiofibular ligament avulsed from tibia, fibula, or both.

---

*The designations in parentheses redefine the fracture, using the previously described terminology.

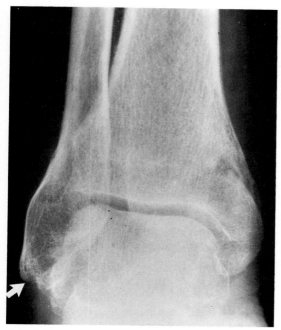

Figure 10–19. Supination-Adduction (Supination-Inversion), 2. There is an avulsion fracture of the lateral malleolus (arrow) and an oblique fracture of the medial malleolus.

Stage 2—oblique spiral fracture of the distal fibula.

Stage 3—fracture of the posterior lip of the tibia.

Stage 4—avulsion fracture of medial malleolus or fracture at the base of medial malleolus.

Pronation-Abduction *(Pronation-Eversion; Figs. 10–22 and 10–23).*

Stage 1—horizontal medial malleolar fracture.

Stage 2—avulsion of anterior and posterior inferior tibiofibular ligaments from tibia.

Stage 3—oblique distal fibula fracture 0.5 to 1 cm above tibial plafond.

Pronation-Eversion *(Pronation–External Rotation; Pronation–Lateral Rotation)*

Stage 1—horizontal medial malleolar fractures (as in Pronation-Abduction, Stage 1).

Stage 2–separation of the tibiofibular syndesmosis.

Stage 3—fracture of the fibula more than 8 to 9 cm proximal to the tip of the lateral malleolus.

Stage 4—posterior tibial fracture (due to avulsion by ligaments and pressure of talus).

This classification seems rather complex. However, the application to most clinical radiographs is not difficult and may be simplified by studying diagrammatic representations of the applied forces and the resulting fractures (Fig. 10–24) and by Wilson's description, summarized in the following section.[51]

Radiological Examination

Ankle injuries are common. Cockshott, Jenkin, and Pui confirmed a prior study showing that radiographs need not be done in cases of ankle injury if no soft tissue swelling is present over the malleoli.[36, 38] In addition, AP and lateral views generally suffice for the detection of ankle fractures, although additional oblique views may show certain fractures to advantage and may help define talar position.

External (Lateral) Rotation Injuries. Fractures due to *lateral rotation* are usually the result of internal rotation of the body when the foot is fixed in pronation or abduction. The combination of lateral rotation and abduction (eversion) is the most frequent mechanism in the production of ankle fractures. The series of events that occurs when an external rotation force is applied is summarized in Figure 10–24.[51] First (when the foot is pronated), either a fracture of the medial malleolus or a rupture of the deltoid ligament occurs. With increasing lateral rotation the anterior tibiofibular ligament tears, or the fibula fractures. A fracture of the posterior tibial tubercle may occur because of compression by

Text continued on page 612

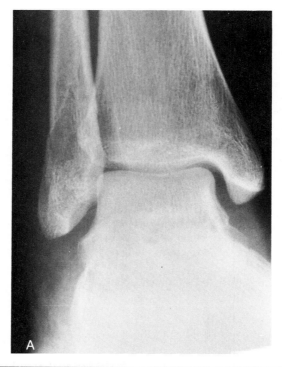

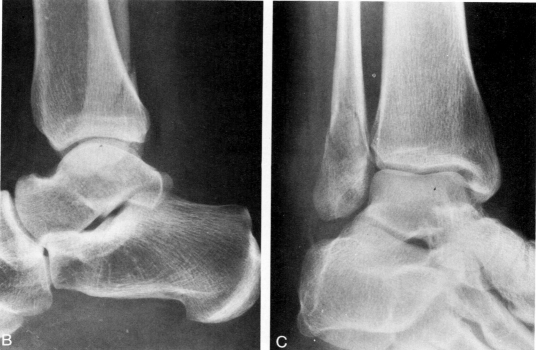

Figure 10–20. Supination-Eversion (Supination–External Rotation; Supination–Lateral Rotation), 2. AP *(A)*, lateral *(B)*, and internal oblique *(C)* views show an oblique fibular fracture that is difficult to see on the frontal views but is well seen on the lateral view, extending from the anterior inferior to the posterior superior aspect of the bone.

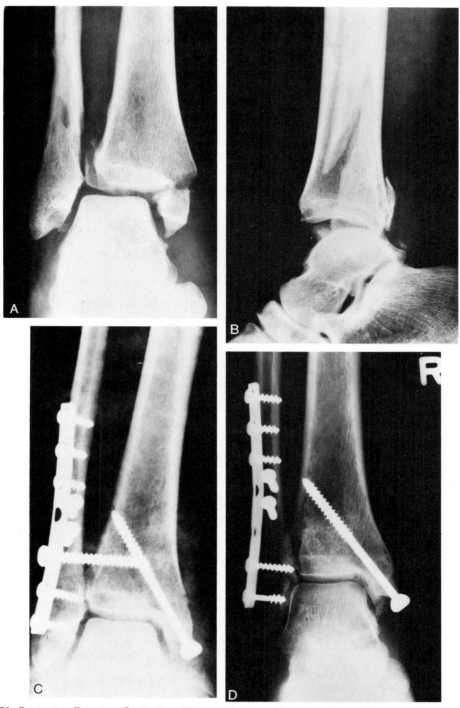

Figure 10–21. Supination-Eversion (Supination–External Rotation; Supination–Lateral Rotation), 4. The AP *(A)* and lateral *(B)* views show an oblique fracture of the fibula extending from its anterior and inferior to its posterior and superior aspects. There is a posterior malleolar fracture and an avulsion fracture of the medial malleolus. The tibiofibular syndesmosis and the anterior joint space are abnormally wide. Anatomical reduction *(C)* with placement of a syndesmotic screw was performed. Six weeks later *(D)* the syndesmotic screw was removed.

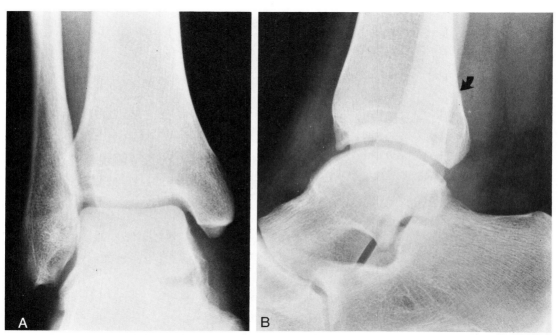

Figure 10–22. Pronation-Abduction, 2. *A,* There is soft tissue swelling medially and slight widening of the medial cartilage space. *B,* The lateral view shows a subtle posterior malleolar fracture (arrow).

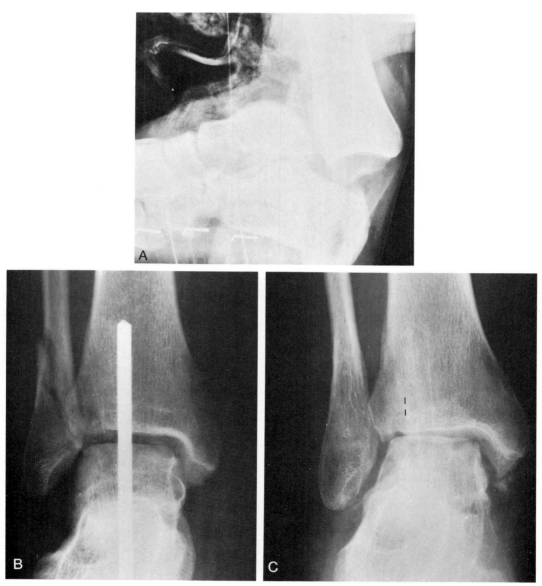

Figure 10–23. Pronation-Abduction, 3. *A,* The initial lateral view shows dislocation of the tibiotalar joint. A lateral malleolar fracture is visible. *B,* After reduction and fixation with a pin through the heel and ankle, the typical oblique fracture of a pronation-abduction injury is seen. Widening of the syndesmosis is noted. *C,* A follow-up film shows marked widening of the syndesmosis as evidenced by the minimal overlap of the tibia and fibula and the greater than 5.5 mm separation between the fibula and the posterior edge of the tibia (lines). There is lateral talar shift (medial cartilage space wider than 4 mm) and severe cartilage-space narrowing. An avulsion fracture of the medial malleolus is now visible.

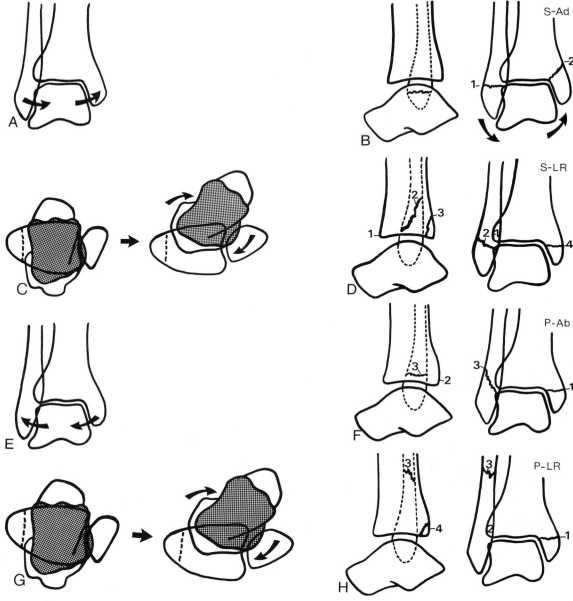

Figure 10–24. Diagrammatic Representation of Lauge-Hansen Classification of Ankle Fractures. *A, B,* Supination-adduction (S-Ad; supination-inversion), stage 1—avulsion fracture of the lateral malleolus, stage 2—medial malleolar fracture. *C, D,* Supination-eversion (supination–lateral rotation; S-LR), stage 1—avulsion of the anterior inferior tibiofibular ligament, stage 2—oblique fracture of the distal fibula, stage 3—fracture of posterior lip of the tibia, stage 4—avulsion fracture medial malleolus. *E, F,* Pronation-abduction (P-Ab; pronation-eversion). stage 1—avulsion fracture of the medial malleolus, stage 2—avulsion of the anterior and the posterior inferior tibiofibular ligaments, stage 3—oblique distal fibular fracture 0.5 to 1 cm above the tibial plafond. *G, H,* Pronation-eversion (pronation–lateral rotation; P-LR), stage 1—avulsion fracture of the medial malleolus, stage 2—separation of the syndesmosis, stage 3—high fibular fracture, stage 4—posterior tibial fracture. (After Arimoto HK, Forrester DM: AJR 135:1057, 1980.)

the talus. The interosseous ligament and membrane may then tear, and, finally, the posterior inferior tibiofibular ligament and the inferior transverse ligament may tear or avulse their attachments to the tibia.

The findings on radiographic examination depend on the severity of injury and on whether or not bony or ligamentous damage has occurred. Findings range from soft tissue swelling to trimalleolar fractures with displacement of the talus. The medial malleolar fracture is of the avulsion type, is transverse, and usually occurs at or below the tibial plafond. The fibular fracture usually involves the distal third, extending obliquely from the anterior inferior to the posterior superior aspect of the fibula (Figs. 10–21 and 10–22). It is seen best or seen only on the lateral view. If the fibular fracture is displaced and if no other fracture is seen, disruption either of the syndesmosis or of the deltoid ligament must be present.[51] The posterior tibial fracture is usually small, caused by avulsion by posterior ligaments or pressure by the fibula.

Maisonneuve fracture refers to an injury produced by external (lateral) rotation of the foot that results in rupture of the anterior tibiofibular ligament and fracture of the proximal third of the fibula (see Fig. 10–16).[46] In addition, rupture of the interosseous ligament, fracture of the posterior tibial tubercle or rupture of the posterior tibiofibular ligament, damage to the anteromedial joint capsule, and rupture of the deltoid ligament or fracture of the medial malleolus may occur. Pankovich noted that Maisonneuve fractures accounted for about 5 per cent of ankle fractures seen at his hospital's emergency room.[46]

Abduction (Eversion) Fracture (Figs. 10–23 and 10–24). Eversion forces first produce injury to the medial malleolus or the deltoid ligament, followed by either fracture of the fibula below the syndesmosis or rupture of the syndesmotic ligaments. If the syndesmosis is disrupted, a fibular fracture occurs above the malleolus, with the fracture level corresponding to the most proximal extent of the interosseous membrane tear. The medial malleolar fracture is typically transverse and usually below the level of the plafond. The fibular fracture is a short, oblique fracture extending from the inferomedial to the superolateral aspect of the fibula, with lateral comminution. If the medial malleolus is not fractured but a displaced fibular fracture and lateral shift of the talus are present, a tear of the

deltoid ligament must also be present. Complete disruption of the tibiofibular syndesmosis is more frequent with this injury than with lateral rotation injuries, which usually spare the posterior ligaments.[51] Compression injuries of the lateral tibial plafond may occur.

Adduction (Inversion) Fracture (Fig. 10–20). With inversion the first injury is either a tear of the lateral collateral ligaments or a transverse fracture of the fibula, usually at or below the level of the plafond. An oblique fracture of the medial malleolus at its junction with the plafond may occur when the talus impacts on the malleolus. Comminution of the medial corner of the tibial plafond frequently occurs.

Compression Fracture. Fractures of the posterior tibia may or may not be caused by compression forces. When vertical compression results in fracture of more than 25 percent of the articular surface, operative reduction may be necessary, since there is a great likelihood that posterior subluxation of the talus and secondary osteoarthritis will ensue.[51] Fractures of the posterior tibial margin that are not due to compression forces usually involve a small segment of the tibia and are the result of avulsion by the posterior tibiofibular ligament and pressure by the rotating talus.[34]

Fractures of the anterior margin of the tibia usually are the result of compression during acute dorsiflexion of the foot. Both anterior and posterior marginal fractures are often comminuted, making anatomical reduction difficult or impossible. Impaction of the corners of the talus on the tibia or fibula may lead to localized areas of cartilage damage (Fig. 10–25).

To facilitate classification into the Lauge-Hansen scheme Arimoto and Forrester published an algorithm, the initial input of which depends on the nature of the fibular fracture (Fig. 10–26).[31]

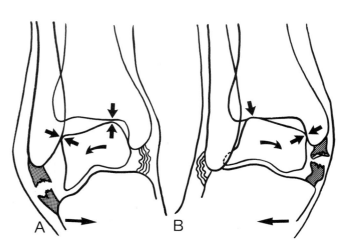

Figure 10–25. Talar Impaction Fracture. Inversion *(A)* or eversion *(B)* of the ankle may result in impingement of the talus on the tibia or fibula, with damage to articular cartilage and subchondral bone.

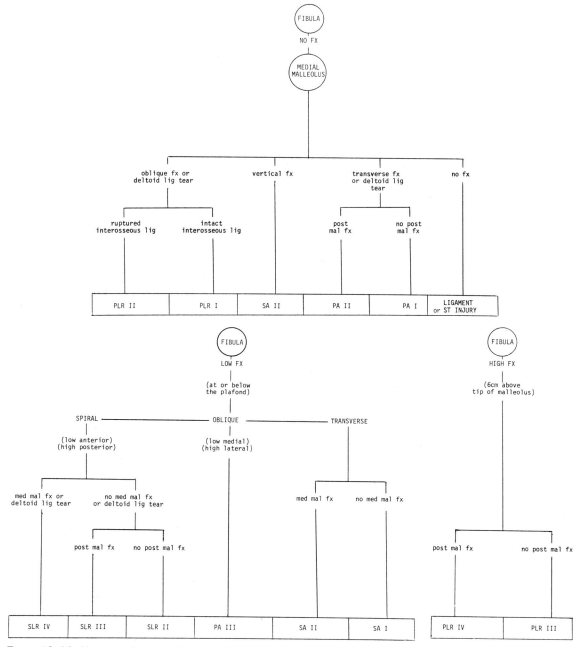

Figure 10–26. Algorithm for Classification of Ankle Fractures. (From Arimoto HK, Forrester DM: AJR 135:1057, 1980, with permission.)

Thus, for example, fractures high in the fibula are seen in pronation–lateral rotation injuries, while spiral fibular fractures that run from inferior and anterior to superior and posterior are seen in supination–lateral rotation injuries. The medial malleolus and the medial side of the ankle mortise are next evaluated, and, finally, the posterior malleolus is studied.

Treatment

As summarized by Wilson, the goals of treatment are the same for all ankle injuries and include (1) anatomical positioning of the talus within the mortise, (2) a joint line that is parallel to the ground, and (3) a smooth articular surface.[51] Films following treatment should be evaluated with these goals in mind. About 85 percent of ankle fractures are stable and need no reduction.[20] Unstable injuries with even a slight talar shift may have significant joint incongruity, leading to secondary degenerative arthritis.[42] Failure to reposition a single malleolus anatomically is less likely to be associated with a poor end result.[51] Pettrone and associates found that anatomical repositioning of both the medial and the lateral malleoli and restoration of the width of the syndesmosis and of the medial tibiotalar cartilage space were all important factors in optimizing treatment results.[47] Careful radiological follow-up is particularly important in unstable fractures treated with closed reduction, since loss of position on follow-up examination is frequent;[41, 42] it has been noted as late as 18 days after injury.[51] Fibular fractures are clinically united long before radiological union occurs.

The primary indication for operative intervention is the inability to obtain or maintain anatomical position of the talus in relation to the tibia; anatomical position of the talus is determined by comparison of the medial cartilage spaces of the involved and the uninvolved sides on the mortise view. Currently, there is a tendency for early operative intervention, with the benefits of anatomical repositioning and internal fixation of fracture fragments making early motion and weight bearing possible. The major contraindication is presence of comminution or of a heavily contaminated wound.[51]

Ankle Fusion (Ankle Arthrodesis)

Technique

Many procedures for ankle fusion have been described, most of which involve resection of the distal surface of the tibia and the proximal surface of the talus, including all articular cartilage.[54–56] The fusion site is held in apposition by staples, bone graft with screws, or a compression device. Graft material may be placed across the joint line and bone chips around the margins. The malleoli are removed, but the tips of the malleoli may be retained.

In the compression arthrodesis described by Charnley no bone graft is used (Fig. 10–27).[55]

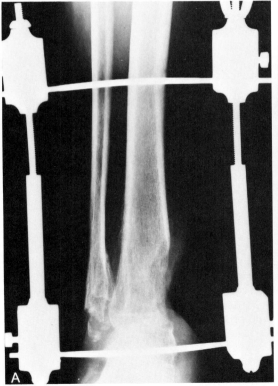
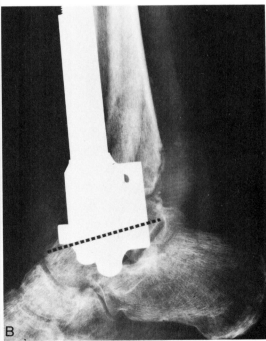

Figure 10–27. Charnley Compression Arthrodesis. *A,* This patient had a history of infection after a fracture, with a large soft tissue defect medially. The medial malleolus had previously been debrided. The lateral malleolus (except its tip) and the articular surfaces of the tibia and the talus have been removed, and the tibial and the talar surfaces are held in apposition by the compression device. The bowing of the pins attests to the compression. The talus is not deviated medially or laterally. *B,* The lateral view shows the foot to be plantar flexed as judged by the axis of the talus (dotted) in relation to the long axis of the tibia. The distal pin of the compression device is placed anterior to the center of motion of the talus so that the compression by the device balances the pull of the Archilles tendon. There is marked patchy osteopenia.

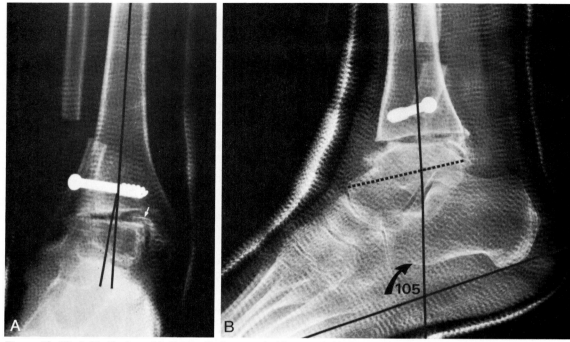

Figure 10–28. Ankle Fusion with Valgus Deformity. *A,* AP view. Ankle fusion has been attempted, with resection of the talar dome but incomplete resection of the tibial plafond (arrow). There is resulting valgus deviation of the foot (measured as the angle between the tibial and talar axes) and a medial gap along the fusion site. There has been osteotomy of the fibula and apposition of the decorticated medial fibula and the tibiotalar joint. *B,* The foot is in about 15 degrees of plantar flexion (115 degrees to the 90-degree neutral position). The axis of the foot can be determined by the plane of the sole or the axis of the talus (dotted line).

The compression device keeps the surfaces together and eliminates shear at the fusion site. After resection of the tibial and the talar surfaces and of the malleoli the compression apparatus is applied. A Steinman pin is inserted through the talus, anterior to its axis of motion and at right angles to the long axis of the tibia on the frontal radiograph. Compression clamps are then attached to the pin and serve as guides for placement of the proximal pin through the lower tibia, parallel to the first pin.

Radiographic Evaluation: Foot Position

Fusion should align the foot parallel to the floor (plantigrade). On frontal views the foot (as judged by the position of the talus) should not be tipped into varus or valgus.[54] The degree to which varus or valgus angulation is present can be measured on the frontal view by noting the angle between the long axis of the tibia and that of the talus. Such angulation (especially varus) is more likely to be associated with postoperative pain than is neutral alignment.[60] External rotation of the foot is matched to the opposite normal side.[63]

Most authors suggest that the foot be fused perpendicular to the tibia or in slight plantar flexion to allow for the height of the heel of a shoe.[53, 55] Morrey and Wiedeman, however, noted that plantar flexion of greater than 10 degrees was more likely to be associated with postoperative pain than was the neutral position or even slight dorsiflexion.[60] The position can be measured on the lateral view by noting the angle formed between the long axis of the tibia and the long axis of the talus or of the sole of the foot (Fig. 10–28). Some authors advocate slight posterior displacement of the talus on the tibia to restore heel contour.[63]

Healing

Clinical stability is noted at 3 months following Charnley compression arthrodesis, but 6 months or more are needed before trabecular continuity across the fusion site is demonstrable on radiographs.[55] Healing may take even longer if other methods of fusion are used. According to Charnley, even if trabecular continuity is not present, bony union should be anticipated at 6 months as long as sclerosis is not apparent, since fibrous union is typically accompanied by sclerosis.[55] Clinically, however, fibrous union may be almost as satisfactory as bony union.[55, 63]

Surprisingly, little disability occurs after ankle fusion if the remainder of the foot is normal.

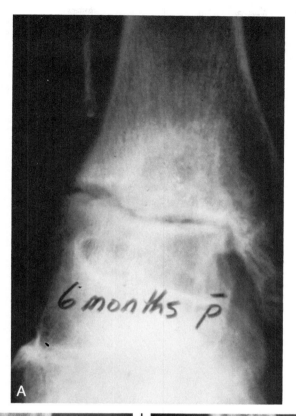

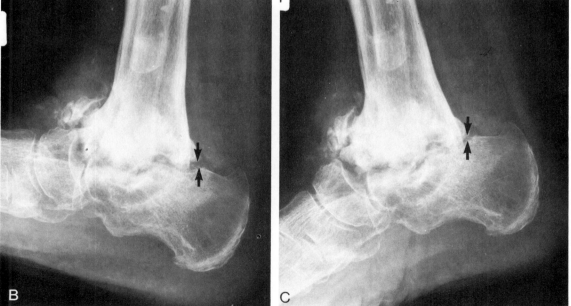

Figure 10–29. Nonunion of Ankle Fusion. *A,* An AP view 6 months after attempted fusion shows a gap remaining at the fusion site and sclerosis of the tibial and the talar surfaces. Reoperation was done. *B, C,* Another patient with pain many months after attempted fusion. Comparison of lateral views in dorsiflexion *(B)* and plantar flexion *(C)* shows motion at the fusion site, most easily demonstrated as a change in the width of the posterior tibiocalcaneal space (arrows). The talus had been resected.

Increased motion at the mid- and hindfoot joints (with the exception of the subtalar joint, in which motion is unchanged or actually decreased) compensates in part for the loss of tibiotalar motion after ankle fusion.[62]

Complications

Nonunion may be defined as motion at the fusion site or radiographic evidence of lack of fusion 12 months after surgery (Fig. 10–29).[60] The incidence of nonunion ranges from 15 to 23 percent.[60, 62]

Residual pain after fusion may occur, and its origin may be difficult to define. In some cases osteoarthritis of the subtalar or talonavicular joints may account for it.[63] However, Morrey and Wiedeman noted a poor correlation between the presence of pain and the presence of radiographic abnormalities at the talonavicular or subtalar joint.[60] Patients with varus or valgus angulation at the fusion site were more likely to have postoperative pain than were patients who had fusion in the neutral position.

Infection around the pin tracts occurred in 10 percent of patients in one series.[60] Heat generated by power-drilling large pins into the tibial cortex may result in local bone and soft tissue injury. A sclerotic ring of bone around the pin tract represents dead bone and may be seen in these cases as well as in cases of infection.[58]

Total Ankle Replacement

Total ankle replacement is not yet as satisfactory a procedure as total hip replacement. Demottaz and co-workers noted complete pain relief in less than 20 percent of patients after total ankle replacement as compared with 75 percent of patients after ankle fusion.[65] Ankle fusion is most satisfactory when the remainder of the foot is normal (as in patients with post-traumatic arthritis) and is least successful when multiple joints are involved (as in those with rheumatoid arthritis). In this latter group total ankle replacement offers the hope of decreased pain and increased mobility.

Two types of prostheses are available—those that allow only flexion-extension motion (e.g., Mayo, Bucholz, Oregon) and those that allow motion in several planes (e.g., Waugh, Smith) (Figs. 10–30 and 10–31).[64, 65] The tibial component is inserted so that it is perpendicular to the long axis of the tibia.[68] The talar component is then positioned parallel to the tibial component, with the foot in neutral position. Thus on standing AP and lateral radiographs a line perpendicular to the superior surface of the tibial component should coincide with the long axis of the tibia, and a line perpendicular to the inferior surface of the talar component should be perpendicular to the weight-bearing surface (Fig. 10–32).

Complications of total ankle replacement include infection (about 3.5 percent) and loosening (about 6.7 percent).[70] Radiographic evidence of loosening includes the development of a wide or increasing cement-bone lucency and documentation of a change in component position (Fig. 10–33). In one series almost 90 percent of patients developed radiolucent zones within the

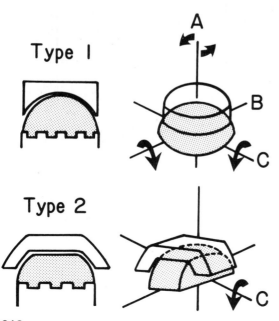

Figure 10–30. Types of Ankle Prostheses. Type 1 prostheses (e.g., Waugh, Smith) allow motion in several planes. Type 2 prostheses (e.g., Mayo, Oregon) allow only flexion-extension motion. (Redrawn from Demottaz JB, Mazur JN, Thomas WH, et al.: J Bone Joint Surg (Am) 61:976, 1979.)

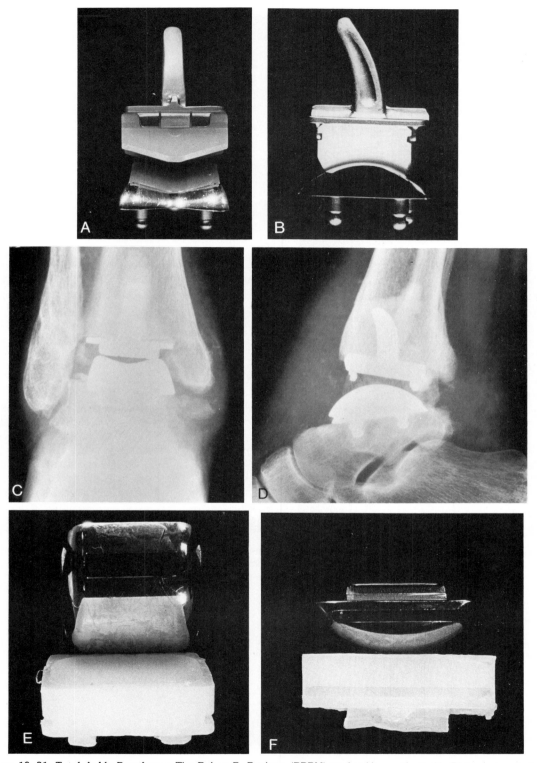

Figure 10–31. Total Ankle Prostheses. The Robert B. Brigham (RBBH) total ankle prosthesis *(A, B)* is semiconstrained and primarily allows flexion and extension motion. AP *(C)* and lateral *(D)* views of the RBBH prosthesis. Exploded frontal *(E)* and lateral *(F)* views of the Mayo total ankle prosthesis. This prosthesis allows only flexion-extension motion (see Fig. 10–32).

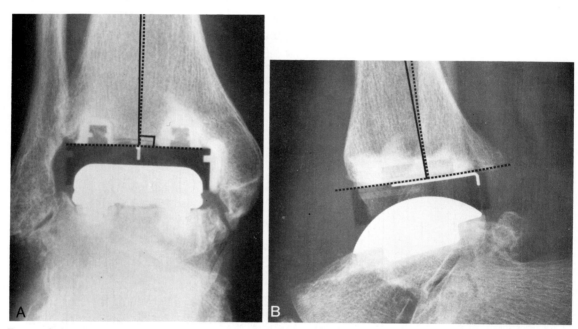

Figure 10–32. Evaluating Component Position. *A,* AP view after insertion of a Mayo total ankle prosthesis shows the tibial component to be almost perpendicular to the long axis of the tibia (solid line). The dashed lines indicate the plane of the tibial component and a perpendicular to this plane. Very thin lucent zones are noted along the cement-bone interfaces. *B,* On lateral view the tibial component is almost ideally positioned—perpendicular to the long axis of the tibia (solid line). Dashed lines indicate the plane of the tibial component and a perpendicular to this plane.

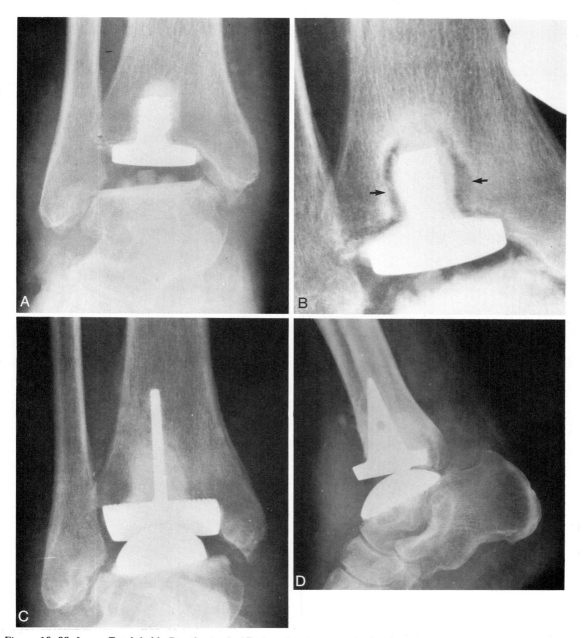

Figure 10–33. Loose Total Ankle Prosthesis. *A,* AP view after insertion of a Smith total ankle prosthesis shows the tibial component to be angled in relation to the talar component and the long axis of the tibia. *B,* Nine months later loosening of the tibial component, with a wide cement-bone lucent zone (arrows), occurred. *C,* Revision was done with insertion of a Waugh total ankle prosthesis. *D,* The lateral view of the Waugh prosthesis shows no evidence of loosening. Moderate postoperative swelling is present anteriorly. (Courtesy Kelley WN, Harris ED, Ruddy S, et al.: Textbook of Rheumatology, Philadelphia, WB Saunders, 1981.)

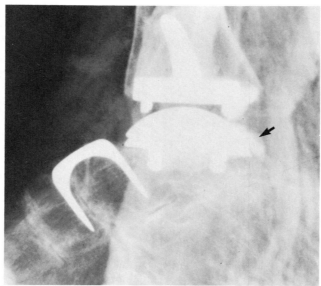

Figure 10–34. Extruded Cement. The immediate postoperative lateral radiograph (through plaster) after insertion of an RBBH total ankle prosthesis shows cement along the posterior joint surface (arrow). Reoperation for cement removal was necessary.

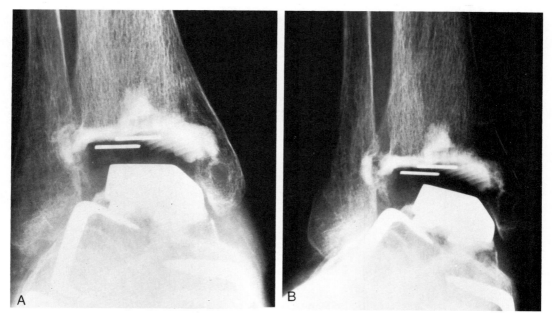

Figure 10–35. Instability After Total Ankle Replacement. *A,* With varus stress the position of the total ankle prosthesis appears good. *B,* With relaxation the foot tips into valgus. (Same patient as in Fig. 10–15.)

first year, and in 10 percent definite loosening, with a change in component position, was noted.[65] Other complications include impingement of the lateral malleolus on the talus, fracture of the medial malleolus during surgery, instability, and heterotopic bone formation (Figs. 10–34 and 10–35).

References

Essential Anatomy

1. Wilson FC: Fractures and dislocations of the ankle. *In* Rockwood CA Jr, Green DP, eds. Fractures. Philadelphia, JB Lippincott, 1975: 1361–1399.
2. Goss CM, ed. Gray's Anatomy of the Human Body. 29th Am ed. Philadelphia, Lea & Febiger, 1973.
3. Heppenstall RB: Fracture Treatment and Healing. Philadelphia, WB Saunders, 1980.

Arthrography

4. Ala-Ketola L, Puranen J, Koivisto E, Puupera M: Arthrography in the diagnosis of ligament injuries and classification of ankle injuries. Radiology 125:63–68, 1977.
5. Arner O, Ekengren K, Hulting B, Lindholm A: Arthrography of the talo-crural joint. Anatomic, roentgenographic and clinical aspects. Acta Chir Scand 113:253–259, 1957.
6. Berridge FR, Bonnin JG: The radiographic examination of the ankle joint including arthrography. Surg Gynecol Obstet 79:383–389, 1944.
7. Brostrom L, Liljeahl SO, Lindvall N: Sprained ankles II. Arthrographic diagnosis of recent ligament ruptures. Acta Chir Scand 129:485–499, 1965.
8. Hansson CJ: Arthrographic studies on the ankle joint. Acta Radiol 22:281–287, 1941.
9. Kaye JJ: The ankle. *In* Freiberger RH, Kaye JJ, eds. Arthrography. New York, Appleton-Century-Crofts, 1979:237–256.
10. Kaye JJ, Bohne WHO: A radiographic study of the ligamentous anatomy of the ankle. Radiology 125:659–667, 1977.
11. Olson RW: Arthrography of the ankle: its use in the evaluation of ankle sprains. Radiology 92:1439–1446, 1969.
12. Sauser DD, Nelson RC, Lavine MH, Wu CW: Acute injuries of the lateral ligaments of the ankle: comparison of stress radiography and arthrography. Radiology 148:653–657, 1983.
13. Spiegel PK, Stapes OS: Arthrography of the ankle joint: problems in diagnosis of acute lateral ligament injuries. Radiology 114:587–590, 1975.
14. Weiss JJ: Anterior tibial nerve palsy after ankle arthrocentesis. Arthritis Rheum 26:573–574, 1983.

Joint Effusion

15. Saunders CG, Weston WJ: Synovial mass lesions in the anteroposterior projection of the ankle joint. J Can Assoc Radiol 22:275–277, 1971.
16. Towbin R, Dunbar JS, Towbin J, Clark R: Teardrop sign: plain film recognition of ankle effusion. AJR 134:985–990, 1980.
17. Weston WJ: Traumatic effusions of the ankle joint and posterior subtaloid joints. Br J Radiol 31:445–447, 1958.
18. Weston WJ, Palmer DG: Soft Tissues of the Extremities. A Radiologic Study of Rheumatic Disease. New York, Springer-Verlag, 1978:91–104.

Ligamentous Injuries

19. Bonnin JG: Injury to the ligaments of the ankle. J Bone Joint Surg (Br) 47:609–611, 1965.
20. Brodie IAOD, Denham RA: The treatment of unstable ankle fractures. J Bone Joint Surg (Br) 56:256–262, 1974.
21. Brostrom L: Sprained ankles. I. Anatomic lesions in recent sprains. Acta Chir Scand 128:483–495, 1964.
22. Brostrom L, Liljeahl SO, Lindvall N: Sprained ankles. II. Arthrographic diagnosis of recent ligament ruptures. Acta Chir Scand 129:485–499.
23. Edeiken J, Cotler JM: Ankle injury: the need for stress films. JAMA 240:1183–1184, 1978.
24. Johnson EE, Markolf KL: The contribution of the anterior talofibular ligament to ankle laxity. J Bone Joint Surg (Am) 65:81–88, 1983.
25. Laurin CA, Ouellet R, St. Jacques R: Talar and subtalar tilt: an experimental investigation. Can J Surg 11:270–279, 1968.
26. Lindstrand A, Mortensson W: Anterior instability in the ankle joint following acute lateral sprain. Acta Radiol [Diagn] (Stockh) 18:529–539, 1977.
27. Neer CS: Injuries of the ankle joint—evaluation. Conn Med 17:580–583, 1953.
28. Protas JM, Kornblatt BA: Fractures of the lateral margin of the distal tibia. The Tillaux fracture. Radiology 138:55–57, 1981.
29. Rubin G, Witten M: The talar-tilt ankle and the fibular collateral ligament: a method for the determination of talar tilt. J Bone Joint Surg (Am) 42:311–326, 1960.
30. Wilson FC: Fractures and dislocations of the ankle. *In* Rockwood CA Jr, Green DP, eds. Fractures. Philadelphia, JB Lippincott, 1975:1361–1399.

Ankle Fractures

31. Arimoto HK, Forrester DM: Classification of ankle fractures: an algorithm. AJR 135:1057–1063, 1980.
32. Ashhurst APC, Bromer RS: Classification and mechanism of fractures of the leg bone involving the ankle. Arch Surg 4:51–129, 1922.
33. Black H: Roentgenographic considerations. Am J Sports Med 5:238–240, 1977.
34. Brostrom L, Liljeahl SO, Lindvall N: Isolated fracture of the posterior tibial tubercle: aetiologic and clinical features. Acta Chir Scand 128:51–56, 1964.
35. Burwell HN, Charnley AD: The treatment of displaced fractures at the ankle by rigid internal fixation and early joint movement. J Bone Joint Surg (Br) 47:634–660, 1965.
36. Cockshott WP, Jenkin JK, Pui M: Limiting the use of routine radiography for acute ankle injuries. Can Med Assoc J 129:129–131, 1983.
37. Coonrad RW: Fracture-dislocations of the ankle joint with impaction injury of the lateral weight-bearing surface of the tibia. J Bone Joint Surg (Am) 52:1337–1344, 1970.
38. DeLacey G, Bradbrooke S: Rationalising requests for x-ray examination of acute ankle injuries. Br Med J 1:1597–1598, 1979.
39. Goergen TG, Danzig LA, Resnick D, Owen CA: Roentgenographic evaluation of the tibiotalar joint. J Bone Joint Surg (Am) 59:874–877, 1977.
40. Helfet AJ, Gruebel Lee, DM: Disorders of the Foot. Philadelphia, JB Lippincott, 1980.
41. Heppenstall RB: Fracture Treatment and Healing. Philadelphia, WB Saunders, 1980:811.
42. Kristensen TB: Fractures of the ankle. VI. Follow-up studies. Arch Surg 73:112–121, 1956.
43. Lauge-Hansen N: Fractures of the ankle. II. Combined

experimental-surgical and experimental-roentgenologic investigations. Arch Surg 60:957–985, 1950.

44. Neer CS: Injuries of the ankle joint—evaluation. Conn Med 17:580–583, 1953.

45. Newberg AH: Osteochondral fractures of the dome of the talus. Br J Radiol 52:105–109, 1979.

46. Pankovich AM: Maisonneuve fracture of the fibula. J Bone Joint Surg (Am) 58:337–342, 1976.

47. Pettrone FA, Gail M, Pee D, Fitzpatrick T, Van Herpe LB: Quantitative criteria for prediction of the results after displaced fracture of the ankle. J Bone Joint Surg (Am) 65:667–677, 1983.

48. Protas JM, Kornblatt BA: Fracture of the lateral margin of the distal tibia. The Tillaux fracture. Radiology 138:55–57, 1981.

49. Purvis GD: Displaced, unstable ankle fractures: classification, incidence and management of a consecutive series. Clin Orthop 165:91–98, 1982.

50. Ramsey PL, Hamilton W: Changes in tibiotalar area of contact caused by lateral talar shift. J Bone Joint Surg (Am) 58:356–357, 1976.

51. Wilson FC: Fractures and dislocations of the ankle. In Rockwood CA Jr, Green DP, eds. Fractures. Philadelphia, JB Lippincott, 1975:1361–1369.

52. Yablon IG, Heller FG, Shouse L: The key role of the lateral malleolus in displaced fractures of the ankle. J Bone Joint Surg (Am) 59:169–173, 1977.

Ankle Fusion

53. Altcheck M: Charnley ankle arthrodesis. J Bone Joint Surg (Am) 50:1255, 1968.

54. Barr JS, Record EE: Arthrodesis of the ankle joint: indications, operative technique and clinical experience. N Engl J Med 248:53–56, 1953.

55. Charnley J: Compression arthrodesis of the ankle and shoulder. J Bone Joint Surg (Br) 33:180–191, 1951.

56. Kennedy JC: Arthrodesis of the ankle with particular reference to the Gallie procedure: a review of fifty cases. J Bone Joint Surg (Am) 42:1308–1316, 1960.

57. Lance EM, Paval A, Fries I, Larsen I, Patterson RL Jr: Arthrodesis of the ankle joint. A follow-up study. Clin Orthop 142:146–158, 1979.

58. Linson MA, Scott R: Thermal burns associated with high-speed cortical drilling. Orthopedics 1:394–396, 1978.

59. Mazur JM, Schwartz E, Simon SR: Ankle arthrodesis: long-term follow-up with gait analysis. J Bone Joint Surg (Am) 61:964–975, 1979.

60. Morrey BF, Wiedeman GP Jr: Complications and long-term results of ankle arthrodeses following trauma. J Bone Joint Surg (Am) 62:777–784, 1980.

61. Said E, Houka L, Siller TN: Where ankle fusion stands today. J Bone Joint Surg (Am) 60:211, 1978.

62. Thomas WH: Reconstructive surgery and rehabilitation of the ankle and foot. In Kelley WN, Harris ED Jr, Ruddy S, Sledge CB, eds. Textbook of Rheumatology. Philadelphia, WB Saunders, 1981:1999–2013.

63. Verhelst MP, Mulier JC, Hoogmartens MJ, Spass F: Arthrodesis of the ankle joint with complete removal of the distal part of the fibula: experience with the transfibular approach and three different types of fixation. Clin Orthop 118:93–99, 1976.

64. Wiedeman GP, Morrey BF: Complications and long-term results of ankle arthrodesis. Orthop Trans 3:347, 1979.

Total Ankle Replacement

65. Demottaz JB, Mazur JM, Thomas WH, Sledge CB, Simon SR: Clinical study of total ankle replacement with gait analysis. A preliminary report. J Bone Joint Surg (Am) 61:976, 1979.

66. Dini AA, Bassett FH III: Evaluation of the early results of Smith total ankle replacement. Clin Orthop 146:228–230, 1980.

67. Newton SE: An artificial ankle joint. Clin Orthop 142:141–145, 1979.

68. Scholz KC: Total ankle replacement arthroplasty. In Bateman JE, ed. Foot Science. Philadelphia, WB Saunders, 1976:106–135.

69. Stauffer RN: Total joint arthroplasty, the ankle. Mayo Clin Proc 54:570–575, 1979.

70. Thomas WH: Reconstructive surgery and rehabilitation of the ankle and foot. In Kelley WN, Harris ED Jr, Ruddy S, Sledge CB, eds. Textbook of Rheumatology. Philadelphia, WB Saunders, 1981:1999–2013.

Chapter 11

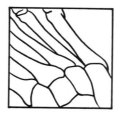

The
FOOT

NORMAL STRUCTURE AND FUNCTION

Essential Anatomy

The foot can be subdivided into three anatomical regions: the hindfoot, including the talus and the calcaneus; the midfoot, including the navic-

ular, the medial, the middle and the lateral cuneiforms, and the cuboid; and the forefoot, consisting of the metatarsals and the phalanges (Fig. 11–1). The joints between the midfoot and the forefoot are collectively termed Lisfranc's joint (Fig. 11–1). Those joints between the hindfoot and the midfoot (the talonavicular and the calcaneocuboid joints) are together termed the midtarsal joints or Chopart's joint.[33]

The contour of the foot includes longitudinal and transverse arches. The medial aspect of the longitudinal arch is higher than the lateral arch and includes the calcaneus, the talus, the navicular, the cuneiforms, and the medial metatarsals. The head of the talus is the keystone between the anterior and the posterior parts of this arch.[16] The transverse arch is formed by the shapes of the cuneiforms. The metatarsals extend anteriorly from this arch, but because of the shapes of these bones, the metatarsal heads all reach the same level above the ground and should therefore share the load during standing.

The calcaneus has a complex contour (Fig. 11–2). The articular surfaces for the cuboid and the talus are all contained in its distal half. The anterior facet for articulation with the talus is sometimes continuous with the middle facet, located on the upper surface of the sustentaculum tali. The posterior facet is separated from these two more anterior facets by the tarsal sinus. The lateral surface of the body of the calcaneus is flat, whereas its medial surface is concave and stronger and continues into the broad sustentaculum tali. The most posterior portion of the calcaneus is called the tuberosity, and its posterior superior corner, the bursal projection. The dorsal lateral margin of the calcaneus serves as the origin for the extensor digitorum brevis and may become the site of an
Text continued on page 629

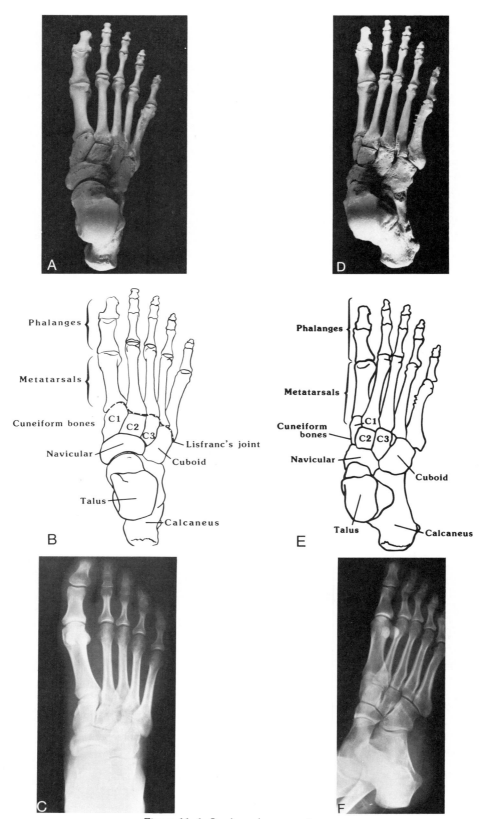

Figure 11–1. *See legend on opposite page.*

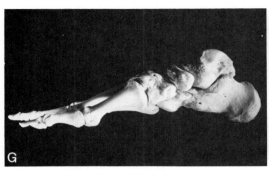

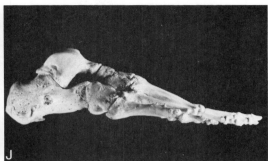

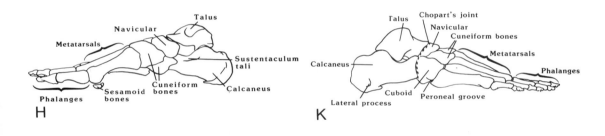

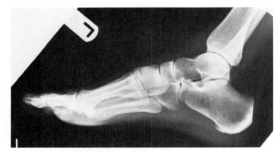

Figure 11–1. Normal Anatomy. Photographic, diagrammatic, and radiographic findings in the PA *(A–C)*, internal oblique *(D–F)*, lateral *(G–K)*.

Legend continued on following page

627

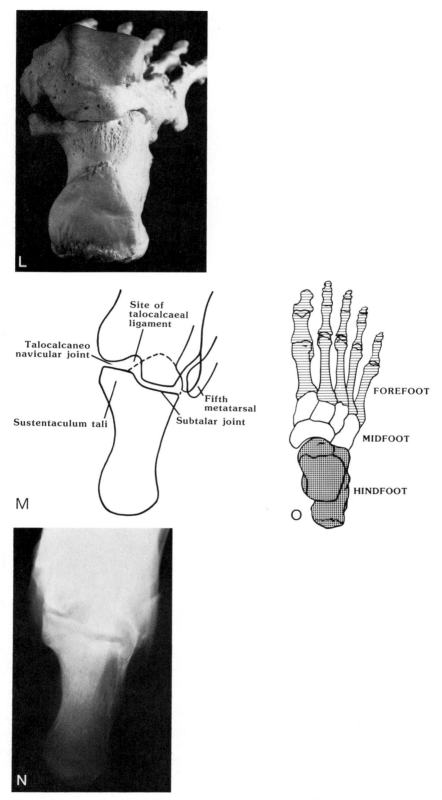

Figure 11–1. Normal Anatomy *Continued.* Tangential calcaneal (Harris; *L–N*) projections. The forefoot, midfoot, and hindfoot are shown.

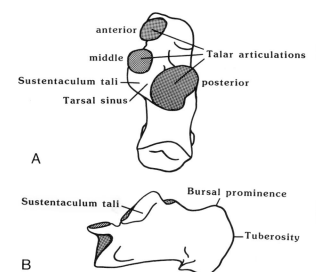

A

B

Figure 11–2. Calcaneal Anatomy. A, As viewed from above, three facets are present for articulation with the talus: anterior, middle (on the sustentaculum tali), and posterior. The tarsal sinus separates the middle and posterior facets. B, The lateral view from the medial side shows the sustentaculum tali.

avulsion fracture in the event of inversion injury.[35] On the plantar surface medial and lateral processes for attachment of the small muscles of the plantar aspect of the foot and the plantar aponeurosis are present.[33]

The distal talus (the head) is directed forward and medially and is supported on its undersurface by the sustentaculum tali. The joint between

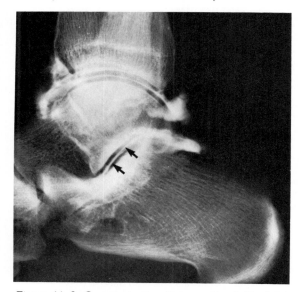

Figure 11–3. Communication Between the Ankle Joint and the Subtalar Joint. Anteriorly, the talocalcaneonavicular joints are continuous. Posteriorly, the talocalcaneal (subtalar) joint is continuous with the ankle joint in about 20 percent of patients. Injection of contrast medium into the ankle joint filled the subtalar joint (arrows) in this patient.

the talus and the calcaneus consists of two articulations: the anterior articulation, in which the joint cavity is continuous with that of the talonavicular joint (these joints are collectively termed the talocalcaneonavicular joint), and the posterior articulation, in which the synovial cavity may be continuous with that of the ankle (Fig. 11–3). Between the anterior and the posterior articulations and bounded inferiorly by the calcaneus is the tarsal sinus. This sinus is a cone-shaped space that opens laterally and is continuous medially with the tube-shaped tarsal canal. In this area a vascular sling is formed by the anastomosis of the artery of the tarsal canal (derived from the posterior tibial artery) and the artery of the tarsal sinus (derived from the perforating peroneal or the anterior tibial artery). Branches from this anastomosis enter the talus and are the major (but not the only) source of its blood supply.[43]

The metatarsal shafts are roughly parallel. The second metatarsal is usually longest and is exposed to increased load as the other metatarsals are unweighted during push-off (Fig. 11–4). The

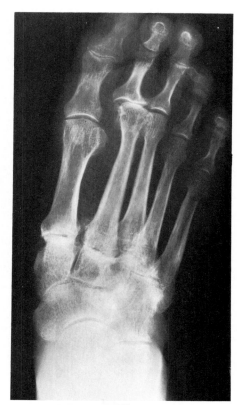

Figure 11–4. Morton's Foot (Metatarsus Primus Atavicus). The first metatarsal is unusually short in relation to the second. Increased stress on the second metatarsal has resulted in osteoarthritis at the second MTP and tarsometatarsal joints.

629

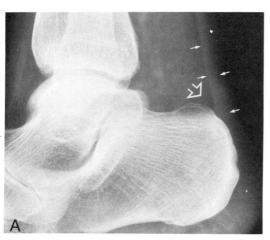

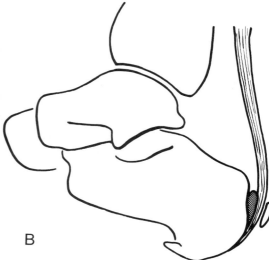

Figure 11–5. Normal Heel. *A,* The normal Achilles tendon shadow (arrows) is seen to its insertion on the posterior calcaneus, about 2 cm distal to the bursal projection of the calcaneus. Fat is present between the tendon and the calcaneus (open arrow). *B,* Diagram showing the position of the subachilles (dotted) and the Achilles tendon (tendo Achillis) bursae.

second metatarsal base is inset between the medial and the lateral cuneiforms and between the first and the third metatarsals. Strong ligaments bind the second and third metatarsals to the tarsals, further increasing the stability of this area. Thus the second and third metatarsals form the stable central portion of the forefoot.

An extensive framework of ligaments unites the arches, anchors the skin to the skeleton, allows passage of important structures through weight-bearing areas, and encloses collections of fat that protect weight-bearing areas.[2] The *plantar aponeurosis* begins on the inferior calcaneus and continues anteriorly in a longitudinal direction to divide into superficial and deep fibers. The superficial fibers insert on the skin of the ball of the foot, to tether it during push-off, and the deep fibers insert on the MTP joint capsules and bind the ends of the longitudinal arch together as the toes are dorsiflexed. The *spring ligament,* or plantar calcaneonavicular ligament, joins the navicular and the sustentaculum tali and supports the head of the talus. The *long plantar ligament* extends from the plantar surface of the calcaneus (anterior to the attachment of the aponeurosis) to the cuboid and acts as a tie beam for the longitudinal arch.[16]

The muscles of the foot consist of an extrinsic group that originates in the calf and an intrinsic group that originates and inserts in the foot.

Normal Radiographic Examination

Anteroposterior (dorsoplantar), internal oblique, and lateral views are usually obtained.

Normal Soft Tissue Anatomy

Most of the information about the soft tissues of the foot is derived from the lateral projection with the foot in neutral position. The Achilles

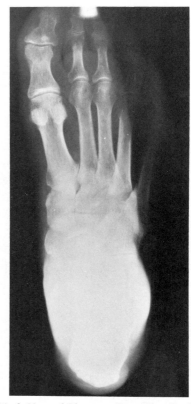

Figure 11–6. Normal Phantom Foot Film. Double exposure, with the ankle extended and then flexed and the tube positioned anteriorly and then posteriorly, allows the hindfoot as well as the forefoot to be evaluated.

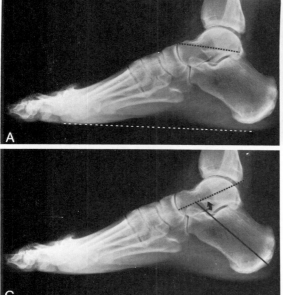

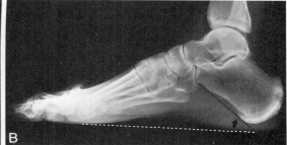

Figure 11–7. Bony Relationships on the Lateral View. *A,* The *diagonal axis* of the talus (dashed black line) should parallel the weight-bearing plane (dashed white line). *B,* *Calcaneal pitch* (arrow); 10 to 20 degrees is low, 20 to 30 degrees intermediate, and more than 30 degrees high. *C,* The *talocalcaneal angle* (arrow) normally measures 15 to 50 degrees, and the longitudinal axis of the talus passes through the first metatarsal shaft.

tendon and its synovial covering are seen as a single soft tissue band outlined anteriorly and posteriorly by fat (Fig. 11–5). This band should measure no more than 8 mm in thickness and should be clearly seen to its insertion on the posterior aspect of the calcaneus, about 2 cm distal to the superior corner (bursal projection) of the bone.[12] Between the Achilles tendon insertion and the posterior calcaneal surface is the small retrocalcaneal bursa. In the normal

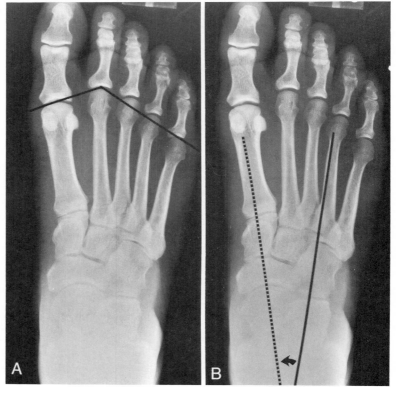

Figure 11–8. Bony Relationships on the Standing AP View. *A,* The metatarsal shafts are roughly parallel. Lines connecting the first, second, and fifth metatarsal heads form an angle of about 136 degrees. *B,* The talar axis extends through the first metatarsal shaft, and the calcaneal axis goes through the fourth metatarsal shaft. The *talocalcaneal* angle (arrow) measures between 15 and 35 degrees in adults.

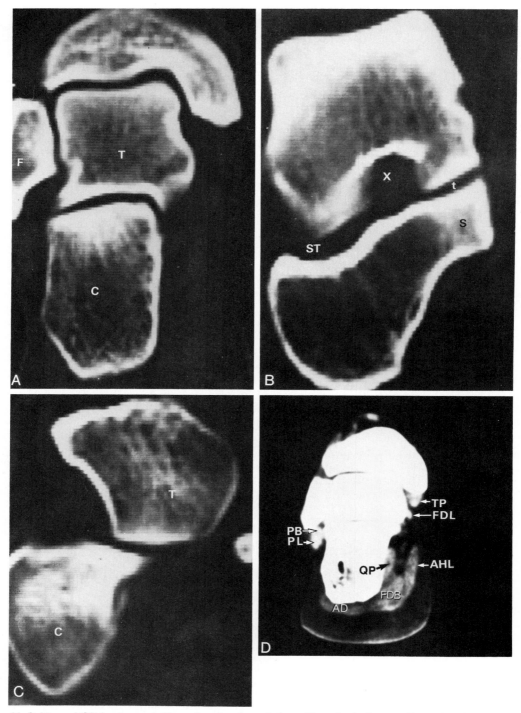

Figure 11–9. Normal CT Anatomy. *A,* Coronal section through the ankle and subtalar joint; T = talus, C = calcaneus, F = fibula. *B,* Further anteriorly, the sustentaculum tali (S), the site of insertion of the talocalcaneal ligament (X), the subtalar joint (ST), and the mid-talocalcaneonavicular joint (t) are seen. *C,* Anterior to the sustentaculum tali, the talus (T) and the calcaneus (C) are seen. *D,* The peroneus brevis (PB), peroneus longus (PL), posterior tibial (TP), and flexor digitorum longus (FDL) tendons are seen. AHL = abductor hallucis longus, FDB = flexor digitorum brevis, QP = quadratus plantae, AD = abductor digiti quinti pedis. This scan is at the level of the posterior aspect of the sustentaculum tali.

situation this bursa is not distended, and its soft tissue density is not visible. Instead, fat is noted to be present above the calcaneus and to extend behind it, distal to the posterior superior margin of the bone, for 2 mm or more. Another (possibly adventitious) bursa is described in the subcutaneous tissues superficial to the Achilles tendon and is termed the tendo Achillis bursa.[9] CT can provide excellent delineation of muscle groups and tendons.

Normal Bony Structures

The bony structures are shown in Figure 11–1. Several observations regarding normal bony relationships have been described. These are best demonstrated on *standing* AP and lateral views. An additional AP view that is double exposed, with the ankle first flexed and then extended, shows the hindfoot to advantage (Fig. 11–6). The structures and relationships that can be evaluated are summarized in the following paragraphs.[15, 17]

Standing Lateral View (Fig. 11–7)

Tarsal Sinus. This sinus is the lucent area that lies above the sustentaculum tali and between the anterior and the posterior talocalcaneal articulations. Identification of the sinus tarsi on lateral views is said to indicate a normal position of the talus and the calcaneus.

Diagonal Axis of the Talus. A line drawn from the anterior superior to the posterior inferior aspect of the talus should be parallel to the weight-bearing plane.

Calcaneal Pitch. This measurement reflects the height of the foot framework and is determined by noting the angle between the inferior aspect of the calcaneus and the weight-bearing surface. Measurements of 10 to 20 degrees are low, 20 to 30 degrees intermediate, and more than 30 degrees high.

The Sustentaculum Tali and the Lateral Tuberosity of the Calcaneus. Sharp definition of these structures indicates normal calcaneal position.

Peroneal Groove of the Cuboid. Normally the groove for the peroneus longus muscle is visible.

Talocalcaneal Angle. The angle of the midtalar and the midcalcaneal axes should measure between 15 and 50 degrees.[15, 17–19]

Longitudinal Arch. The shape of the arch is measured by constructing lines along the inferior margins of the calcaneus and the fifth metatarsal. The measured angle normally is between 150 and 175 degrees.[17, 19]

Smooth Curve of Chopart's Joint. The talonavicular and the calcaneocuboid joint spaces form a smooth curve (Fig. 11–1).

Alignment of the Talus. The central longitudinal axis of the talus passes through the first metatarsal shaft.

Anteroposterior View (Fig. 11–8)

Metatarsal Length. The second metatarsal is usually longest, with the lengths of the third, fourth, and fifth metatarsals gradually and progressively decreasing. An angle of about 136 degrees is made by lines connecting the first, second, and fifth metatarsal heads. The metatarsal shafts are roughly parallel.[18]

Midline of the Foot. The midline is represented by a line from the center of the calcaneus to the medial aspect of the third metatarsal. Normally, the midaxis of the talus is 15 degrees medial to this line. The lateral border of the foot is parallel to the midline, and the transverse axis of the navicular is perpendicular to it.

Talocalcaneal Angle. Normally, a line drawn through the axis of the talus extends through the first metatarsal shaft, and a line through the axis of the calcaneus goes through the fourth metatarsal shaft.[15, 17] The angle between these two axes (the midtalar-midcalcaneal angle) measures between 15 and 35 degrees in adults.[17–19]

Chopart's Joint. A smooth curve is formed by the talonavicular and calcaneocuboid joints (Fig. 11–1).

Coronal CT. The normal computed tomographic anatomy of the hindfoot is shown in Figure 11–9.

ABNORMAL CONDITIONS

Soft Tissue Abnormalities

Retrocalcaneal (Subachilles) Bursitis

Retrocalcaneal bursitis refers to inflammatory changes that occur in the bursa located between the Achilles tendon insertion and the posterior aspect of the calcaneus. Rheumatoid arthritis, ankylosing spondylitis, psoriatic arthritis, and Reiter's syndrome may be associated with both bursitis and tendinitis in this area. Retrocalcaneal bursitis is documented radiographically on the lateral projection by noting obliteration of the fat density that normally intervenes between the superior posterior aspect of the calcaneus and the Achilles tendon (Fig. 11–10). With enough

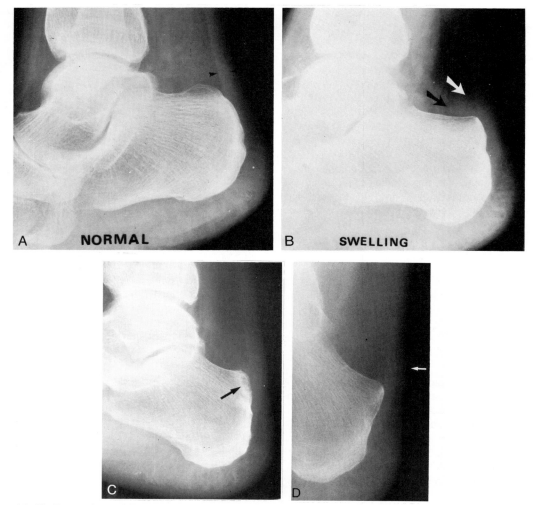

Figure 11–10. Retrocalcaneal Bursitis. *A,* The Achilles tendon (arrowheads) inserts distal to the posterior angle (bursal prominence) of the calcaneus. Fat is interposed between the Achilles tendon and the bone. *B,* Retrocalcaneal bursitis. The soft tissue density of the distended bursa (arrows) obliterates the normally present fat. *C,* Calcaneal erosion. Long-standing retrocalcaneal bursitis has led to erosion (arrow) of the posterior calcaneus. *D,* Pump bump. There is swelling behind the Achilles tendon (arrow).

distension the rounded soft tissue density representing the distended bursa itself may be seen elevating this collection of fat. Inflammatory changes in the retrocalcaneal bursa may eventually result in erosion of the posterior or the superior aspect of the calcaneus or both, and in patients with ankylosing spondylitis, psoriatic arthritis, or Reiter's syndrome new bone formation may also occur.

Pump Bumps

Swelling behind the Achilles tendon insertion associated with the wearing of high-heeled shoes (pumps) has been termed pump bumps (Fig. 11–10). A closely fitted shoe counter, together with a prominent posterior superior calcaneus, is thought to be the cause. These factors result in the formation of either a painless callus or a painful tendo Achillis bursitis.

Clinical examination documents swelling just above the insertion of the Achilles tendon, with either a palpable fluid collection (bursitis) or a diffuse swelling, sometimes with skin changes.

On radiographic examination soft tissue swelling is seen to be localized in the soft tissues behind the Achilles tendon, just above its insertion. The retrocalcaneal bursa is not enlarged; therefore, the normal collection of fat is seen between the Achilles tendon and the calcaneus.

The Haglund syndrome is a painful condition of the heel characterized radiographically by a combination of retrocalcaneal bursitis, Achilles tendinitis, superficial tendo Achillis bursitis, and a prominent posterior superior corner of the calcaneus.[10] The prominence of this bursal projection of the calcaneus can be determined in two ways. The first uses the posterior calcaneal angle, described by Fowler and Philip, in which the angle formed by the intersection of lines along the base of the calcaneus and the posterior surface of the bursal projection and the posterior tuberosity is measured (Fig. 11–11). An angle of greater than 75 degrees is abnormal.[7, 10]

The second method is that suggested by Pavlov and co-workers in which a baseline is drawn along the inferior margin of the calcaneus. A perpendicular to this baseline, extending to the posterior limit of the talar articular facet of the calcaneus, is then constructed. From this point a line is drawn parallel to the baseline. An abnormally prominent bursal projection protrudes above this higher line.[10]

Achilles Tendinitis

Both Achilles tendinitis and retrocalcaneal bursitis may occur in association with rheumatoid arthritis or the rheumatoid variant disorders. In Reiter's syndrome, in particular, tendinitis may be prominent (Fig. 11–12).

A number of other disorders are also associated with Achilles tendon abnormalities. Owing to xanthomatous deposits, bilateral thickening of the Achilles tendons may be seen in type II hyperlipoproteinemia (Fig. 11–13). No calcifications are seen, but bilateral nodular cylindrical thickening is typical.[8] Infections, such as tuberculous peritendinitis, may also produce nodular widening of the Achilles tendon.

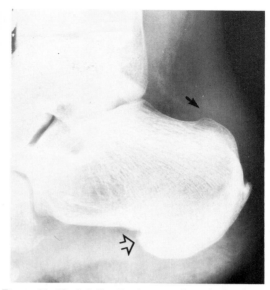

Figure 11–12. Achilles Tendinitis in Reiter's Syndrome. Sub-Achilles bursitis (arrow) and diffuse swelling of the distal Achilles tendon and of the superficial soft tissues are present. A small plantar calcaneal spur with erosion (open arrow) and calcaneal sclerosis are also seen.

Calcific Tendinitis

Calcific tendinitis analogous to that occurring in the shoulder may occur in the feet. A case of bilateral involvement of the peroneal tendons was reported in a house painter who braced his legs against the sides of a ladder.[54] In addition to the peroneal tendons, the dorsum of the foot or other sites may be involved (Figs. 11–14 and 11–15).[56]

Bony Abnormalities

Calcaneal Spurs

Bony projections may arise at the insertions of the attachment of the plantar aponeurosis, at the more anterior and medial attachment of the long plantar ligament,[13] or at the Achilles tendon insertion. In a study of 100 "normal" lateral heel radiographs spurs were noted in 22 percent. These spurs are smooth in outline, well corticated, and small (Fig. 11–16A). In patients with rheumatoid arthritis, psoriatic arthritis, ankylosing spondylitis, or Reiter's syndrome similar small spurs are more frequent. In addition, however, larger and more irregular spurs occur in patients with these conditions and are typically associated with bone erosion and soft tissue swelling. New bone formation may be prominent, particularly in patients with ankylosing spondylitis, psoriatic arthritis, and Reiter's syndrome (Fig. 11–16B). In patients with Reiter's

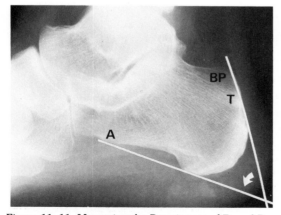

Figure 11–11. Measuring the Prominence of Bursal Projection. The angle (arrow) between lines along the anterior tubercle (A) of the calcaneus and along the posterior aspect of the bursal projection (BP) and tuberosity (T) is measured. Angles of greater than 75 degrees suggest a prominent bursal projection.

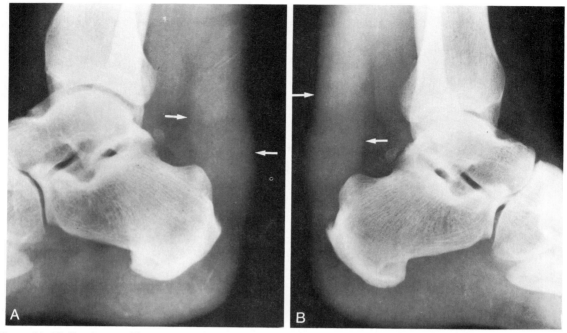

Figure 11–13. Xanthomas. There is marked bilateral enlargement of the Achilles tendons (arrows) in this patient with type II hyperlipoproteinemia. *A*, Right; *B*, left.

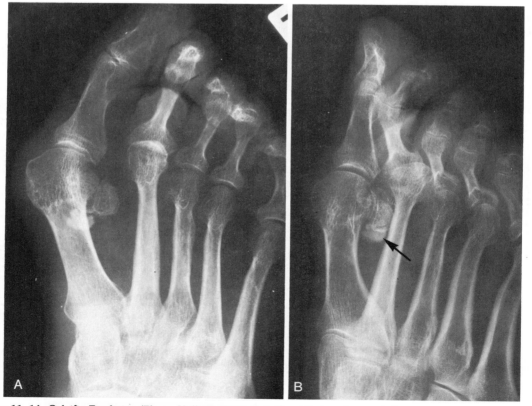

Figure 11–14. Calcific Tendinitis (Flexor Hallucis Brevis). *A*, The AP view shows calcification adjacent to the proximal border of the medial sesamoid, the site of insertion of the flexor hallucis brevis. Hallux valgus deformity is noted. *B*, The oblique view confirms the location of the calcification (arrow).

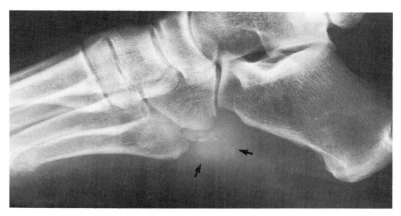

Figure 11–15. Calcific Tendinitis. There is calcification and soft tissue swelling (arrows) along the course of the flexor hallucis longus tendon.

syndrome some healing of the spurs, producing a more benign appearance, has been noted.[12]

Structural Abnormalities

Many foot abnormalities are identified in childhood or in adolescence. Nonetheless, the terminology used to describe major foot deformities is important to physicians dealing exclusively with an adult population. An overview of these terms is therefore included.[14–19]

Heel valgus. The position of the heel is described as though viewed from behind. When the Achilles tendon and the calcaneus deviate laterally, heel valgus is present. The long axis of

the talus then lies medial to the first metatarsal, and the midfoot and the forefoot are adducted to some degree. On both PA and lateral views the talocalcaneal angle is increased.

Heel varus. This deformity results from medial rotation of the calcaneus under the talus. The midtalar line is lateral to the first metatarsal shaft. The talus and the calcaneus are superimposed on the AP view, and the midtalar and the midcalcaneal lines become parallel on the lateral view. The talocalcaneal angle may be normal or decreased.

Equinus deformity. Equinus position refers to elevation of the posterior calcaneus. The talar and the calcaneal lines are parallel on the lateral

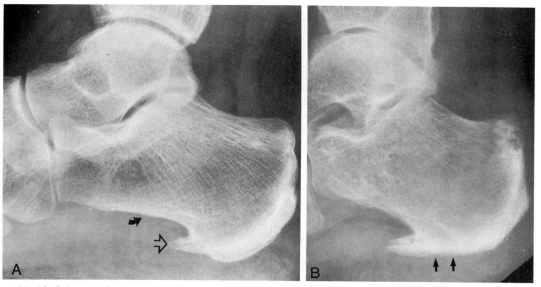

Figure 11–16. Calcaneal Spurs. *A,* The normal plantar spur (open arrow) has smooth margins, no sclerosis or erosion, and no adjacent soft tissue swelling. Very small spurs are present at the insertions of the long plantar ligament (arrow) and the Achilles tendon. *B,* Reiter's syndrome. The plantar spur and adjacent bone are dense, and there is erosion of the undersurface of the calcaneus (arrows). There is sub-Achilles bursitis, diffuse enlargement of the tendon shadow, and erosion and new bone production at the bursal projection.

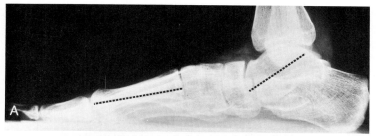

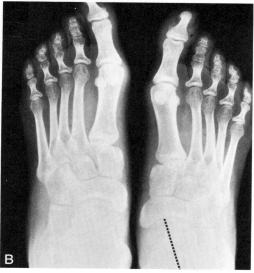

Figure 11–17. Pes Planovalgus. *A,* Standing lateral view of the right foot shows many of the features of this condition, including the narrowed distance between the calcaneus and the weight-bearing surface, overlap of more than one third of the cuboid by the talus, and plantar deviation of the axis of the talus in relation to the axis of the first metatarsal (dashed lines). *B,* The standing AP view shows medial rotation of the heads of the tali, indicating bilateral heel valgus (dashed line = talar axis).

projection. The angle formed between the inferior calcaneus and the fifth metatarsal is greater than 175 degrees.

Calcaneus deformity. This term refers to a positional abnormality in which the posterior calcaneus is directed plantarward. The angle between the inferior calcaneus and the fifth metatarsal is decreased to less than 150 degrees on the lateral view, and the talocalcaneal angle is increased to more than 50 degrees.

Cavus deformity. Cavus deformity is seen on the lateral view as upward angulation of a line from the midtalus to the first metatarsal. Normally, this line is straight.

Planus deformity. This condition is the opposite of cavus deformity. There is downward angulation of the midtalar–first metarsal line on the lateral view (Fig. 11–17).

Forefoot adduction (metatarsus varus). The midshafts of the metatarsals are angled toward the midline, and the midcalcaneal line is lateral to the fourth metatarsal (heel valgus).

Forefoot abduction (metatarsus valgus). The metatarsals are directed away from the midline, and the line through the central axis of the calcaneus is medial to the fourth metatarsal.

Flat Foot (Pes Planus)

This term refers to a longitudinal arch that is flatter than normal on weight bearing. About one third of adults have this abnormality.[16]

Mobile Flat Foot. Mobile flat foot is usually due to ligamentous laxity. This condition is termed congenital pes planus, and it persists into adulthood with the possibility that secondary osteoarthritis of the midtarsal joints may supervene.[16] Flat-foot deformity may also be associated with or caused by other anatomical abnormalities besides ligamentous laxity, including poor development of the intrinsic musculature of the feet. Congenital pes planus is characterized on standing views by the following (Fig. 11–15):[22]

1. Abnormal calcaneal position and shape. The inferior anterior aspect of the calcaneus is closer to the weight-bearing surface than is normal. This abnormality may be defined as a decrease of the angle between the weight-bearing surface and the undersurface of the calcaneus (decreased calcaneal pitch). The anterior inferior calcaneal cortex is thickened.

2. Adduction of the talus. The head of the talus is rotated medially. Despite this, Chopart's

joint (between the talus and the navicular and the calcaneus and the cuboid) remains normal.

3. The metatarsals and the toes are abducted.

4. The tarsometatarsal joints are spread.

Spasmodic Flat Foot. In contrast with the mobile flat foot, stiff flat foot is the result of a fixed bony abnormality. Spasmodic flat foot (peroneal spastic flat foot) is the term used when flat-foot deformity is associated with congenital fibrous, cartilaginous, or bony fusion (coalition) between the tarsals.[20, 24, 25] At birth the fusion is fibrous or cartilaginous, but ossification occurs later, further limiting motion.[26] In the normal foot external rotation at the subtalar joint compensates for the internal rotation of the tibia that occurs with each step, but in the foot with tarsal coalition subtalar motion is limited, and the calcaneus is forced into valgus, with consequent flattening of the arch and gradual shortening of the peroneal tendons. Painful contraction of

these tendons occurs when inversion of the foot is attempted.

Symptoms usually begin in adolescence. It should be noted, however, that the radiographic demonstration of tarsal coalition may be incidental, unassociated with pes planus, peroneal muscle spasm, or symptoms.[20]

Radiographic Examination. In *calcaneonavicular* coalition the bony bar may be seen only on internal oblique views (Fig. 11–18). When fusion is fibrous or cartilaginous, rather than bony, there will be irregularity and poor definition of the opposing cortical margins. The head of the talus may be hypoplastic.

Talocalcaneal coalition may be even more difficult to demonstrate. The bony fusion is most likely to involve the sustentaculum tali, but the anterior or posterior portions of the subtalar joint may be involved. Plain film findings include the following (Figs. 11–19 and 11–20):

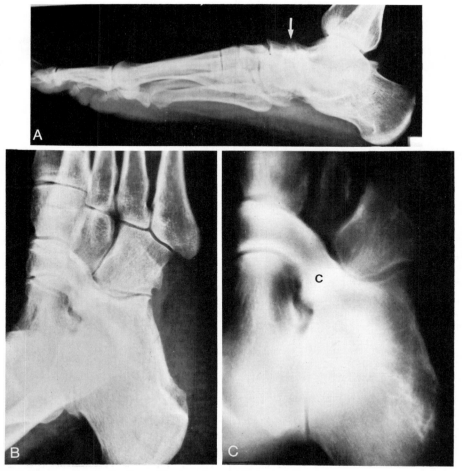

Figure 11–18. Calcaneonavicular Coalition. The lateral view *(A)* shows flattening of the longitudinal arch and a talar beak (arrow). An internal oblique view *(B)* and subsequent tomogram *(C)* confirm bony bridging *(C)* between the calcaneus and the navicular. No talocalcaneal coalition was demonstrated, although that is a more likely cause of talar beaking.

639

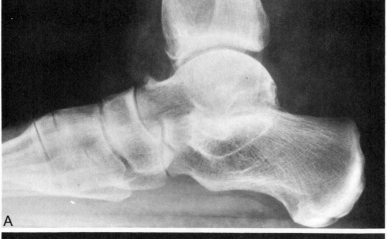

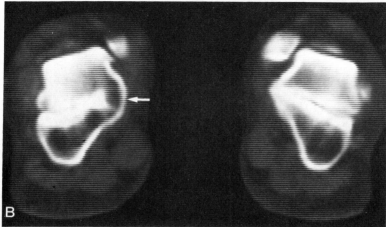

Figure 11–19. Talocalcaneal Coalition. *A,* The lateral view of the right foot shows a beak at the site of insertion of the joint capsules on the talus. The usual, more distal, talar beaking is absent. The subtalar joint is obscured. *B,* CT section through the subtalar joints on each side show complete bony bridge between the right talus and the calcaneus (arrow). The pointed shapes of the sustentaculum tali and of the adjacent talus on the left suggest a fibrous coalition.

1. Talar beaking. A bony spur from the anterior superior aspect of the talus is typical and is thought to result from the limited subtalar motion that forces the navicular to override the head of the talus, providing traction on the periosteum of the anterior aspect of the talus.[26] This spur is located more distally than that arising at the site of capsular insertion on the talus. The latter spur is of no clinical consequence.[29]

2 There is broadening of the lateral process of the talus.

3. There is narrowing of the posterior subtalar joint, which is a nonspecific finding seen in long-standing cases.

An appearance suggesting a bony bridge between the talus and calcaneus can occasionally be seen on the lateral view in normal individuals if the foot is abducted or inverted (Fig. 11–21). Since true talocalcaneal coalition is apparent only on axial views or on tomography and since no secondary radiographic signs of coalition will be present, this positioning artifact should be distinguishable from true coalition. A true lateral projection will confirm normal appearances.[28]

In symptomatic patients recognition of the secondary signs of talocalcaneal coalition should be confirmed by additional studies. Axial views with 30, 40, and 45 degree tube angulation or tomography in the lateral projection may be done, but for confirming the diagnosis more emphasis is currently being placed on computed tomography.[21] The coronal projection that can be obtained with the knees flexed and the feet flat on the CT table provides a cross-sectional view of the sustentaculum tali and an optimal view of any bar across it (Fig. 11–19).

Arthrography. Kaye and associates have used arthrography combined with multiple tangential views to document the presence of talocalcaneal coalition.[27] The talosustentacular and talonavicular joints normally communicate; therefore, contrast medium injected into the talonavicular joint should fill the talosustentacular joint. Failure to fill this joint indicates coali-

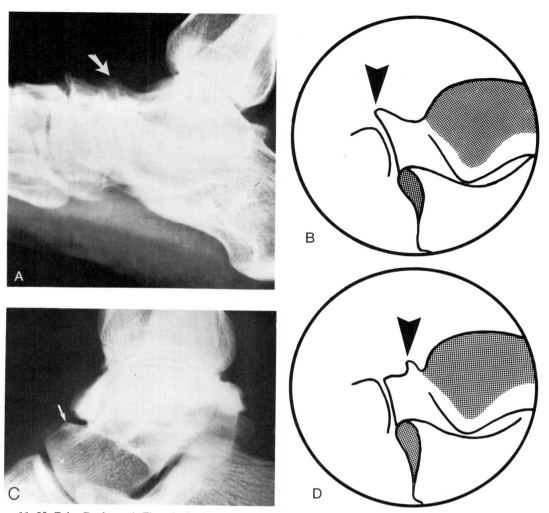

Figure 11–20. Talar Beaking. *A*, The talar beak associated with tarsal coalition (arrowhead) arises at the talonavicular joint (same patient as in Figure 11–16). *B*, Diagram of *A*. *C*, The normal talar beak (arrow) arises at the area of capsular insertion. Contrast material from a prior arthrogram is present in the ankle joint. *D*, Diagram of *C*.

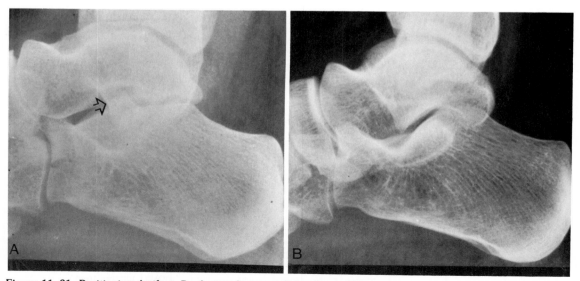

Figure 11–21. Positioning Artifact, Producing Apparent Talocalcaneal Fusion. *A*, An off-lateral view shows apparent bony bridging, owing to overlapping of the lateral process of the talus (arrow) and the calcaneus. *B*, The true lateral view shows no abnormality.

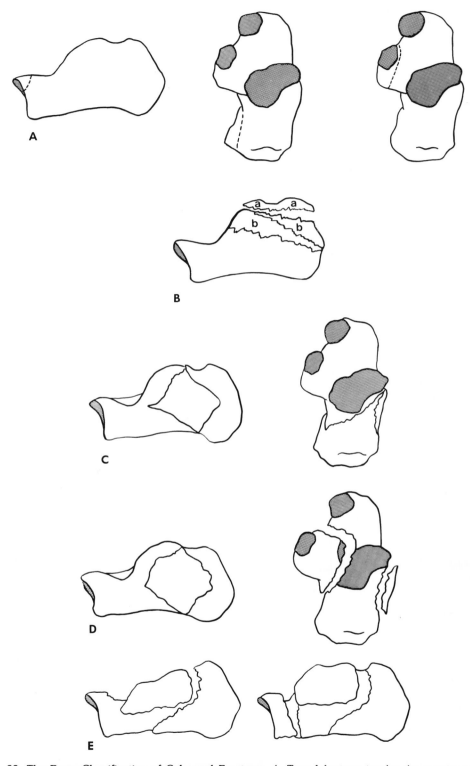

Figure 11–22. The Rowe Classification of Calcaneal Fractures. *A,* Type I fractures involve the anterior process, the tuberosity, or the sustentaculum tali. *B,* Type II fractures are beak (a) fractures or avulsion (b) fractures of the Achilles tendon. *C,* Type III fractures are oblique and do not involve the subtalar joint. *D,* Type IV fractures involve the subtalar joint. *E,* Type V fractures are centrally depressed and comminuted. (Redrawn from Rowe CR, Sakellarides HT, Freeman PA, et al.: JAMA 184:920, 1963.)

tion.[27] An advantage of this technique is the ability to demonstrate cartilaginous or fibrous as well as bony coalition.

Bone Scanning. The radionuclide bone scan may be a useful screening method in patients suspected of having talocalcaneal coalition. The combination of increased isotope uptake in the subtalar area and the superior talus or talonavicular regions is said to be specific for the diagnosis.[23] Occasionally, however, only the subtalar area of affected patients exhibits increased isotope uptake. A negative scan should obviate the need for more invasive testing.

Treatment. Several modes of therapy have been used for treating painful tarsal coalition.[25a, 26] Jayakumar and Cowell note that resection of a cartilaginous calcaneonavicular bar is indicated in a young individual with foot pain and limited subtalar motion.[26] An ossified fusion site is said to be a relative contraindication to resection, since secondary osteoarthritic changes may have occurred in adjacent joints. The presence of a talar beak suggests a talocalcaneal coalition and is another contraindication to resection of a calcaneonavicular bar. These authors suggest conservative therapy for talocalcaneal coalition. If this fails, triple arthrodesis is preferred to resection of the bar, since resection removes much of the weight-bearing area of the subtalar joint and shifts stress to the other joints.[26]

Fractures and Dislocations

Calcaneal Fractures

Fractures of the calcaneus account for 60 percent of all major tarsal injuries.[32] These are

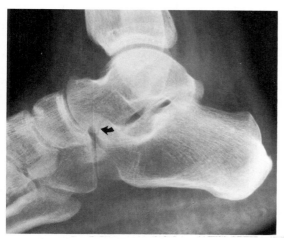

Figure 11–23. Anterior Process Fracture. There is a fracture (arrow) through the anterior process of the calcaneus.

problematical fractures; because of the complex contour of the calcaneus, multiple radiographic views are often necessary for full evaluation, and there is disagreement over the method of treatment of those injuries, particularly of intraarticular fractures.

Classification. Two major classifications, that of Rowe and colleagues and that of Essex-Lopresti, are used.[33, 39] Giannestras and Summarco recommend using the Rowe classification for extraarticular fractures and the Essex-Lopresti classification for intraarticular fractures.[34]

The Rowe Classification. Rowe and coworkers classified calcaneal fractures into five groups based on analysis of 146 patients (154 fractures) (Figs. 11–22 and 11–23).

Type I (21 percent)
Fractures of tuberosity
Fractures of sustentaculum tali
Fractures of anterior process

Type II (3.8 percent)
Beak fractures
Avulsion fractures of Achilles tendon insertion

Type III (19.5 percent)
Oblique fractures not involving the subtalar joint

Type IV (24.7 percent)
Fractures involving the subtalar joint

Type V (31 percent)
Central depression with varying degrees of comminution

Types I, II, and III do not involve the subtalar joint. Types IV and V do involve this joint and, as shown, composed 56 percent of all fractures in this series.

The Essex-Lopresti Classification. In 1951, Essex-Lopresti classified fractures into two main categories, those sparing the subtalar joint (25 percent of his patients) and those involving this joint (75 percent of patients). The discussion of intraarticular fractures presents mechanical, pathological, and radiological material and is suggested to interested readers. According to Essex-Lopresti, the force generated at the time of injury is carried along the tibia, through the talus, and then by two routes to the calcaneus. These two routes are (1) an *outer route*—invoked when the subtalar joint is forced to evert and the sharp, lateral spike of the talus is driven into the crucial angle of the calcaneus, producing a fracture—and (2) an *inner route*—invoked when, after the outer fracture, the force is directed through the anterior subtalar joint to the sustentaculum tali. The sustentaculum tali and

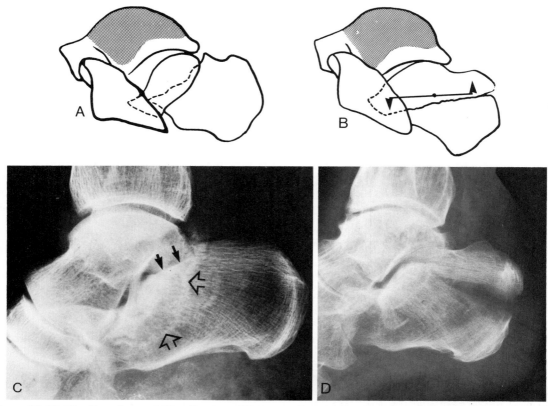

Figure 11–24. The Essex-Lopresti Classification of Fractures. Fractures involving the subtalar joint are subdivided into joint depression *(A)* and tongue *(B)* types. Severe examples are shown. *C,* Joint-depression fracture. There is depression of the subtalar articular surface (arrows), with flattening of Böhler's angle. Overlapping and impacted fracture lines are seen (open arrows). *D,* Tongue-type fracture. The horizontal fracture line extends into the posterior portion of the subtalar joint. *(A* and *B* after Essex-Lopresti P: Br J Surg 39:395, 1952.)

the medial third or half of the posterior subtalar joint may be separated from the remainder of the calcaneus.

Continued force will produce either of two types of fracture (Fig. 11–24): (1) *tongue fracture,* in which the secondary fracture line runs straight back to the posterior border of the tuberosity (the anterior part of this tongue may be pushed down and the tuberosity forced up and back, resulting in loss of the normal tuber angle [Böhler's angle]); and (2) *joint depression* fracture, in which the secondary fracture line runs across the body of the calcaneus just behind the subtalar joint (the fragment thus created consists of the bone and the articular cartilage of the outer half to two thirds of the posterior subtalar joint). Joint depression occurs more frequently than tongue displacement.

Radiographic Examination. Standard radiographic examination consists of lateral and axial views of the calcaneus and an AP view of the foot on the involved side. However, when the articular facets of the calcaneus are involved, Giannestras and Sammarco suggest multiple ad-

ditional views (see Oblique Views, in the following section) and note the necessity for high-quality radiographs. Films of the dorsal and lumbar spine and the ankle should be done almost routinely, since spinal fractures have been noted to accompany calcaneal fractures in about 10 percent of patients and since fractures of the tibia and fibula or the tibia alone have been noted in 9 percent. Calcaneal fractures may be bilateral (about 5 percent of patients in one series), and it has been recommended that views of both feet be obtained in order to exclude bilateral injury and to have a normal examination for comparison with the affected side.[34] Extensive soft tissue injury occurs with all calcaneal fractures.

Lateral View. The lateral view is the primary film used to establish a diagnosis of calcaneal fracture. On the lateral view of the normal foot the calcaneus is noted to consist largely of cancellous bone. A strong, thick area of cortical bone on the upper outer margin of the calcaneus extends from the anterior calcaneus to the posterior margin of the subtalar joint (Fig. 11–25).

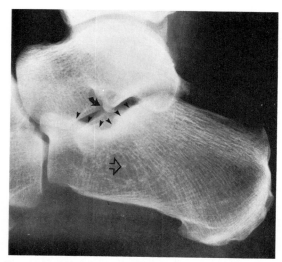

Figure 11–25. Crucial Angle. On this lateral view arrowheads point to an area of strong, thick cortical bone (the crucial angle) that supports the lateral spur of the talus. In this case there is some deformity of the lateral spur of the talus (arrow), presumably from prior injury. Incidental note is made of a normal vascular foramen (open arrow) and a normal zone of relative lucency around it.

This area supports the lateral spur of the talus and is concave superiorly under the talus, forming the crucial angle.[33]

Lorenz Böhler described the tuber-joint angle (now called Böhler's angle), in which a line drawn between the posterior superior aspect of the calcaneus and the highest point of the posterior subtalar articular surface intersects a line drawn from the highest point of the anterior process to the posterior margin of the subtalar articular surface to form an angle of 30 to 35 degrees (Fig. 11–26).[31] Depression of the sub-

talar joint, usually caused by an intraarticular fracture, results in a decrease in this angle (see Fig. 11–28). Some fractures of the body that do not involve the subtalar joint may also decrease Böhler's angle, and this observation may lead to recognition of otherwise radiographically occult fractures. Intraarticular involvement accounts for the poorer prognosis noted when Böhler's angle is flat as compared with those cases in which this angle is maintained.[34]

Axial Views. Radiography in the axial projection is essential for evaluation of the subtalar joint and the width of the calcaneus. The appearance of the subtalar joint and the length of the posterior calcaneus will depend on the angle at which the x-ray is taken as well as the anatomy of the calcaneus itself. The sustentaculum tali is seen as a shelf extending from the inner side of the calcaneus (see Fig. 11–1).

Normally, the calcaneus is 30 to 35 mm in width.[31] Widening as a consequence of fracture may result in impingement of the calcaneus against the fibula, with entrapment of the peroneal tendons. Widening can also be documented on the anteroposterior view of the ankle if the lateral border of the calcaneus extends up to or beyond the tip of the lateral malleolus.[34]

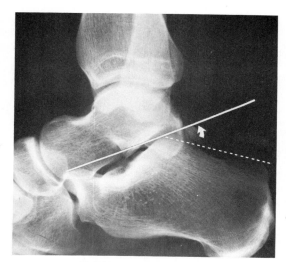

Figure 11–26. Böhler's Angle. Normally, this angle is between 30 and 35 degrees.

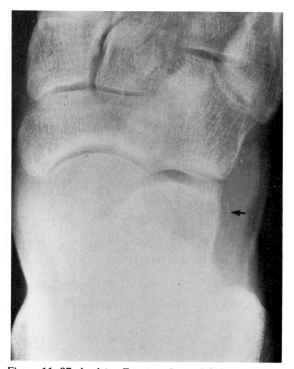

Figure 11–27. Avulsion Fracture, Lateral Calcaneus. Localized soft tissue swelling and tenderness were present over the lateral aspect of the foot. A small linear bone fragment (arrow) indicates an avulsion fracture at the site of insertion of the extensor digitorum brevis.

AP View. This view is necessary for evaluating the calcaneocuboid joint. Avulsion fractures of the anterior lateral aspect of the calcaneus may be demonstrated on this view (Fig. 11–27).[36]

Oblique Views. Multiple oblique views have been suggested. They are of considerable help in demonstrating both fractures extending into the articular surfaces and the loss of parallelism of joint surfaces.[30] When fractures are thought to involve the subtalar joint, Giannestras and Sammarco suggest the following additional views:[34]

1. The lateral oblique view. The foot is placed with the medial side against the cassette and with an angle of 35 degrees between the cassette and the sole of the foot.

2. Axial medial oblique view. The foot is internally rotated to an angle of 60 degrees with the cassette, and the tube is centered over the talocalcaneal joint.

3. Axial lateral oblique view. The foot is externally rotated to make an angle of 30 degrees with the cassette.

Computed Tomography. CT is an excellent technique for the evaluation of calcaneal fractures, since involvement of the subtalar joint can be clearly appreciated (Fig. 11–28). Optimal evaluation of calcaneal widening is provided by CT.

Peroneal Tenography. Contrast agent injection into the common sheath of the peroneus brevis and the peroneus longus as it descends behind the lateral malleolus may be useful for evaluating persistent pain after calcaneal fracture (Fig. 11–29). Compression of the sheath with partial or complete obstruction of the flow of contrast medium, tendon displacement, or rupture may be demonstrated.[38] Aspiration of the contrast material followed by injection of anesthetic should provide temporary relief of pain in these patients and should document the origin of symptoms.

Treatment. The prognosis for fractures that spare the subtalar joint is almost always good. Fractures in which there is marked comminution, widening of the calcaneus, loss of the normal tuber-joint angle, or deformity of the subtalar joint are associated with the poorest prognosis.[32]

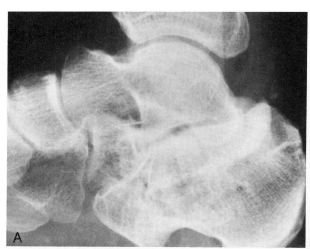

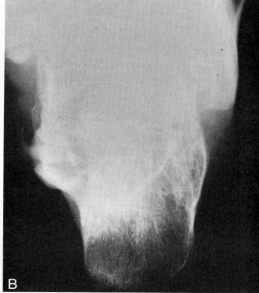

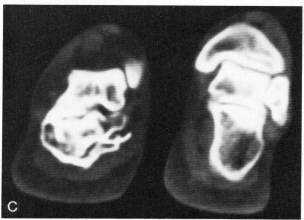

Figure 11–28. Calcaneal Fracture. *A,* A lateral view years after a calcaneal fracture shows residual flattening of Böhler's angle and an abnormal plantar contour. *B,* Multiple attempts at obtaining the axial view were unsuccessful in showing the subtalar joint. Bony spurs project from the medial calcaneus. *C,* Computed tomography better shows marked compression and widening of the calcaneus and marked depression of the subtalar articular surface.

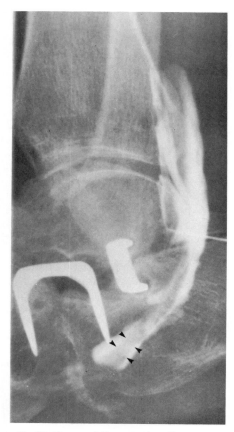

Figure 11–29. Peroneal Tenography. Contrast agent injected into the common sheath of the peroneus brevis and the peroneus longus muscles failed to outline completely the peroneus brevis, suggesting scarring of the sheath, in this case apparently the result of prior surgery. The peroneus longus tendon (arrowheads) can be seen.

Type I fractures (tuberosity fractures, sustentaculum tali fractures, and anterior process fractures) are generally treated conservatively, with union of fracture fragments occurring by about 8 weeks. Nonunion may result after fractures of the sustentaculum tali if premature weight bearing is allowed, but no treatment is required if this nonunion is asymptomatic. Surgical excision of the fragment may be indicated in cases of painful nonunion.

Type II fractures involve avulsion injury of the tuberosity by the Achilles tendon. This is an uncommon injury and is treated conservatively if the fragment is not displaced or by open reduction if it is displaced.[34]

Type III fractures (fractures of the body that do not involve the subtalar joint) are treated conservatively, with early active exercise but no weight bearing until union is solid, usually by 8 to 12 weeks. If the fracture is displaced and Böhler's angle is flattened, controversy exists regarding whether reduction of the fragments is desirable. Giannestras and Sammarco suggest manipulative reduction in cases in which Böhler's angle is 10 degrees or less.[34]

Intraarticular fractures are treated by a variety of means, including treatment without reduction, closed reduction, open reduction, and primary subtalar fusion or triple arthrodesis.

The period of recuperation after calcaneal fracture is long, sometimes lasting 18 to 24 months. Continued pain may be due to post-traumatic subtalar osteoarthritis, compression of the peroneal tendons between the fibula and the calcaneus, deformity of the plantar surface of the heel, and the increased pressure on the soft tissues of the heel that accompanies flattening of Böhler's angle.

Talar Fractures and Dislocations

Fractures of the talus are the second most frequent tarsal bone fracture.[34] Injury may involve the head, neck, body, or posterior process of the talus, but the neck is the most vulnerable site.

Chip and avulsion fractures may involve the superior surface of the neck or lateral, medial, or posterior parts of the body (Fig. 11–30).[45] A large medial fragment that includes part of the articular surface and the groove for the flexor hallucis longus tendon may interfere with motion and necessitate surgical intervention.[41]

Fractures of the talar dome may present a clinical picture similar to that of a moderate or severe ankle sprain.[46] The fractures result from impaction of the superior margin of the talus on the ankle mortise. Thus, with an inversion injury the superomedial aspect of the talus impinges

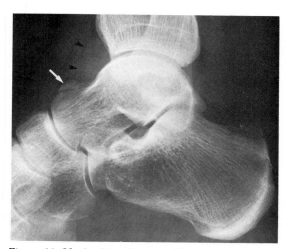

Figure 11–30. Avulsion Fracture. There is elevation of a small superior fragment (arrow) at the site of capsular insertion on the talus. An ankle effusion (arrowheads) is present.

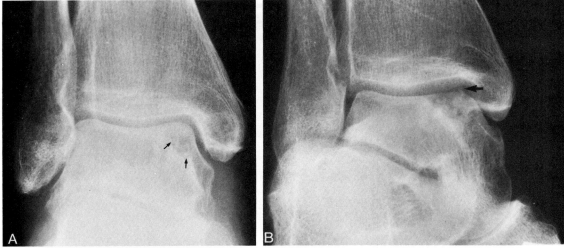

Figure 11–31. Compression Injury of the Talus. *A,* The AP view shows a lucency with a sclerotic margin and small central densities (arrows) in the superomedial aspect of the talus . *B,* The mortise view suggests a loose body (arrow).

on the tibia, and the superolateral aspect strikes the fibula. The exact site of talar damage depends on the degree of flexion or extension of the ankle at the time of injury.

On radiographs these fractures may be subtle (Figs. 11–31 and 11–32). When critically evaluated, the mortise view shows abnormalities in the talus medially, laterally, or in both areas, consisting of small fractures in the subchondral cortex and the adjacent cancellous bone and areas of subchondral lucency, increased density, or irregularity. Smith and associates suggest that

the marginal location of these abnormalities differentiates them from typical avascular necrosis or osteochondritis dissecans.[46] Pluridirectional tomography, especially in the lateral projection, best demonstrates and localizes the abnormality. Associated compression of a portion of the tibial plafond can be evaluated at the same time. Single- or double-contrast arthrography with tomography permits evaluation of the overlying articular cartilage.

Fractures of the neck of the talus are usually the result of a force from below pushing the

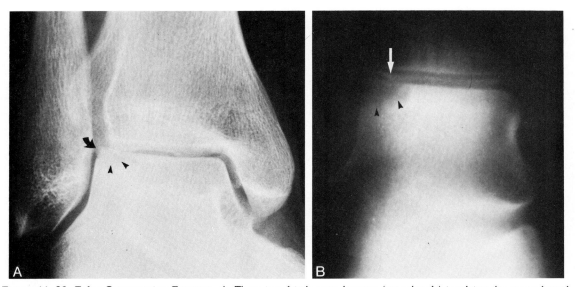

Figure 11–32. Talar Compression Fracture. *A,* There is a faintly seen lucency (arrowheads) involving the superolateral aspect of the talus, with irregularity of the overlying subchondral cortex and a possible loose body (arrow). *B,* An AP tomogram after single-contrast arthrography shows the lucent defect in the talus (arrowheads) with irregularity of the overlying cartilage (arrow) but no loose body. Lateral tomography should also be done in these cases, although in this instance no additional information was provided by that view.

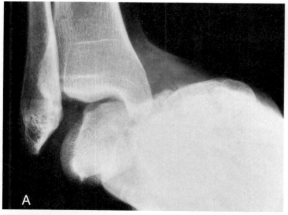

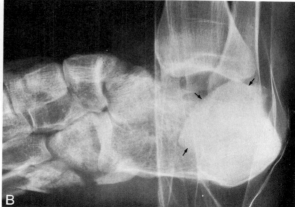

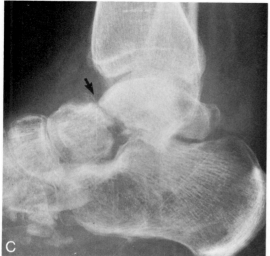

Figure 11–33. Talar Dislocation with Avascular Necrosis. *A,* AP view of the ankle shows abnormal rotation of the talus in relation to the tibia, with dislocation at the tibiotalar and subtalar joints. *B,* The lateral view shows a fracture through the neck of the talus. The proximal talus (arrows) has rotated and is dislocated from its normal tibial and calcaneal articulations. Overlap of bone at the calcaneocuboid joint indicates dislocations here, too. There is a comminuted fracture of the base of the fifth metatarsal. *C,* Follow-up radiograph months after reduction and pinning (note vertical pin tract in calcaneus) shows incomplete reduction of dislocation with the calcaneus anteriorly displaced in relation to the talus. Despite the osteoporosis of the other bones, there is increased density of the talus, indicating avascular necrosis. The talar fracture (arrow) has not united.

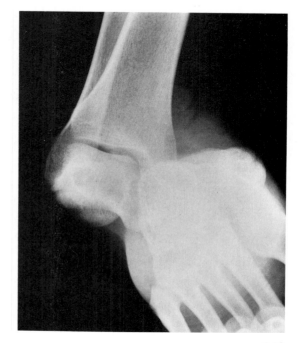

Figure 11–34. Medial Subtalar Dislocation. The AP view shows the talus in position under the tibia, but there is medial displacement of the calcaneus and the remainder of the foot. There were no associated fractures.

talus upward—the mechanism operative in aviator's astragalus, when during a plane crash the rudder bar is pressed into the instep of the foot.[41] Damage to the anterior tibia that may be seen radiographically attests to this mechanism of forced dorsiflexion.

These fractures may be associated with subtalar dislocation or with posterior dislocation of the body of the talus from its normal relationship with either the foot or the tibia (Fig. 11–33). Subtalar dislocation accompanying fractures of the neck of the talus may be subtle, and to make the diagnosis careful inspection of the lateral radiograph for obliteration of the subtalar joint by the overlapping talus and calcaneus is

necessary. The type of subtalar dislocation is named according to the position of the foot relative to the talus; thus in a medial dislocation the talus is displaced laterally (Figs. 11–34 and 11–35). Associated avulsion fractures of the malleoli or the tarsals may occur.

Fractures of the body of the talus are the third most common talar fractures. They may be followed by osteonecrosis.[34] Fracture of the neck and the body of the talus unite in about 8 weeks.

Dislocation without major fracture may occur at the subtalar joint or the midtarsal joints, and major complications after reduction are unusual (Figs. 11–34 and 11–35).[42] Marginal fractures

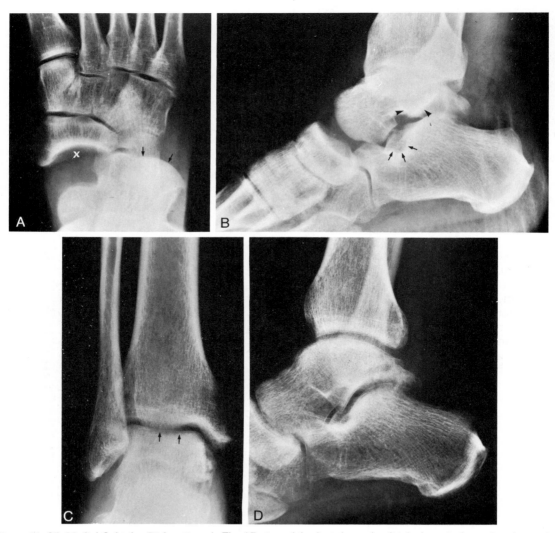

Figure 11–35. Medial Subtalar Dislocation. *A,* The AP view of the foot shows the distal talar articular surface (arrows) to be laterally displaced. The "empty" navicular fossa (x) is seen. *B,* Lateral view shows the abnormal separation between the talus and the navicular. The subtle displacement of the talus on the calcaneus is confirmed by noting the posterior position of the lateral process of the talus (arrowheads) in relation to the "crucial angle" (small arrows) of the calcaneus. The AP *C* and lateral *(D)* views of the ankle weeks after reduction show osteoporosis with subchondral rarefaction (arrows). This is reassuring evidence that circulation to the talus is intact.

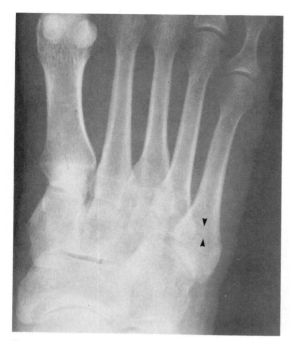

Figure 11–36. Jones's Fracture. A barely visible fracture line (arrowheads) is present.

may, however, predispose to degenerative joint disease.[45] Total talar dislocation at all three talar articulations is a severe injury, and avascular necrosis is expected (Fig. 11–33). The talus is displaced forward and laterally.[41]

Osteonecrosis (Avascular Necrosis) After Fractures or Dislocations. The body of the talus is most often the site of avascular necrosis after injury. Blood supply to the talus is actually derived from all three major arteries to the leg (the anterior and posterior tibials and the peroneal). Branches reach the talus through the superior and inferior surfaces of the neck, the anterior and medial aspects of the body, and the posterior tubercle. The major blood supply is from the inferior aspect of the neck, through an anastomotic sling in the tarsal sinus and the tarsal canal.[44]

Kelly and Sullivan noted osteonecrosis in 6.2 percent of patients after fusions involving the subtalar joint and attributed this low incidence to the collateral blood supply from periosteal vessels.[44] A higher incidence of osteonecrosis is noted after trauma and may be attributed to damage to intraosseous vessels. In Coltart's series of patients osteonecrosis did not occur after uncomplicated fractures of the neck of the talus or after simple dislocation at the subtalar joint.[41] However, one third of patients with both fracture of the neck of the talus and subtalar dislocation had this complication. Radiographic evidence of osteonecrosis was apparent in these cases by 8

weeks after injury (Fig. 11–31). The development of osteoporosis, manifested by a subchondral lucency in the talar dome (Hawkins's sign), is evidence that disuse osteoporosis is occurring and, therefore, that the blood supply is intact (Fig. 11–33).[43]

Fifth Metatarsal (Jones's) Fractures

Robert Jones suffered a fracture of the fifth metatarsal while dancing and reported this and additional cases in 1902.[48] This injury is an avulsion fracture resulting from plantar flexion and inversion stress, with contraction of the peroneus brevis muscle. The fracture is usually not displaced and may be difficult to see on radiographs (Fig. 11–36). Localized soft tissue swelling will be present, and the fracture line, unlike the longitudinal lucency that defines a nonunited proximal ossification center, will be noted to run obliquely or transversely through the proximal fifth metatarsal (Fig. 11–37). Nearby accessory ossicles are distinguished by their smooth, dense margins and often by their bilateral presence. To avoid missing a Jones's fracture, the base of the fifth metatarsal should be included on all radiographs of the ankle.

Treatment is conservative, with strapping for nondisplaced fractures and casting for displaced fractures and for transverse fractures at the base

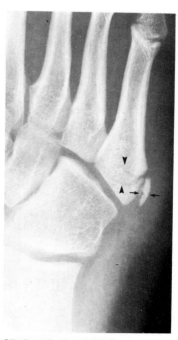

Figure 11–37. Jones's Fracture. There is an oblique fracture (arrowheads) of the fifth metatarsal base of a child. The longitudinal orientation of the proximal ossification center (arrows) helps to make the distinction between this normal finding and a fracture fragment.

of the metatarsal.[47] Nondisplaced fractures unite by the end of 4 weeks.

Tarsometatarsal (Lisfranc's) *Fracture-Dislocations*

Dislocation at the tarsometatarsal (Lisfranc's) joints may be a radiographically subtle diagnosis (Figs. 11–38 and 11–39). Most often, the entire forefoot is dislocated laterally and dorsally. The first and second metatarsals may be spread; the first metatarsal may be deviated in the same direction as or the opposite direction from the other metatarsals, or it may not be deviated at all. Lateral views usually show dorsal displacement of the involved metatarsals. Associated fractures are common.

Several normal tarsometatarsal relationships have been described so that minor degrees of dislocation can be detected.[52] The most constant relationship on frontal or oblique films is the alignment of the medial margin of the second metatarsal with the medial edge of the second cuneiform. The other relationships between the metatarsals and the tarsals occasionally deviate

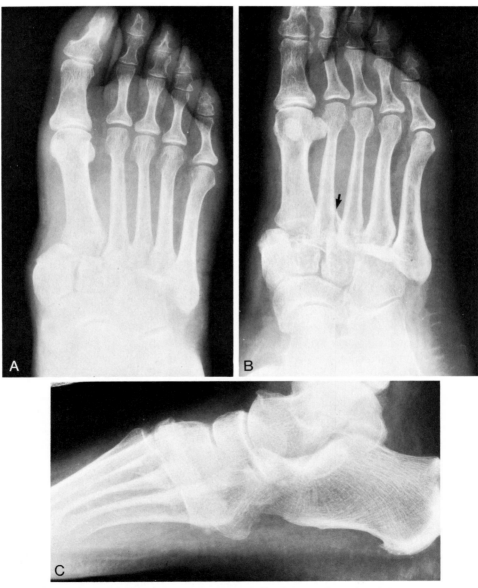

Figure 11–38. Lisfranc's Fracture-Dislocation in a Diabetic. *A*, The PA view shows lateral dislocation of the bases of the first through fifth metatarsals. *B*, The loss of parallelism of the lateral tarsometatarsal joints is seen. There is a fracture of the second metatarsal (arrow). *C*, The lateral view shows the first and second metatarsal bases elevated and abnormal overlap of tarsals and metatarsals.

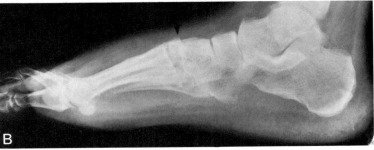

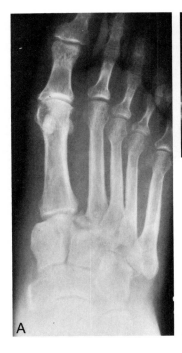

Figure 11–39. Lisfranc's Fracture-Dislocation. *A,* The AP view shows separation of the first and second metatarsals due to lateral subluxation of the second through fifth metatarsals. Note the offset between the medial side of the second metatarsal and the middle cuneiform and between the lateral edge of the fifth metatarsal articular surface and the lateral cuboid. There is a fracture of the base of the second metatarsal. *B,* The lateral view confirms superior displacement of the metatarsals (arrow).

by a few millimeters, but for the detection of asymmetry comparison views of the opposite foot may help. Normally, the medial aspect of the base of the fourth metatarsal is aligned with the medial edge of the cuboid, the fifth metatarsal notch (indicating the end of the articular surface) is aligned with the lateral cuboid, and the lateral aspect of the first metatarsal is aligned with the corresponding edge of the medial cuneiform.

Lisfranc's fracture-dislocations have been noted to occur in patients with diabetes mellitus or other conditions causing sensory neuropathy (Figs. 11–36 and 11–37). Giesecke and co-workers noted that the presence of such a dislocation in the absence of a history of an acute traumatic event should suggest the diagnosis of a neuropathic foot.[53] In one of their patients the diagnosis of diabetes mellitus had not been made previously.

To establish normal relationships and to avoid vascular compromise in acute traumatic cases reduction by closed or open methods is necessary.[51]

Foot Stabilization Procedures

Fusion of the subtalar, the talonavicular, or both of these joints may be done to relieve pain caused by joint incongruity (such as that occurring after calcaneal fracture with subtalar involvement), as part of an operative procedure to correct deformity, or in both cases. Some

general points regarding these procedures may be made. First, stability of the ankle is a prerequisite for these surgical procedures, and varus-valgus stress views may be required to confirm stability preoperatively. In addition, after surgery to correct deformity the medial border of the foot should be straight, the first and fifth metatarsals and the heel should lie on the same plane, and the heel should be in neutral or in mild valgus, but not in varus position.[60]

Triple Arthrodesis

This procedure includes resection of articular surfaces and adjacent bone from the calcaneocuboid, talonavicular, and subtalar joints and from the sustentaculum tali (Fig. 11–40).[61] Wedges of bone may be removed to correct deformity (Fig. 11–41). The resected bone margins are apposed, and any removed bone may be used as graft. Metal staples across the fusion sites help maintain position during healing. Postoperative AP and internal oblique views of the foot and AP and lateral views of the ankle should show close contact between the resection margins. Solid bony union is expected by 12 weeks.[60]

Several modifications of this procedure are used, including (1) the *Dunn* arthrodesis, in which the navicular is removed (the head of the talus will be next to the cuneiforms), and (2) the *Hoke* arthrodesis, in which the head of the talus is removed, denuded of cartilage, and a portion replaced between the navicular and the body of

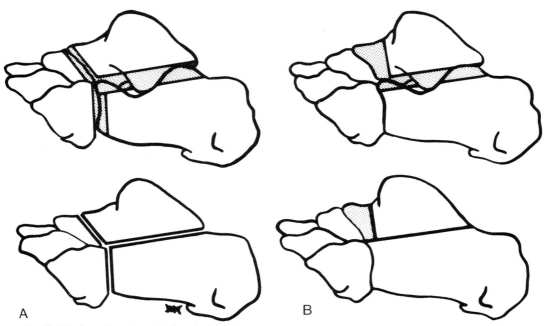

Figure 11–40. Triple Arthrodesis. *A,* Standard triple arthrodesis. *B,* Hoke modification. Stippled areas represent sites of bone resection.

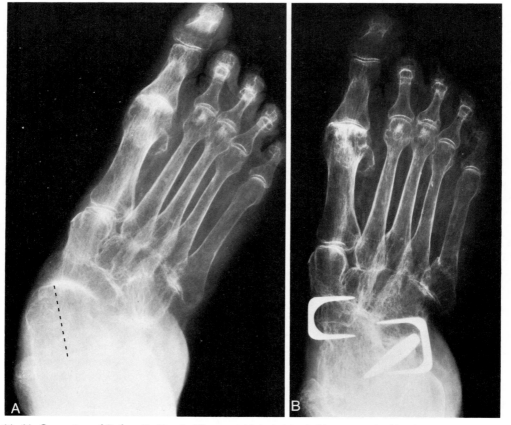

Figure 11–41. Correction of Deformity Due to Rheumatoid Arthritis. *A,* There is marked heel valgus, with the talar axis (dashed line) deviated medially. There is severe osteopenia and cartilage-space narrowing in the mid- and hindfoot articulations. *B,* A wedge of bone has been removed from the medial aspect of the foot, allowing the foot to be realigned. The more normal alignment is confirmed by alignment of the first metatarsal and the talar axes and straightening of the medial border of the foot. As part of the attempted fusion, staples are present across the talonavicular, the calcaneocuboid, and the subtalar joints.

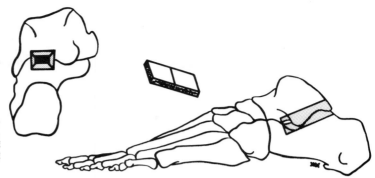

Figure 11–42. The Gallie Subtalar Fusion. Bone is removed from the subtalar joint, and bone graft is inserted into the resulting tunnel. (After Gallie WE: J bone Joint Surg 25:731, 1943.)

the talus (Fig. 11–40). The talocalcaneal and often the calcaneocuboid joints are also fused.[61]

Complications of triple arthrodesis include (1) osteonecrosis of the body of the talus;[60] (2) secondary osteoarthritis in the ankle as a result of increased stress on this joint;[60] (3) pseudarthrosis, which occurs in as many as one quarter of fusions and in almost 90 percent of patients involves the talonavicular joint;[61] (4) residual or recurrent deformity; and (5) anterior subluxation of the talus resulting from ligamentous damage (especially of the anterior talofibular ligament), which sometimes occurs at the time of surgery.[62]

Subtalar Arthrodesis

In this procedure the surfaces of the subtalar joint are removed. More bone may be taken from the medial side of the joint to correct eversion of the calcaneus.[60]

The Gallie subtalar fusion involves removal of a tunnel of bone from the posterior subtalar joint and insertion of bone graft from the tibia or the ilium into the defect (Fig. 11–42). The procedure is less difficult than the standard technique of subtalar fusion, but no correction of varus or valgus deformity is possible.

Grice noted that triple arthrodesis was unsuit-

able for use in young children, since subsequent growth disturbance would occur.[59] He proposed that children with marked valgus flat-foot deformity caused by poliomyelitis could have the deformity corrected and the position held by insertion of a wedge of bone into the tarsal sinus. This extraarticular method of fusion (the *Grice procedure*) is expected to interfere very little with growth. Healing at the graft site occurs at 10 to 12 weeks.

The *Thomas* arthrodesis is a modification of the Grice procedure (Figs. 11–43 and 11–44). A tunnel is made by removing bone from the talar and calcaneal margins of the tarsal sinus through a lateral approach. A full-thickness graft from the iliac crest is inserted into the defect.

Talonavicular Arthrodesis

The talonavicular joint is the most frequently involved hindfoot joint in patients with rheumatoid arthritis. In some of these patients pain can be relieved and deformity corrected by fusion of this damaged joint alone. The tubercle of the navicular is removed, the talonavicular joint surfaces are excised down to cancellous bone, and—with the foot held in the corrected position—bone graft is inserted across the me-

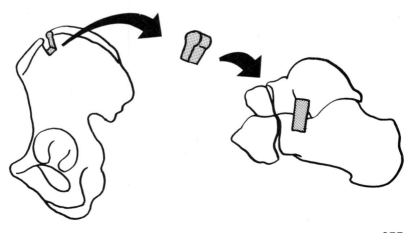

Figure 11–43. The Grice Procedure (Thomas modification). A wedge of bone is inserted into the tarsal sinus. (Redrawn from Thomas FB: J Bone Joint Surg (Br) 49:93, 1967.)

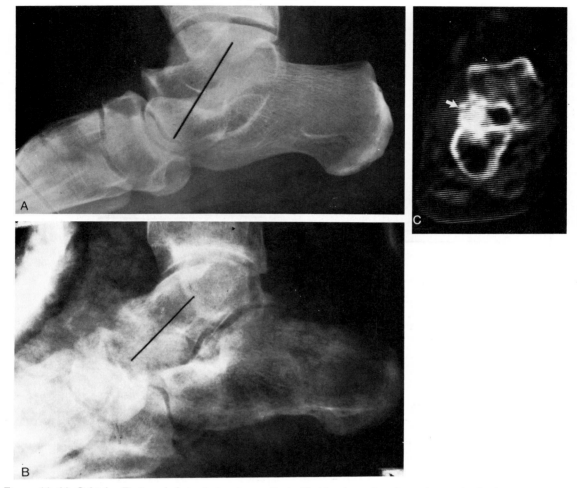

Figure 11–44. Subtalar Fusion. *A*, Lateral view in a patient with talocalcaneal coalition shows talar beaking and plantar deviaiton of the talar axis. *B*, Postoperative lateral view in plaster, after attempted correction of deformity and subtalar fusion, shows improvement in the talar axis. *C*, The CT scan shows graft (arrow) in the subtalar joint.

dial aspect of the joint and held with a metal staple. Union occurs in 10 to 12 weeks (Fig. 11–45).[63]

Toe Deformities and Arthritis

Hallux Valgus

Some degree of valgus positioning of the great toe is normally seen. With increased angulation (hallux valgus) stretching of the medial collateral ligament and consequent lateral subluxation of the proximal phalanx may result. Bony proliferation occurs along the medial aspect of the first metatarsal head, apparently as a consequence of inflammation at the insertion of the medial collateral ligament. A bursa develops in the subcutaneous tissue over the medial aspect of the first metatarsal head, and although its development is a protective reaction, the bursa

may become inflamed and may consequently be the source of additional symptoms. Secondary metatarsophalangeal osteoarthritis may also develop. Pressure from the deviated first toe commonly results in deformity of the other toes, and hammer-toe deformity of the second toe is typical.

Hallux valgus deformity is more frequent in women. It may be familial and may be associated with other deformities, such as flat foot, in which heel valgus and the associated inward rolling of the foot (pronation) shifts stress onto the medial side of the great toe.[67] Medial deviation of the first metatarsal (metatarsus primus varus) often accompanies hallux valgus. In these patients an angle of more than 10 degrees between the long axes of the first and second metatarsals is noted on standing views.[70]

Radiographic Findings. The position of the great toe can be measured by noting the angle

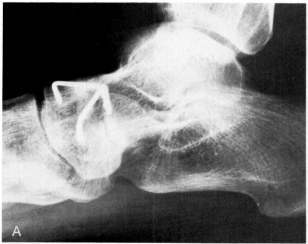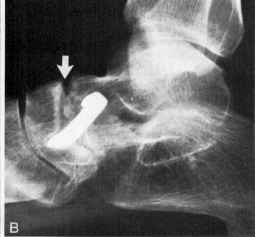

Figure 11–45. Bilateral Talonavicular Fusion with Nonunion on One Side. *A.* In the view·of the left side the talonavicular cartilage space is completely obliterated. (Film is oriented to compare with *B. B,* One year after attempted right talonavicular fusion, a gap remains between the talus and the navicular (arrow), indicating nonunion.

made between lines drawn through the axes of the first metatarsal and the proximal phalanx (Fig. 11–46). Normally, this angle is no greater than 10 degrees.[22] As deviation of the great toe increases, lateral subluxation of the proximal phalanx may develop. This is evaluated by noting the amount of the first metatarsal joint surface that is uncovered, with "deviation" of the phalanx present if less than 30 percent of the articular surface is uncovered and with "subluxation" present if more than 30 percent of the metatarsal head is uncovered.[22] Hallux valgus may be accompanied by rotation of the toe. Other associated radiographic findings include

periosteal new bone along the medial aspect of the first metatarsal head, lateral notching of the first metatarsal head, and lateral shifting of the sesamoids.

Surgical Procedures. Surgical correction is done to relieve pain, to improve appearance, or for both reasons. The choice of surgical procedures depends on the age of the patient, on the presence or absence of varus of the first metatarsal, and on the presence or absence of osteoarthritis at the first MTP.

Excision of the medial bony prominence of the metatarsal head alone may be done. However, although the overlying bursitis may be

Figure 11–46. Measuring Hallux Valgus Deformity. On the left the angle of intersection of the long axes of the proximal phalangeal and the first metatarsal shafts is 40 degrees. Normally, this angle is no greater than 10 degrees. On the right there is rotation of the great toe and lateral subluxation of the proximal phalanx, leaving about one half of the articular surface of the metacarpal uncovered. The angle of the first and second metatarsal shafts (solid lines) is 22 degrees. On standing views angles of greater than 10 degrees indicate metatarsus primus varus. (Same patient as in Fig. 11–14.)

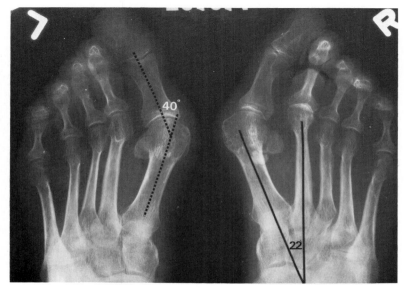

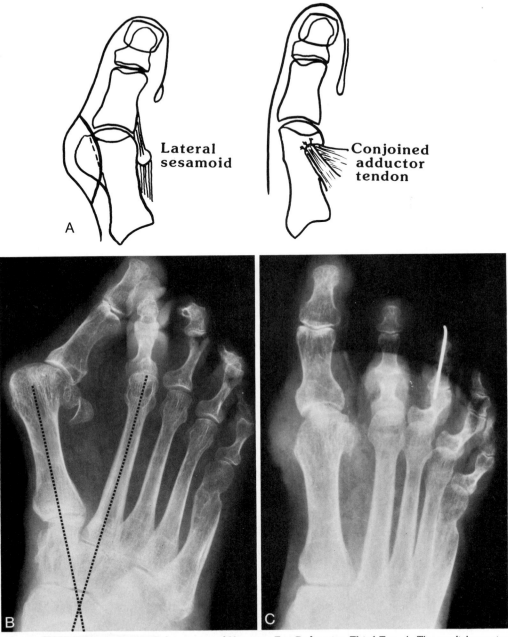

Figure 11–47. McBride Bunionectomy; Correction of Hammer Toe Deformity, Third Toe. *A*, The medial prominence of the metatarsal head is excised. The lateral sesamoid and the conjoined adductor tendons are exposed. The sesamoid is excised, and the conjoined adductor tendon·is sutured to the metatarsal neck. *B*, The preoperative slightly oblique radiograph shows severe hallux valgus deformity, with subluxation of the proximal phalanx laterally and toward the sole. The degree of metatarsus primus varus is indicated (dashed lines). The sesamoids are displaced laterally. There is flexion of the third toe DIP and of the second toe PIP. *C*, The medial aspect of the first metatarsal has been removed and soft tissue reconstruction done, resulting in correction of the valgus alignment to mild varus and of the metatarsus primus varus from 30 degrees to 10 degrees. The third toe DIP joint has been removed for correction of deformity, and the position is held by a K-wire. There has been resection of the distal portion of the second toe proximal phalanx. (After Stewart, M: Miscellaneous affections of the foot. *In* Edmonson AS, Crenshaw AH, eds. Campbell's Operative Orthopedics. St. Louis, CV Mosby, 1980.)

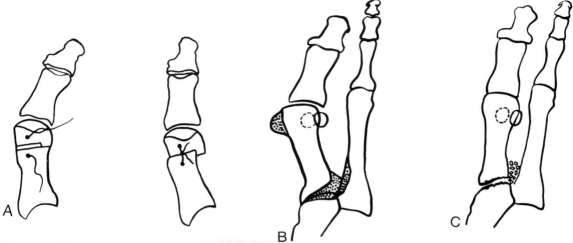

Figure 11–48. Metatarsal Osteotomy. *A,* Mitchell osteotomy is done at the metatarsal neck, and the metatarsal head is shifted laterally and slightly toward the sole. *B, C,* In the Lapidus operation the tarsometatarsal joint of the great toe is fused to the second metatarsal, and the varus position of the first metatarsal is corrected. The bony prominence of the metatarsal head is resected. (*A,* redrawn from Mitchell CL, Fleming JL, Allen R, et al.: J bone Joint Surg (Am) 40:41, 1958; *B,* redrawn from Stewart M: *In* Edmonson AS, Crenshaw AH, eds. Campbell's Operative Orthopedics. St Louis, CV Mosby, 1980.)

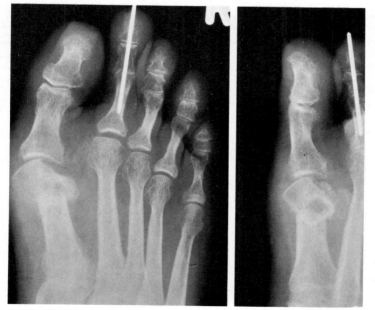

Figure 11–49. Mitchell Osteotomy. There has been an osteotomy at the base of the first metatarsal neck and the distal fragment has been shifted laterally. The distal fragment is rotated medially and more dorsally than usual. Fusion of the third toe PIP was done to correct a flexion deformity.

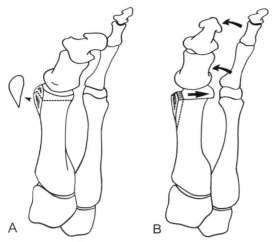

Figure 11–50. Chevron Osteomy. The medial eminence of first metatarsal head is removed, and a V-shaped osteotomy is done through the metatarsal head. The metatarsal head is then displaced laterally, and excess bone is removed medially.

relieved, deformity may progress and osteoarthritis develop, necessitating a second operative procedure.[67]

Soft Tissue Reconstruction. Removal of this medial bony prominence and soft tissue revision

(i.e., the *McBride* procedure) may be done (Fig. 11–47).

Osteotomy of First Metatarsal.[66, 67, 70] Osteotomy of the first metatarsal (to correct the varus position of the first metatarsal) may be combined with removal of the medial bony prominence of the metatarsal head. The *Mitchell* osteotomy is done at the level of the metatarsal neck, and the head is shifted laterally and plantarward (Figs. 11–48 and 11–49). The *Chevron* osteotomy is a modification of this procedure (Figs. 11–50 and 11–51).[68] Osteotomy at the metatarsocuneiform joint (the *Lapidus* osteotomy) may also be done.

Postoperative malposition (dorsal displacement or marked shortening of the metatarsal shaft) may shift stress onto the other metatarsal heads, producing severe pain (Fig. 11–52). Postoperative hypertrophy of the second metatarsal and the proximal phalangeal shafts attests to the shift in stress.[75] Nonunion may occur.

MTP Joint Resection. The Keller arthroplasty consists of excision of the base of the proximal phalanx of the great toe and of the medial prominence of the metatarsal head (Fig. 11–53).[69] A fibrous joint forms around the metatarsal head and the resected proximal phalanx.

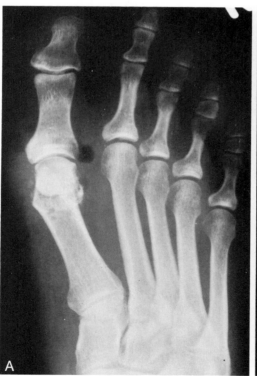
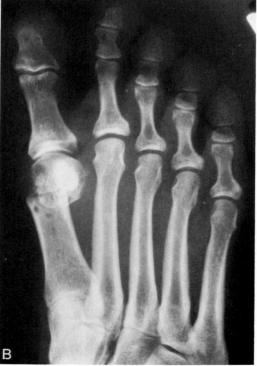

Figure 11–51. Chevron Osteotomy. AP *(A)* and oblique *(B)* immediate postoperative views show that the medial bony prominence of the first metatarsal has been removed. The metatarsal head is shifted laterally and plantarward. Small holes for attachment of soft tissues can be seen. Gas in the area is noted .

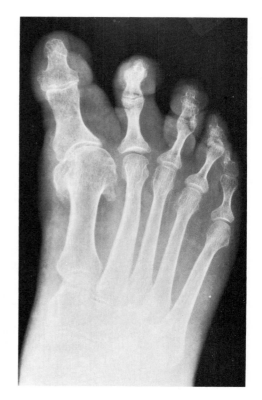

Figure 11–52. Varus Deformity after Surgery for Hallux Valgus. Soft tissue reconstruction had been performed, but overcorrection has resulted in varus deformity.

Complications include excessive shortening of the great toe (which may then require additional surgery) and its displacement or rotation. Some loss of weight-bearing function of the great toe may result, particularly if more than 1 cm of the proximal phalanx is excised, and this loss predisposes to pain over the other metatarsals.[78] Currently, the Keller arthroplasty is usually supplemented by insertion of a silicone prosthesis.

Proximal Phalangeal Osteotomy. This procedure includes varus osteotomy through the proximal phalanx, sometimes combined with soft tissue reconstruction.

Fusion of the First Metatarsophalangeal Joint. The MTP is positioned in slight dorsiflexion and in valgus to maintain weight bearing on the first metatarsal (see Fig. 11–57).[78]

Hallux Rigidus

This term describes the limited motion of the great toe that may occur when chronic trauma (such as that caused by ill-fitting shoes) results in inflammatory and, later, degenerative arthritis of the first MTP. Cartilage-space narrowing, subchondral sclerosis, flattening of the metatarsal articular surface, and osteophytes are noted on

Text continued on page 666

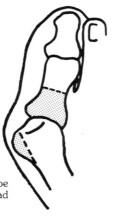
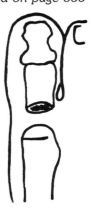

Figure 11–53. The Keller Arthroplasty. The base of the great toe proximal phalanx and the medial prominence of the metatarsal head are excised. A silicone prosthesis may be inserted.

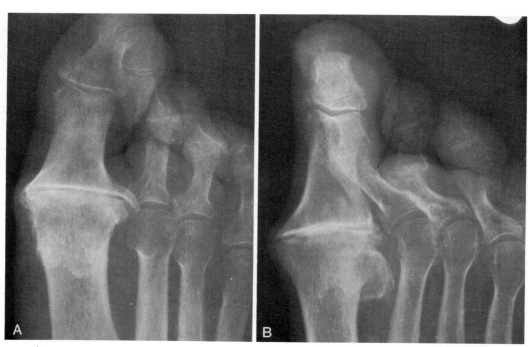

Figure 11–54. Hallux Rigidus. The PA *(A)* and oblique *(B)* views of the great toe MTP show the marked cartilage loss, flattening of articular surfaces, and hypertrophic lipping that resulted in severe loss of motion.

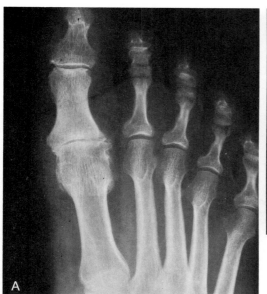

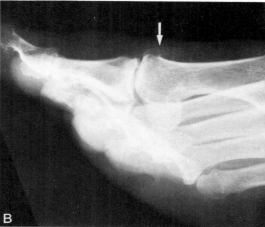

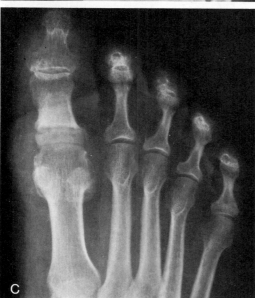

Figure 11–55. Hallux Rigidus. *A,* PA view shows marked narrowing of the great toe metatarsophalangeal joint. *B,* An off-lateral view documents flattening of articular surfaces and a large dorsal osteophyte (arrow). *C,* PA view immediately after replacement of the base of the proximal phalanx with a stemmed silicone prosthesis.

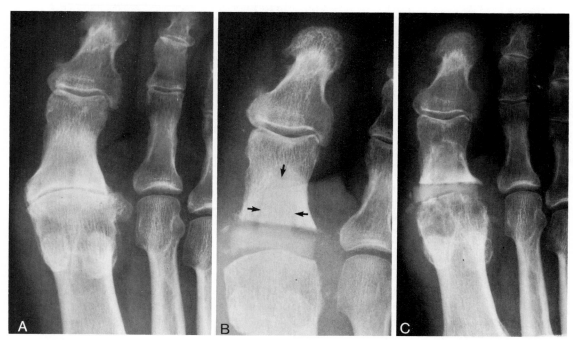

Figure 11–56. Hallux Rigidus, Silicone Prosthesis with Deformity. *A,* There is cartilage-space narrowing and hypertrophic lipping at the great toe MTP. *B,* The osteophytes have been removed, the base of the proximal phalanx resected, and a single-stemmed (arrows) silicone prosthesis inserted. *C,* One year later there is flattening of the silicone and irregularity of the subchondral bone of the metatarsal head.

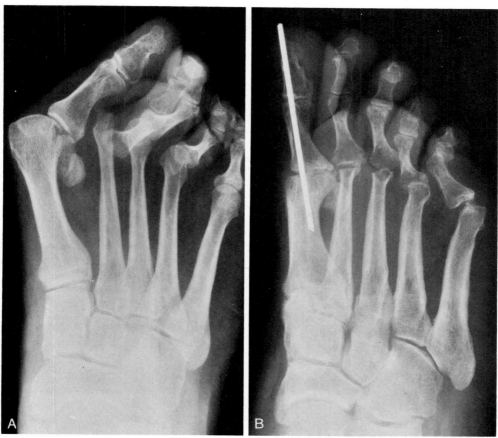

Figure 11–57. Rheumatoid Arthritis with Hallux Valgus and Cock-up Deformities, Treated with Fusion of the Great Toe MTP and Metatarsal Head Resections. *A,* The preoperative AP radiograph shows severe hallux valgus deformity, with rotation and lateral subluxation of the toe. There is erosion of the second metatarsal head and cock-up deformity of the second and probably the third and fourth toes. *B,* An oblique view after surgery shows that the great toe MTP joint has been resected and a threaded K-wire inserted to maintain the slightly dorsiflexed position of the great toe. The second to fifth metatarsal heads have been resected, with improvement in alignment of the toes and with palpable improvement in the prominence of the metatarsal heads. Less of the fourth and fifth metarsal heads has been removed than is often done.

THE FOOT

radiographs (Fig. 11–54). Extension motion is limited by the abnormal contour of the metatarsal head and by the dorsally placed metatarsal osteophytes. Surgical excision of a part of the joint (e.g., the Keller procedure), joint fusion, or partial or complete joint replacement (Figs. 11–55 and 11–56) are possible alternatives.[68]

Hammer Toes

This term is commonly used for all flexion deformities of the toes. In congenital hammer toe deformity the toe is proximally straight, but the distal phalanx is flexed. Abnormalities at the MTP joints are not part of the hammer toe deformity. Subluxation at the MTPs is however a frequent accompaniment of toe flexion in rheumatoid arthritis and is termed cock-up deformity to differentiate it from routine hammer toe deformity (Fig. 11–57). Deformity in the second to fifth toes may be corrected by resection of the PIP joints (see Fig. 11–47).[66]

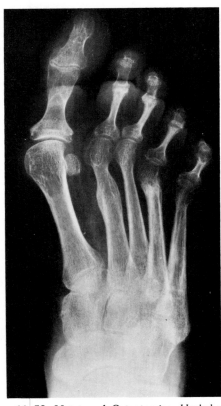

Figure 11–58. Metatarsal Osteotomies. Healed second and fourth metatarsal osteotomies, with resultant shortening, are noted. The dorsal position of these metatarsal heads is not shown here but could be evaluated on a standing lateral view. There has been resection of the ends of the second through fifth proximal phalanges at the PIP joints to correct flexion deformities.

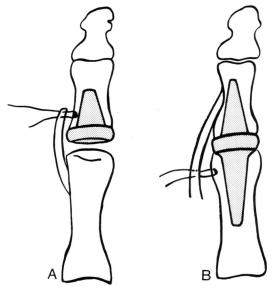

Figure 11–59. Silicone Prosthesis for the MTP Joint. *A,* Single-stemmed prosthesis. *B,* Double-stemmed prosthesis. The soft tissues are held with a suture that passes through the bone. (After Swanson AB, Lumsden RM, Swanson G: Clin Orthop 142:30, 1979.)

Other Surgical Procedures

Metatarsal Osteotomy.[70] Metatarsal osteotomy may be performed to relieve pain from calluses that form beneath prominent metatarsal heads. The procedure includes osteotomy at the head-neck junction and manual dorsal displacement of the metatarsal head (Fig. 11–58). Dorsal subluxation at the MTPs that is not fixed will be improved by this change in metatarsal head position, but fixed subluxation will require an alternative procedure, such as metatarsal head resection. Radiographic evidence of healing may take 6 to 10 weeks.

Metatarsal Head Resection. Metatarsal head resection is considered when severe disability is present as a consequence of fixed MTP subluxation or dislocation. This is most often the result of severe rheumatoid arthritis. When more than two or three metatarsals are severely involved, all four of the lesser metatarsals are excised (Fig. 11–57). When the great toe metatarsal head is involved, it, too, is resected at the level of the second metatarsal.[78]

Postoperative radiographs should show that no metatarsal head is unusually prominent, so that weight-bearing forces are distributed evenly.[78] The resected ends of the lesser metatarsals should form a shallow curve. Insufficient resection of bone or an irregular line of resection, with prominence of a metatarsal head, may result in postoperative pain.[71, 72]

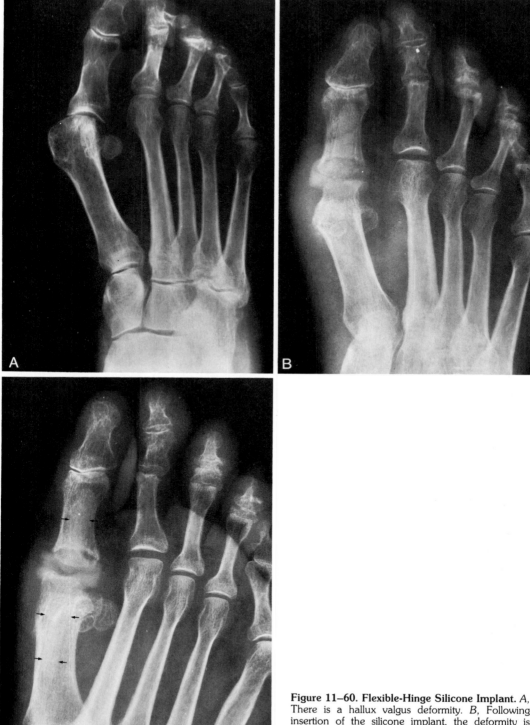

Figure 11–60. Flexible-Hinge Silicone Implant. *A,* There is a hallux valgus deformity. *B,* Following insertion of the silicone implant, the deformity is improved. *C,* The oblique view shows the stems of the prosthesis (arrows). The concave aspect of the hinge faces dorsally.

Implant Arthroplasty.[81, 82] Single- or double-stemmed silicone prostheses have been developed for use at the great toe MTP joint. The single-stemmed prosthesis replaces the base of the proximal phalanx and has been used in treating mild-to-moderate hallux valgus and hallux rigidus. The stem of the implant is inserted into the medullary canal with the base of the prosthesis flush against the resected margin of bone (Figs. 11–55, 11–56 and 11–59). In contrast with the single-stemmed prosthesis, the double-stemmed implant has a flexible hinge between the stems and is used in patients with greater deformity, greater bone damage, or both. The metatarsal head is resected at its widest point, and the base of the proximal phalanx is removed. The stems of the prosthesis are introduced into the medullary canals so that the concavity of the central hinge portion faces dorsally (Figs. 11–59 and 11–60). Complications include infection, inflammatory reaction, implant damage, osteonecrosis of the metatarsal head, and recurrent or postoperative deformity (see Fig. 11–56).

Freiberg's Infraction[79, 80]

This disorder is characterized clinically by acute pain, tenderness, and swelling of one or several metatarsal heads and radiologically by typical findings of osteonecrosis of the involved bones.

The acute phase of this disorder usually affects girls in childhood or adolescence, but the resulting deformity persists into adulthood. The second metatarsal head is involved in about two thirds of patients, the third metatarsal in most of the remainder, and the fourth metatarsal on occasion. It is suggested that this distribution relates to the distribution of weight-bearing stress on the metatarsals, a theory supported by the frequency of associated metatarsal stress fracture.

Radiographic findings are those of osteonecrosis, with eventual flattening of the metatarsal head and cartilage-space widening (Fig. 11–61). Later, secondary osteoarthritis and cartilage-space narrowing may supervene.

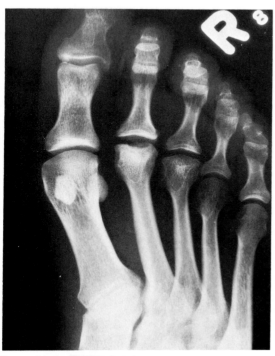

Figure 11–61. Freiberg's Infraction. There is splaying and flattening of the second and third metatarsal heads. The sclerosis and irregularity of the second metatarsal head strongly suggests avascular necrosis. Some secondary hypertrophic changes are present at the second MTP.

References

Normal Structure and Function

1. Eisenberg RL, Hedgcock MW, Williams EA, Lyden BJ, Akin JR, Gooding GA, Ovenfors CO: Optimum radiographic examination for consideration of compensation awards: III. Knee, hand and foot. AJR 135:1075–1078, 1980.
2. Bojsen-Moller F: Anatomy of the forefoot, normal and pathologic. Clin Orthop 142:10–18, 1979.
3. Morris JM: Biomechanics of the foot and ankle. Clin Orthop 122:10–17, 1977.
4. Resnick D: Radiology of the talocalcaneal articulations. Anatomic considerations and arthrography. Radiology 111:581–586, 1974.

Achilles Tendinitis and Bursitis

5. Bywaters EGL: Heel lesions of rheumatoid arthritis. Ann Rheum Dis 13:42–51, 1954.
6. Dickinson PH, Coutts MB, Woodward EP, Handler D: Tendo achillis bursitis. Report of twenty-one cases. J Bone Joint Surg (Am) 48:77–81, 1966.
7. Fowler A, Philip JF: Abnormality of the calcaneus as a cause of painful heel. Its diagnosis and operative treatment. Br J Surg 32:494–498, 1944–1945.
8. Gerster JC, Hauser H, Fallet GH: Xeroradiographic techniques applied to assessment of Achilles tendon in inflammatory or metabolic diseases. Ann Rheum Dis 34:479–488, 1975.
9. Keck SW, Kelly PJ: Bursitis of the posterior part of the heel: evaluation of surgical treatment of eighteen patients. J Bone Joint Surg (Am) 47:267–273, 1965.
10. Pavlov H, Heneghan MA, Hersh A, Goldman AB, Vigorita V: The Haglund syndrome: initial and differential diagnosis. Radiology 144:83–88, 1982.
11. Resnick D, Shaul SR, Robins JM: Diffuse idiopathic skeletal hyperostosis (DISH): Forestier's disease with extraspinal manifestations. Radiology 115:513–524, 1975.
12. Resnick D, Feingold ML, Curd J, Niwayama G, Goergen TG: Calcaneal abnormalities in articular disorders. Rheumatoid arthritis, ankylosing spondylitis, psoriatic arthritis and Reiter syndrome. Radiology 125:355–366, 1977.
13. Resnick D, Niwayama G: Entheses and enthesopathy. Anatomical, pathological, and radiological correlation. Radiology 146:1–9, 1983.

Terminology of Structural Abnormalities

14. Freiberger RH, Hersh A, Harrison MO: Roentgen examination of the deformed foot. Semin Roentgenol 5:341–353, 1970.
15. Gamble FO, Yale I: Clinical Foot Roentgenology. An Illustrated Handbook. New York, Robert E. Krieger, 1975.
16. Helfet AJ et al: Disorders of the Foot. Philadelphia, JB Lippincott, 1980.
17. Meschan I: Radiology of the normal foot. Semin Roentgenol 5:327–340, 1970.
18. Ritchie GW, Keim HA: Major foot deformities: their classification and x-ray analysis. J Can Assoc Radiol 19:155–166, 1968.
19. Templeton AW, McAlister WH, Zim ID: Standardization of terminology and evaluation of osseous relationships in congenitally abnormal feet. AJR 93:374–381, 1965.

Flat Foot

20. Conway JJ, Cowell HR: Tarsal coalition: Clinical significance and roentgenographic demonstration. Radiology 92:799–811, 1969.
21. Deutsch AL, Resnick D, Campbell G: Computed tomography and bone scintigraphy in the evaluation of tarsal coalition. Radiology 144:137–140, 1982.
22. Gamble FO and Yale I: Clinical Foot Roentgenology. New York, Robert E. Krieger, 1975:271–277.
23. Goldman AB, Pavlov H, Schneider R: Radionuclide bone scanning in subtalar coalitions: differential considerations. AJR 138:427–432, 1982.
24. Harris RI: Follow-up notes on articles previously published in the journal. Retrospect—peroneal spastic flat foot (rigid valgus foot). J Bone Joint Surg (Am) 47:1657–1667, 1965.
25. Harris RI, Beath T: Etiology of peroneal spastic flat foot. J Bone Joint Surg (Br) 30:624–634, 1948.
25a. Herzenberg J, Goldner JL, Korobkin M, Martinez S: Tarsal coalition—the role of CT scan in diagnosis and surgical treatment. Orthop Trans 7:158, 1982.
26. Jayakumar S, Cowell HR: Rigid flatfoot. Clin Orthop 122:77–84, 1977.
27. Kaye JJ, Ghelman B, Schneider R: Talocalcaneonavicular joint arthrography for sustentacular-talar tarsal coalitions. Radiology 115:730–731, 1975.
28. Shaffer HA Jr, Harrison RB: Tarsal pseudocoalition—a positional artifact. J Can Assoc Radiol 31:236–237, 1980.
29. Keats TE, Harrison RB: Hypertrophy of the talar beak. Skeletal Radiol 4:37–39, 1979.
29a. Resnick D: Talar ridges, osteophytes, and beaks: a radiologic commentary. Radiology 151:329–332, 1984.

Calcaneal Fractures

30. Anthosen W: An oblique projection for roentgen examination of the talo-calcanean joint, particularly regarding intra-articular fracture of the calcaneus. Acta Radiol 24:306–310, 1943.
31. Böhler L: Diagnosis, pathology, and treatment of fractures of the os calcis. J Bone Joint Surg 13:75–89, 1931.
32. Cave EF: Fracture of the calcis: the problem in general. Clin Orthop 30:64–66, 1963.
33. Essex-Lopresti P: The mechanism, reduction technique and results in fractures of the os calcis. Br J Surg 39:395–419, 1952.
34. Giannestras NJ, Sammarco GJ: In Rockwood CA Jr, Green DP, eds. Fractures, Vol. 2. Philadelphia, JB Lippincott, 1975.
35. Harty M: Anatomic considerations in injuries of the calcaneus. Orthop Clin North Am 4:179–183, 1973.
36. Norfray JF, Rogers LF, Adamo GP, Groves HC, Heiser WJ: Common calcaneal avulsion fracture. AJR 134:119–123, 1980.
37. Parkes JC II: Injuries of the hindfoot. Clin Orthop 122:28–36, 1977.
38. Resnick D, Goergen TG: Peroneal tenography in previous calcaneal fractures. Radiology 115:211–213, 1975.
39. Rowe CR, Sakellarides HT, Freeman PA, Sorbie C: Fractures of the os calcis: a long-term follow-up study of 146 patients. JAMA 184:920–923, 1963.
40. Warrick CK, Bremner AE: Fractures of the calcaneum: with an atlas illustrating the various types of fracture. J Bone Joint Surg (Br) 35:33–45, 1953.

Talar Fractures and Dislocations

41. Coltart WD: "Aviator's astragalus." J Bone Joint Surg (Br) 34:545–566, 1952.
42. El-Khoury GY, Yousefzadeh DK, Mulligan GM, Moore TE: Subtalar dislocation. Skeletal Radiol 8:99–103, 1982.
43. Hawkins LG: Fractures of the neck of the talus. J Bone Joint Surg (Am) 52:991–1002, 1970.
44. Kelly PJ, Sullivan CR: Blood supply of the talus. Clin Orthop 30:37–44, 1963.
45. Pennal GF: Fractures of the talus. Clin Orthop 30:53–63, 1963.
46. Smith GR, Winquist RA, Allan TNK, Northrop CH: Subtle transchondral fractures of the talar dome: a radiological perspective. Radiology 124:667–673, 1977.

Fifth Metatarsal Fractures

47. Giannestras NJ, Sammarco GJ: Fractures and dislocations in the foot. In Rockwood CA Jr, Green DP, eds. Fractures. Philadelphia, JB Lippincott, 1975.
48. Jones R: Fracture of the base of the fifth metatarsal bone by indirect violence. Ann Surg 35:697–700, 1902.
49. Peltier LF: Eponymic fractures: Robert Jones and Jones's fracture. Surgery 71:522–526, 1972.

Tarsometatarsal (Lisfranc's) Fracture-Dislocations

50. Anderson LD: Injuries of the forefoot. Clin Orthop 122:18–27, 1977.
51. Cassebaum WH: Lisfranc fracture-dislocations. Clin Orthop 30:116–129, 1963.
52. Foster SC, Foster RR: Lisfranc's tarsometatarsal fracture-dislocation. Radiology 120:79–83, 1976.
53. Giesecke SB, Dalinka MK, Kyle GC: Lisfranc's fracture-dislocation: a manifestation of peripheral neuropathy. AJR 131:139–141, 1978.

Calcific Tendinitis

54. Miller CF: Occupational calcareous peritendinitis of the feet. A case report. AJR 61:506–510, 1949.
55. Weston WJ: Peroneal tendinitis calcarea. Br J Radiol 32:134–135, 1959.
56. Weston WJ: Tendinitis calcarea on the dorsum of the foot. Br J Radiol 32:495, 1959.

Foot Stabilization Procedures

57. Gallie WE: Subastragalar arthrodesis in fractures of the os calcis. J Bone Joint Surg 25:731–736, 1943.
58. Grice DS: An extra-articular arthrodesis of the subastragalar joint for correction of paralytic flat feet in children. J Bone Joint Surg (Am) 34:927–940, 1952.
59. Grice DS: Further experience with extra-articular arthrodesis of the subtalar joint. J Bone Joint Surg (Am) 37:246–259, 1955.
60. Smith H: Malunited fractures. In Monson A, Crenshaw

AH, eds. Campbell's Operative Orthopaedics, 6th ed. St. Louis, CV Mosby, 1980:714–760.

61. Patterson RL Jr, Parrish FF, Hathaway EN: Stabilizing operations on the foot: A study of the indications, techniques used, and end results. J Bone Joint Surg (Am) 32:1–26, 1950.

62. Pyka RA, Coventry MB, Moe JH: Anterior subluxation of the talus following triple arthrodesis. J Bone Joint Surg (Am) 46:16–23, 1964.

63. Thomas FB: Arthrodesis of the subtalar joint. J Bone Joint Surg (Br) 49:93–97, 1967.

64. Thomas WH: Reconstructive surgery and rehabilitation of the ankle and foot. In Kelley WN, Harris ED, Ruddy S, Sledge CB, eds. Textbook of Rheumatology. Philadelphia, WB Saunders, 1981:1999–2012.

65. Thompson TC: Foot stabilization. The physical and physiological principles and a comparison of operative methods. Bull Hosp Special Surg 2:6–42, 1959.

Hallux Valgus and Hallux Rigidus

66. Stewart M.: Miscellaneous affections of the foot. In Edmonson AS, Crenshaw AH, eds. Campbell's Operative Orthopaedics, 6th ed. St. Louis, CV Mosby, 1980:1703–1731.

67. Helfet AJ, Gruebel Lee DM: Disorders of the Foot. Philadelphia, JB Lippincott, 1980:117–131.

68. Johnson KA, Cofield RH, Morrey BF: Chevron osteotomy for hallux valgus. Clin Orthop 142:44–47, 1979.

69. Keller WL: The surgical treatment of hallux valgus and bunions. NY State J Med 80:741–742, 1904.

70. Mitchell CL, Fleming JL, Allen R, Glenney C, Sanford GA: Osteotomy-bunionectomy for hallux valgus. J Bone Joint Surg (Am) 40:41–60, 1958.

Metatarsal Osteotomy and Metatarsal Head Resection

71. Amuso SJ, Wissinger HA, Margolis HM, Eisenbeis CH Jr, Stolzer BL: Metatarsal head resection in the treatment of rheumatoid arthritis. Clin Orthop 74:94–100, 1971.

72. Barton NJ: Arthroplasty of the forefoot in rheumatoid arthritis. J Bone Joint Surg (Br) 55:126–133, 1973.

73. Bateman JE: Pitfalls in forefoot surgery. Orthop Clin North Am 7:751–777, 1976.

74. Fowler AW: A method of forefoot reconstruction. J Bone Joint Surg (Br) 41:507–513, 1959.

75. Frede TE, Lee JK: Compensatory hypertrophy of bone following surgery on the foot. Radiology 146:347–348, 1983.

76. Giannestras NJ: Shortening of the metatarsal shaft in the treatment of plantar keratosis; an end-result study. J Bone Joint Surg (Am) 40:61–71, 1958.

77. Lipscomb PR, Benson GM, Sones DA: Resection of proximal phalanges and metatarsal condyles for deformities of the forefoot due to rheumatoid arthritis. Clin Orthop 82:24–31, 1972.

78. Thomas WH: Reconstructive surgery and rehabilitation of the ankle and foot. In Kelley WN, Harris ED, Ruddy S, Sledge CB, eds. Textbook of Rheumatology. Philadelphia, WB Saunders, 1981.

Freiberg's Infraction

79. Gauthier G, Elbaz R: Freiberg's infraction: a subchondral bone fatigue fracture. A new surgical treatment. Clin Orthop 142:93–95, 1979.

80. Smillie IS: Freiberg's infraction. (Köhler's second disease.) J Bone Joint Surg (Br) 39:580, 1957.

Total Joint Replacement

81. Johnson KA: Total joint arthroplasty. The foot. Mayo Clin Proc 54:576–578, 1979.

82. Swanson AB, Lumsden RM, Swanson G: Silicone implant arthroplasty of the great toe. A review of single stem and flexible hinge implants. Clin Orthop 142:30–43, 1979.

INDEX

Note: Page numbers in *italics* refer to illustrations; numbers followed by t refer to tables.

671